A modern epidemic

Expert perspectives on obesity and diabetes

Edited by Louise A Baur, Stephen M Twigg
and Roger S Magnusson

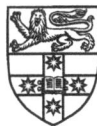

SYDNEY UNIVERSITY PRESS

Published 2012 by Sydney University Press

SYDNEY UNIVERSITY PRESS
University of Sydney Library
sydney.edu.au/sup

Reproduction and Communication for other purposes

Sydney University Press
Fisher Library F03
University of Sydney NSW 2006 AUSTRALIA
Email: sup.info@sydney.edu.au

National Library of Australia Cataloguing-in-Publication entry

Title: A modern epidemic : expert perspectives on obesity and
          diabetes / edited by Louise A. Baur, Stephen M. Twigg and Roger S. Magnusson.
ISBN: 9781920899851 (pbk.)
Notes: Includes bibliographical references and index.
          Subjects: Obesity--Social aspects.
          Diabetes--Social aspects.
          Health--Social aspects--21st Century.
Other Authors/Contributors:
          Baur, Louise.
          Twigg, Stephen M.
          Magnusson, Roger S.
Dewey Number: 362.196398

Book Project Manager Kerrie Legge
Cover design by Miguel Yamin, University Publishing Service, the University of Sydney

Contents

The physiological level

Specific risk groups and settings

Preface

The start of 2012 is marked by the establishment of the Charles Perkins Centre at the University of Sydney, with Professor Stephen J Simpson as Academic Director, to support research and education programs that will lead to real-world solutions for obesity, diabetes and cardiovascular disease. The centre is the result of a remarkable conversation where groups of diverse researchers and educators have come together to consider how they might combine forces and contribute real-world solutions to mitigate the growing impacts of these chronic diseases that are of increasing global concern.

The conversation was stimulated in part by the commitment of the University, with a A$95m grant from the Australian Government, to a A$395m infrastructure investment that will provide state-of-the-art education and research facilities that will serve the centre. The year 2011 was marked by some memorable milestones in support of this compelling vision. We broke ground on the new 45,000 square metre building that will become the hub for the academic program, which is now under construction in a strategic position next to the Royal Prince Alfred Hospital and Centenary Institute. We celebrated the sale of Picasso's portrait of Marie-Thérèse Walter at Christie's auction house. The funds (A$20.3m) generated through the generous act of an anonymous donor will support chair appointments in disciplines supporting the academic program's strategic goals.

A series of workshops including 'The mind-body interface', 'E-health and social media', and 'Corporate social responsibility and obesity, diabetes and cardiovascular disease' have brought focus to the conversation in high priority areas. More than 300 academics worked together during the genesis of our centre, led by Professor David Ian Cook with support from many, but especially from Professor Warwick Britton and Dr Mark Ainsworth. These researchers created the first draft strategic plan for what has become a truly University-wide academic program – bringing together the excellence and breadth needed to realise an ambitious and timely vision.

This volume is the product of the passion and commitment of the contributing researchers to push forward the frontier of knowledge, and ensure the new knowledge impacts on the health and quality of life for individuals and our communities in the future.

Jill Trewhella
Deputy Vice-Chancellor (Research)

About the contributors

Brooke Adam is clinical psychologist at the Boden Institute of Obesity, Nutrition, Exercise and Eating Disorders, the University of Sydney, where she is currently working on an National Health and Medical Research Council (NHMRC) trial examining the efficacy of psychological treatment for obese patients. In addition, Brooke is clinical psychologist at the Eating Disorders Day Program at Royal Prince Alfred Hospital, Sydney. Brooke has a strong research interest in obesity, as well as the psychological correlates between obese individuals and patients with 'traditional' eating disorders.

Shirley Alexander is clinical lecturer with the Discipline of Paediatrics and Child Health, Sydney Medical School, the University of Sydney and a general paediatrician, currently working as a staff specialist in the Weight Management Services (WMS) at the Children's Hospital at Westmead. The WMS is a multidisciplinary service working with families of children and young people with overweight and obesity. Shirley has published broadly on the topic of child and adolescent obesity and is a sub-editor for the *Journal of Paediatrics and Child Health*.

Geoffrey Ambler is paediatric endocrinologist and diabetologist at the Children's Hospital at Westmead, where he is co-head of the Institute of Endocrinology and Diabetes. He is also a clinical professor at the University of Sydney. He has a longstanding clinical and research interest in insulin resistance and obesity as well as clinical management of type 1 and type 2 diabetes, particularly the use of insulin pump therapy and other new technologies.

Carol Armour is professor of pharmacology at the Woolcock Institute of Medical Research, the University of Sydney. She is internationally recognised for her work in asthma research in terms of basic mechanisms of the disease and has had continuous funding from the NHMRC since 1982. More recently she has developed the evidence base for community pharmacy services in both asthma and diabetes, and has been successful in receiving tenders to test the implementation of these services in primary care.

Adrian Bauman is Sesquicentenary Professor of public health (behavioral epidemiology and health promotion) at the Sydney School of Public Health, the University of Sydney. He is also director of the Prevention Research Collaboration and of the Physical Activity, Nutrition and Obesity Research Group, both at the University of Sydney. Adrian is a world-renowned expert in physical activity and public health.

Louise A Baur is professor in the Discipline of Paediatrics and Child Health, Sydney Medical School, the University of Sydney, and also holds a conjoint appointment as professor in the Sydney School of Public Health, where she is co-director of the Prevention Research Collaboration. She is a consultant paediatrician and director of Weight Management Services at the Children's Hospital at Westmead and Obesity team leader for the Charles

Perkins Centre, the University of Sydney. Louise researches in the areas of the prevention of childhood obesity, the antecedents of obesity and the metabolic syndrome in childhood and adolescence, the complications of paediatric overweight and obesity, and the effective management of obesity and related disorders in a variety of clinical settings.

Jennie Brand-Miller AM is professor of human nutrition at the School of Molecular Bioscience and the Boden Institute of Obesity, Nutrition, Exercise and Eating Disorders, the University of Sydney. Jennie is currently a co-investigator on several nationally competitive grants, including an NHMRC project grant to reduce the risk of adverse pregnancy outcomes in women with gestational diabetes. She is a past president of the Nutrition Society of Australia and immediate past chair of the National Committee on Nutrition of the Australian Academy of Science.

Alex Brown is an Indigenous doctor and head of the Baker IDI Heart and Diabetes Institute in Central Australia. He has developed a leading national profile in Indigenous cardiovascular and metabolic disease research and policy development. He is a chief investigator in the Kanyini Vascular Collaboration and represents Aboriginal issues on key national committees and forums including the National Aboriginal and Torres Strait Islander Health Equality Council.

Stacy M Carter is senior lecturer in qualitative research in health at the Sydney School of Public Health, the University of Sydney and the Centre for Values, Ethics and the Law in Medicine, the University of Sydney. Stacy's expertise is in qualitative methodology and the ethics of public health, especially health promotion. Together with Lucie Rychetnik and Ian Kerridge, she is currently researching how health promotion professionals across NSW intervene in population weight. Stacy was the inaugural academic coordinator and director of the Master of Qualitative Health Research program at the University of Sydney, the first of its kind in Australia. She held a University of Sydney Thompson Fellowship in 2011, and holds an NHMRC Career Development Fellowship (2012–2015).

Alan Cass is senior director of the Renal and Metabolic Division at the George Institute for Global Health and a professor at the Sydney Medical School, the University of Sydney. He is a chief investigator in the Kanyini Vascular Collaboration and holds a National Health and Medical Research Council Principal Research Fellowship. He undertakes clinical research, intervention research in Aboriginal health, studies of the economic burden of chronic disease and implementation research focusing on translating research evidence into practice. He regularly works with governments and NGOs to develop strategies for chronic disease prevention and management.

Ian Caterson is currently Boden Professor of Human Nutrition and foundation director of the Boden Institute of Obesity, Nutrition, Exercise and Eating Disorders, the University of Sydney. He has had a long interest and involvement in the causes, prevention and management of obesity. He has been involved in many prevention initiatives, including government committees and groups dealing with obesity. He has received funding from the NHMRC and other government agencies for many clinical trials.

Betty Chaar is lecturer in pharmacy practice and professional ethics at the Faculty of Pharmacy, the University of Sydney. Her publications and ongoing research are in the areas of pharmacy practice, moral reasoning, ethical decision-making, professional ethics in practice, misconduct, and ethics in the context of the practice in pharmacy, as well as the pharmaceutical industry. Her interest in obesity and weight management is from a community pharmacy perspective. She has investigated the types of services offered in pharmacy, what pharmacists would like to offer and what evidence there is for effectiveness. She is currently working with the Boden Institute of Obesity, Nutrition, Exercise and Eating Disorders, the University of Sydney in this area.

Natalie Chilko is research assistant at the Sydney Nursing School, the University of Sydney, and at the Dementia Collaborative Research Centre, the University of New South Wales. Natalie's research interests include obesity, healthy ageing, and the behavioural and psychological symptoms of dementia.

Maria Craig is paediatric endocrinologist at the Children's Hospital at Westmead and St George Hospital, associate professor at the School of Women's and Children's Health, University of New South Wales and associate professor in the Discipline of Paediatrics and Child Health, Sydney Medical School, the University of Sydney. Her main research focus is childhood diabetes, including epidemiology, evidence-based medicine, the association between enteroviruses and diabetes, and microvascular complications. She holds an NHMRC career development award. She was co-chair of the NHMRC-approved Australian National Evidence Based Clinical Practice Guidelines for Type 1 Diabetes in Children, Adolescents and Adults (2011).

Michael J Dibley is a nutritional epidemiologist and associate professor in international public health at the Sydney School of Public Health, the University of Sydney. Over the last 20 years, Michael has explored the 'double burden of under and over nutrition' found in many countries in the Asia-Pacific region. In Vietnam and China he has collaborated on research assessing the magnitude of childhood and adolescent obesity, and investigated a wide range of environmental, social and behavioural risks factors associated with excess weight gain. He is currently participating in a cohort study of 800 adolescents in Ho Chi Minh City, Vietnam, which is examining the role of diet, physical activity and environmental change on the risk for adolescent overweight and obesity.

Kim Donaghue holds a conjoint appointment as professor in the Discipline of Paediatrics and Child Health, Sydney Medical School, the University of Sydney, and senior staff endocrinologist at the Children's Hospital at Westmead. She is co-head of Institute of Endocrinology and Diabetes and Head of Diabetes Services which also coordinates paediatric diabetes outreach services in rural NSW. Her major research interest is evidence-based medicine, and prevention of diabetes and its complications. She is editor of the 2012 *Global IDF/ISPAD Guideline for Diabetes in Childhood and Adolescence*. She served as Foundation Chair of Education and Training for Australasian Paediatric Endocrine Group in 2006–10.

Maria Fiatarone Singh holds the John Sutton Chair of Exercise and Sports Science at the Discipline of Exercise and Sports Science, Faculty of Health Sciences, the University of Sydney, and is professor of medicine at the Sydney Medical School, the University of Sydney. She is convenor of Exercise, Health and Rehabilitation Faculty Research Group and also director of the Exercise Division at the Boden Institute of Obesity, Nutrition, Exercise and Eating Disorders, the University of Sydney.

Nick Finer is consultant in obesity medicine at University College Hospital, London and a member of the Vascular Physiology Unit at Great Ormond Street Hospital for Sick Children. He is honorary professor in the Department of Medicine, University College London, visiting professor at the University of Sydney and Robert Gordon University, Aberdeen. Nick chairs the International Association for the Study of Obesity Education and Management Task Force, is past chair of the UK Association for the Study of Obesity and editor-in-chief of *Clinical Obesity*. His research focuses on clinical aspects of obesity and associated endocrine disease.

Murray Fisher is associate professor and director of Preregistration Programs in the Sydney Nursing School, the University of Sydney. Murray is currently the chief investigator on a number of research projects investigating the relationship of masculinity to men's health. Murray has an extensive publications record and has contributed to committees of professional organisations and discipline-specific regulatory bodies.

Klaus Gebel is research associate at the Sydney School of Public Health, the University of Sydney. He has master degrees in exercise science from the German Sport University Cologne and Victoria University, Melbourne, where he specialised first on exercise for rehabilitation and then on physical activity and public health. From 2005 to 2009 he did his PhD at the Sydney School of Public Health, the University of Sydney. Klaus has studied and worked at six universities in three countries and has received multiple scholarships and awards. His main research interests are in environmental determinants of physical activity and obesity and in the health benefits of physical activity.

Christian M Girgis received his graduate medical qualifications in 2004 from the University of New South Wales. He is currently in his final year of advanced physician training in the field of endocrinology and has recently commenced postgraduate studies in insulin resistance and vitamin D at the Garvan Institute of Medical Research, Sydney. He is a PhD student in the Sydney Medical School, the University of Sydney.

Jenny Gunton is the head of the Diabetes and Transcription Factors Group at the Garvan Institute of Medical Research, Sydney. The main interest of her lab is beta-cell function. She is also an endocrinologist at Westmead Hospital. She is the current vice-president of the Australian Diabetes Society. Jenny is a conjoint senior lecturer in the Sydney Medical School, the University of Sydney.

Connie Ha is a PhD candidate in the School of Molecular Bioscience, the University of Sydney. She has been investigating the diversity of gut microbial community under the supervision of Associate Professor Andrew Holmes. Connie is currently researching the dietary factors that promote changes in the gut microbiota and the role of diet responsive microbes in host health.

Andrew Holmes is associate professor in microbiology in the School of Molecular Bioscience, the University of Sydney. His research interests revolve around applied microbial ecology with particular emphasis on the development of tools to enable management of the gut microbial ecosystem for health. He was the recipient of the 2006 Fenner Prize from the Australian Society for Microbiology. He is currently an editor of *Microbiology*, and a member of the editorial boards of *Applied and Environmental Microbiology* and *The ISME Journal*.

Tony Keech is professor of medicine, cardiology and epidemiology in the Sydney Medical School, the University of Sydney. He is consultant cardiologist at Royal Prince Alfred Hospital, Sydney, Principal Research Fellow of the NHMRC, and deputy director of the NHMRC Clinical Trials Centre. He is an expert in clinical trials research and has been involved in many large randomised trials undertaken in cardiovascular disease treatment and prevention. Impacts on clinical practice of his trials have been particularly important in treatments for acute myocardial infarction and lipid management to reduce morbidity and complications in type 2 diabetes mellitus.

Bridget Kelly is research dietitian in the Prevention Research Collaboration, the Sydney School of Public Health, the University of Sydney with both research and teaching responsibilities in public health nutrition. Her research focuses on the development of public policy to support healthy eating, in particular on food marketing and its effect on childhood weight and obesity.

Ian Kerridge is director and associate professor in bioethics at the Centre for Values, Ethics and the Law in Medicine, the University of Sydney and staff haematologist/bone marrow transplant physician at Royal North Shore Hospital, Sydney. He has published widely in ethics and medicine/haematology and is the author of over 150 papers in peer-reviewed journals and five textbooks of ethics, most recently *Ethics and law for the health professions* (Federation Press, 2009). He is chair of the Australian Bone Marrow Donor Registry Ethics Committee and a member of the NSW Health Department's Clinical Ethics Advisory Panel. His current research interests include the philosophy of medicine, public health ethics, evidence-based medicine, stem cells, end-of-life care, synthetic genomics, identity formation in illness, research ethics, organ donation and transplantation, and the pharmaceutical industry.

Lesley King is adjunct senior lecturer in the Prevention Research Collaboration, the Sydney School of Public Health, the University of Sydney, and the executive officer of the NSW Physical Activity Nutrition Obesity Research Group (PANORG) funded by NSW government to undertake policy-relevant research. Lesley has expertise in health promotion, chronic disease prevention and public health policy, with a focus on the design and implementation of community-based programs, and the dissemination of research into policy and practice. Lesley has had prior experience as a senior manager of health promotion in government and non-government organisations. She has published academic papers on topics related to obesity prevention.

Ines Krass is professor in pharmacy practice at the Faculty of Pharmacy, the University of Sydney. Her research has focused on disease state management, screening and health promotion, and quality use of medicines in diabetes, asthma and cardiovascular disease. She has built a worldwide reputation in health services research in community pharmacy evidenced through significant competitive funding success, an extensive publication record, visiting professorships, invitations to speak at national and international conferences and contribute to subject reviews.

Yan Lam is Postdoctoral Research Fellow in the Boden Institute of Obesity, Nutrition, Exercise and Eating Disorders, the University of Sydney. Yan is currently undertaking an NHMRC-funded project which investigates the relationships between gut health, visceral fat inflammation and metabolic dysfunction. Yan has a unique background having trained in both clinical nutrition, and basic cell and molecular biology, which underpins both basic research into mechanisms of disease and translational work into the clinical setting.

Mu Li is associate professor in the Sydney School of Public Health, the University of Sydney. Mu's research interests include micronutrient deficiencies disorders, international program evaluation and childhood obesity. Mu is currently a co-chief investigator of a study in China to investigate the feasibility and acceptability of using mobile phone short messages to promote breastfeeding and healthy infant feeding in new mothers, in order to prevent early childhood obesity.

Roger S Magnusson is professor of health law and governance at the Sydney Law School, the University of Sydney. His research interests are in public health law and governance, health law and bioethics, global health and health development. His publications include *Angels of death: exploring the euthanasia underground* (Melbourne University Press, 2002) which reported on the practice of illicit, physician-assisted suicide and euthanasia among health professionals working in HIV/AIDS healthcare. His current research focuses on the opportunities for law and regulation in responding to chronic, non-communicable diseases, including those caused by tobacco use, obesity and poor diet.

Marg McGill is adjunct associate professor at the Sydney Medical School (Central Clinical School) and the Sydney Nursing School, the University of Sydney. She was appointed Australia's first paediatric diabetes educator in 1978. She has been manager of the Diabetes Centre at Royal Prince Alfred Hospital, Sydney for more than two decades. Marg was elected vice-president of the International Diabetes Federation (IDF) in 2003 and was senior vice-president from 2006 to 2009. She was chair of the IDF Consultative Section on Diabetes Education (DECS) for nine years. During this time she made significant contributions to improving the status of diabetes education as a profession as well as developing initiatives to assist in building the skills of physicians and health professionals working in diabetes care globally. Her clinical and research interests and publications are focused on the assessment and management of diabetic complications. She was named in the 2011 Australia Day Honours List with the award of Member of the Order of Australia (AM) for her contribution to diabetes nationally and overseas.

Susan V McLennan is principal hospital scientist at Royal Prince Alfred Hospital, Sydney and associate professor in medicine at the Sydney Medical School, the University of Sydney. Her principal area of expertise is the role of the MMP/TIMP system in extracellular matrix turnover, with a focus in diabetes on microvascular complications, liver disease, cardiomyopathy and wound healing. She has been investigating the role of the MMP/TIMP system in regulation of fibrosis, including the effects of high glucose and advanced glycation regulation of extracellular matrix turnover in diabetic kidney disease, and the development of methods for the collection of fluids from human diabetic wounds to study bacterial growth and wound fluid MMP concentrations. Susan is a basic scientist who is committed to linking clinical and laboratory based research in order to rapidly progress from bench to bedside.

Rohan Miller is senior lecturer in marketing and marketing communications in the University of Sydney Business School. He was formerly an an advertising practitioner and now consults to industry, government and peak industry groups. Rohan's research investigates negative effects of consumption, advertising to children, and public policy.

Michael Murray is professor of pharmacogenomics at the Faculty of Pharmacy, the University of Sydney. After a postdoctoral period at Cornell University, US he returned to Westmead Hospital, was appointed as an NHMRC Research Fellow in 1987, and was promoted in 1989 and 1994 to Senior and Principal Research Fellow, respectively. In 1995 he received a DSc from the University of Sydney. Michael is the author of 168 publications and has presented 70 symposia and seminars. In 2002 he was the ASCEPT visitor to the British Toxicology Society.

Philip O'Connell is clinical professor of medicine, the University of Sydney at Westmead Hospital. He is director of transplantation and medical director of the National Pancreas Transplant Unit. Philip is co-chief investigator on a number of national and internationally competitive reseach grants, including grants from the NHMRC and the NIH. He is a chief investigator on an NHMRC program grant for the prevention and cure of type 1 diabetes. His major research interest is in islet transplantation and he is director of the Australian Islet Transplant Consortium which has introduced clinical islet transplantation for selected patients in Australia with type 1 diabetes.

Jenny O'Dea is a dietitian, health and nutrition education researcher and professor in nutrition and health education in the Faculty of Education and Social Work, the University of Sydney. Jenny is currently working on two large Australian Research Council studies investigating body image, weight issues, self-concept, self-esteem, and eating issues. Jenny is well known for her contributions to the international media and public debate about food, nutrition, body image, obesity and has authored many scientific research publications as well as five books including *Everybody's different: a positive approach to teaching about health, puberty, body image, nutrition, self-esteem and obesity prevention* (ACER Press, 2007) and *Childhood obesity prevention: international research, controversies and interventions* (Oxford University Press, 2010).

Jane Overland is clinical associate professor at the Sydney Nursing School, the University of Sydney. She has worked in chronic disease management for over 20 years and she speaks widely in the area of diabetes and healthcare delivery to a range of healthcare professionals, both nationally and internationally. She is an active researcher, attracting over $500,000 in research grants during her career and successfully publishing in a range of peer-reviewed journals. She has acted as a consultant to both government and non-government health related bodies. She has also successfully supervised postgraduate students from a variety of health-related faculties.

Philayrath Phongsavan is senior lecturer with the Prevention Research Collaboration, the Sydney School of Public Health, the University of Sydney. Philayrath's research specialises in social epidemiology, behavioural science, and disease prevention and health promotion program evaluation. Her other research interest is evaluating the impact of redesign of urban public open spaces in socially disadvantaged areas and the effect on residents' physical activity behaviour, obesity, and sense of community and safety.

David Raubenheimer is professor of nutritional ecology at the Institute of Natural Sciences, Massey University, Auckland, New Zealand. Born in South Africa, David was based at Oxford University for 16 years, where he obtained his DPhil, before moving to New Zealand in 2004. In a long-term collaboration with Stephen J Simpson, David has developed the geometric framework for nutrition, and used it to address a wide range of problems in biology. His current research focus is on developing nutritional geometry for use in field studies, an extension that is being applied to a range of study systems spanning marine fish, birds, dolphins, large predators (tigers and snow leopards) and primates including humans. David has been Visiting Fellow at the Smithsonian Institute, a Fellow of the Institute for Advanced Study (Wissenschaftskolleg) in Berlin, distinguished lecturer in behavioural and brain sciences at Cornell University, Fellow at the Institute for Advanced Study in Oslo, and Visiting Research Fellow at the University of Sydney. He heads the Nutritional Ecology Research Group at Massey University, and is senior associate member of the New Zealand Institute for Advanced Study.

Elizabeth Rieger is associate professor and clinical psychologist in the Department of Psychology, Australian National University. Elizabeth has published widely in the area of eating and weight disorders, and is currently chief investigator on a randomised controlled trial funded by the NHMRC to investigate the effectiveness of motivational enhancement therapy for obese patients and their support network.

Chris Rissel is professor of public health at the Prevention Research Collaboration, the Sydney School of Public Health, the University of Sydney. His main research interests focus on obesity prevention and active travel, particularly cycling advocacy. He is one of the authors of the national report 'Cycling: getting Australia moving. Barriers, facilitators and interventions to get more Australians physically active through cycling.' He has just completed a three-year grant to promote increased use of cyclepaths in south-west Sydney

– 'Cycling connecting communities', and is currently involved in an ARC grant looking at safer cycling.

Lucie Rychetnik is Senior Research Fellow at the Sydney School of Public Health, the University of Sydney. Her main areas of interest and expertise are the appraisal, translation and application of evidence for public health and health promotion policy and practice. From 2000 to 2009 Lucie was senior associate at the Sydney Health Projects Group (SHPG), an academic consulting group in the Sydney School of Public Health, the University of Sydney whose primary role was to translate research evidence for a wide range of public health policy and practice settings. She joined the School of Public Health, Screening and Test Evaluation Program (STEP) in September 2009, where she primarily conducts qualitative research to complement and enhance the established program of quantitative research. In March 2010 she joined the Centre for Values, Ethics and the Law in Medicine (VELIM), the University of Sydney as chief investigator on an NHMRC project – 'Reconceptualising health promotion: the role of values, ethics and evidence in obesity intervention'. Prior to completing her MPH (1996) and PhD (2001) she worked in the health sector as a clinical dietitian and community nutritionist in Oxford, London and Sydney, and as a health promotion officer with the (then) Southern Sydney Area Health Service.

Amanda Sainsbury is conjoint associate professor in the Sydney Medical School, the University of Sydney. She leads a research team at the Garvan Institute of Medical Research, Sydney investigating how the brain and diet interact to control body weight and body composition. Her research is funded by a Career Development Award and competitive grants from the NHMRC, and spans studies with transgenic mice to randomised controlled clinical weight-loss trials in humans. Amanda disseminates her research findings to the wider community by lecturing to students in science, medicine, nursing and human movement, and she has authored two books and given seminars on weight management for health professionals and the public.

Alexandra Sharland is senior lecturer in transplantation immunobiology in the Collaborative Transplantation Research Group, the University of Sydney. Her research encompasses innate immunity and inflammation in brain death and ischaemia-reperfusion injury, autoimmunity, and the mechanisms by which these factors promote transplant rejection and interfere with the development of transplantation tolerance. She is a former councillor of the Transplantation Society of Australia and New Zealand, and chair of the TSANZ Scientific Advisory Committee.

Stephen J Simpson is the Academic Director of the Charles Perkins Centre and an Australian Research Council Laureate Fellow in the School of Biological Sciences, the University of Sydney, having returned to Australia in 2005 as an ARC Federation Fellow after 22 years at Oxford where he was professor of entomology and curator of the University Museum of Natural History. Stephen has pioneered developments at the interface of nutritional physiology, ecology, and behaviour. Together with David Raubenheimer, he developed state-space models for nutrition (the geometric framework), which were devised and tested using insects but have since been applied to a wide range of animals and problems, from aquaculture and conservation biology to the dietary causes of human obesity. His research on locusts has led to an understanding of locust swarming that links chemical events in the brains of individual insects to landscape-scale mass migration. Stephen has been visiting professor at Oxford, a Fellow of the Institute for Advanced Study (Wissenschaftskolleg) in Berlin, Distinguished Visiting Fellow at the University of Arizona, and guest professor at the University of Basel. In 2007 he was elected a Fellow of the Australian Academy of Science, in 2008 he was awarded the Eureka Prize for Scientific Research, in 2009 he was named NSW Scientist of the Year, and in 2010 he was named as the Wigglesworth Medallist by the Royal Entomological Society of London.

Paul Snelling is senior staff specialist in nephrology at Royal Prince Alfred Hospital, Sydney. He has extensive experience in renal service delivery to Indigenous Australians and was previously director of Renal Services in the Northern Territory. He provides crucial clinical input and understanding to a broad range of Aboriginal health and kidney health research programs and has worked closely with government in the development of strategies for renal service provision.

Kate Steinbeck is the Medical Foundation Chair of Adolescent Medicine, the University of Sydney and is an adolescent endocrinologist and physician. She has significant experience in the management of secondary obesity, including post-craniopharyngioma obesity and the Prader-Willi syndrome. Her research interests include the longitudinal effects of puberty hormones on weight and body composition, and obesity management in the transition from adolescence to young adulthood.

Stephen M Twigg is professor in medicine at the Sydney Medical School, the University of Sydney, Diabetes theme leader for the Charles Perkins Centre, the University of Sydney, and deputy head of Department of Endocrinology and medical head of the Endocrinology Research Laboratories at Royal Prince Alfred Hospital, Sydney. His research focuses on the prevention and management of diabetes complications including pathogenic growth factors and tissue fibrosis, as well as optimisation of quality and length of life in people with diabetes. As a physician-scientist, he is dedicated to optimising healthcare delivery in diabetes, finding scientific solutions to the medical problems related to diabetes and its complications, and mentoring and training advanced clinical trainees in clinical skills, and laboratory students and fellows in the scientific method. He is the immediate past president of the Australian Diabetes Society, and a past honorary board member of Diabetes Australia.

Hidde P van der Ploeg is Senior Research Fellow in the Sydney School of Public Health, the University of Sydney. He has a masters degree in human movement science, a postgraduate degree in epidemiology and a PhD in physical activity and public health, all from the Vrije Universiteit Amsterdam in the Netherlands. His main research interest is in the development and evaluation of physical activity programs for people with chronic disease.

Introduction

In 2006, Sydney University Press and Sydney University Research Portfolio began a collaboration to produce a series of books containing multidisciplinary perspectives on issues of global importance. Because diabetes, obesity and their related diseases place a high burden on individuals, the community and the healthcare system, this topic was an obvious choice for the second book in this series. In this book, researchers and clinicians from the University of Sydney and beyond have joined forces to tackle this major health challenge.

Type 2 diabetes and obesity share common risk factors, including insufficient physical activity, and the over-consumption of energy-dense, nutrient poor foods. Obese individuals are at an increased risk of developing chronic health problems including cardiovascular disease and type 2 diabetes. These diseases are not just problems for the individual, but create psychological and relational problems within families, reflect environmental problems within communities, and ultimately carry economic consequences for entire nations. The solutions, therefore, need to be equally wide-ranging, and accessible to all.

As well as affecting the adult population, obesity and diabetes are increasingly seen in childhood and adolescence. Obesity is associated with a range of psychosocial problems such as depression and low self-esteem, and discrimination. Often an individual does not perceive their weight accurately and tends to either over- or underestimate it. However the solutions to the diabetes and obesity epidemic require more than just changes in the perceptions and behaviours of individuals. Obesity and diabetes are environmental health problems and effective solutions will require policies that target the entire population, regardless of their current health status. Cultural differences, food production and supply, urban design and transportation are important factors to consider. In addition, new kinds of interventions will be needed in key settings including schools, workplaces, primary healthcare, pharmacies and hospitals.

Acknowledging this, the authors write about risks, causes and consequences, as well as prevention and treatment: how to identify and mitigate the risk factors, deliver targeted and effective healthcare, and formulate national and global strategies to ultimately turn the tide on some of the 21st-century's most devastating diseases. Contributors to this book are necessarily diverse and include endocrinologists, pharmacists, haematologists, biologists, paediatricians, psychologists, health policy experts, lawyers, nutritional scientists, nurses, health promotion experts, exercise and sports scientists, and dietitians. By drawing from a range of specialties these authors present new insights and hope to present a more holistic understanding of the challenges faced by individuals and societies.

This book brings together new research in obesity and diabetes from a range of perspectives. Drawing from the fields of medicine, the biological sciences, health science, business, law, social sciences, pharmacy, education and nursing, the authors first define the nature and scale of the obesity and diabetes crisis, and then explore possible solutions. In the first section, researchers explore the problems of obesity and diabetes at the cellular or physiological level. The issues that these conditions raise are not the same for everyone. Hence, in the second section, the authors turn to specific risk groups and settings. The third section considers options for regulatory approaches as well as the ethics of policy interventions. Finally, in section four, researchers discuss treatment, prevention and management strategies for both diseases.

Some important findings presented in the book include the following:

- Healthy behaviours established in young people tend to translate into healthy habits in adulthood, which are subsequently modelled and passed on to the following generations.

- Eating according to hunger results in loss of excess weight.

- An individual genetically predisposed to obesity requires an obesogenic diet in order to manifest the genetic blueprint via gene-environment interactions. Epigenetics suggests that obesogenic diets not only render individuals incapable of losing excess weight, but may also have adverse impacts on the health of future generations.

- Discrimination against obese individuals is evident in all areas of life including social life, parenting practices, education, employment and healthcare. The stress which obese individuals are exposed to as a result of negative societal attitudes and behaviours can lead to further weight gain, and worse health outcomes.

- Regular physical activity and exercise, independent of weight loss, are effective in both prevention and treatment of diabetes. Prolonged sitting time might be associated with the risk of developing type 2 diabetes, independent of leisure-time physical activity.

- Obesity is linked to changes in the nutritional balance of our diet, with a primary role for protein appetite driving excess energy intake. Small changes in the percentage of protein in the diet can potentially yield big effects on intake, with consequences – both good and bad – for weight management.

- In considering approaches to the prevention of obesity, there are distinct and overlapping ethical concerns at both individual and population levels; at both levels moral compromise is necessary.

- School-based health promotion programs can have a positive and lasting impact on body image, eating behaviours, attitudes, and the self -image of adolescents. So promoting a healthy body image, establishing positive food habits and encouraging involvement in sport and physical activity at school can be catalysts for behavioural changes to improve health globally and reduce healthcare costs.

- Diabetes complications occur to some degree in practically every person who develops diabetes, although severe complications occur in only a minority. Because it has a high prevalence in Australia however, diabetes is the single commonest cause of end-stage kidney disease and the commonest cause of working-age blindness. Evidence from clinical trials indicates that by using current healthcare and therapy standards, much can be done to prevent the onset and progression of diabetes complications. Prospective therapies to prevent and treat complications in diabetes include the agent fenofibrate and stem cells to treat diabetes and the organ affected by complications.

- A considerable body of evidence highlights the significant adverse health-related impact of childhood and adolescent obesity. Moreover, childhood obesity may track into adulthood, with further increased obesity-related morbidity and mortality.

- Organised high-quality diabetes care needs to be accessible and affordable to an increasing number of people with diabetes. Community pharmacists are a valuable resource of trained healthcare professionals that can be utilised to provide prevention and care services as part of an integrated primary care sector approach.

- Childhood obesity has become a major public concern in developing countries where the absolute number of children who are overweight or obese is now much higher than in developed countries.

- A holistic approach that considers how an individual configures their masculinity or femininity may assist in promoting and maintaining weight loss in obese individuals as it addresses the struggle in society experienced by many obese people. Weight-loss approaches that recognise the individual struggle with gender and the influence of other social structures may be an alternative to current, largely unsuccessful treatments of obesity.

- While weight loss can be achieved, the major issue in the treatment of obesity remains weight maintenance. Those individuals who lose weight and successfully keep it off undertake lifestyle changes that includes high levels of physical activity, eating breakfast and regular meals, and a diet that is low in fat. Self-monitoring is an important way of catching 'slips' early and correcting them.

- Promising societal and environmental responses to overweight and obesity include redesigning the built environment, providing active transport options, promoting the availability and accessibility of healthy food choices, restricting promotion of unhealthy foods, and implementing ongoing social marketing strategies to influence sustained healthy eating and physical activity behaviours. Achieving these things is a massive challenge. Government leadership, social planning and urban renewal that engages communities, businesses and other relevant stakeholders are fundamental to the process.

Editors: Louise A Baur, Stephen M Twigg and Roger S Magnusson
Book Project Manager: Kerrie Legge

The physiological level

1

The biology of weight control

Amanda Sainsbury[1,2,3]

Many clinical and commercial weight-loss programs use external controls such as kilojoule allowances to reduce energy intake. While this results in weight loss, it is not necessarily suitable for people prone to disordered eating, nor is it feasible for public health initiatives opposing obesity. In this chapter I cover the endogenous biological systems that enable humans to attain and maintain a healthy body weight – without kilojoule counting – and how genetic variations and our obesogenic environment can compromise them. These endogenous weight-control mechanisms allow individuals who don't respond well to external controls about how much to eat, to lose excess weight and keep it off, provided that the endogenous signals are heard and heeded, and the environment is conducive to doing so. These mechanisms are also suitable for community interventions.

When it comes to losing excess weight, many people utilise methods such as 'kilojoule counting' and weighing or measuring portion sizes in order to reduce their energy intake. For people not inclined to count or measure their food, structured programs are available that provide 'pre-counted' reduced energy intakes, such as specific diet menus, meal replacement programs and home-delivered meals. These are all examples of weight reducing diets in which energy intake is externally prescribed. For many people, the clear directives about what and how much to eat provided by such regimes impart knowledge about healthy foods choices and reasonable portion sizes. This is particularly important in the current obesogenic environment, where default food choices, portion sizes and the physical environment have led many adults to become overweight or obese. Weight-loss programs with externally prescribed energy intakes have helped many people to lose excess weight efficiently and – in a proportion of cases – sustainably. In fact, a recent study showed that a commercial weight-loss program involving food counting outperformed individualised attention from general practitioners in terms of helping overweight and obese adults to reduce body weight over a one-year period [1].

Despite their effectiveness for a proportion of people, weight-reducing diets with externally prescribed energy intakes are not suitable for everyone. Examples include people with

---

1 Neuroscience Research Program, Garvan Institute of Medical Research, Sydney.

2 Sydney Medical School, University of Sydney.

3 School of Medical Sciences, University of New South Wales.

higher or lower energy requirements than those stipulated by the diet, or those prone to disordered eating. For these reasons, in addition to the high level of support required for adherence to such diets, they are not suitable for community initiatives against obesity. In this chapter I explore an alternate solution for weight management in these people, drawing on the function of biological weight-control systems. Because these endogenous weight management systems appear to be intact in a significant proportion of people, they are potentially amenable to community-level interventions against obesity.

One size never fits all

Most clinical and commercial weight-loss programs use standardised energy intakes, with some programs offering two or three options for people with lower or higher energy requirements (eg diets providing 1200, 1500 or 1800 kilocalories per day). However, many people have energy requirements for weight loss that are different from these standardised levels, at least at times, due to intra- and inter-individual variations in factors such as body size and composition, age, sex, physical activity levels, phase of the menstrual cycle, as well as prevailing climatic conditions. This means that, for a proportion of people, weight-reducing diets with defined levels of energy intake are either ineffective or unsustainable, as outlined below.

When dietary energy intake is too high

> I found that in order to eat all of the allocated food on that diet's menu plan, I was often eating when I wasn't hungry, and I actually gained weight. (Maria, 49 years of age and 1.52 metres tall)

Losing body fat is a question of consuming less energy than the amount of energy used for basal metabolic processes, digestion, adaptive thermogenesis and physical activity. Some people's energy requirements are so low that even adherence to a 1200 kilocalorie per day diet will not result in weight loss. It is not uncommon to hear of people who started and apparently followed a weight-loss diet with a defined energy intake, only to achieve either very slow or no weight loss. While it is often assumed that the person 'must be doing something wrong', the standardised energy intakes of many weight-loss diets can be too high to produce negative energy balance in people with low energy requirements, as in older women with low muscle mass and a low level of physical activity, for example.

When dietary energy intake is too low

> With uni study, social life and trying to exercise regularly, it was not possible for me to 'diet' and 'live' at the same time. (Sabrina, 21 years of age)

A more common limitation of weight-loss diets with standardised kilojoule allowances is that people with higher energy requirements – such as younger, larger or more active individuals – can be left with inadequate energy with which to live full and active lives. A woman once told me that she often stopped going to the gym when following a commercial weight-loss program because she felt she didn't have enough energy for the vigorous workouts she otherwise enjoyed. This may be due to physical and psychological effects.

Physical effects of energy deficit

Energy deficit is known to cause adaptive responses that inhibit ongoing weight loss and which promote fat regain [2]. Emerging evidence suggests that the greater the deficit between energy requirements and intake, the greater the magnitude of these adaptive responses [3–5]. Such adaptations have been observed in overweight and obese humans and animals in response to even moderate energy restriction, and include increased appetite, reduced energy expenditure [2], a possible reduction in spontaneous physical activity [2, 5–8], and an increase in skeletal muscle work efficiency [9]. Additional adaptations include changes in endocrine status that would tend to promote the accretion of fat (particularly visceral fat) at the expense of muscle and bone, as recently reviewed [10]. For instance, energy deficit has been shown to decrease circulating levels of thyroid hormones, sex hormones, insulin like growth factor-1 and gut-derived satiety hormones such as peptide YY, in addition to increased circulating cortisol levels [10].

As larger energy deficits appear to induce stronger adaptive responses [3–5], and as the magnitude of the deficit-induced increase in appetite [11, 12] or decrease in energy expenditure [11–14] predicts subsequent weight regain, the widespread use of standardised energy intakes in weight-reducing diets could be inadvertently promoting a situation where the large get larger. For instance, a 1500 kilocalorie per day diet would produce a greater energy deficit in a woman weighing 100 kgs than in a woman weighing 80 kgs, all other things being equal. As such, the more overweight woman could be expected to exhibit a greater adaptive response to weight loss in response to the standardised diet, potentially putting her at greater risk of rebound weight gain.

Psychological effects of energy deficit

As well as having effects on physical predictors of weight regain, notably appetite and energy expenditure, energy deficit affects psychological determinants of feeding behaviour. For instance, energy restriction in rodents up-regulates hypothalamic brain expression of dynorphins [15, 16], which are endogenous opioids that induce dysphoria (an emotional state characterised by anxiety, depression, or unease). Moreover, blocking endogenous opioids with non-specific opioid antagonists such as naloxone or naltrexone has been shown to reduce binge-eating behaviour and food intake in bulimia nervosa [17] and in obese women [18]. These findings suggest that energy deficit may be contributing to changes in the brain that promote binge eating. In keeping with this, restricting energy intake to levels dictated by external factors rather than physiological needs (as in dieting) contributes to binge eating and other eating disorders in some people. Indeed, 100% of patients with bulimia and anorexia nervosa have followed restrictive diets in the past, and abstaining from such practices is part of the established treatment for eating disorders.

In light of the limitations of weight-reducing diets with standardised energy intakes, as well as the impracticality of determining energy requirements tailored to the individual needs of millions of people who need to lose excess weight, what are the alternatives?

Tapping into biological weight-control systems for individual and community solutions

Many members of the public and health practitioners alike do not realise that mammals such as humans are equipped with physiological systems that enable individuals to attain and maintain an optimum weight – without the need to follow externally prescribed kilojoule allowances – provided that the types of foods eaten are generally healthy, and provided that the endogenous hunger and satiety signals about when and how much to eat are heeded. In this and the next section I will outline how these physiological weight-management systems work, as well as the evidence that they function even in modern society, where the current obesity epidemic might suggest otherwise. An advantage of tapping into these endogenous weight-management systems is that they offer the potential for personalised solutions, where energy intake can be automatically matched to the optimal level for weight loss in each individual every day, without the need to measure actual energy requirements. These biological weight-control systems are also amenable to community interventions against obesity because – when combined with population-wide strategies facilitating healthy food and activity choices – the associated public health message could be reduced to a single instruction: eat according to your physical needs.

Pathways that prevent excessive weight gain

When an individual consistently consumes a greater number of kilojoules than that which is used by the body, the result is storage of excess energy, predominantly in the form of triglycerides (fat) in white adipose tissue. When total body energy stores exceed the level that the body defends (often referred to as the 'set point'), physiological changes that promote restoration of the set point ensue. These changes include decreased appetite, increased physical activity, enhanced energy expenditure and hormonal alterations, as evidenced below. While the appetite-inhibiting effects of energy excess are easy to override, as described later in this chapter, research suggests that these adaptive responses to energy excess occur nonetheless in up to 84% of individuals [19], making them potential targets for community-based interventions against obesity.

Positive energy balance reduces appetite

The most obvious sign of the adaptive responses opposing excessive weight gain is a reduction in appetite. Anecdotally, many people notice this after a spate of particularly heavy eating or inactivity or both (eg after holiday overindulgences), when they may not feel as drawn to as abundant or as rich foods as usual. This phenomenon has been measured in clinical trials. When healthy young male volunteers were instructed to overeat by 4200 kilojoules (1000 kilocalories) a day for three weeks and were then asked to eat *ad libitum*, they voluntarily consumed 2000 kilojoules (480 kilocalories) fewer per day than they were consuming before the experiment began [20]. Moreover, they voluntarily chose to eat foods that were lower in fat than those they normally ate [20]. Similar results have been observed in lean rodents, which exhibit spontaneous reductions in food intake in response to exposure to a high-fat diet [21], probably driven by changes in the hypothalamus of the brain as described below. Further research is required to determine whether the effect of short-term energy excess to inhibit appetite is also apparent in all people, particularly those who are overweight or obese, as a recent study has suggested that this response may be impaired in some [22].

Positive energy balance increases physical activity

In addition to reducing appetite, energy excess increases physical activity, the amount of energy used to perform physical activity, or both [8, 9, 23], thereby helping to allay fat accumulation. Lean volunteers were asked to overeat by 4200 kilojoules (1000 kilocalories) each day for eight weeks [23]. They were specifically instructed *not* to increase the amount of exercise they did during the experiment, and they stringently maintained a low level of voluntary physical activity throughout the eight-week overfeeding period. Remarkably, the volunteers displayed a massive increase in non-exercise activities such as spontaneous muscle contractions, posture maintenance and fidgeting. In fact, the average increase in energy spent on these types of non-volitional physical activities – termed non-exercise activity thermogenesis, or NEAT – added up to 1425 kilojoules (340 calories) a day. One volunteer even burnt up 2900 additional kilojoules (700 calories) a day, which he achieved without meaning to by pacing for about 15 minutes of every waking hour. This spontaneous increase in the amount of energy expended on physical activity in response to energy excess has been confirmed in other studies in humans [9]. It is a change that has been suggested to oppose weight gain, because spontaneous physical activity in mice and rhesus monkeys negatively correlates with weight gain, consistent with human epidemiological data [24]. Not only does energy excess increase the volume of physical activity performed, it also appears to decrease muscle work efficiency in humans [9], thereby further increasing the amount of energy expended on physical activity and decreasing that available for storage.

Positive energy balance may increase energy expenditure

In addition to decreasing appetite and stimulating the amount of energy expended on physical activity, some studies have shown that energy excess leads to an increase in total daily energy expenditure or basal metabolic rate in humans [22, 25–27], albeit this has not been observed in all studies, as recently reviewed [28]. Such a change would be expected to further increase energy dissipation and help to prevent weight gain.

Neuroendocrine responses to positive energy balance

The changes in food intake, physical activity and possibly also total energy expenditure that occur in response to energy excess are likely to be mediated by associated effects on neuroendocrine status. For instance, feeding rodents a high-fat diet for eight weeks reduces expression of orexigenic peptides that promote food intake, notably neuropeptide Y (NPY) [21]. As NPY has been shown to stimulate feeding, reduce physical activity and decrease metabolic rate [2], such a change in its hypothalamic expression could contribute to effects of energy excess on appetite, physical activity and energy expenditure.

While it is not possible to measure dynamic changes in hypothalamic peptide expression in response to energy excess in humans, investigation of human body fluids or peripheral tissues provides indirect evidence of similar brain changes to those that have been measured in rodents. For instance, overfeeding increases activity of both the hypothalamo-pituitary thyroid axis and the sympathetic nervous system in humans, as evidenced by measurements of serum thyroid hormone and catecholamine levels [29] or muscle sympathetic nerve activity [30]. Both of these changes would be expected to result from decreases in orexigenic peptide expression in the hypothalamus of the brain [10, 31], and could in turn contribute to the adaptive changes opposing weight gain in response to energy excess. For instance, induction of hyperthyroidism in rats leads to an increase in physical activity and NEAT [8, 32]. Additionally, thyroid hormones are classically known for their effect to stimulate energy expenditure by acting on peripheral tissues to directly influence cellular metabolism [33], and they have recently been shown to act in the hypothalamus of the brain to stimulate sympathetic nervous activity [34], which in turn is known to stimulate energy expenditure [35].

Changes in gut hormone secretion could also contribute to the effects of energy excess on energy intake and expenditure. Short-term energy excess in lean, overweight and obese males increases circulating concentrations of the gut-derived satiety hormone peptide YY (PYY) [36]. As PYY has been shown to reduce appetite and food intake in lean and obese humans and rodents [37–39], this change could contribute to the associated reduction in appetite seen after energy excess. Increased PYY levels could also contribute to observed increases in energy expenditure during energy excess, since PYY has been shown to increase energy expenditure in lean and obese men [40], and to decrease energy efficiency and increase core body temperature in rodents [41].

Evidence that biological weight-control systems can lead to loss of excess weight

In light of adaptive responses to energy excess such as those described above, it would be expected that eating according to individual physical hunger and satiety signals would result in reversal of past overindulgences. Energy intake would be reduced on account of the associated reduction in appetite, and increases in physical activity levels or the energy cost of physical activity, combined with a possible increase in total energy expenditure, would further facilitate loss of excess weight and restoration of the defended 'set point'. But what is the evidence that eating according to individual hunger and satiety cues – without external prescriptions on energy intake – does indeed result in loss of excess weight in lean, overweight and obese people?

Effectiveness of biological weight-control systems in lean people

In a classic overfeeding study [42], 12 pairs of lean young identical male twins were instructed to stop exercising and to overeat by 4200 kilojoules (1000 kilocalories) a day, six days a week, for 12 weeks. Every single man gained weight during the study, with a mean weight gain of 8.1 kg. As might be expected based on anecdotal observations that some people can 'gain weight just by looking at food' and others 'can eat anything they want and never gain weight', the range of weight gain was wide (4.3 to 13.3 kg), and there was a markedly greater similarity within each twin pair than among pairs with respect to weight gain. This finding shows that genetics play a significant role in determining the ability of endogenous weight-control systems to cope with energy excess. Intriguingly, despite this wide range of weight gain among twin pairs, when the volunteers resumed their regular lives at the end of the study, *all* of them spontaneously returned to within one kilogram of their original weight within four months [42, 43]. This finding provides indirect evidence that even those individuals with a genetic propensity to gain the most weight during periods of energy excess can reverse those excesses by eating according to appetite, without the need for diets with an externally prescribed energy intake.

Similar spontaneous returns to initial body weight have been seen in men from Cameroun after four to six months of fattening by massive carbohydrate overconsumption for the traditional Guru Walla session [44]. However, a recent study of 12 lean men and six lean women showed that a four-week period of hyper-alimentation and limited physical activity resulted in increases in body weight and adiposity that were almost – albeit not completely – reversed within 12 months of return to *ad libitum* food intake and usual activity patterns [22]. It is thus likely that the homeostatic control mechanisms that contribute to reversal of energy excesses are not impervious, at least in some individuals.

Effectiveness of biological weight-control systems in overweight and obese people

It might be expected that lean young men and women would reverse energy excesses reasonably efficiently without the need for fixed energy intake prescriptions. However, evidence that homeostatic regulatory systems can also contribute to reversal of excess weight in overweight, obese or severely obese people comes from weight-loss studies involving *ad libitum* intake of a modified diet. When obese [45] or severely obese [46] men and women limited carbohydrate intake without restricting consumption of fat and protein, they lost at least as much weight after six to 12 months (~4% to 7% of body weight) as people in a control arm who consciously restricted total daily energy intake via calorie counting. Additionally, overweight or obese young men and women lost an average of ~5% of their body weight in a 12-week intervention involving the instruction to 'eat to appetite', choosing from lists of appropriate meals and snacks that would result in modification of glycaemic load and/or protein intake [47]. Similar effects on body weight are seen when the fat intake of the diet is modified without prescribing energy intake [48]. Indeed, the Clinical Practice Guidelines for the Management of Overweight and Obesity in Adults from the National Health and Medical Research Council (NHMRC) of Australia provides evidence that low-fat diets consumed *ad libitum* can lead to weight and waist circumference losses of 2–6 kg and 2–5 cm after one year, and that these diets – if intensively monitored – may be more effective for maintaining weight loss than more prescriptive low-energy diets [48].

Potential significance for the treatment of overweight and obesity

It has been estimated that these endogenous weight regulatory mechanisms are effective in up to 84% of people [19]. This number is derived from observations that up to 84% of people tested in several independent overfeeding studies gained less weight than expected, indicating adaptive metabolic processes that dissipated part of the energy excess [19]. This means that for situations where rigid prescriptions of energy intake are impractical or contraindicated, it can still be possible for people to lose excess weight and keep it off, provided that endogenous signals of hunger and satiety are heard and heeded, and provided that healthy foods are easily accessible and chosen. Such situations include people who eat outside the home frequently or who have a propensity for disordered eating, as well as for community interventions where it is unfeasible to mass-prescribe kilojoule allowances. There are, however, circumstances that appear to render these biological weight-control systems ineffective, at least in some people, and these are discussed below.

Factors that interfere with biological weight-control systems

There are multiple factors that interfere with the body's innate ability to defend a healthy set point weight. These include congenital disorders associated with increased appetite, such as Prader Willi syndrome, or mutations of critical genes involved in the regulation of body weight, such as leptin, the leptin receptor or the melanocortin 4 receptor. Additionally, certain medications such as cortisol and insulin can interfere with the function of endogenous weight-control systems, leading to increased hunger and weight gain unless energy intake is deliberately restrained. In this section however, I will deal with two situations that threaten the functionality of endogenous weight-control systems in the majority of – if not all – people living in obesogenic environments such as Australia. The first of these involves situations that encourage people to eat when they are not hungry, and the second involves the types of foods that are available to most people.

Environmental triggers for non-hungry eating

Availability of food in excess

In modern society, eating often occurs independently of biological hunger and satiety signals. With so many delicious, varied and affordable foods and beverages readily available, how many people stop to question whether they are physically hungry before hoeing in? We often eat irresistible foods at the moment they are offered to us. I for one find it exceedingly difficult to save a biscuit, bun or chocolate for later if a colleague brings one to my office when I am not hungry. We often eat meals simply because it is mealtime, regardless of whether or not we have an appetite. And people commonly eat out of pure boredom, joy or other emotional triggers, even in the complete absence of physical hunger. These are all examples of non-hungry eating, an everyday occurrence for most people. As such, the ability of biological weight-control systems to work effectively is compromised, even in people in whom the appetite-reducing effects of these systems are perfectly functional.

In addition to increasing the number of eating and drinking episodes per day, our environment readily offers excessively large portions at each sitting, and this appears to compromise the satiety signals that tell us when to stop eating. Research volunteers were invited to eat from a bowl of soup until they felt satisfied [49]. Unbeknown to any of the volunteers, some of them were eating soup from bowls that were slowly and imperceptibly refilling as their contents were consumed. Uncannily, these people ate a massive *73% more* than volunteers who had eaten from normal soup bowls. What is even more fascinating is that the volunteers who had eaten from the surreptitiously rigged bowls didn't feel any more satisfied or oversatisfied than those who had eaten from normal bowls, demonstrating that we use visual as well as physical cues to determine when we have had enough to eat. This effect of larger portion sizes appears to be prolonged. When normal-weight and overweight adults were served 50% larger portions for 11 days, they ate an average of 423 additional kilocalories per day over the 11-day test period compared to an 11-day control period two weeks earlier or later in which they ate standard-sized portions [50]. This consistently increased energy intake occurred despite the fact that the volunteers reported feeling significantly less hungry and significantly more satiated during the overfeeding period than during the control period [50]. These results collectively imply that unless deliberate attempts are made to control portion sizes and heed endogenous hunger and satiety signals, then even if an individual is in energy excess with a subsequently reduced appetite, they will eat more than their physical needs dictate, and their biological weight-control systems will not have the opportunity to function optimally in the defence against excessive weight gain.

Health messages that inadvertently discourage eating according to physical hunger

It may seem obvious that our obesogenic environment pushes people to overeat when not hungry. However, even amongst people who are trying to lose weight, there is a disconnect between eating and biological hunger.

> The diet specified that you have to eat at least six times a day, as this is supposed to keep the metabolism of premenopausal women high. (Maria, 49 years of age and 1.52 metres tall)

People wishing to lose excess weight frequently seek knowledge about how to do so from the media, from books and from gyms. Unfortunately, these avenues often provide weight-loss directives that can inadvertently encourage non-hungry eating. Examples of such directives include 'eat little and often to keep your metabolism high' and 'you must eat within 30 minutes after a workout to build muscle' or 'never skip a meal'. While the importance of regular consumption of nutritious foods is acknowledged, it must be balanced with the likelihood that many people seeking to lose excess weight will have a reduced appetite due to effects of their biological weight-control systems. Encouraging eating without regard to hunger signals prevents these people from listening to the innate systems that could actually help them to lose excess weight, if heeded.

Diets high in sugar and/or fat

It is well accepted in the scientific literature that feeding rodents a diet high in sugar and fat (or high in fat) for several months results in approximately 30% of animals becoming apparently *permanently obese* [12, 51–53]. When switched to an *ad libitum* low-fat diet, these diet-induced obese rodents maintain the same elevated body weight. When placed on an energy-restricted low-fat diet, they lose weight, but once *ad libitum* access is reinstated, body weight rebounds to the elevated level. Whereas these animals would never have become obese if they had not been fed the obesogenic diet – as indicated by the fact that littermate controls maintained on the low-fat diet remain lean throughout life – the high-fat diet induces a shift in 'set point' such that a higher body weight is defended.

Genes load the gun, the environment pulls the trigger. (Quote attributed to George Bray)

Genetic blueprint is a major determinant of whether or not an individual animal will be susceptible or resistant to diet-induced obesity. However, having the genes for obesity is not enough; an individual genetically predisposed to obesity requires an obesogenic diet in order to manifest this genetic blueprint via gene–environment interactions. So what are the effects of obesogenic diets on biological weight-control systems? This question has been addressed in studies in which diets that are either high in fat, or high in fat and sugar, have been fed to animals.

Obesogenic diets induce leptin resistance

One clear effect of long-term exposure to an environment rich in dietary fat is the development of leptin resistance [21, 54–56]. The hormone leptin is a key regulator of biological weight-control systems. It is secreted in large part from white adipose tissue (body fat). Under normal circumstances, a gain in body fat leads to an increase in circulating concentrations of leptin, which in turn acts on the hypothalamus of the brain to contribute to effects of energy excess as discussed above, namely inhibition of appetite, stimulation of physical activity and enhancement of energy expenditure. However, after several months on a high-fat diet, there is a decrease in the ability of leptin to induce its effects, possibly via changes such as a decrease in the number of leptin receptors in the brain. This change in turn leads to ineffectiveness of the endogenous weight-control mechanisms, with subsequently accelerated weight gain.

Obesogenic diets induce changes resembling 'food addiction'

Constant exposure to, and overconsumption of, a high fat–high sugar diet triggers similar changes in the brain to those seen in drug addiction. These changes can override the biological weight-control systems, driving the development of compulsive overeating and excessive weight gain. When adult rats were given unlimited access to bacon, sausages, cheesecake, pound cake, frosting and chocolate (as well as normal low-fat chow) for about 20 hours a day for 40 days, they rapidly developed a preference for the high-fat foods [57]. Moreover, the rats exhibited compulsive-like feeding behaviour, demonstrated by the fact that they kept eating even in adverse conditions that normally cause rats to cease eating. At the end of 40 days, the animals had gained significant amounts of excess weight. Genetic techniques revealed that this drive to eat 'compulsively' was likely due to a decrease in the amount of dopamine D2 receptors in the striatum, a part of the brain involved in the development of addictive behaviours [57]. Dopamine is a neurotransmitter that is released in the brain in response to pleasurable stimuli such as eating, sex, or use of addictive drugs like cocaine. By acting on dopamine D2 receptors, dopamine induces changes in mood. Intriguingly, this reduction in dopamine D2 receptors in the brain is also seen in the brains of people who are addicted to drugs, as well as in people who have a body mass index in the obese range [57]. These findings may help to explain the observation that despite the presence of endogenous weight-control systems, many people overeat in our current obesogenic environment, where foods such as sausages, pound cake and frosting are easier – and cheaper per kilojoule – to procure than fruits and vegetables.

Reversibility – or not – of diet-induced brain changes that predispose to obesity

A plethora of studies such as the ones cited above unanimously show that overconsumption of a diet high in sugar and/or fat leads to changes in the brain that compromise the functionality of biological weight-control systems, at least in animals. What is not known from this research is whether such changes occur in people who have been exposed to similarly obesogenic diets for a long time, and whether any such changes are reversible in humans or animals, particularly in those with a genetic propensity for diet-induced obesity.

New evidence points to the possibility that at least some of the effects of a high-fat diet on the brain may be reversible. In one study, the severe leptin resistance seen in the hypothalamus of mice on a high-fat diet was reversed after two weeks on a low-fat diet [56]. Exercise has also been shown to alleviate the effects of a high-fat diet on the defended set point. As mentioned above, diet-induced obese rats with a strong genetic propensity for weight gain lose weight when put on a low-fat/low-energy diet, but they regain their pre-diet weight within eight weeks of *ad libitum* access to low-fat food [52]. In contrast, diet-induced obese rats that ran on a treadmill for half-an-hour a day, six days a week, regained significantly less weight than the sedentary control rats, weighing approximately 10% less, and having approximately 13% less body fat, than non-exercising controls [52]. In fact, the total body fat of the exercising rats was no different from that of lean rats that had never been obese in their lives. This beneficial effect of exercise was due to inhibition of the drive to eat rather than an increase in energy expenditure. Circumstantial evidence also suggests that effects of obesogenic diets on addiction-like changes in the brain may be reversible. Just as the low levels of the dopamine D2 receptor in the brain of people who are addicted to drugs appear to be increased upon abstinence from the drug to which they are addicted, the low levels of D2 receptor seen in postmortem brains of obese people are not apparent in brains from formerly obese people who had lost weight following gastric surgery [57]. Collectively, these findings raise the hopeful possibility that environmental and behavioural changes leading to a better diet, increased physical activity and weight loss can reverse the brain changes that compromise the effectiveness of biological weight-control systems.

More research into the potential reversibility – or not – of diet-induced brain changes is urgently needed. Of particular concern is the observation that a high-fat diet has been shown to cause epigenetic changes in the gene for leptin [58]. Epigenetic changes are changes to the DNA structure that are not encoded by the DNA sequence itself but which are nonetheless transmitted to subsequent generations. Examples include the addition of methyl groups to regions of the DNA, resulting in alterations to the expression of nearby genes. Feeding lean rats a high-fat diet resulted in methylation of DNA in the promotor region controlling the expression of leptin [58]. The link between epigenetic changes and obesity is an expanding area of research. It raises the troubling possibility that obesogenic diets not only render individuals incapable of losing excess weight, but they can also lumber ensuing generations with residual environmentally induced problems. Circumstantial evidence for this comes from the finding that the sons and grandsons of men who had been exposed to overabundant food at around the time of puberty in Overkalix, an isolated region in Sweden, lived significantly shorter lives than the progeny of men who had not been exposed to a rare period of food overabundance in their pre-pubertal development [59].

Implications for human obesity

With these rodent diet-induced obesities in mind, it is deeply concerning to see people consuming high-fat or high-fat and high-sugar diets – with little fruits and vegetables – from an early age onwards. Is our environment robbing their bodies of the natural ability to guard against excess weight, thereby setting them and their progeny up for permanent obesity? Outstanding research questions are listed below. Sadly, we will probably have the answers to these questions when the first generation of children who have grown up almost exclusively on junk food come of age.

- Does overconsumption of an obesogenic diet induce brain changes in humans that predispose to overeating and obesity, as has been observed in rodents?
- If so, how many months or years on an obesogenic diet are required to induce such brain changes in humans?
- Are such effects of an obesogenic diet on the brain permanent, or can switching to a healthy diet, exercising and losing weight reverse them?
- What are the genotypes or epigenotypes that increase the susceptibility to diet-induced obesity in humans?
- Can we identify diagnostic biomarkers to identify children with such genotypes or epigenotypes, so that they can be protected from obesogenic diets, just as children with nut allergies are vehemently protected from nuts in the environment?

Conclusion

In modern society, the process of eating is becoming increasingly disconnected from the physical need to replenish fuel supplies. We consume highly palatable foods and beverages because they are readily available in large quantities, and lack of physical hunger is all too rarely an impediment to eating. When weight gain ensues, many people and their health practitioners resort to external directives about what, when and how much to eat. While this approach – where energy intake is determined externally – helps a proportion of people to lose excess weight and keep it off, it also results in a proportion of people eating too little or too much for effective weight loss, potentially exacerbating their overweight or obese conditions. Moreover, such methods are not suitable for everyone, especially people whose lifestyles do not afford the rigidity required to count or measure foods or eat separate meals to their family and friends, and those prone to eating disorders. Additionally, such weight-loss strategies are not suited to public health campaigns to promote healthy weight.

The body is equipped with endogenous systems to control excess weight. There is evidence that these biological weight-control systems are active in the majority of people and can enable loss of excess weight and/or maintenance of a healthy weight if the signals are heard and heeded. These biological control systems allow for individualised solutions to weight management, because energy intake is tailored to each person's individual needs at any particular time. However, unless public health measures are implemented to improve food supply and portion sizes, and thus allow these systems to work as effectively as they are able, it will be difficult for many people to listen to the signals. This is particularly true of people with a genetic propensity for obesity. Moreover, continuation of the current obesogenic environment may lead to irreparable brain changes that make it impossible for certain people to lose excess weight, with changes potentially being transmitted to subsequent generations. While intense lobbying to change our environment via public health measures continues, benefits could be obtained now by helping people to learn to eat according to internal hunger and satiety signals. This could be achieved via commercial weight-loss programs, health practitioners, or potentially also via public health campaigns, thus enabling more people to benefit from the biological systems that naturally control body weight.

Acknowlegement

Amanda Sainsbury is supported by a Career Development Award from the National Health and Medical Research Council (NHMRC) of Australia.

Disclosure

Amanda Sainsbury is the author of two books: *The don't go hungry diet* (Bantam, 2007) and *Don't go hungry for life* (Bantam, 2011).

References

1. Jebb SA, Ahern AL, Olson AD, Aston LA, Holzapfel C, Stoll J, et al. (2011). Primary care referral to a commercial provider for weight loss treatment, relative to standard care: an international randomised controlled trial. *The Lancet,* DOI:10.1016/50140-6736(11)61344-5.

2. Sainsbury A & Zhang L (2010). Role of the arcuate nucleus of the hypothalamus in regulation of body weight during energy deficit. *Molecular and Cellular Endocrinology,* 316(2): 109–19.

3. Wing RR & Jeffery RW (2003). Prescribed 'breaks' as a means to disrupt weight control efforts. *Obesity Research,* 11(2): 287–91.

4. Sweeney ME, Hill JO, Heller PA, Baney R & DiGirolamo M (1993). Severe vs moderate energy restriction with and without exercise in the treatment of obesity: efficiency of weight loss. *American Journal of Clinical Nutrition,* 57(2): 127–34.

5. Sullivan EL & Cameron JL (2010). A rapidly occurring compensatory decrease in physical activity counteracts diet-induced weight loss in female monkeys. *American Journal of Physiology: Regulatory, Integrative and Comparative Physiology,* 298(4): R1068–R74.

6. Martin CK, Das SK, Lindblad L, Racette SB, McCrory MA, Weiss EP, et al. (2011). Effect of calorie restriction on the free-living physical activity levels of nonobese humans: results of three randomized trials. *Journal of Applied Physiology,* 110(4): 956–63.

7. Martin CK, Heilbronn LK, de Jonge L, DeLany JP, Volaufova J, Anton SD, et al. (2007). Effect of calorie restriction on resting metabolic rate and spontaneous physical activity. *Obesity,* 15(12): 2964–73.

8. Novak CM & Levine JA (2007). Central neural and endocrine mechanisms of non-exercise activity thermogenesis and their potential impact on obesity. *Journal of Neuroendocrinology,* 19(12): 923–40.

9. Rosenbaum M, Vandenborne K, Goldsmith R, Simoneau JA, Heymsfield S, Joanisse DR, et al. (2003). Effects of experimental weight perturbation on skeletal muscle work efficiency in human subjects. *American Journal of Physiology Regulatory Integractive Comparitive Physiology,* 285(1): R183–R92.

10. Sainsbury A & Zhang L (2011). Role of the hypothalamus in the neuroendocrine regulation of body weight and composition during energy deficit. *Obesity Reviews,* DOI:10.1111/j.1467-789X.2011.00948.x.

11. Pasman WJ, Saris WH & Westerterp-Plantenga MS (1999). Predictors of weight maintenance. *Obesity Research,* 7(1): 43–50.

12. MacLean PS, Higgins JA, Johnson GC, Fleming-Elder BK, Peters JC & Hill JO (2004). Metabolic adjustments with the development, treatment, and recurrence of obesity in obesity-prone rats. *American Journal of Physiology: Regulatory, Integrative and Comparative Physiology,* 287(2): R288–R97.

13. Goran MI (2000). Energy metabolism and obesity. *Medical Clinics of North America,* 84(2): 347–62.

14. Dulloo AG & Girardier L (1990). Adaptive changes in energy expenditure during refeeding following low-calorie intake: evidence for a specific metabolic component favoring fat storage. *The American Journal of Clinical Nutrition,* 52(3): 415–20.

15. Berman Y, Devi L, Spangler R, Kreek MJ & Carr KD (1997). Chronic food restriction and streptozotocin-induced diabetes differentially alter prodynorphin mRNA levels in rat brain regions. *Molecular Brain Research,* 46(1–2): 25–30.

16. Herve C & Fellmann D (1997). Changes in rat melanin-concentrating hormone and dynorphin messenger ribonucleic acids induced by food deprivation. *Neuropeptides,* 31(3): 237–42.

17. Jonas JM & Gold MS (1988). The use of opiate antagonists in treating bulimia: a study of low-dose versus high-dose naltrexone. *Psychiatry Research,* 24(2): 195–99.

18. Atkinson RL (1982). Naloxone decreases food intake in obese humans. *Journal of Clinical Endocrinology and Metabolism,* 55(1): 196–98.

19. Stock MJ (1999). Gluttony and thermogenesis revisited. *International Journal of Obesity and Related Metabolic Disorders,* 23(11): 1105–17.

20. Roberts SB, Young VR, Fuss P, Fiatarone MA, Richard B, Rasmussen H, et al. (1990). Energy expenditure and subsequent nutrient intakes in overfed young men. *American Journal of Physiology,* 259(3 Pt 2): R461–R9.

21. Lin S, Storlien LH & Huang X (2000). Leptin receptor, NPY, POMC mRNA expression in the diet-induced obese mouse brain. *Brain Research,* 875(1–2): 89–95.

22. Ernersson A, Nystrom FH & Lindstrom T (2010). Long-term increase of fat mass after a four week intervention with fast food based hyper-alimentation and limitation of physical activity. *Nutrition and Metabolism (London),* 7: 68.

23. Levine JA, Eberhardt NL & Jensen MD (1999). Role of nonexercise activity thermogenesis in resistance to fat gain in humans. *Science,* 283(5399): 212–14.

24. Sullivan EL, Koegler FH & Cameron JL (2006). Individual differences in physical activity are closely associated with changes in body weight in adult female rhesus monkeys (Macaca mulatta). *American Journal of Physiology: Regulatory, Integrative and Comparative Physiology,* 291(3): R633–R42.

25. Leibel RL, Rosenbaum M & Hirsch J (1995). Changes in energy expenditure resulting from altered body weight. *New England Journal of Medicine,* 332(10): 621–28.

26. Wijers SL, Saris WH & van Marken Lichtenbelt WD (2009). Recent advances in adaptive thermogenesis: potential implications for the treatment of obesity. *Obesity Reviews,* 10(2): 218–26.

27. Rising R, Alger S, Boyce V, Seagle H, Ferraro R, Fontvieille AM, et al. (1992). Food intake measured by an automated food-selection system: relationship to energy expenditure. *American Journal of Clinical Nutrition,* 55(2): 343–49.

28. Joosen AM & Westerterp KR (2006). Energy expenditure during overfeeding. *Nutrition and Metabolism (London),* 3: 25.

29. Rosenbaum M, Hirsch J, Murphy E & Leibel RL (2000). Effects of changes in body weight on carbohydrate metabolism, catecholamine excretion, and thyroid function. *American Journal of Clinical Nutrition,* 71(6): 1421–32.

30. Gentile CL, Orr JS, Davy BM & Davy KP (2007). Modest weight gain is associated with sympathetic neural activation in nonobese humans. *American Journal of Physiology: Regulatory, Integrative and Compatative Physiology,* 292(5): R1834–R8.

31. Sainsbury A, Cooney GJ & Herzog H (2002). Hypothalamic regulation of energy homeostasis. *Best Practice & Research Clinical Endocrinology and Metabolism,* 16(4): 623–37.

32. Levine JA, Nygren J, Short KR & Nair KS (2003). Effect of hyperthyroidism on spontaneous physical activity and energy expenditure in rats. *Journal of Applied Physiology,* 94(1): 165–70.

33. Silva JE (2003). The thermogenic effect of thyroid hormone and its clinical implications. *Annals of Internal Medicine,* 139(3): 205–13.

34. Lopez M, Varela L, Vazquez MJ, Rodriguez-Cuenca S, Gonzalez CR, Velagapudi VR, et al. (2010). Hypothalamic AMPK and fatty acid metabolism mediate thyroid regulation of energy balance. *Nature Medicine,* 16(9): 1001–08.

35. Wijers SL, Schrauwen P, van Baak MA, Saris WH & van Marken Lichtenbelt WD (2011). Beta-adrenergic receptor blockade does not inhibit cold-induced thermogenesis in humans: possible involvement of brown adipose tissue.*The Journal of Clinical Endocrinology and Metabolism,* 96(4): E598–E605.

36. Cahill F, Shea JL, Randell E, Vasdev S & Sun G (2011). Serum peptide YY in response to short-term overfeeding in young men. *The American Journal of Clinical Nutrition,* 93(4): 741–47.

37. Batterham RL, Cohen MA, Ellis SM, Le Roux CW, Withers DJ, Frost GS, et al. (2003). Inhibition of food intake in obese subjects by peptide YY3–36. *New England Journal of Medicine,* 349(10): 941–48.

38. Pittner R, Moore C, Bhavsar S, Gedulin B, Smith P, Jodka C, et al. (2004). Effects of PYY[3–36] in rodent models of diabetes and obesity. *International Journal of Obesity*, 28: 963–71.

39. Chelikani PK, Haver AC, Reeve JR Jr, Keire DA & Reidelberger RD (2006). Daily, intermittent intravenous infusion of peptide YY(3–36) reduces daily food intake and adiposity in rats. *American Journal of Physiology: Regulatory, Integrative and Comparative Physiology*, 290(2): R298–R305.

40. Sloth B, Holst JJ, Flint A, Gregersen NT & Astrup A (2007). Effects of PYY1–36 and PYY3–36 on appetite, energy intake, energy expenditure, glucose and fat metabolism in obese and lean subjects. *American Journal of Physiology: Endocrinology and Metabolism*, 292(4): E1062–E68.

41. Boey D, Lin S, Enriquez RF, Lee NJ, Slack K, Couzens M, et al. (2008). PYY transgenic mice are protected against diet-induced and genetic obesity. *Neuropeptides*, 42(1): 19–30.

42. Bouchard C, Tremblay A, Despres JP, Nadeau A, Lupien PJ, Theriault G, et al. (1990). The response to long-term overfeeding in identical twins. *The New England Journal of Medicine*, 322(21): 1477–82.

43. Ukkola O, Tremblay A, Sun G, Chagnon YC & Bouchard C (2001). Genetic variation at the uncoupling protein 1, 2 and 3 loci and the response to long-term overfeeding. *European Journal of Clinical Nutrition*, 55(11): 1008–15.

44. Pasquet P & Apfelbaum M (1994). Recovery of initial body weight and composition after long-term massive overfeeding in men. *The American Journal of Clinical Nutrition*, 60(6): 861–63.

45. Foster GD, Wyatt HR, Hill JO, McGuckin BG, Brill C, Mohammed BS, et al. (2003). A randomized trial of a low-carbohydrate diet for obesity. *The New England Journal of Medicine*, 348(21): 2082–90.

46. Samaha FF, Iqbal N, Seshadri P, Chicano KL, Daily DA, McGrory J, et al. (2003). A low-carbohydrate as compared with a low-fat diet in severe obesity. *The New England Journal of Medicine*, 348(21): 2074–81.

47. McMillan-Price J, Petocz P, Atkinson F, O'Neill K, Samman S, Steinbeck K, et al. (2006). Comparison of 4 diets of varying glycemic load on weight loss and cardiovascular risk reduction in overweight and obese young adults: a randomized controlled trial. *Archives of Internal Medicine*, 166(14): 1466–75.

48. National Health and Medical Research Council. Clinical Practice Guidelines for the Management of Overweight and Obesity in Adults. Canberra: Commonwealth of Australia, 2003.

49. Wansink B, Painter JE & North J (2005). Bottomless bowls: why visual cues of portion size may influence intake. *Obesity Research*, 13(1): 93–100.

50. Rolls BJ, Roe LS & Meengs JS (2007). The effect of large portion sizes on energy intake is sustained for 11 days. *Obesity (Silver Spring)*, 15(6): 1535–43.

51. Levin BE (2007). Why some of us get fat and what we can do about it. *Journal of Physiology*, 583(Pt 2): 425–30.

52. MacLean PS, Higgins JA, Wyatt HR, Melanson EL, Johnson GC, Jackman MR, et al. (2009). Regular exercise attenuates the metabolic drive to regain weight after long-term weight loss. *American Journal of Physiology - Regulatory, Integrative and Comparative Physiology*, 297(3): R793–R802.

53. Hariri N & Thibault L (2010). High-fat diet-induced obesity in animal models. *Nutrition Research Reviews*, 23(2): 270–99.

54. Lin S, Thomas TC, Storlien LH & Huang XF (2000). Development of high fat diet-induced obesity and leptin resistance in C57Bl/6J mice. *International Journal of Obesity and Related Metabolic Disorders*, 24(5): 639–46.

55. El-Haschimi K, Pierroz DD, Hileman SM, Bjorbaek C & Flier JS (2000). Two defects contribute to hypothalamic leptin resistance in mice with diet-induced obesity. *Journal of Clinical Investigation*, 105(12): 1827–32.

56. Enriori PJ, Evans AE, Sinnayah P, Jobst EE, Tonelli-Lemos L, Billes SK, et al. (2007). Diet-induced obesity causes severe but reversible leptin resistance in arcuate melanocortin neurons. *Cell Metabolism*, 5(3): 181–94.

57. Johnson PM & Kenny PJ (2010). Dopamine D2 receptors in addiction-like reward dysfunction and compulsive eating in obese rats. *Nature Neuroscience*, 13(5): 635–41.

58. Milagro FI, Campion J, Garcia-Diaz DF, Goyenechea E, Paternain L & Martinez JA (2009). High fat diet-induced obesity modifies the methylation pattern of leptin promoter in rats. *Journal of Physiology and Biochemistry*, 65(1): 1–9.

59. Bygren LO, Kaati G & Edvinsson S (2001). Longevity determined by paternal ancestors' nutrition during their slow growth period. *Acta Biotheoretical*, 49(1): 53–59.

2

The geometry of human nutrition[1]

Stephen J Simpson[2] and David Raubenheimer[3]

This chapter is an excerpt from a forthcoming book, titled 'The nature of nutrition: a unifying framework from animal adaptation to human obesity' by Stephen J Simpson and David Raubenheimer (Princeton University Press, 2012). In the book we present a graphical approach, the 'geometric framework', which we believe can help to integrate nutrition into the broader biological sciences and introduce generality into the applied nutritional sciences. In the present chapter we use this approach to show that the epidemic of human obesity and metabolic disease is linked to changes in the nutritional balance of our diet, with a primary role for protein appetite driving excess energy intake on a modern Western diet.

The modern human nutritional dilemma

It is conservatively estimated that more than one billion people worldwide are overweight or obese. Rates of obesity are increasing, notably among the young, and the associated disease burden is immense [1–3]. Figure 1A plots the relative risk of dying prematurely as an adult against body mass index (BMI), which approximates to body fatness and is calculated as body mass in kilograms divided by the square of height in metres. Clinicians categorise adults as underweight if they have a BMI of less than 18.5, as overweight if they have BMI values between 25 and 30, and as obese if they exceed 30. The curve is U-shaped, with the risk of dying prematurely increasing at both low and high values of BMI, and the target zone for health and longevity lying in between.

The relationship between body fat content and risk of premature death in humans is very similar to what we have observed in the locust, Figure 1B. This is a species that defends a target intake of macronutrients [4], and Figure 1B suggests a reason why that target is defended: because doing so minimises the risk of dying early. We have encountered similar 'nutritional wisdom' in caterpillars, as well as fruit flies and field crickets [4].

1   We are grateful to Princeton University Press for permission to include this chapter from the author's forthcoming book: Simpson SJ and Raubenheimer D (2012). *The nature of nutrition: a unifying framework from animal adaptation to human obesity*, Princeton: Princeton University Press.

2   School of Biological Sciences and Charles Perkins Centre, University of Sydney.

3   Institute of National Sciences, Massey University, Auckland, New Zeland.

Regrettably, the same cannot be said for our own species. Take as an example the US, where approximately 65% of adults are overweight or obese, while 30% are clinically obese. And the US is not atypical – the same trend is seen in all developed countries and increasingly in developing countries, too. Why have we gone so badly wrong? The answer lies in the interplay between the nutritional environment and regulatory physiology.

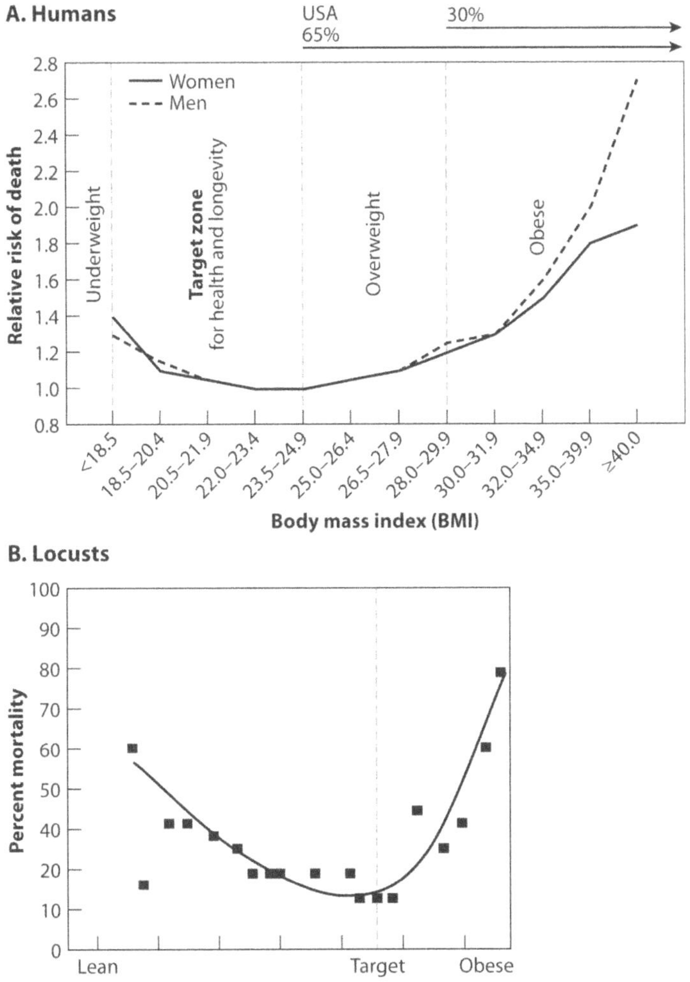

Figure 1A. The relative risk of dying prematurely as an adult against body mass index (BMI) in US adults (based on Calle et al. [72]); and B. an equivalent plot for locusts [73].

As summarised in Figure 2, the human nutritional environment has changed considerably over the past 35,000 years since the Upper Palaeolithic. Anthropologists and archaeologists have reconstructed the nutritional ecology of our forebears during this period [5]. The main conclusion is that people then were probably energy-limited, because sources of simple sugar, fat and starch were rare. In contrast, protein was relatively abundant in the form of lean game animals. Skeletal analyses indicate that people were large, lean and healthy under such an environment [5].

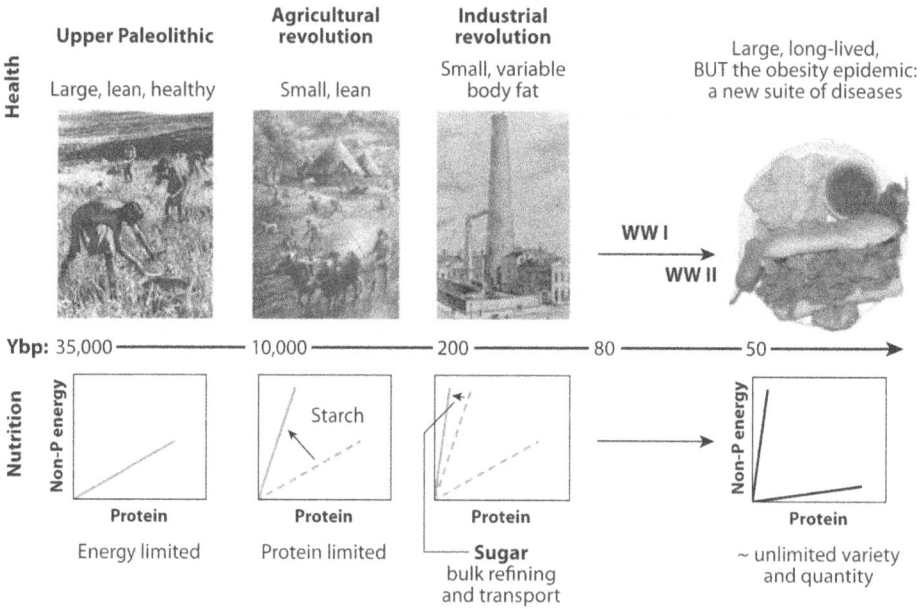

Figure 2. A summary timeline for the changing human nutritional environment since the Paleolithic.

A major transition in human nutrition occurred with the shift from hunter-gatherer lifestyle to agriculture. This took place at different times in different parts of the world, but the results were similar: there was an increase in the amount of readily available carbohydrate, particularly starch from grains, in the diet. This may have been associated with protein limitation and also micronutrient imbalances, and probably led to increased problems of famine as well as a greater disease burden as populations became more concentrated and sedentary [6–8]. As a result, people were, on average, smaller than in the Upper Palaeolithic, lean and less healthy.

The incorporation of carbohydrate into the diet increased further during the Industrial Revolution, due to the bulk refining and efficient transport of grains and sugar. Around that time, most people were small and lean, with corpulence being largely restricted to the wealthy few.

Since the Industrial Revolution, there has been a further major nutritional transition, between and following the two world wars. Today in the developed world, we have an unprecedented general access to all manner of foods and nutrients. We in the Western world are large and live long, but are also suffering the obesity epidemic and an upsurge in a new set of chronic diseases associated with our modern lifestyle.

In contrast to the changing nutritional environment, our physiology seems to have remained much more constant over the same timescale. There is evidence of genetic adaptation in human populations to changed patterns of food availability since the Upper Palaeolithic [8] – for example, the evolution of lactose tolerance among human populations with the advent of dairy herding and, possibly also the selection of genes that confer resistance to diabetes [9]. However, the pace at which our nutritional environment has changed is considerably faster than the rate at which our metabolism can evolve: we are caught in a time lag, in which our physiology is poorly adapted to our lifestyle.

If we are to understand how our 'outdated' physiology interacts with our changed nutritional environment, we must answer three fundamental questions:

1. Do humans regulate intake of multiple nutrients to an intake target (*sensu* Simpson and Raubenheimer [4])?
2. How do humans balance eating too much of some nutrients against too little of others when faced with an imbalanced diet – ie what is the rule of compromise for humans (*sensu* Simpson and Raubenheimer [4])?
3. How do humans deal with nutrient excesses?

We will deal with these questions in turn, restricting our discussion to the three macronutrients – protein, carbohydrate and fat. Of these nutrients, we argue that protein has played a pivotal role in the development of the obesity epidemic.

Do humans regulate to an intake target?

As yet, no properly controlled geometric experiment, along the lines described in [4] for numerous other animals, has been published for humans. Partly for this reason, it remains contentious whether humans are able to regulate their intake of different macronutrients [10–12]. There are, nonetheless, three sources of information that suggest that we can regulate the intake of specific nutrients.

1. Comparative data from rodents and other omnivores

Rodents are widely used as models for human nutritional physiology. From a nutritional perspective, there is some rationale to this because, like humans, rodents are broad-scale food generalists. Reinterpreting published data on rats showed convincingly that these mammals have the capacity to regulate their intake of protein and carbohydrate [13]. An example is shown in Figure 3A, in which we replotted data collected by Theall et al. [14]. Rats were provided with one of eight different complementary food pairings, and in every case converged on the same intake of protein and carbohydrate, indicating that these animals regulated their intake of both macronutrients. Subsequently, Sørensen and colleagues [15] conducted a full geometric analysis of protein and carbohydrate regulation in another model rodent, the mouse, and showed unequivocally that mice, too, regulate protein and carbohydrate to an intake target (Figure 3B).

2. Studies on human macronutrient appetite

There are data which indicate that we have some capacity to regulate our intake of macronutrients, notably protein, despite the extreme complexity of our social and nutritional environments [12, see 16]. It appears that macronutrient-specific feedbacks operate over a period of one to two days, and that, at least for protein, we subliminally learn to associate foods with the nutritional consequences of eating them [17, 18].

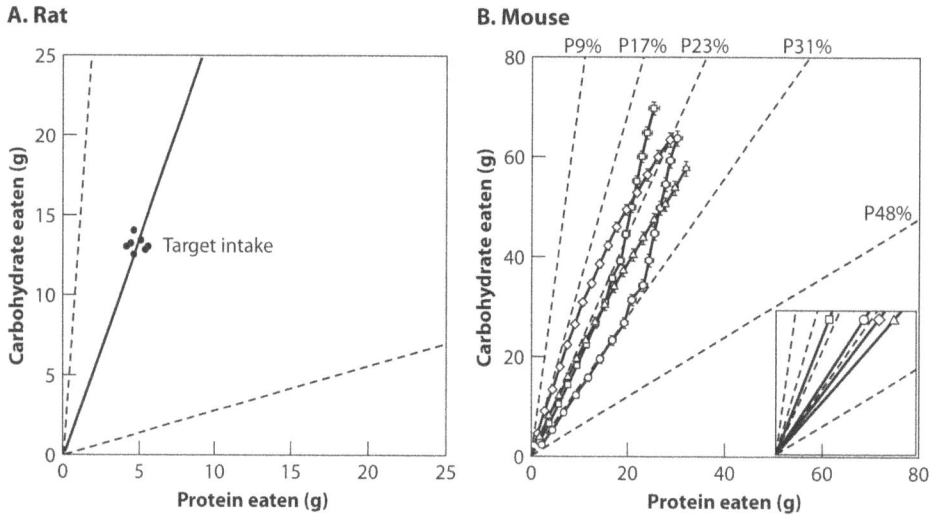

Figure 3. Rats and mice possess separate appetites for protein and carbohydrate. A. Data for rats provided with one of eight different complementary food pairings (food rails not marked except for the two most extreme ratios). Rats converged on a point of protein–carbohydrate intake, indicating tight regulation of both macronutrients to an intake target. (Data from Theall et al. [14], reanalysed in Simpson and Raubenheimer [13]). B. Cumulative protein–carbohydrate intake trajectories for mice offered one of five food pairings. Mice converged significantly relative to a common (target) intake trajectory. Had they fed indiscriminately between foods in each pairing, trajectories would have diverged markedly, as shown in the lower insert. (From Sørensen et al. [15], with permission).

3. Population-level data

A striking feature of the human diet is that the proportion of protein in the diet is highly consistent across populations and across time, comprising around 15% of total energy, whereas fat and carbohydrate vary [19] (Figure 4). And not only the proportion of protein, but also the amount is consistent, at least in some populations. Figure 5 plots estimates for per capita intake for the UK population from 1961 until 2000, taken from the Food and Agriculture Organization of the United Nations (FAOSTAT) database [20]. According to these data (which are based on nutrient supply rather than measures of actual intake), intake of protein and also fat and carbohydrate have remained remarkably stable since 1961. Not only that, they appear to have been 'defended'. If we first take the case of dietary fat supply and break down the total into fats derived from animal and vegetable sources, it is apparent that during the mid 1980s intake of animal fats fell precipitously, presumably in response to the public health campaign urging people to eat less of these fats. Thus, at this time there was a perturbation in the nutritional environment – was there a compensatory change to counterbalance this? Yes – as can be seen in Figure 5, the intake of vegetable fats rose in direct proportion to falling intake of animal fats, leading to maintenance of total fat intake at a constant level. Similar substitutions between food groups were also seen over the same period for protein and carbohydrate. Sugar intake fell and was compensated for by increasing consumption of complex carbohydrates (starches, fruit and vegetables). Declining consumption of beef, pork and lamb was compensated by increased poultry consumption, reflecting increasing availability and cheapness of the latter with increased industrialisation of poultry production.

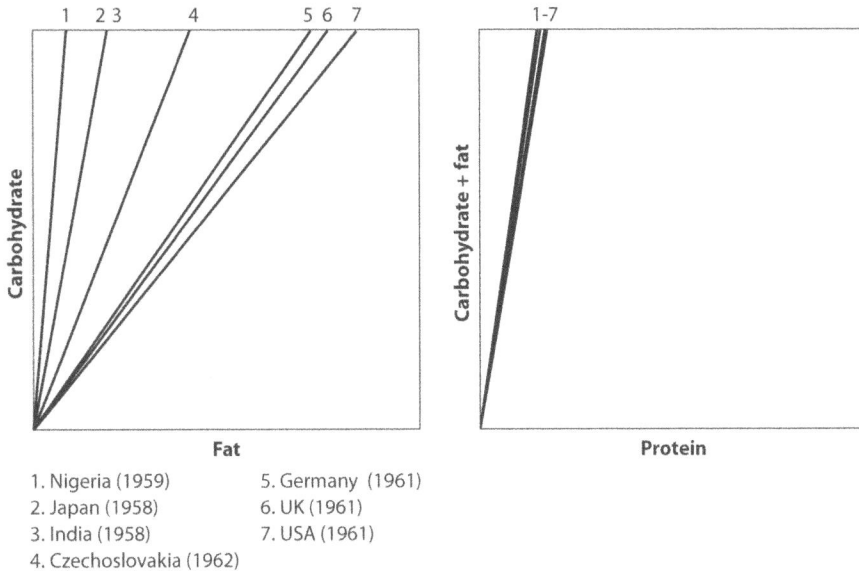

1. Nigeria (1959)   5. Germany (1961)
2. Japan (1958)   6. UK (1961)
3. India (1958)   7. USA (1961)
4. Czechoslovakia (1962)

Figure 4. Ratios of average macronutrient intake (scaled in units of energy) in various human societies during the late 1950s and early 1960s. (Based on data from Westerterp-Plantenga [19] and the FAOSTAT database [20]).

But regulation of macronutrient intake is not always perfect, as strikingly illustrated by the US, where carbohydrate and fat intake (as again estimated from FAOSTAT data) have risen substantially over the period 1961 to 2000 (Figure 6). However, protein intake has risen to a lesser degree over the same period. As a result, in the US there has been a shift in diet composition towards a lower ratio of protein to carbohydrate and fat, with protein comprising 12.5% as compared with 14% of total energy intake. Almost certainly this shift has been away from the intake target ratio. Data from the National Health and Nutrition Examination Survey (NHANES) in America indicate a similar pattern: a small decline in percent dietary protein, caused largely by increasing fat and especially, carbohydrate intake [21, see also 22, 23]. Understanding the effect of such a change requires knowledge of the rule of compromise.

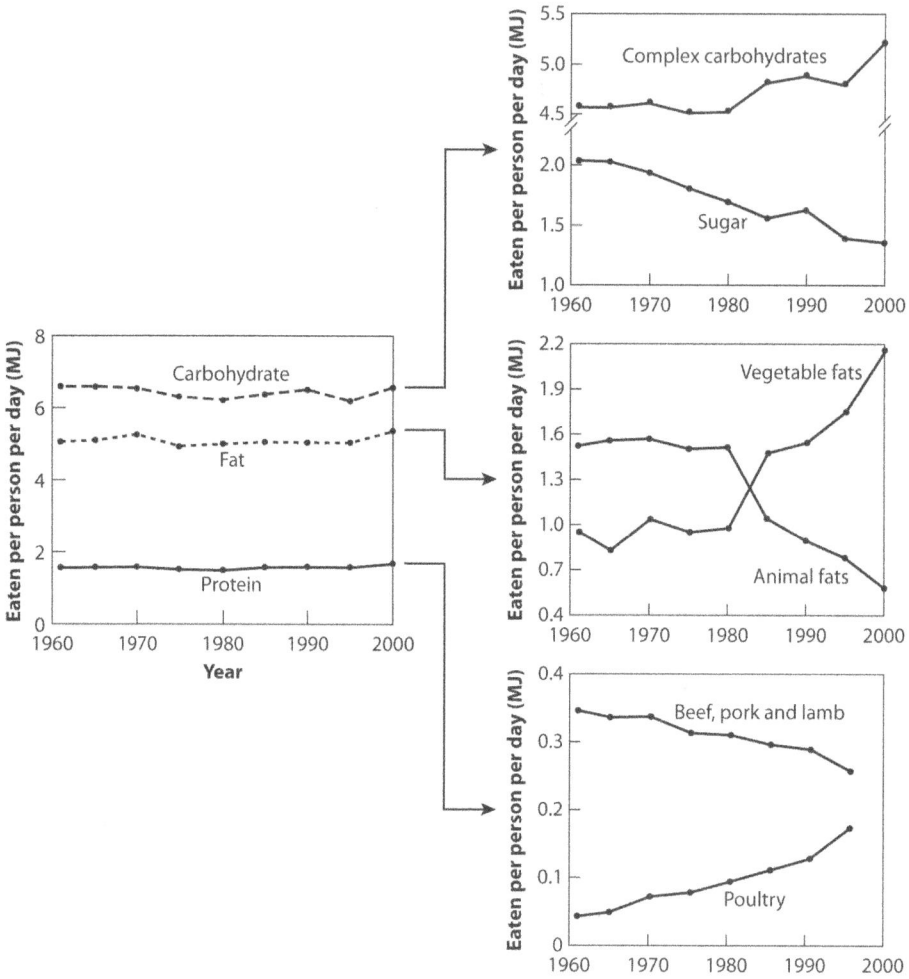

Figure 5. Changing patterns of macronutrient supply (from which intake can be approximated) in the UK from 1961 to 2000, based on FAOSTAT data. Macronutrient intake remained stable and seemingly regulated. See text for interpretation.

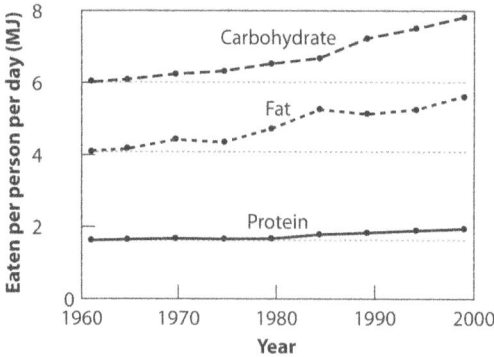

Figure 6. Data as in Figure 5, for the US. Intake of carbohydrate and fat rose faster than that for protein and as a result the percentage of protein in the daily diet fell.

What is the human rule of compromise?

To address this question, we used the geometric framework to explore the human rule of compromise [16]. Our initial study was a short-term experiment, involving ten subjects incarcerated in a chalet in the Swiss Alps, focusing on intake of protein vs carbohydrate and fat combined. We decided to treat fat and carbohydrate as a single dimension (carbohydrate and fat) scaled in energy units since the existing evidence from humans, rodents and other omnivorous animals suggested that the key interaction was between protein and non-protein energy in the diet.

Subjects were housed together for six days. For the first two days, they were provided with the opportunity to select their breakfast, lunch, afternoon snack and dinner from a buffet of items comprising a wide range of macronutrient compositions. Everything they ate was weighed and their macronutrient intake was estimated from food composition tables. For the next two days, one group of subjects (treatment 1) was restricted to foods that were high in protein and low in carbohydrate and fat, while the remaining subjects in treatment group two were provided with only low-protein, high-fat + carbohydrate items. For the final two days of the experiment (days five and six), all subjects were given the same free choice of foods as on days one and two. The results are summarised in Figure 7. The overriding message of the experiment was that when subjects were restricted to a diet that contained either a higher (treatment 1) or lower (treatment 2) ratio of protein to carbohydrate and fat than they had self-selected during days one and two, they maintained their intake of protein at the expense of the regulation of carbohydrate and fat intake. Thus, treatment group one underingested carbohydrate and fat rather than overate protein, while treatment group 2 overate carbohydrate and fat to gain limiting protein.

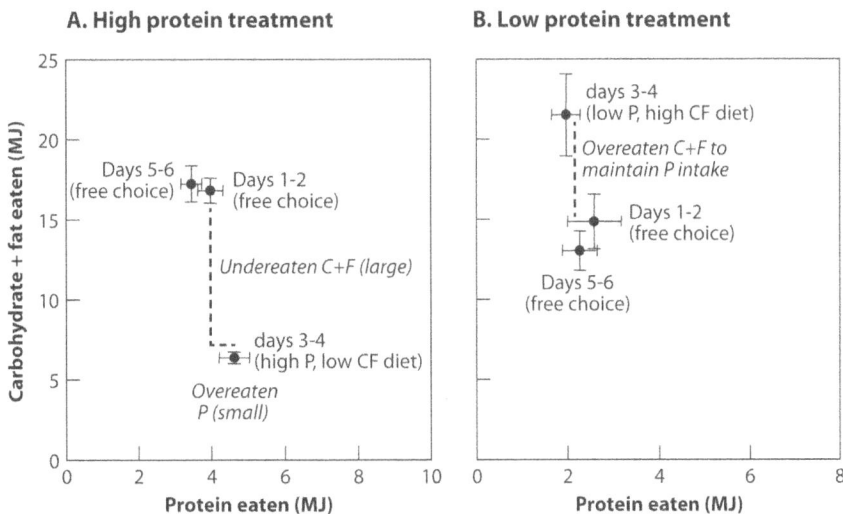

Figure 7. Results from our Swiss study [16]. See text for details. (After Simpson et al. [16], with permission).

From these data, we derived an indication of the form of the human rule of compromise for protein vs carbohydrate and fat, which is that, when forced to trade off intake of protein vs carbohydrate and fat, humans prioritise protein intake. We termed this the 'protein leverage hypothesis' [24].

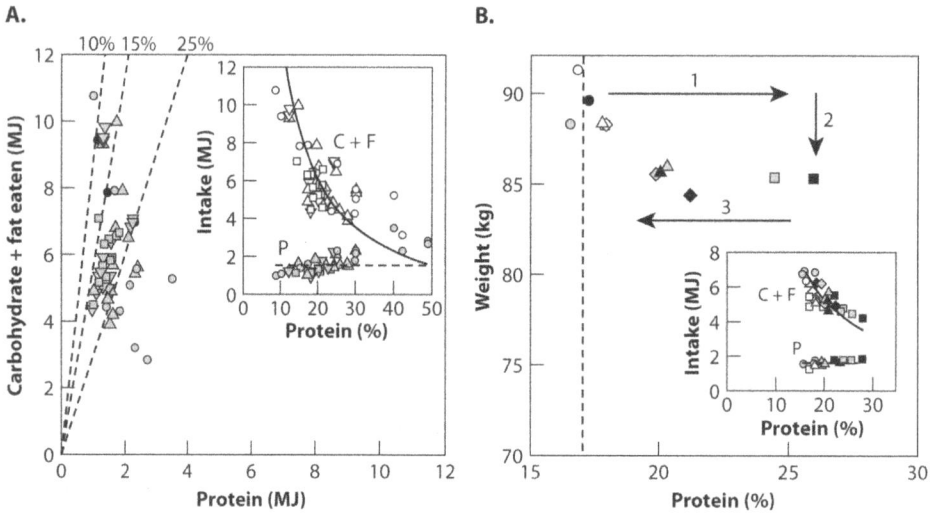

Figure 8A. Protein intake is more tightly regulated than non-protein intake in humans. Protein versus non-protein intakes from a meta-analysis of 23 studies measuring *ad libitum* daily intake on diets of different macronutrient compositions for time periods ranging from less than two months (circle), two to four months (upwards triangle), six to eight months (downwards triangle) and 12 months (square). The rails represent 10%, 15% and 25% protein diets. The inset shows that as the percentage of protein in the diet increases, non-protein (carbohydrate and fat) intake decreases but protein intake remains relatively constant. The dashed line is the mean protein intake for all studies (1.52 MJ). The solid line is calculated as the non-protein (carbohydrate and fat) intake given the percent protein intake in each study but assuming protein intake was equal to the mean (1.52 MJ); in other words, the case where protein leverage is complete and regulation of absolute protein intake dominates total energy consumption. B. Three published weight-loss studies, each showing changes in weight between baseline (circle), two months (square), six months (diamond) and 12 months (triangle). In each study participants were prescribed one of the following weight-loss regimes: the Atkins (black); Zone (grey); and Ornish (white) diets. Percent of dietary protein vs weight (kg) was plotted for each time point in each study. As percent of protein of the diet increases as a result of the Atkins and Zone regimes during the first two months (1) body weight decreases (2). Between six and 12 months the weight loss that occurred on the Atkins and Zone diets is maintained but no further weight loss occurs (3). The inset shows percent dietary protein vs (i) protein intake (dashed line: mean of protein intakes) or (ii) carbohydrate and fat (non-protein; solid line calculated as above) intake information for the three studies. From Gosby et al., unpublished.

To examine whether other experimental data supported this result, we plotted the data from our experiment along with data recast from several earlier experiments. The signature pattern of protein leverage emerged [24]. A more recent update including 23 separate studies measuring *ad libitum* intake on diets of different macronutrient compositions for time periods ranging from several days to 12 months, shows the pattern very strongly indeed (Figure 8). As predicted by the protein leverage hypothesis, in cases where subjects were restricted to a diet comprising a fixed ratio of protein to carbohydrate and fat, either in the short or long term, they maintained daily protein intake at a more constant level than that of the other two macronutrients.

Two other notable features appeared from the compilation of data in Figure 8. First, stable patterns of energy intake in response to altered dietary protein develop within one to two days and persist over at least 70 days thereafter (eg the study by Weigle et al. [18]). Second, there is evidence of an asymmetry in protein leveraging in humans. Hence, humans appear to be more willing to overeat low-protein diets to gain limiting protein than to limit intake to avoid ingesting excess protein [25]. This asymmetry may reflect the fact that the evolutionary costs of eating too little protein exceed those of eating too much. Hence, underconsumption is costly because protein is the only macronutrient to contain nitrogen, which is essential for growth and reproduction. On the other hand, excess protein consumption has been shown to have associated performance costs in some animals [eg 26, 27] – and perhaps also in humans, and suggested risks include increased insulin resistance, kidney damage, bone decalcification, ketoacidosis, cardiovascular disease and some cancers [28–31].

Also consistent with the protein leverage hypothesis are comparative data from rodents and other omnivores such as chickens and pigs [13, 15, 32–34] – and even from herbivorous and omnivorous insects such as locusts and cockroaches. Hence, rats and mice confined to a diet containing a lower protein–to–carbohydrate ratio than at the intake target, maintained protein intake near constant and in so doing overeat carbohydrate. In contrast, rodents provided with a high-protein diet did not substantially overeat protein to gain their intake target level of carbohydrate (although the asymmetry in protein leverage, alluded to above for humans, is apparent) (Figure 9). More strikingly still, data for another primate, the spider monkey, show the signature of extreme protein leverage in which protein intake is maintained near constant and non-protein energy intake allowed to vary freely to attain the protein target [35].

An acid test of protein leverage: disguising the macronutrient composition of the diet

All of the studies summarised in Figure 8 involved offering subjects diets composed of varying numbers of types of familiar foods. There was therefore the possibility that changes in the proportion of protein in the diets were confounded by other factors, such as differences in the palatability of the treatment foods, the variety of options available within each treatment, and prior experience. An acid test of the protein leverage hypothesis requires that these potentially confounding effects are controlled for. Recently, Gosby and colleagues [36, 37] set out to do just that.

A. Rat

B. Mouse

C. Chicken

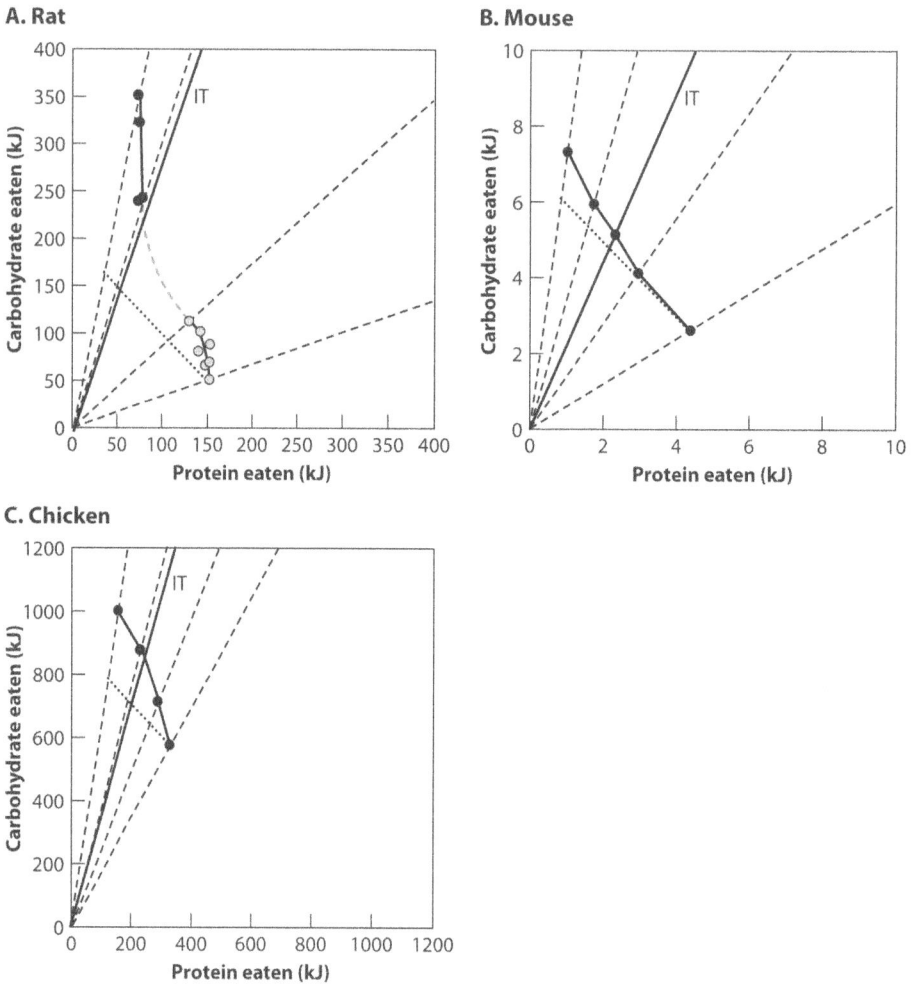

Figure 9. The rule of compromise in rats, mice and chicken. These omnivores prioritise protein intake when confined to diets (dashed rails) requiring them to tradeoff protein versus non-protein energy intake. IT indicates the position of the intake target ratio, as derived from experiments in which animals were offered one of eight (A), five (B) or four (C) complementary food pairings and demonstrated tight convergence to a nutrient intake point. The dotted line indicates isocaloric intakes, to emphasise the point that as percent of dietary protein fell, total daily energy intake rose (ie the intake arrays have slopes steeper than –1). A. After Simpson and Raubenheimer [13], derived from data by Theall et al. [14], with extra data (grey points) added from a study by Tews et al. [74]. The grey dashed curve is an interpolation between the two experiments. B. From Sørensen et al. [15]. C. From Raubenheimer and Simpson [34], based on data from Shariatmadari and Forbes [75].

A.

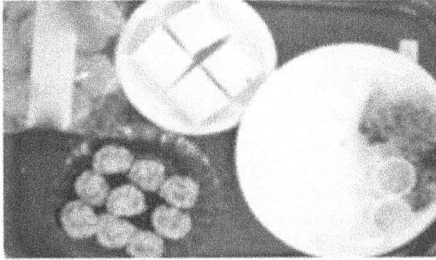

10% protein lunch

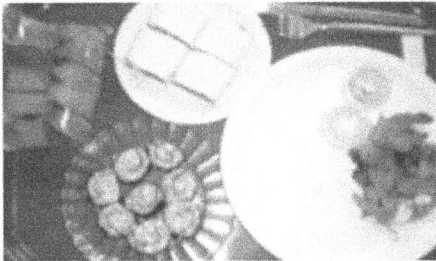

25% protein lunch

B.

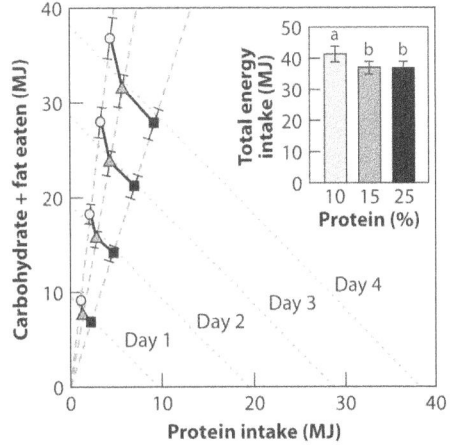

C. Savory

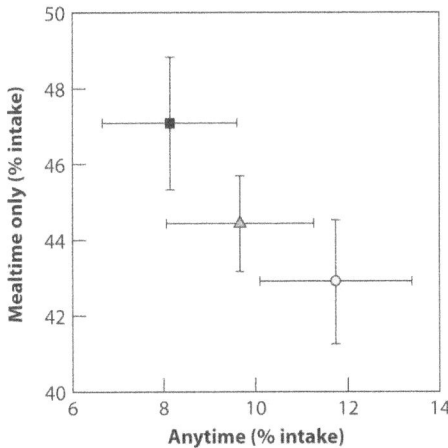

D. Sweet

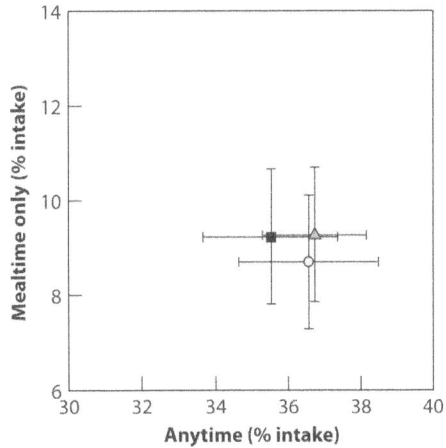

Figure 10. The Sydney protein leverage trial in which subjects were confined to four-day menus in which protein content of all foods was the same but disguised. Each participant spent three four-day periods in the trial. In one, all foods for the period contained 10% protein, in another all foods were 15% protein and in the third they were all 25% protein. Foods were matched for pleasantness and variety. A. An example of a lunch from the 10% protein week and its equivalent in the 25% protein week. Participants were provided with a selection of sweet (apple crumble muffins) and savory (Teriyaki sushi rolls and Mexican wraps) foods to choose from as well as a serving of salad leaves and dressing. Participants were asked to eat until they felt comfortably full. B. Cumulative daily bi-coordinate means for protein and non-protein (carbohydrate and fat) intake (MJ) for participants during the four-day 10% (light-grey circles), 15% (grey triangles) and 25% (black squares) protein study

periods. The dashed lines represent the nutrient rails participants were restricted to during the 10%, 15% and 25% study periods. The dotted lines represent intakes that may occur on the 10%, 15% and 25% foods if intake was regulated to energy requirements. The inset shows total energy intake (MJ) for participants over the four-day 10% (white), 15% (grey) and 25% (black) periods. Bi-coordinate means for 'anytime' and 'meal time' savory (C) and sweet (D) foods as a percent of total intake for participants over the four-day 10% (white circles), 15% (grey triangles) and 25% (black squares) *ad-libitum* study periods. As the percent of protein in the diet fell, not only did total energy intake rise, also the proportion of intake from savory snack foods rose, indicating protein-seeking behaviour (From Gosby et al. [37], with permission).

We began by designing a series of experimental foods that were disguised in their macronutrient composition. The recipes were manipulated to produce three versions of each food, containing 10%, 15% or 25% protein. Dietary fat was kept constant at 30%, and carbohydrate was adjusted to be 60%, 55% or 45% of total energy. Some of these foods were designed to be sweet, others savoury; some were to be presented as part of a main meal (breakfast, lunch or dinner) and others available between meals. Volunteers were recruited to taste-test the foods to make sure that the 10%, 15% and 25% protein versions of each food were equally palatable. As a result, we ended up with three versions of a four-day menu comprising 28 foods. For one version, all foods contained 10% protein, another 15% protein and the third 25% protein. An example of a 10% and the equivalent 25% protein lunch is shown in Figure 10A.

Lean adult subjects were next recruited who spent three four-day periods confined in an apartment at the Woolcock Institute Sleep Study Centre at the University of Sydney. Subjects were given breakfast, lunch and dinner each day and also offered free access to snack foods throughout the day. For one of the four-day periods every food eaten contained 10% protein; during another all foods contained 15% protein; and for the third period all foods were 25% protein. Subjects could eat as much as they liked and their food intake was measured. Because macronutrient composition was disguised and palatability, availability, variety and sensory aspects of foods were matched between treatment periods, the experiment provided a strong test of the effect of protein leverage on energy intake.

As predicted by the protein leverage hypothesis, reducing the protein content of the diet from 15% to 10% resulted in subjects increasing total energy intake. The extent of the increase was 12% over the four-day trial (Figure 10B); which if continued, would be expected to promote an increase in body fat of one kilogram per month. The increased energy intake was already evident within the first day and was mainly due to eating more of foods available between meals (Figure 10 C, D), with a predilection for savoury over sweet-tasting foods (although remember that all foods were actually the same in their macronutrient composition within the four-day trial). This preference for savoury-flavoured foods is strongly suggestive of protein-seeking behaviour.

In contrast to previous studies using undisguised foods (Figure 8), increasing the percent protein from 15% to 25% did not result in a lowering of energy intake (Figure 10B). This result suggested that continual access to a variety of energy-dense foods may counteract the inhibition of energy intake due to elevated dietary protein [37]. We return to this important point below.

What are the implications of protein leverage?

The implications of such a rule of compromise are considerable when considering the modern nutritional dilemma. To illustrate this, we will consider four scenarios for the case of a 45-year-old, moderately active adult male 1.8 ms tall and stably weighing 76 kg (BMI 23.5). His total daily energy requirements to remain in energy balance are 10 700 kJ. Achieving a diet comprising 14% protein requires him to eat 1500 kJ per day of protein and 9200 kJ of carbohydrate and fat combined. This represents a daily intake of 88 g protein and a total mass of carbohydrate and fat eaten that will depend on the relative proportions between the two in the diet, given that fat has twice the energy density of carbohydrate. As before, we will combine fat and carbohydrate into a single value for energy, since their relative contributions are not germane to the logic of our argument.

The four scenarios are:

1. There is a shift to a diet containing a higher percentage of carbohydrate and fat

This could occur where fat- and/or carbohydrate-rich foods are more accessible, more affordable, in greater variety, or more palatable than alternatives [3, 38], leading to people being effectively trapped on a suboptimal diet. Under such circumstances, maintaining the amount of protein eaten requires overconsumption of carbohydrate and fat.

Since protein is a minor component of the total diet, only a small decrease in the percentage of protein results in a substantial excess of carbohydrate and fat eaten: the protein leverage effect. Let us return to the above example of the US (Figure 6), where the FAOSTAT data suggest that, since 1961, the average diet composition has changed from 14% protein: 86% carbohydrate and fat to 12.5% protein: 87.5% carbohydrate and fat [20]. Maintaining protein intake under these circumstances required a 14% increase in the carbohydrate and fat eaten (Figure 11A). The implications for body weight regulation are clear: unless the excess carbohydrate and fat ingested to maintain protein intake is removed through increased physical or metabolic activity, body weight will rise, predisposing to obesity.

One important caveat that must be considered here is that the opportunity to overeat carbohydrate and fat to an extent sufficient to reach the protein intake target will depend on the energy density of the foods available. Where the ratio of protein to carbohydrate and fat is lower than the intake target ratio, but nutrient density is low (eg in the diets of macrobiotic vegetarians), physical bulk may inhibit reaching the protein intake target [see 39], thus leading to cessation of intake before the protein target is reached. In contrast, the fact that modern packaged and convenience foods are often energy-dense makes it easy to achieve the protein target on a diet with a lower than optimal ratio of protein to carbohydrate and fat.

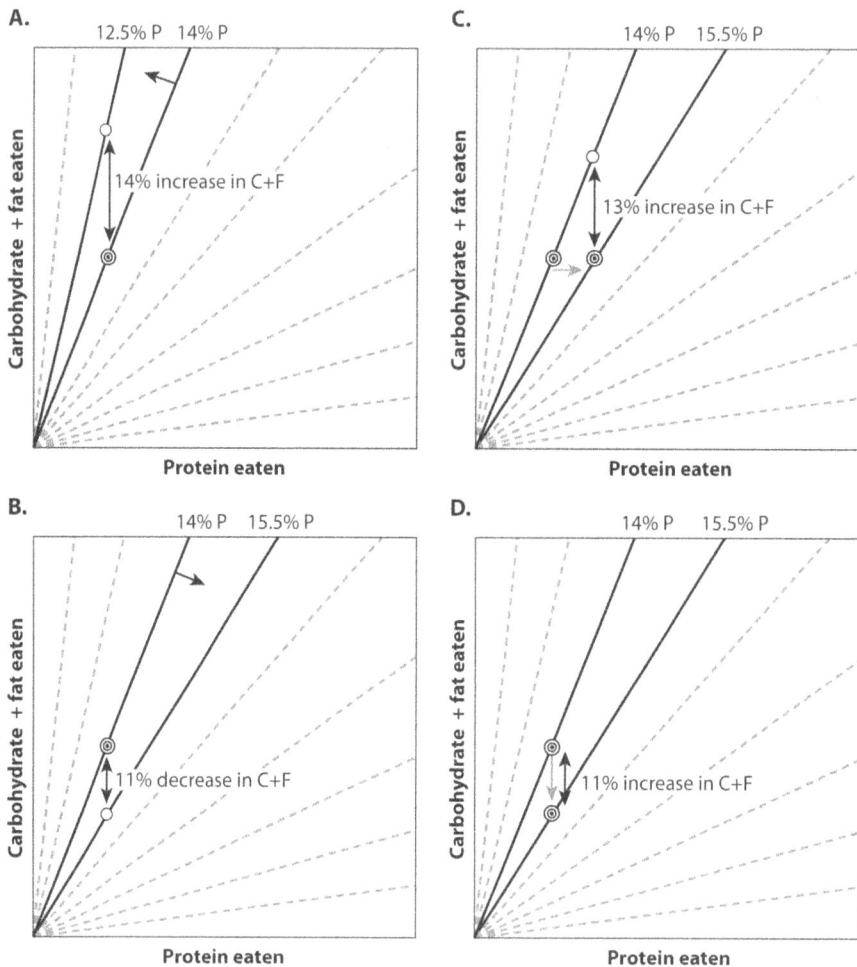

Figure 11. The consequences of four nutritional scenarios, given a rule of compromise that is to maintain protein intake. See text for details.

Additionally, having 24-hour access to food in the modern world, rather than restricting food to meal times, allows people the opportunity to 'snack' and 'graze', ie to increase the number of eating episodes in a day [40]. Hence, in the study by Alison Gosby et al. [37], subjects achieved greater consumption of the 10% protein diet not by eating more during main meals, but by increasing intake between meals (Figures 10C, D). In free-living individuals in the US the number of eating episodes per day is on the increase [41]. To make matters worse, increased food variety may also play a role in helping reach the protein target by stimulating increased intake on low-protein diets [37]. Variety can increase total energy intake independently of macronutrient composition [42], which may be an evolved response to ensure that we eat enough different foods to achieve our requirements for various micronutrients [43] and to overcome boredom effects and 'sensory specific satiety' [44–46].

2. There is a shift to a diet containing a higher percentage of protein

If humans are restricted to a diet that contains a higher percentage of protein, yet the absolute amount of protein eaten were regulated to the intake target, the result will be that carbohydrate and fat intake would fall, bringing the body into energy deficit and promoting weight loss. For example, a 1.5% increase in dietary protein from 14% to 15.5% would result in an 11% decrease in the carbohydrate and fat eaten (Figure 11B). As seen in Figure 8, available data suggest that some overconsumption of protein is tolerated, but not sufficient to maintain carbohydrate and fat intake. This explains why high-protein diet regimes promote weight loss and improve weight-loss maintenance [29, 30, 47–49]. It also explains why the most successful fad diets in terms of proponents and product sales over recent years have been those containing an elevated percentage of protein. Irrespective of the supposedly scientific claims made, and whether these diets promote omitting carbohydrates, reducing fat intake, or both, the primary reason why they encourage weight loss is simply because people eat less.

Perhaps then, augmenting the proportion of protein in the daily diet offers a means of ameliorating obesity by taking advantage of the inhibition of intake once the protein target is reached? Three things take some of the gloss from this optimistic suggestion. First, as we mentioned above, Gosby et al. [37] (Figure 10) did not find a decrease in intake when the diet contained 25% rather than 15% protein and concluded that

> it appears that the benefits of protein leverage – reduced intake on high percent protein diets – may be circumvented in [W]esternised countries in which the variety and availability of foods, especially snack foods, is greater than it has ever been in our evolutionary history [37]

Consistent with this conclusion, it is commonly reported that when subjects begin on a high-protein dietary regime they initially lose weight as a result of eating less, but over time the temptations of the modern nutritional environment lead to a gradual reduction in the percentage of protein in the diet, with associated cessation of weight loss (Figure 8B).

A second difficulty with increasing dietary protein is that, as well as the benefits in terms of weight loss, eating too much protein (even though this is resisted by protein regulatory feedbacks) may come at a cost to health (see above). A third problem is that increasing the proportion of protein in the diet has economic and potentially also environmental costs.

Brooks et al. [38] conducted an analysis of the economic costs of macronutrients in relation to the biology of protein leverage. We partitioned the energy content of supermarket foods and demonstrated that increasing overall energy content only modestly raises the cost of foods, largely because carbohydrate and fat are cheap. In fact, *lower* food prices were associated with *higher* carbohydrate content; whereas higher food prices were associated with increased protein content. It follows that the different costs of protein and carbohydrates may bias consumers – especially those on limited incomes [2, 50] – towards diets higher in carbohydrate and lower in protein energy content, which will then cause them to eat excessive energy to meet their dietary protein needs via the protein leverage effect. It also follows that there is economic pressure on processed food manufacturers to substitute protein in their products with cheaper energy sources, thereby driving increased energy intake in consumers via protein leverage. Such an economic pressure acts not only upon the manufacturers of human foods, but also upon those producing feeds for domestic animals [4]. In the case of food animal production, the result is to further increase the lipid content of the human diet through production of fatty meat.

Brooks et al. [38] used estimates of the strength of protein leverage from a compilation of published studies (an earlier version of Figure 8, from Simpson and Raubenheimer [24] and analysed further by Cheng et al. [25]) to estimate the extent to which dietary protein would need to be augmented to achieve a reduction in levels of obesity in a population, and the cost of this to the economy. Under the assumptions used (which in light of the results of Gosby et al. [37] may have overstated the inhibitory effect of protein on long-term intake), the cost of providing the extra protein needed to reduce intake was substantially less than the health costs of obesity.

There are, of course, important environmental implications for raising protein supply, especially when that comes from animal sources. However, an increase in dietary percentage of protein may be more effectively achieved by reducing consumption, and therefore production, of non-protein energy, rather than by increasing intake and production of protein. For example, taxation of foods rich in sugar (or starch or fat) but poor in protein could simultaneously reduce the need for large increases in protein production and reduce the land used for sugar (or starch or oil) crops, therefore helping to offset the environmental costs of increasing protein supply [38].

3. There is an increase in the requirement for protein

If diet composition remains unchanged, yet protein requirements increase, then overconsumption of carbohydrate and fat will result (Fig 11C). For example, shifting the intake target ratio from 14% to 15.5% protein in the diet leads to a 13% increase in the carbohydrate and fat eaten – with attendant risks of weight gain. But under what circumstances might this occur?

One source of protein loss is hepatic gluconeogenesis, whereby amino acids are used in the liver to produce glucose. This is inhibited by insulin, as is the breakdown of muscle proteins to release amino acids, and therefore usually occurs mainly during periods of fasting. However, inhibition of gluconeogenesis and protein catabolism is impaired when insulin release is abnormal, insulin resistance occurs, or free fatty acids circulate in the blood at high levels. These are interdependent conditions that are associated with overweight and obesity and are especially pronounced in type 2 diabetes [51, 52]. The result is an increased requirement for ingested protein. Unless either more high-protein, low-carbohydrate and fat items are included in the diet (ie scenario 2 above) or rates of removing excess co-ingested carbohydrate and fat are increased, weight gain will occur. And the system becomes unstable – the increased fat deposits (especially abdominal fat [51]) will further increase protein needs, which will in turn drive even greater weight gain [24, 27] (Figure 12). Data from rodents also support such a scenario – a vicious cycle to morbid obesity

[53, 54]. Further evidence in support of our 'vicious cycle' come from Newgard et al. [55], who discovered that obese humans are distinguished from lean subjects by a metabolic signature indicating elevated protein catabolism.

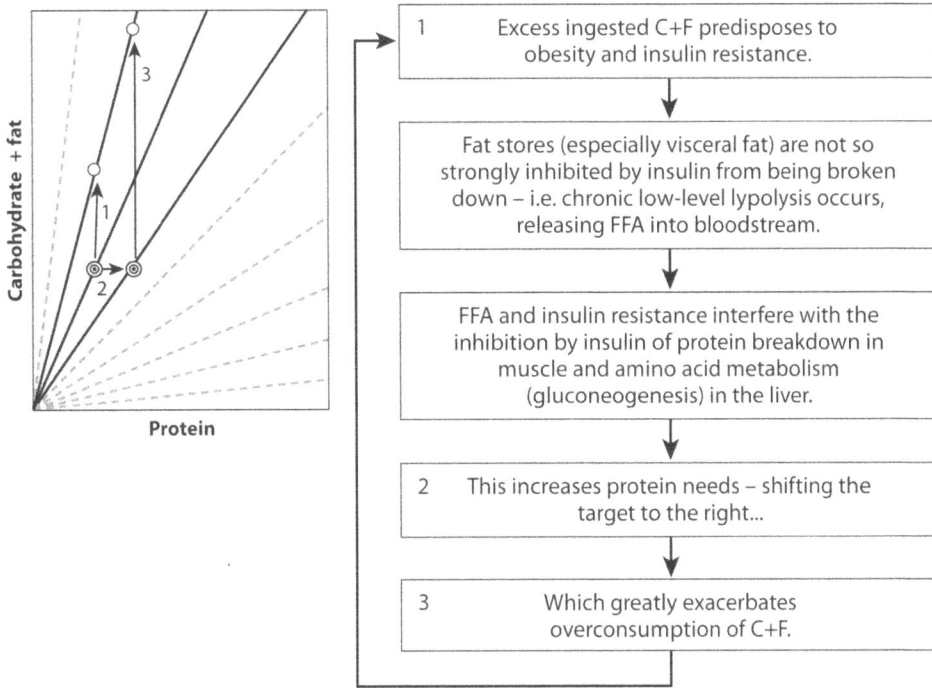

Figure 12. The vicious cycle by which protein appetite may drive obesity.

Another reason why protein needs may increase is during periods of lean muscle growth, for example during adolescence, accompanying weight training, or after a period of starvation. The effect of an increased protein requirement will depend on the extent to which requirements for non-protein energy change as well, but if the net movement of the target is to the right on a carbohydrate + fat vs protein intake plot (as in Figure 11 C), placing such a person onto a low-protein diet would predispose to excessive energy consumption and weight gain. This might help explain the 'yo-yo' diet effect, whereby subjects regain weight rapidly following a period on a crash diet [56]; and perhaps also why some athletes are prone to weight gain once they cease training.

A corollary is that we might predict that individuals and populations with an elevated intake target for protein should be more prone to developing obesity on a low-protein diet than those with a lower protein target [24]. Organisms evolve such that their intake target reflects the composition of their natural diet [4]. Humans too adapt to their current diet, genetically, developmentally and culturally [7, 57–59]. Perhaps populations that have traditionally eaten a high-protein diet have an elevated protein target, and therefore suffer increased susceptibility to obesity and metabolic disease when making the transition to a modern Western diet in which carbohydrate-rich foods are cheap and abundant [24]? The prevalence of obesity and type 2 diabetes among Oceanic populations is particularly telling, since such populations have until recently remained on a protein-rich marine-based diet, rather than having shifted like many others to terrestrial agriculture in the Neolithic with a consequent increase in dietary carbohydrate [60–62].

A particularly striking example is the Kosrae district of Micronesia, where nearly 90% of adults are overweight and 53% are obese. Here, the recent development of a wage-based economy has led to altered eating habits from a traditional diet high in fish, fruit and vegetables to a diet based on imported packaged food [39, 62].

4. Diet remains unchanged but energy expenditure declines

We must take account of changes to the demand side of the energy budget when considering the implication of protein leverage. Because much of our metabolic fuel comes from carbohydrate and fat, the result of lowered levels of exercise and other forms of energy expenditure is, in effect, to lower the position of the intake target on the carbohydrate and fat axis (Figure 11D). Unless the diet changes towards a higher percentage of protein, the result will be weight gain.

As we discussed above, unlike the US where intake has risen (Figure 6), in the UK macronutrient and energy intake appear to have remained relatively stable over the period from 1960 to 2000 (Figure 5); yet obesity rose rapidly, in direct correlation with causes of declining activity levels, such as the use of cars and television viewing [50]). As well as spending more time inactive, many of us now live (and drive around) within temperature controlled environments – cooled during summer and warmed during winter – with consequent metabolic savings for thermoregulation, especially in higher latitudes [8].

To make matters worse, as well as lowering the demand for fuel, decreasing the level of exercise has a direct influence on metabolic physiology, associated with increased resistance to insulin and thus enhanced gluconeogenesis [63]. As we saw above (scenario 3), insulin resistance and its consequences will cause an increased need for protein, shifting the intake target towards an even higher percentage of protein that results from the lowered need for carbohydrate and fat to fuel metabolism under a low-exercise regime.

And to compound matters, while humans respond by increasing intake following high levels of energetic expenditure, we tend not to compensate fully by eating less when our energy needs fall [63]. Possibly our intake target has evolved to 'assume' a certain level of energy expenditure based on our ancestral lifestyle, and we may therefore be 'hard wired' to eat that amount, even if we do not use it [24].

Interacting consequences

The scenarios introduced above interact with one another. Either shifting the diet composition to a lower percentage of protein (scenario one), or effectively doing the same by having low levels of energy expenditure (scenario four), will result in overconsumption of energy to maintain protein intake. This in turn will predispose towards weight gain and insulin resistance, leading to disinhibition of protein breakdown and gluconeogenesis, which will increase protein demand (scenario three). Unless this increased demand is met by shifting to a higher percentage protein diet, protein appetite will drive increased energy intake, resulting in further weight gain, and so on in a vicious cycle leading to obesity, metabolic disease and associated pathologies (Figure 12).

One nagging question remains. If humans do regulate protein intake, why do we not simply select protein-rich foods to rebalance our diet, as a locust would? It seems that we are led astray by our sweet tooth. For most of our evolutionary history the human diet consisted of a high proportion of animal foods [64–66]. Simple sugars were rare, and wild animals typically have much lower fat content than modern commercial meat (4 g compared with 20 g fat per 100 g meat) [67, 68]. Hence, hunter-gatherer peoples around the world go to considerable risks to collect honey from tall trees and cliff faces, and fat is highly prized. A history of short supply of simple sugars and fat has been proposed as an explanation for their high palatability, which may predispose towards the overconsumption of fat and carbohydrate-rich foods even when these are not required [69]. Similar arguments have been put to explain aspects of human metabolic physiology, most notably the ease with which we store rather than eliminate excess ingested energy [70] (see below). Because it appears that we have limited evolutionary experience of excess carbohydrates (especially simple sugars) or fats, it seems reasonable to infer that natural selection against their overconsumption would not have been strong.

These evolutionary predispositions interact with the modern nutritional environment to misdirect our regulatory physiology. As we have seen, highly energy-dense, fat- and carbohydrate-rich foods are constantly available and affordable, and levels of energy expenditure are lower than it is anticipated by our ancestral physiology. It is also telling that taste stimuli naturally associated with protein-rich foods, such as sodium and umami stimulants, are extensively used in low-protein processed foods, and may as a result subvert protein regulatory systems and lead to overconsumption of fat and carbohydrates [24]. For example, Americans increased intake of salty snack foods between 1977 and 1996 [71] – perhaps as part of a subliminal effort to gain protein, but in fact exacerbating the problem.

How do humans deal with nutrient excesses?

We return finally, and briefly, to the third of our initial questions: having eaten excess energy, what happens to it? The extent to which weight gain occurs following ingestion of excess nutrients depends on what happens to such excesses once they enter the body. There is a clear relationship between the priority with which surplus nutrients are voided from the body through being metabolised and excreted, and the extent to which they are stored [10]. Excess carbohydrates are readily metabolised and excreted, and stores are minimal (in the form of glycogen in the liver and muscles). Surplus protein is also metabolised and excreted with high efficiency and little if any is stored. In marked contrast, ingested fat is the last fuel to be burned, and excesses are mostly stored in adipose tissue – a store with virtually unlimited capacity. These metabolic patterns are consistent with our having evolved in an environment where energy was limited and periods of food scarcity were not uncommon, especially since the post-agricultural era [7].

Conclusions

An analysis of the modern human nutritional dilemma using the geometric framework leads to the following conclusions.

1. The intake target

The available evidence suggests that humans can regulate macronutrient intake, but that the intake target contains a built-in component for fat storage. This has probably evolved to 'anticipate' energetic demands for activity and thermoregulation, and also periods of food shortage. Failure to use this stored fat promotes obesity.

2. Rule of compromise

When faced with imbalanced diets, protein intake is prioritised. Therefore, on low-protein/high-carbohydrate and fat diets, carbohydrate and/or fat are overeaten; and on high-protein/low-carbohydrate and fat diets, carbohydrate and/or fat are undereaten. When the ratio of protein to carbohydrate in the diet is lower than optimal, it is easier to gain the required amount of protein – and hence overconsume fat and carbohydrate – when foods are high in energy density, present in great variety, and easily available throughout the day. These are defining features of the modern Western nutritional environment. Regarding dietary causes of obesity, most emphasis in research over the past 40 years or more has been on changing patterns of fat and carbohydrate consumption. In contrast, the role of protein has largely been ignored because it typically comprises only 15% of dietary energy and protein intake has remained near constant within and across populations throughout the development of the obesity epidemic. We have shown that, paradoxically, these are precisely the two conditions that provide protein with the leverage both to drive the obesity epidemic through its effects on food intake and potentially (with caveats) to assuage it.

3. Post-ingestive regulation

Regulation of nutrient intake has evolved 'assuming' a higher level of energetic expenditure than is usual today. Energy limitation in our ancestral nutritional environment may well explain our predisposition to store fat and poor ability to void excesses. The combined consequences of the interactions between our regulatory physiology and our changing nutritional environment can be seen in Figure 1.

Whereas it is not our intention here to give detailed dietary recommendations, our hope is that we have provided an awareness of the unconscious appetites that shape our feeding behaviour. Managing diet and health, whether at the level of individuals, societies or nations, requires such an understanding if we are to work with, rather than against, biology; otherwise, biology will always win. The evidence indicates that efforts to fight our powerful protein appetite will be bound to fail. As can be seen in Figure 11, small changes in the percentage of protein in the diet can potentially yield big effects on intake, with consequences – both good and bad – for weight management. Diluting protein with fat and sugar will drive excess energy intake and promote weight gain, because more must be eaten to reach the protein target. In the extreme, sugary beverages (carbonated drinks or fruit juice) and many high-fat and carbohydrate snack foods take the consumer up the Y-axis in Figure 11 to infinity and no closer to the protein intake target, leaving the protein appetite unsatisfied. In contrast, a modest reduction in fat, sugar and other readily digested carbohydrates in the diet will make it far easier to limit energy intake and lose weight, by effectively concentrating protein in the diet and allowing the protein target to be achieved at lower total energy intake.

References

1. Must A, Spadano J, Coakley EH, Field AE, Colditz G & Dietz WH (1999). The disease burden associated with overweight and obesity. *Journal of the American Medical Association*, 282(16): 1523–29.

2. Björntorp P (Ed) (2001). *International textbook of obesity*. Chichester: John Wiley and Sons.

3. Hill JO, Wyatt HR, Reed GW & Peters JC (2003). Obesity and the environment: where do we go from here? *Science*, 299(5608): 853–55.

4. Simpson SJ & Raubenheimer D (2012). The nature of nutrition: a unifying framework from animal adaptation to human obesity. Princeton: Princeton University Press (in press).

5. Eaton SB, Eaton III SB, Konner MJ & Shostak M (1996). An evolutionary perspective enhances understanding of human nutritional requirements. *Journal of Nutrition*, 126(6): 1732–40.

6. Prentice AM (2001). Fires of life: the struggles of an ancient metabolism in a modern world. *British Nutrition Foundation Nutrition Bulletin*, 26(1): 13–27.

7. Prentice AM, Hennig BJ & Fulford AJ (2008). Evolutionary origins of the obesity epidemic: natural selection of thrifty genes or genetic drift following predation release? *International Journal of Obesity*, 32: 1607–10.

8. Wells JCK (2010). *The evolutionary biology of human body fatness*. Cambridge: Cambridge University Press.

9. Gibson G (2007). Human evolution: thrifty genes and the dairy queen. *Current Biology*, 17(8): R295–96.

10. Stubbs RJ (1998). Appetite, feeding behaviour and energy balance in human subjects. *Proceedings of the Nutrition Society*, 57: 141–56.

11. Friedman MI (2000). Too many choices? A critical essay on macronutrient selection. In H-R Berthoud & RJ Seeley (Eds). *Neural and metabolic control of macronutrient intake* (pp11–18). Boca Raton: CRC Press.

12. Berthoud H-R & Seeley RJ (Eds) (2000). *Neural and metabolic control of macronutrient intake*. Boca Raton: CRC Press.

13. Simpson SJ & Raubenheimer D (1997). The geometric analysis of feeding and nutrition in the rat. *Appetite*, 28(3): 201–13.

14. Theall CL, Wurtman JJ & Wurtman RJ (1984). Self-selection and regulation of protein:carbohydrate ratios in foods adult rats eat. *Journal of Nutrition*, 114: 711–18.

15. Sørensen A, Mayntz D, Raubenheimer D & Simpson SJ (2008). Protein-leverage in mice: the geometry of macronutrient balancing and consequences for fat deposition. *Obesity*, 16(3): 566–71.

16. Simpson SJ, Batley R & Raubenheimer D (2003). Geometric analysis of macronutrient intake in humans: the power of protein? *Appetite*, 41(2): 123–40.

17. de Castro JM (1999). What are the major correlates of macronutrient selection in western populations? *Proceedings of the Nutrition Society*, 58(4): 755–63.

18. Weigle DS, Breen PA, Matthys CC, Callahan HS, Meeuws KE, Burden VR, et al. (2005). A high-protein diet induces sustained reductions in appetite, ad libitum caloric intake, and body weight despite compensatory changes in diurnal plasma leptin and ghrelin concentrations. *American Journal of Clinical Nutrition*, 82(1): 41–48.

19. Westerterp-Plantenga MS (1994). Nutrient utilization and energy balance. In MS Westerterp-Plantenga, EWHM Fredrix, AB Steffens & HR Kissileff (Eds). *Food intake and energy expenditure* (pp311–19). Boca Raton: CRC Press.

20. FAOSTAT database (2002). Food Balance Sheets [Online]. Available: faostat.fao.org/site/368/default. aspx#ancor [Accessed 31 August 2011].

21. Austin GL, Ogden LG & Hill JO (2011). Trends in carbohydrate, fat, and protein intakes and association with energy intakes in normal-weight, overweight, and obese individuals: 1971–2006. *American Journal of Clinical Nutrition*, 93(4): 836–43.

22. Fulgoni III VL (2008). Current protein intake in America: analysis of the National Health and Nutrition Examination Survey, 2003–2004. *American Journal of Clinical Nutrition*, 87(5): 1554S–1557S.

23. Swinburn BA, Sacks G, Lo SK, Westerterp KR, Rush EC, Rosenbaum M, et al. (2009). Estimating the changes in energy flux that characterize the rise in obesity prevalence. *American Journal of Clinical Nutrition*, 89(6): 1723–28.

24. Simpson SJ & Raubenheimer D (2005). Obesity: the protein leverage hypothesis. *Obesity Reviews*, 6(2): 133–42.

25. Cheng K, Simpson SJ & Raubenheimer D (2008). A geometry of regulatory scaling. *American Naturalist*, 172(5): 681–93.

26. Lee KP, Simpson SJ, Clissold FJ, Brooks R, Ballard JWO, Taylor PW, et al. (2008). Lifespan and reproduction in *Drosophila*: new insights from nutritional geometry. *Proceedings of the National Academy of Sciences of the United States of America*, 105(7): 2498–2503.

27. Simpson SJ & Raubenheimer D (2009). Macronutrient balance and lifespan. *Aging*, 1(10): 875–80.

28. Metges CC & Barth CA (2000). Metabolic consequences of a high dietary-protein intake in adulthood: assessment of the available evidence. *Journal of Nutrition*, 130(4): 886–89.

29. Freedman MR, King J & Kennedy E (2001). Popular diets: a scientific review. *Obesity Research*, 9(11): 1S–40S.

30. Elsenstein J, Roberts SB, Dallal G & Salzman E (2002). High-protein weight-loss diets: are they safe and how do they work? A review of the experimental and epidemiologic data. *Nutrition Reviews*, 60(7 Pt 1): 189–200.

31. Weickert MO, Roden M, Isken F, Hoffmann D, Nowotny P, Osterhoff M, et al. (2011). Effects of supplemented isoenergetic diets differing in cereal fiber and protein content on insulin sensitivity in overweight humans. *American Journal of Clinical Nutrition*, 94(2): 459–71.

32. Kyriazakis I & Emmans GC (1991). Diet selection in pigs: dietary choices made by growing pigs following a period of underfeeding with protein. *Animal Production*, 52: 337–46.

33. Webster AJF (1993). Energy partitioning, tissue growth and appetite control. *Proceedings of the National Academy of Sciences of the United States of America*, 52(1): 69–76.

34. Raubenheimer D & Simpson SJ (1997). Integrative models of nutrient balancing: application to insects and vertebrates. *Nutrition Research Reviews*, 10(1): 151–79.

35. Felton AM, Felton A, Raubenheimer D, Simpson SJ, Foley WJ, Wood JT, et al. (2009). Protein content of diets dictates the daily energy intake of a free–ranging primate. *Behavioral Ecology*, 20(4): 685–90.

36. Gosby AK, Campbell C, Badaloo A, Soares-Wynter S, Antonelli M, Hall R, et al. (2010). Design and testing of foods differing in protein to energy ratios. *Appetite*, 55(2): 367–70.

37. Gosby AK, Conigrave AD, Lau N, Hall R, Jebb SA, Brand-Miller J, et al. (2011). Testing the protein leverage hypothesis in lean humans. *PLoS ONE,* 6(10): e25929.

38. Brooks RC, Simpson SJ & Raubenheimer D (2010). The price of protein: combining evolutionary and economic analysis to understand excessive energy consumption. *Obesity Reviews*, 11(12): 887–94.

39. Rolls BJ (2000). The role of energy density in overcomsumption of fat. *Journal of Nutrition*, 130(2): 268S–271S.

40. Levitsky DA, Halbmaier CA & Mrdjenovic G (2004). The freshman weight gain: a model for the study of the epidemic of obesity. *International Journal of Obesity and Related Metabolic Disorders*, 28: 1435–42.

41. Popkin BM & Duffey KJ (2010). Does hunger and satiety drive eating anymore? Increasing eating occasions and decreasing time between eating occasions in the United States. *American Journal of Clinical Nutrition*, 91(5): 1342–47.

42. Stubbs RJ, Johnstone AM, Mazlan N, Mbaiwa SE & Ferris, S. (2001). Effect of altering the variety of sensorially distinct foods, of the same macronutrient content, on food intake and body weight in men. *European Journal of Clinical Nutrition*, 55(1): 19–28.

43. Maillot M, Vieux F, Ferguson EF, Volatier J-L, Amiot MJ & Darmon N (2009). To meet nutrient recommendations, most French adults need to expand their habitual food repertoire. *Journal of Nutrition*, 139(9): 1721–27.

44. Norton GN, Anderson AS & Hetherington MM (2006). Volume and variety: relative effects on food intake. *Physiology & Behavior*, 87(4): 714–22.

45. Brondel L, Romer M, Van Wymelbeke V, Pineau N, Jiang T, Hanus C, et al. (2009). Variety enhances food intake in humans: role of sensory-specific satiety. *Physiology & Behavior*, 97(1): 44–51.

46. Nolan LJ & Hetherington MM (2009). The effects of sham feeding-induced sensory specific satiation and food variety on subsequent food intake in humans. *Appetite*, 52(3): 720–25.

47. Astrup A (2005). The satiating power of protein: a key to obesity prevention? *American Journal of Clinical Nutrition*, 82(1): 1–2.

48. Larsen TM, Dalskov S-M, van Baak M, Jebb SA, Papadaki A, Pfeiffer AFH, et al. (2010). Diets with high or low protein content and Glycemic Index for weight-loss maintenance. *New England Journal of Medicine*, 363(22): 2102–13.

49. Ludwig DS & Ebbeling CB (2010). Weight-loss maintenance – mind over matter? *New England Journal of Medicine*, 363(22): 2159–61.

50. Prentice AM & Jebb SA (1995). Obesity in Britain: gluttony or sloth. *British Medical Journal*, 311: 437–39.

51. Saltiel AR & Kahn CR (2001). Insulin signaling and the regulation of glucose and lipid metabolism. *Nature*, 414: 799–806.

52. Boden G (2003). Effects of free fatty acids on gluconeogenesis and glycogenolysis. *Life Sciences*, 72(9): 977–88.

53. Zhou Q, Du J, Hu Z, Walsh K & Wang XH (2007). Evidence for adipose-muscle crosstalk: opposing regulation of muscle proteolysis by adiponectin and fatty acids. *Endocrinology*, 148(12): 5696–5705.

54. Quinn LS (2008). Interleukin-15: A muscle-derived cytokine regulating fat-to-lean body composition. *Journal of Animal Science*, 86(Suppl. 14): E75–E83.

55. Newgard CB, An J, Bain JR, Muehlbauer MJ, Stevens RD, Lien LF, et al. (2009). A branched-chain amino acid-related metabolic signature that differentiates obese and lean humans and contributes to insulin resistance. *Cell Metabolism*, 9(4): 311–26.

56. Westerterp-Plantenga MS, Lejeune MPGM, Nijs I, van Ooijen M & Kovacs EMR (2004). High protein intake sustains weight maintenance after body weight loss in humans. *International Journal of Obesity and Related Metabolic Disorders*, 28(1): 57–64.

57. Harris M & Ross EB (Eds) (1987). *Food and evolution*. Philadelphia: Temple University Press.

58. Barker DJP (1998). *Mothers, babies and health in later life*. 2nd edn. London: Churchill Livingstone.

59. Diamond J (2003). The double puzzle of diabetes. *Nature*, 423: 599–602.

60. Richards MP, Schulting RJ & Hedges REM (2003). Sharp shift in diet at onset of Neolithic. *Nature*, 425: 366.

61. Ulijaszek SJ (2003). Trends in body size, diet and food availability in the Cook Islands in the second half of the 20th century. *Economics & Human Biology*, 1(1): 123–37.

62. Cassels S (2006). Overweight in the Pacific: links between foreign dependence, global food trade, and obesity in the Federated States of Micronesia. *Global Health*, 2: 10.

63. International Agency for Research on Cancer (IARC) (2002). *Weight control and physical activity. IARC handbook of cancer prevention*, vol. 6. Lyon: World Health Organization Press.

64. Brand-Miller JC & Colagiuri S (1999). Evolutionary aspects of diet and insulin resistance. *World Review of Nutrition and Dietetics*, 84: 74–105.

65. Cordain L, Miller JB, Eaton SB & Mann N (2000). Macronutrient estimations in hunter-gatherer diets. *American Journal of Clinical Nutrition*, 72(6): 1589–90.

66. Milton K (2003). The critical role played by animal source foods in human (*Homo*) evolution. *Journal of Nutrition*, 133(11 Suppl. 2): 3886S–3892S.

67. Speth JD (1991). Protein selection and avoidance strategies of contemporary and ancestral foragers: unresolved issues. *Philosophical Transactions of the Royal Society B: Biological Sciences*, 334(1270): 265–70.

68. Eaton SB, Eaton III SB & Konner MJ (1997). Paleolithic nutrition revisited: a twelve-year retrospective on its nature and implications. *European Journal of Clinical Nutrition*, 51(4): 207–16.

69. Galef BG (1996). Food selection: problems in understanding how we choose foods to eat. *Neuroscience & Biobehavioral Reviews*, 20(1): 67–73.

70. Lev-Ran A (2001). Human obesity: an evolutionary approach to understanding our bulging waistline. *Diabetes/Metabolism Research and Reviews*, 17(5): 347–62.

71. Nielsen SJ, Siega-Riz AM & Popkin BM (2002). Trends in energy intake in US between 1977 and 1996: similar shifts seen across age groups. *Obesity Research*, 10(5): 370–78.

72. Calle EE, Thun MJ, Petrelli JM, Rodriguez C & Heath Jr. CW (1999). Body-mass index and mortality in a prospective cohort of US adults. *New England Journal of Medicine*, 341(15): 1097–1105.

73. Raubenheimer D & Simpson SJ (1993). The geometry of compensatory feeding in the locust. *Animal Behaviour*, 45(50): 953–64.

74. Tews JK, Repa JJ & Harper AE (1992). Protein selection by rats adapted to high or moderately low levels of dietary protein. *Physiology & Behavior*, 51(4): 699–712.

75. Shariatmadari F & Forbes JM (1993). Growth and food intake responses to diets of different protein contents and a choice between diets containing two concentrations of protein in broiler and layer strains of chicken. *British Poultry Science*, 34(5): 959–70.

3

Insulin resistance pathogenesis in visceral fat and gut organisms

Yan Lam,[1] Connie Ha[2] and Andrew Holmes[2]

Epidemiological work has shown that visceral adiposity is strongly related to metabolic disorders including insulin resistance. What regulates visceral fat deposition and why it is so metabolically deleterious remains largely unclear. Recent data suggest that the gastrointestinal tract may be a central player in the development of visceral fat accumulation and metabolic syndrome. An impaired gut barrier function, as a consequence of inflammation and/or altered microbiota composition, increases the leak of microbial molecules and their metabolites to the adjacent mesenteric fat resulting in hypertrophy and inflammation of the fat depot. Subsequently, the increased efflux of fatty acids and pro-inflammatory factors in the portal vein leads to liver dysfunction and systemic insulin resistance.

Obesity is a condition in which fat accumulation in adipose tissue is in excess to an extent that health may be impaired. Obese individuals are at an increased risk of developing chronic health problems including cardiovascular disease, type 2 diabetes, hypertension, non-alcoholic fatty liver disease and certain cancers [1]. A subset of obese individuals, classified as 'metabolically healthy obese' (MHO) account for ~20% of the obese population, remain insulin-sensitive and appear to be less susceptible to obesity-related metabolic complications [2]. It has been estimated that type 2 diabetes and cardiovascular disease is six- and twofold respectively more common in 'at-risk' obese as compared to MHO individuals [3]. An important feature of MHO individuals is they have proportionally less visceral fat (the abdominal fat within the visceral cavity). This is consistent with recent data suggesting that regional fat distribution is an important determinant of insulin sensitivity and metabolic risk [4]. What regulates visceral fat deposition and why it is so metabolically dangerous remains largely unclear. This article summarises literature on underlying mechanisms of visceral adipose dysfunction and the emerging role of the gut, and its resident microbes, as a central player in metabolic disorders (Figure 1).

---

1 Boden Institute of Obesity, Nutrition, Exercise and Eating Disorders, University of Sydney.

2 School of Molecular Bioscience, University of Sydney.

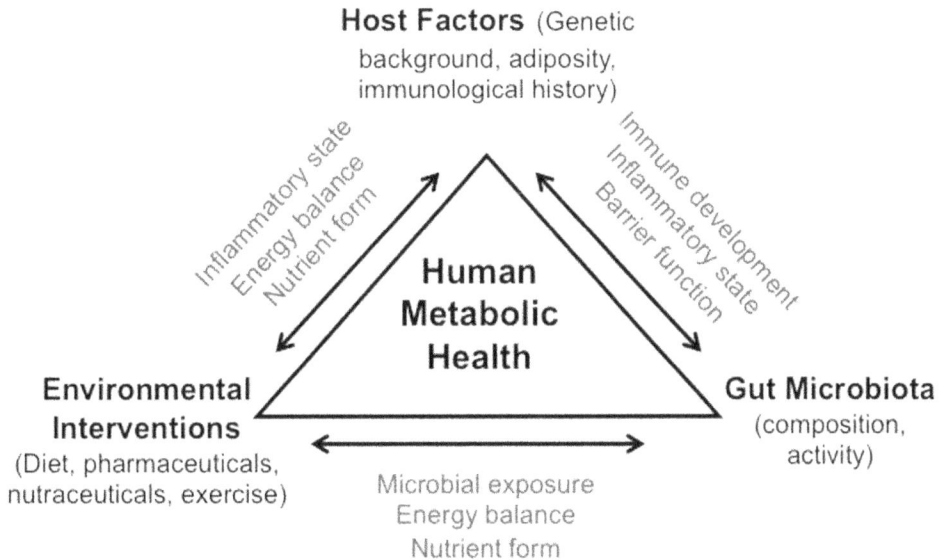

Figure 1. Overview of interconnections between lifestyle factors, host factors and gut microbiota in metabolic health. Refer to the text for a more detailed explanation and description of terms used.

Regional fat distribution

The distribution of adipose tissue varies considerably among individuals even with similar total body fat. What regulates regional fat deposition is not entirely clear but is at least known to be affected by gender, age and ethnicity. Men tend to have more visceral fat and have at least twice the proportion of fat localised in the intra-abdominal depot as compared to women [5, 6]. The gender-specific difference in fat distribution, however, appears to diminish in older age as females tend to develop central adiposity after menopause [7]. Ethnicity also affects regional adiposity. Aboriginal men and women in Australia have been shown to have greater waist-to-hip ratio as compared to their European Australian counterparts and the difference is observed across all BMI levels up to 30 kg/m^2 [8]. Central obesity is also more common in Hispanic as compared to white women in early adulthood [9].

Epidemiological data suggest a relationship between central adiposity and metabolic risk factors including elevated blood pressure, fasting plasma glucose and triglycerides [10]. Visceral fat accounts for ~50% of the variance in insulin sensitivity [11, 12] and has been shown to be a predictor for future insulin resistance [13]. The accumulation of visceral fat is strongly related to reduced insulin responsiveness irrespective of adiposity [6, 14]. Conversely, the association between visceral fat reduction and improved insulin sensitivity has been consistently demonstrated in obese [15], glucose intolerance-impaired [16] and type 2 diabetic [17] individuals.

In contrast to visceral fat, the relationship between subcutaneous fat and metabolic risk is less clear-cut. Wagenknechi and co-workers [18] reported that both visceral and subcutaneous adiposity were inversely associated with insulin sensitivity; Cnop et al. [19] estimated that subcutaneous fat only accounted for 5% of the variance in insulin sensitivity; in patients with type 2 diabetes, Miyazaki and colleagues [20] reported that insulin-stimulated glucose disposal was inversely correlated with visceral but not subcutaneous fat area; data from the Framingham Heart Study even suggested a protective effect of subcutaneous fat against metabolic and cardiovascular risk in individuals in the highest tertile of visceral adiposity [21]. Some attributed the inconsistent relationship between subcutaneous fat and insulin sensitivity to different metabolic effects of the subdivisions of the fat depot [22], with the deep subcutaneous adipose tissue exhibiting a secretory profile similar to that of visceral fat [22]. It has also been proposed that once the accumulation of visceral adipose tissue exceeds a certain threshold, the contribution of the depot to insulin resistance would overwhelm that of abdominal subcutaneous fat regardless of subdivisions [23].

It is logical to hypothesise that the intrinsic difference(s) between visceral and subcutaneous adipocytes (fat cells) may contribute to the region-specific metabolic effects of fat depots. Indeed, visceral adipocytes are shown to be both structurally and functionally distinct. For example, they are larger in size, less insulin-sensitive and have a greater lipolytic activity as compared to subcutaneous adipocytes (for details please refer to a comprehensive review by Ibrahim [24]). These characteristics, however, do not appear to completely account for the deleterious nature of visceral fat.

Obesity, inflammation and insulin resistance

Over the past decade it has been increasingly recognised that adipose tissue is a complex endocrine organ secreting, inter alia, a range of cytokines [25]. Together with the well-characterised state of low-grade chronic inflammation in obesity [26], this points to an entirely novel angle to investigate regional metabolic effects of fat depots. Adipose tissue produces a range of protein factors including cytokines, chemokines and growth factors. Leptin and adiponectin increase insulin sensitivity; tumor necrosis factor (TNF)-alpha, interleukin (IL)-1beta, IL-6, IL-8 and monocyte chemoattractant protein (MCP)-1 are pro-inflammatory, either by direct activation of the inflammatory signalling pathway or by promoting the migration of immune cells; IL-10, which inhibits the production of pro-inflammatory cytokines, is one of the main adipose-derived anti-inflammatory factors.

Epidemiological data indicate an association between chronic inflammation and decreased insulin sensitivity. Circulating levels of inflammatory markers are increased in individuals with type 2 diabetes, insulin resistance or the metabolic syndrome [27]. In a prospective case-control study, elevated plasma levels of IL-6 and C-reactive protein were shown to be associated with an increased risk of developing type 2 diabetes independent of BMI, physical activity and other lifestyle factors [28]. The role of inflammation in the pathogenesis of insulin resistance is further supported by the effect of high-dose aspirin, an anti-inflammatory drug commonly used to treat rheumatoid arthritis, in reducing fasting blood glucose and improving insulin-stimulated peripheral glucose uptake in type 2 diabetic patients [29].

More importantly, there is evidence supporting inflammation as the major determinant of the deleterious metabolic effects of visceral fat. Compared to people with normal fat distribution, the plasma concentrations of inflammatory mediators are up to ~50% higher in centrally obese individuals [30]. Direct comparison of cytokine production using adipose tissue explants *in vitro* revealed that visceral fat released higher concentrations of pro-inflammatory cytokines including IL-6, IL-8 and TNF-alpha as compared to subcutaneous fat [31, 32]. Using adipose tissue-conditioned media, we provided direct evidence for visceral fat induction of insulin resistance in skeletal muscle *in vitro* [33]. Individual pro-inflammatory cytokines, specifically IL-6 [33] IL-1beta [34] and TNF-alpha [35], have been shown to inhibit insulin signalling. Further, our data suggest that the sequential activation of nuclear factor kappa B (NFκB) and mammalian target of rapamycin complex 1 (mTORC1) may be the common pathway which mediates visceral fat-induced insulin resistance [33]. Briefly, pro-inflammatory cytokines phosphorylates inhibitor of kappa B kinase (IKK) and activates mTORC1. Ribosomal S6 kinase 1, a downstream effector of mTORC1, phosphorylates insulin receptor substrate-1 and inhibits its interaction with the insulin receptor and/or p85 subunit of phsophatidylinositol 3-kinase. Also, activated IKK degrades inhibitor protein inhibitor kappa B. The subsequent nuclear translocation of NFκB induces the transcription of pro-inflammatory cytokines and therefore provides a positive feedback to the inflammation cascade.

Macrophage infiltration in adipose tissue

Ameliorating fat inflammation has thus become a major focus in both prevention and treatment of type 2 diabetes. It is now recognised that in adipose the majority of cytokines originate from 'non-fat' cells [36]. Obesity is characterised by an increased accumulation of adipose tissue macrophages (ATMs) [37] which have been identified as the major contributor of both pro- and anti-inflammatory cytokines. Further, Harman-Boehm et al. [38] reported that the number of ATM was approximately two- to fourfold higher in omental (a major visceral fat depot in human) as compared to subcutaneous fat irrespective of levels of adiposity. A causal relationship between ATM infiltration and insulin resistance has been demonstrated in animal studies. Attenuating ATM infiltration, by genetic modification or pharmacological treatment, partially improved glucose homeostasis and insulin sensitivity in diet-induced obese mice, an effect associated with reduced expression of pro-inflammatory cytokines [39]. Conversely, over-expression of MCP-1, a major chemokine which promotes macrophage infiltration, in adipocytes increased ATM abundance and induced insulin resistance without affecting adipose tissue weight [40].

Mechanisms of macrophage infiltration

The mechanisms by which ATM infiltration occurs, however, are not entirely clear. It has long been proposed that macrophage infiltration is part of an immune response to adipose dysfunction in obesity. A credible hypothesis is that chronic energy excess and increased lipid accumulation leads to adipocyte hypertrophy. Limited lipid storage capacity then induces oxidative stress, which results in necrotic-like cell death and subsequently triggers an inflammatory response [41].

The increased susceptibility of visceral adipocytes to cell death may lead to differential ATM infiltration. The majority of ATMs aggregate around dead adipocytes and form the characteristic 'crown-like structures' (CLS). In genetically (ob/ob and db/db) and diet-induced obese mice, both dead adipocytes and CLS are more abundant in visceral as compared to subcutaneous fat [42, 43]. A linear correlation between adipocyte size and CLS density has been demonstrated in all fat depots, suggesting that visceral adipocytes may have a smaller critical size triggering death and therefore promotes the migration of macrophages into this fat depot [43].

Adipocyte hypertrophy: the role of extracellular matrix

It is tempting to hypothesise that ATM infiltration, and therefore the associated deleterious metabolic consequences, may be preventable if the fat depots could expand indefinitely. The ability of adipocytes to expand is partly restricted by the extracellular matrix (ECM) and the abundance of ECM proteins determines the physical limit to cell growth. An increased area of fibrosis has been shown in adipose tissue from obese individuals as compared to lean controls [44]. More importantly, the mRNA (Messenger RNA) expression of collagen VI alpha3-subunit, the predominant ECM component in adipose tissue, is positively correlated with visceral fat content but no such relationship exists with the subcutaneous depot [45]. Khan and colleagues [46] used a genetic model of collagen VI disruption and demonstrated that the weakening of ECM structure allowed 'stress-free' expansion of adipocytes during high-fat feeding, an effect associated with a reduction in ATM infiltration and an improvement in glucose tolerance. In support, correlation between collagen VI and macrophage expression in adipose tissue and their inverse relationship with insulin sensitivity has also been recently demonstrated in humans [46].

The fact that obesity is characterised by both an increase in adipocyte size and ECM protein abundance in the adipose tissue, however, is intriguing and appears to work against the above-mentioned hypothesis. It is possible that, in the case of obesity, the increase in ECM component is a secondary effect from the already hypertrophic adipocytes in an attempt to restrict further lipid accumulation in the tissue. Mere adipocyte expansion is not physiologically viable in the long term due to excessive demands on the endoplasmic reticulum (ER) for protein folding, lipid esterification and nutrient-sensing results in ER stress [47]. This triggers an inflammatory response including the activation of the mitogen-activated protein kinase (MAPK) signalling pathway which has been linked to insulin resistance [48]. Further, unresolved ER stress and elevated intracellular levels of free fatty acids generate oxidative stress in the mitochondria which further impairs cellular function of adipocytes and may eventually induce apoptotic and/or necrotic cell death [49].

ECM regulates adipocyte size, and there is some evidence that 'healthy' hypertrophy may ameliorate adipose inflammation and obesity-associated insulin resistance. Thus, modulating ECM may provide some benefits during early obesity – when intervention precedes the stage at which adipocyte expansion becomes dangerous. However, such an approach would only achieve maximal long-term benefits when treatments to prevent further energy surplus and adipose expansion are in place.

Phenotypic switching of macrophages

The metabolic effects of ATMs are specific to their phenotypes. Macrophages are broadly classified as M1 (classically activated) or M2 (alternatively activated) based on the expression of cell surface markers. M1 macrophages produce primarily pro-inflammatory cytokines, eg IL-1beta, IL-6 and TNF-alpha, whereas M2 macrophages (which may be further subdivided into M2a, M2b and M2c) are generally responsible for tissue remodelling and down-regulation of an inflammatory response [50]. Obese mice exhibited an increased M1:M2 ATM ratio in visceral as compared to subcutaneous fat [51] and similar findings have also been reported in humans [52], suggesting the predominant effect of M1 ATMs in the pro-inflammatory nature of visceral fat. Recent data, however, challenge the simple M1/M2 classification system. For instance, CD11c has long been recognised as a typical M1 marker. In a study by Li and colleagues [50] in which mice were switched from a high-fat to a normal chow diet, the abundance of CD11c[+] ATMs remained unchanged despite a reduction in the release of pro-inflammatory cytokines. Similar alterations in gene expression profile of CD11c[+] ATMs have also been observed during the course of high-fat feeding [53], suggesting that such macrophages may exhibit a spectrum of functionality. Accordingly, the increased ATM infiltration in visceral fat does not necessarily, by itself, result in a 'pro-inflammatory' fat depot.

What further complicates our understanding of ATMs is their plasticity. The secretory function of macrophages is dependent on the specific microenvironment. It has been shown that macrophages activation, as defined by the expression of both cell surface markers and chemokines, is plastic and fully reversible depending on the presence and withdrawal of specific stimuli [54]. As in the case of chronic systemic inflammation in viscerally obese individuals, this would implicate the presence of factors that activate and maintain the ATMs in the pro-inflammatory phenotype. The nature and range of these factors is currently only poorly understood.

The role of gut in metabolic dysfunction

From leaky gut to visceral adipose expansion

The role of the gut in adipose physiology has long been recognised in patients with Crohn's disease (a condition characterised by severe gut inflammation). These patients have an increased ratio of intra-abdominal to total abdominal fat as compared to healthy individuals [55]. The excess accumulation of mesenteric fat around the inflamed gut, known as 'fat wrapping', is associated with the prognosis of the disease [56] and is characterised by the increased infiltration of immune cells (eg macrophages and T-cells) and production of pro-inflammatory factors (eg IL-6 and MCP-1) [57]. Data from experimental models suggest causality between gut inflammation and mesenteric fat dysfunction – rats with induced colitis have 35% more mesenteric fat as compared to controls [58]. Using a similar model, Thomaz and colleagues [59] showed that mesenteric fat in the colitis animals had increased expression of F4/80 (a macrophage marker) and TNF-alpha. Importantly, it has been shown that the effect of gut inflammation on adipose tissue is localised [58] and therefore implicates anatomical proximity as important for gut-visceral fat interactions.

Indeed, there is some evidence suggesting that gut-induced adipose dysfunction may be a consequence of the direct 'leakage' of luminal antigens, microbiota and their metabolites through the gut wall into the adjacent mesenteric fat. Gut barrier integrity is normally maintained by multiple mechanisms. First, tight-junction proteins (eg zona occludens [ZO]-1, occludins and claudins) form multi-protein complexes to seal the space between neighbouring epithelial cells and therefore act as a physical barrier [60]. Second, intestinal epithelial cells produce a wide range of anti-microbial peptides, including defensins and cathelicidins, which serve as an immunological barrier to protect the mucosal surface from microbial pathogens [61]. Inflammation impairs gut barrier function, as evident by the increased gut permeability in patients with Crohn's disease [62] and animal models of induced inflammation [63]. *In vitro*, activation of the inflammatory NFκB pathway (eg by TNF-alpha [64] and IL-1beta [65]) has been shown to disrupt tight-junction integrity by increasing the expression and activity of myosin light chain kinase, leading to the contraction of peri-junctional actin-myosin filaments and opening of the tight-junctions. This may result in a 'leak' of bacteria and their products, as demonstrated by the translocation of bacteria into the mesenteric fat in mice with induced-gut inflammation [63].

Mesenteric fat, therefore, is left to cope with an increased microbial load from the 'leaky' gut. Lipopolysaccharides (LPS), a major bacterial cell component derived from the cell wall of Gram-negative bacteria, induce insulin resistance in adipocytes [66]. Further, LPS induces the release of MCP-1 and pro-inflammatory cytokines in adipocytes [67, 68] and promotes the 'pro-inflammatory' polarisation of macrophages (ie increase production of IL-1, IL-6 and TNF-alpha and reduce that of the anti-inflammatory IL-10 [69]) and, therefore results in an inflamed fat depot. The chronic stimulation from the bacterial antigens also leads to activation and the subsequent enlargement of lymph nodes [70, 71], which together with the direct effect of bacterial stimuli on activating peroxisome proliferator-activated receptor-γ and then on to adipogenesis [71], results in mesenteric hypertrophy and/or hyperplasia. Mesenteric fat expansion as a consequence of the microbial leak from the inflamed gut however, may be an important defensive mechanism to prevent further translocation of bacteria and/or their products into the visceral cavity, which in extreme cases, can be fatal.

From leaky gut to systemic dysfunction

Unfortunately the metabolic consequences of a leaky gut do not stop at visceral adipose dysfunction. Following on from the inflamed and hypertrophic mesenteric fat, more pro-inflammatory factors and free fatty acids (as a result of increased lipolysis of insulin-resistant adipocytes) enter the portal circulation and subsequently lead to an inflamed, steatotic and insulin-resistant liver [72]. The deleterious effects of a diseased liver on carbohydrate and lipid homeostasis are obvious – reduced glucose uptake, impaired suppression of postprandial glucose release and over-production of fatty acids [73].

There is also the effect of bacterial components and metabolites on systemic host metabolism when they enter the circulation. Under normal circumstances, only a very small amount of endotoxins (primarily LPS) pass through the gut barrier and reach the liver in which they are detoxified [74]. An impaired gut barrier function, however, will see an increased delivery of LPS into the liver. This may saturate the hepatic detoxification capacity and result in an 'overflow' of LPS into the systemic circulation [75]. A study by Pastor Rojo et al. [76] showed that 48% of patients with Crohn's disease had an increased serum concentration of endotoxins. Recently, there is also some evidence for an elevated circulating level of endotoxins in overweight/obese individuals [77] and patients with type 2 diabetes [78]. This phenomenon, often referred to as 'metabolic endotoxemia', is associated with insulin resistance, chronic systemic inflammation and increased cardiovascular risk [79]. The metabolic consequence of endotoxemia is directly demonstrated in a study by Mehta and co-workers [80], in which intravenous LPS administration in healthy humans resulted in elevated plasma concentrations of inflammatory markers and a 35% reduction in insulin sensitivity. The molecular pathways by which LPS induces inflammation are detailed in a comprehensive review by Lu and colleagues [81]. Briefly, LPS is first recognised in the circulation by the LPS-binding protein and is then transported to the target cells, where LPS binds to CD14 and the toll-like receptor (TLR)-4/MD-2 receptor complex. After interacting with a series of adaptor proteins including myeloid differentiation primary response gene (MyD)-88, the net response to LPS is activation of both the NFκB and the MAPK signalling pathways and subsequently induction of the expression of pro-inflammatory cytokines. It should be noted that TLR4 is ubiquitously expressed in insulin-targeting tissues, eg adipose tissue, liver, skeletal muscle and pancreatic beta-cells, and there is evidence for TLR4-induced inflammation to inhibit insulin signal transduction (for details please refer to a review by Kim and Sears [82]).

In summary, the initially 'localised' inflammation of the gut may have deleterious consequence on whole-body metabolism. Inflammation and the associated insulin resistance, eg in liver, adipose tissue and skeletal muscle, will then stimulate insulin secretion from the beta-cells and subsequently results in peripheral insulin resistance and a vicious cycle of systemic metabolic dysfunction. This inflammatory response involves interaction with the gut microbiota.

Gut microbiota

Available evidence indicates that gut microbiota influence metabolic health in a variety of ways. The gastrointestinal tract (GIT) harbours a large microbial community (total of ca 10^{14} cells) with very high microbial cell densities in the ileum and large intestine [83, 84]. Many of the processes that occur in the GIT are either encoded by microbial genomes, or strongly influenced by microbial activity, and our physiology is a convergent of human and microbial traits [85, 86]. Accordingly, we need to consider the role of gut microbial community in the pathogenesis of metabolic disorders. Each individual's gut microbiota is unique. While 80%–90% of the gut bacteria belong to the phyla *Firmicutes* and *Bacteroidetes*, the species involved and their relative abundances vary from person to person [87]. This variation in microbiota composition is widely accepted to be a contributing factor to differences in host physiological outcomes.

Gut microbiota and barrier function

Functional disruptions to the epithelial lining of GIT is characterised by an altered microbial community. In fact, epithelial cells and resident bacteria are thought to be synergistic partners in modulating gut barrier function. Gut microbiota contributes to barrier function through three different mechanisms. Firstly, normal mucosal resident bacteria competitively exclude other, potentially pathogenic bacteria, from attachment to the epithelial mucosa. Secondly, some gut bacteria have been shown to promote tight-junction integrity by inducing the expression levels of tight-junction-related genes [88] and/or by promoting the localisation of proteins (eg ZO-1 and occludin) in the tight-junctions [89]. Thirdly, gut bacteria produce substrates for the maintenance of enterocytes. Butyrate, for example, is the primary energy source for colonic epithelial cells. In germ-free mouse models, the absence of microbial butyrate resulted in the depletion of ATP level and induced autophagy, an effect reversed by introducing exogenous butyrate or by colonising germ-free mice with butyrate-producing bacteria [90]. These data support the notion that gut microbes are directly involved in the normal functioning of epithelial cells and maintenance of gut barrier integrity.

It has long been postulated that the beneficial effect of gut bacteria is not universal but is confined to specific species with other species being detrimental. To date only very few species are thoroughly investigated. Initial studies focused on organisms commonly isolated from the gut epithelium, eg *Lactobacillus* and *Bifidobacterium*. In gnotobiotic studies, *Lactobacillus acidophilus* has been shown to inhibit cell association and the invasion of flagellated bacteria, therefore ameliorating inflammation and improving gut barrier function [91]. Similarly, *Bifidobacterium infantis* increased epithelial integrity and was protective against inflammation-induced impaired gut barrier function both *in vitro* and in an experimental model of spontaneous colitis [92]. The effect of the described species (and strains) on maintaining epithelial barrier integrity in simple models (eg mono-associated gnotobionts), however, does not necessarily translate to physiological benefits in the natural gut system with its complex community. *Lactobacillus* and *Bifidobacterium* only account for a small proportion of the gut microbial community and therefore their metabolic effects may be relatively minor as compared to that of the more abundant genera such as *Clostridium*.

Recent studies have focused on investigating the function of gut microbiota at a systems level. Using real-time quantitative polymerase chain reaction (PCR), Cani and colleagues [93] measured gut bacterial populations in ob/ob mice which also exhibited impaired gut permeability. They demonstrated an association between systemic metabolic dysfunction (including endotoxemia and inflammation) and alternations in the abundances of *Bifidobacterium*, *Lactobacillus* and *Clostridium coccoides-Eubacterium rectale* cluster. Importantly, this study identified the relationship between Clostridia and metabolic dysregulation, which has not been previously noted in monocolonisation studies. The role of Clostridia in gut inflammation and barrier function is further substantiated by metagenomic analysis which examines the genomic profile of the entire gut microbial community. Metagenomic studies of gut microbiota showed that patients with inflammatory bowel disease had a lower relative abundance of Clostridial cluster IV and XIVa as compared to healthy controls [94]. This suggests that the absence of these Clostridial clusters may enhance gut permeability and subsequently increase host susceptibility to chronic inflammation. There is also some evidence suggesting that bacteria in Clostridial cluster IV and XIVa are potent inducers of gut regulatory CD4 T cells, which are important modulators in the initiation of immune responses [95].

In summary, numerous studies revealed the role of certain gut microbes in modulating intestinal permeability. The effect of bacteria on gut health appears to be highly species- and even strain-specific. Identifying beneficial strains will be important for developing nutraceutical, and even pharmaceutical, interventions to improve gut health.

Gut microbiota and energy homeostasis

Gut microbiota influence host energy metabolism by modulating nutrient absorption and energy storage. There is some evidence suggesting that gut bacteria stimulate angiogenesis in the small intestine epithelium and therefore increase the efficiency of nutrient absorption [96]. It is also well documented that gut microbiota ferments dietary compounds, which are otherwise indigestible by the host, and therefore increases energy harvest.

The effect of gut microbiota on host energy homeostasis is primarily a consequence of short-chain fatty acids (SCFAs) production. Bacterial enzymes, eg glycoside hydrolases, break down dietary polysaccharides to SCFAs such as butyrate, acetate and propionate [97]. While butyrate is the primary energy substrate for colonocytes and is important for fortification of the GIT epithelial barrier, acetate and propionate are delivered to the liver for de novo lipogenesis through acetyl-CoA carboxylase and fatty acid synthase. The direct effect of gut microbiota on hepatic lipid metabolism is demonstrated in conventionalisation studies, in which the colonisation of germ-free mice with cecal content of conventionally raised animals increased fatty acid and triglyceride synthesis in the liver and promoted peripheral fat storage [98]. Bacterial SCFAs may also directly modulate the signalling pathways involved in host fat storage. SCFAs are specific ligands for at least two G protein coupled receptors, GPR 41 and GPR 43, which when deficient ameliorate microbe-associated energy harvest [99] and diet-induced obesity [100].

It is important to note that the interactions between gut microbiota, GIT and liver are part of the normal physiological processes in the host. Disturbances or alterations to the microbial community (collectively known as microbial dysbiosis) however, are likely to shift the energy balance in favour of nutrient recovery and storage. This notion is best illustrated in a series of studies by Turnbaugh, Gordon and colleagues. Germ-free mice receiving an obesity-associated microbiota (OAM, from diet-induced obese mice) had increased fat deposition as compared to those transplanted with a lean-associated microbiota (LAM) [101]. Further, it has also been shown that OAM is enriched for genes that encode enzymes involved in starch, sucrose, and galactose metabolism to breakdown otherwise indigestible polysaccharides [102]. These data suggest that OAM has a higher energy harvesting potential. The increased influx of SCFAs into the systemic and, more importantly, the portal circulation may increases lipid load in the liver and predispose hepatic insulin resistance.

The research of gut microbiota currently focuses on unravelling microbial populations affected in microbial dysbiosis and the associated metabolic sequelae. A feature of many human [103] and experimental models of obesity [104], is that an OAM is characterised by a lower *Bacteroidetes:Firmicutes* ratio as compared to an LAM. Whether this is a generic trend across the obesity-associated metabolic disorders is not entirely clear. For example, patients with type 2 diabetes have been shown to have similar *Bacteroidetes:Firmicutes* ratio as healthy controls but the proportion of bacteria represented within *Bacteroidetes* differed in the two cohorts [105]. To date there is limited evidence suggesting the predominant role of a particular microbe or a specific group of bacterial species in the events leading up to metabolic disorders. Experimental data however, strongly indicate that the composition of gut microbiota is an important aspect of host metabolic phenotype. Microbial dysbiosis, therefore, should be considered as an additional risk factor in the pathogenesis of insulin resistance and systemic metabolic dysregulations.

Future directions: focus on immune and gut systems

The discovery of the involvement of the immune and gut systems in obesity-related metabolic dysfunctions identify a subset of at-risk individuals who would benefit from novel immune- and gut-targeted therapies to improve metabolic health. Here we highlight some recent data to identify potential therapeutic targets.

Immunomodulators

A logical approach to prevent inflammation-associated metabolic sequelae is to block the initiation of an immune response. The chronic use of agents which non-selectively antagonise the key pro-inflammatory pathways (eg glucocorticoids), however, are often associated with immunosuppression-related side effects [106]. Attempts to develop interventions to reduce localised inflammation have also proven to be impractical. In the gut system, inhibiting the signalling of specific TLRs interferes with mucosal repair [107] and has even been shown to induce 'hallmark features of metabolic syndrome' including insulin resistance, hyperlipidemia and increased adiposity [108, 109]. It then becomes apparent that a specific TLR functional deficiency is compensated by the activation of other TLRs [108]. Further, this feedback loop appears to modulate gut microbiota profile [109] and therefore may subsequently lead to metabolically deleterious phenotypes.

Promoting resolution has recently been appreciated as an alternative way to minimise the deleterious effects of inflammation. Rather than directly interfering with the inflammatory signalling pathways, pro-resolving mediators reduce the infiltration and, at the same time, enhance the clearance of immune cells at the site of inflammation [106]. Accordingly, these mediators promote tissue recovery and therefore prevent unnecessarily prolonged inflammation. Resolvins are a family of endogenous pro-resolution molecules which have received much of the attention. N-3 polyunsaturated fatty acids have long been recognised as anti-inflammatory due to the preferential production of less inflammatory eicosanoids [110]. The recent discovery of the D- and E-series of resolvins, derived from docosahexaenoic acid (DHA; 22:6n-3) and eicosapentaenoic acid (EPA; 20:5n-3) respectively, suggests that the pro-resolving nature is another important aspect of n-3 polyunsaturated fatty acids to modulate inflammation. Human clinical trials of resolvins to treat inflammatory diseases including rheumatoid arthritis and inflammatory bowel disease are already underway. Consistent with the further role of inflammation in obesity/ diabetes, resolvin D1 administration has recently been shown to reduce CLS-localised ATMs in visceral adipose tissue and improve insulin sensitivity in db/db mice [111]. Taken with the protective effect of fish oil feeding against LPS-induced inflammation and insulin resistance [112], these results also point to the potential of resolvins as a pharmacological target for obesity and diabetes.

Probiotics, prebiotics and resistant starches

The compelling evidence of the role of gut microbiota in gut functions and energy metabolism clearly indicates manipulating the microbial community as an important avenue to improve metabolic health. Probiotic supplementation, which involves the ingestion of live micro-organisms, is the most direct way to introduce specific beneficial bacteria into the gut system. Strains of several species of *Lactobacillus* and *Bifidobacteria*, eg *L. plantarum* [113] and *B. bifidum* [114] are probiotics with consistently demonstrated health benefits. There is an emerging literature supporting the use of probiotics supplementary to standard treatment for inflammatory bowel disease [115] and irritable bowel syndrome [116]. Dietary probiotic supplements and food fortified with probiotics (eg dairy products and infant formulas) are also widely available for general consumption. There have been concerns however, about the efficacy of probiotic supplementation as the effective dose of beneficial bacteria reaching the GIT may be highly variable and it is likely to account for only a relatively small proportion of the entire microbial population. Also little is known about the duration of effect so dosage may be critical for long-term health benefits.

Supplementation of prebiotics in combination with resistant starch is an alternative way to manipulate gut microbiota profile. Prebiotics are oligosaccharides which serve as substrates for specific gut microbes. For example inulin is a fructan preferentially used by *Lactobacillus* and *Bifidobacteria* [117]. Resistant starch is defined as starch and/or products of starch degradation, which are not absorbed in the small intestine, and therefore enters the colon with butyrate as a predominant product from microbial fermentation [118]. While each bacterial genus or species has its own preferential substrates, prebiotics and resistant starch promote the growth of specific beneficial bacterial populations and subsequently shifts the balance of microbial communities in a way that favours gut and metabolic health.

The use of food ingredients to manipulate gut microbiota composition is advantageous to probiotics supplementation. Bioavailability becomes less of an issue, but perhaps what makes prebiotics and resistant starch a really appealing option is their ability to modify, long term, autochthonous microbial communities and therefore increase the likelihood of having persisting health benefits. There is also the possibility of engineering dietary components to facilitate colonisation of specific microbial populations and/or to produce specific species of SCFAs to serve particular therapeutic purposes. Rats fed with diet containing 10% butyrylated high-amylose maize starch, for example, had increased total SCFAs and in particular butyrate content in the colon as compared to those which consumed non-butyrylated carbohydrates [119]. Finally, the notion of synbiotics (a combination of probiotics and prebiotics), which potentially introduce and, at the same time, maintain beneficial microbes in the gut system, may well be the most promising intervention to modify gut microbiota profile and achieve maximal health benefits.

Gut mucosal defence

Strengthening the innate defence mechanisms against pathogens is critical to maintain gut health. The gastrointestinal tract is coated with a mucus layer, as the first line of defence, to protect the epithelium from both physical and chemical damage. Mucins, the major component of the overlaying mucus layer, are glycoproteins produced primarily by goblet cells. The highly complex oligosaccharide side-chains of mucins form a viscous lining which interacts with and trap microbes and subsequently prevent direct contact of epithelial surface with pathogens [120]. The interaction between mucins and bacteria has also been shown to facilitate specific patterns of bacterial colonisation [134]. A study by An et al. [121] provided direct evidence for the role of mucins in gut function, in which mice deficient in the biosynthesis of core 3 O-glycans (the predominant component of mucins) had increased gut permeability and were more susceptible to experimental colitis and colorectal adenocarcinoma. Similarly, mice deficient in Muc2 (the most abundant mucin) exhibited signs of spontaneous colitis and growth retardation [122].

Dietary supplementations to induce mucins expression may be important to ameliorate metabolic sequelae associated with gut inflammation. Probiotics (eg specific strains of *Lactobacillus*) have been shown to increase mRNA levels of mucins in colonic cells *in vitro* [123, 124]. There is also some evidence for the ability of probiotic administration to induce gene expression of mucins in animal models of colitis [125]. Similarly, dietary supplementation of amino acids specific to mucins production restores the colonic protein level of mucins to that in the controls and promotes epithelial repair in rats with experimental colitis [126].

Trefoil factors (TFF) are another group of important proteins involved in the maintenance of the mucosal barrier. Among this family of small peptides, TFF3 is one of the most abundant secretory products from goblet cells. TFF3 works synergistically with mucins to strengthen the structural integrity of the intestinal mucosal barrier [120]. TFF3 is also critical in aiding epithelial repair following injury by promoting epithelial restitution via the TGF-beta-dependent pathway [127]. When subjected to experimental colitis, mice deficient in TFF3 are more susceptible to mortality and exhibit delayed mucosal healing as a consequence of inhibited anti-apoptosis during acute inflammation [128].

TFF3 serves as a critical molecular link between microbiota and intestinal integrity. Commensal bacteria activate many members of the TLR family (eg TLR2 and TLR4), which subsequently induce the expression of TFF3 via the Ras/MEK/MAPK and PI3K/Akt pathways [120]. Accordingly, TFF3 is the downstream effector of the microbiota-initiated innate immune response. Manipulating TLRs, as we have argued earlier, might be a dangerous impairment of the innate immune system. However, modulating TFF3 may offer an alternate opportunity to develop interventions to improve gut health while bypassing the upstream effects of microbiota and inflammatory and/or stress-activated pathways on epithelial function. This notion is best-illustrated in a study by Podolsky and colleagues [128], in which administration of a TLR2 agonist in TFF3$^{-/-}$ mice and oral supplementation of recombinant TFF3 in TLR2$^{-/-}$ mice both confer protection of the intestinal mucosa during experimental colitis.

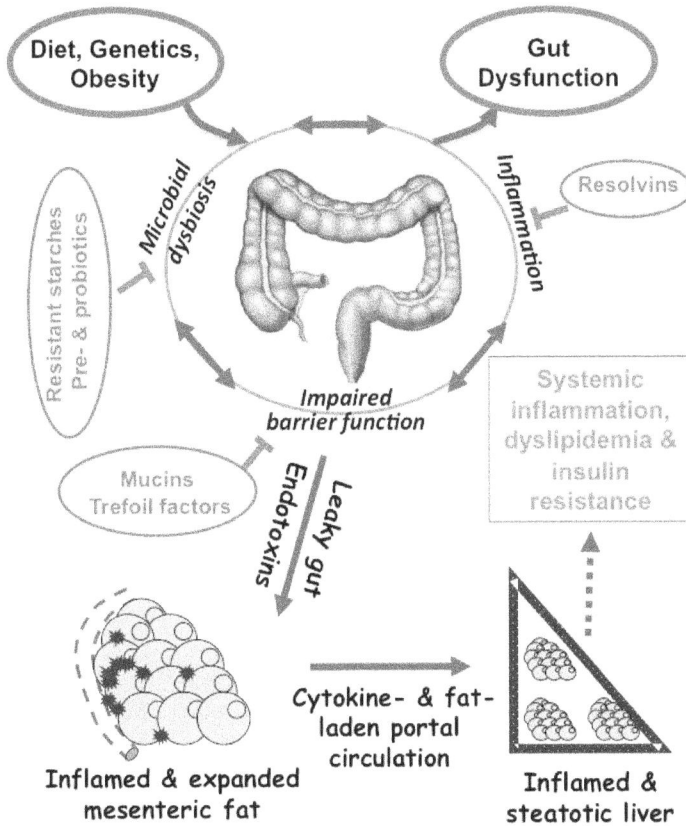

Adapted from Lam et al, Obesity 2011

Figure 2. The role of gut in the development of systematic inflammation and metabolic dysfunctions.

Conclusion

Insulin resistance is central to obesity-associated metabolic dysfunctions. The little success we have in reversing the insulin-resistant state clearly suggest the need to focus on preventative measures to achieve maximal metabolic health. Recent advances in understanding the metabolic sequelae of visceral fat deposition and gut dysfunction, summarised in Figure 2, provide unprecedented opportunities to both prevent and treat metabolic disorders. What is critical now is to develop biomarkers for large-scale population screening to identify individuals with high metabolic risk and offer early preventative interventions. Dietary modifications via the development of fortified and functional foods, perhaps in combination with novel pharmaceuticals, are also promising avenues to improve metabolic health at the population level.

References

1. Reaven G (2005). All obese individuals are not created equal: insulin resistance is the major determinant of cardiovascular disease in overweight/obese individuals. *Diabetes and Vascular Disease Research*, 2(3): 105–12.

2. Rasouli N, Molavi B, Elbein SC & Kern PA (2007). Ectopic fat accumulation and metabolic syndrome. *Diabetes, Obesity and Metabolism*, 9(1): 1–10.

3. Meigs JB, Wilson PW, Fox CS, Vasan RS, Nathan DM, Sullivan LM, et al. (2006). Body mass index, metabolic syndrome, and risk of type 2 diabetes or cardiovascular disease. *The Journal of Clinical Endocrinology and Metabolism*, 91(8): 2906–12.

4. Weiss R (2007). Fat distribution and storage: how much, where, and how? *European Journal of Endocrinology*, 157(Suppl. 1): S39–45.

5. Bjorntorp P (1990). 'Portal' adipose tissue as a generator of risk factors for cardiovascular disease and diabetes. *Arteriosclerosis*, 10(4): 493–96.

6. Wajchenberg BL (2000). Subcutaneous and visceral adipose tissue: their relation to the metabolic syndrome. *Endocrine Reviews*, 21(6): 697–738.

7. Ito H, Ohshima A, Ohto N, Ogasawara M, Tsuzuki M, Takao K, et al. (2001). Relation between body composition and age in healthy Japanese subjects. *European Journal of Clinical Nutrition*, 55(6): 462–70.

8. Piers LS, Rowley KG, Soares MJ & O'Dea K (2003). Relation of adiposity and body fat distribution to body mass index in Australians of Aboriginal and European ancestry. *European Journal of Clinical Nutrition*, 57(8): 956–63.

9. Casas YG, Schiller BC, DeSouza CA & Seals DR (2001). Total and regional body composition across age in healthy Hispanic and white women of similar socioeconomic status. *The American Journal of Clinical Nutrition*, 73(1): 13–18.

10. Fox CS, Massaro JM, Hoffmann U, Pou KM, Maurovich-Horvat P, Liu CY, et al. (2007). Abdominal visceral and subcutaneous adipose tissue compartments: association with metabolic risk factors in the Framingham Heart Study. *Circulation*, 116(1): 39–48.

11. Kelley DE, Thaete FL, Troost F, Huwe T & Goodpaster BH (2000). Subdivisions of subcutaneous abdominal adipose tissue and insulin resistance. *American Journal of Physiology – Endocrinology and Metabolism,* 278(5): E941–48.

12. Cnop M, Landchild MJ, Vidal J, Havel PJ, Knowles NG, Carr DR, et al. (2002). The concurrent accumulation of intra-abdominal and subcutaneous fat explains the association between insulin resistance and plasma leptin concentrations: distinct metabolic effects of two fat compartments. *Diabetes,* 51(4): 1005–15.

13. Hayashi T, Boyko EJ, McNeely MJ, Leonetti DL, Kahn SE & Fujimoto WY (2008). Visceral adiposity, not abdominal subcutaneous fat area, is associated with an increase in future insulin resistance in Japanese Americans. *Diabetes,* 57(5): 1269–75.

14. Karelis AD, St-Pierre DH, Conus F, Rabasa-Lhoret R & Poehlman ET (2004). Metabolic and body composition factors in subgroups of obesity: what do we know? *The Journal of Clinical Endocrinology and Metabolism,* 89(6): 2569–75.

15. Lien LF, Haqq AM, Arlotto M, Slentz CA, Muehlbauer MJ, McMahon RL, et al. (2009). The STEDMAN project: biophysical, biochemical and metabolic effects of a behavioral weight loss intervention during weight loss, maintenance, and regain. *OMICS,* 13(1): 21–35.

16. Carr DB, Utzschneider KM, Hull RL, Kodama K, Retzlaff BM, Brunzell JD, et al. (2004). Intra-abdominal fat is a major determinant of the National Cholesterol Education Program Adult Treatment Panel III criteria for the metabolic syndrome. *Diabetes,* 53(8): 2087–94.

17. Ibanez J, Izquierdo M, Arguelles I, Forga L, Larrion JL, Garcia-Unciti M, et al. (2005). Twice-weekly progressive resistance training decreases abdominal fat and improves insulin sensitivity in older men with type 2 diabetes. *Diabetes Care,* 28(3): 662–67.

18. Wagenknecht LE, Langefeld CD, Scherzinger AL, Norris JM, Haffner SM, Saad MF, et al. (2003). Insulin sensitivity, insulin secretion, and abdominal fat: the Insulin Resistance Atherosclerosis Study (IRAS) Family Study. *Diabetes,* 52(10): 2490–96.

19. Cnop M, Landchild MJ, Vidal J, Havel PJ, Knowles NG, Carr DR, et al. (2002). The concurrent accumulation of intra-abdominal and subcutaneous fat explains the association between insulin resistance and plasma leptin concentrations: distinct metabolic effects of two fat compartments. *Diabetes,* 51(4): 1005–15.

20. Miyazaki Y, Glass L, Triplitt C, Wajcberg E, Mandarino LJ & DeFronzo RA (2002). Abdominal fat distribution and peripheral and hepatic insulin resistance in type 2 diabetes mellitus. *American Journal of Physiology – Endocrinology and Metabolism,* 283(6): E1135–43.

21. Porter SA, Massaro JM, Hoffmann U, Vasan RS, O'Donnel CJ & Fox CS (2009). Abdominal subcutaneous adipose tissue: a protective fat depot? *Diabetes Care,* 32(6): 1068–75.

22. Walker GE, Verti B, Marzullo P, Savia G, Mencarelli M, Zurleni F, et al. (2007). Deep subcutaneous adipose tissue: a distinct abdominal adipose depot. *Obesity,* 15(8): 1933–43.

23. Ross R, Freeman J, Hudson R & Janssen I (2002). Abdominal obesity, muscle composition, and insulin resistance in premenopausal women. *The Journal of Clinical Endocrinology and Metabolism,* 87(11): 5044–51.

24. Ibrahim MM (2010). Subcutaneous and visceral adipose tissue: structural and functional differences. *Obesity Reviews*, 11(1): 11–18.

25. Rabe K, Lehrke M, Parhofer KG & Broedl UC (2008). Adipokines and insulin resistance. *Molecular Medicine*, 14(11–12): 741–51.

26. Gregor MF & Hotamisligil GS (2011). Inflammatory mechanisms in obesity. *Annual Review of Immunology*, 23(29): 415–45.

27. Crook M (2004). Type 2 diabetes mellitus: a disease of the innate immune system? An update. *Diabetic Medicine*, 21(3): 203–07.

28. Hu FB, Meigs JB, Li TY, Rifai N & Manson JE (2004). Inflammatory markers and risk of developing type 2 diabetes in women. *Diabetes*, 53(3): 693–700.

29. Hundal RS, Petersen KF, Mayerson AB, Randhawa PS, Inzucchi S, Shoelson SE, et al. (2002). Mechanism by which high-dose aspirin improves glucose metabolism in type 2 diabetes. *The Journal of Clinical Investigation*, 109(10): 1321–26.

30. Panagiotakos DB, Pitsavos C, Yannakoulia M, Chrysohoou C & Stefanadis C (2005). The implication of obesity and central fat on markers of chronic inflammation: The ATTICA study. *Atherosclerosis*, 183(2): 308–15.

31. Krysiak R, Labuzek K & Okopien B (2009). Effect of atorvastatin and fenofibric acid on adipokine release from visceral and subcutaneous adipose tissue of patients with mixed dyslipidemia and normolipidemic subjects. *Pharmacological Reports*, 61(6): 1134–45.

32. Bruun JM, Lihn AS, Madan AK, Pedersen SB, Schiott KM, Fain JN, et al. (2004). Higher production of IL-8 in visceral vs subcutaneous adipose tissue. Implication of nonadipose cells in adipose tissue. *American Journal of Physiology – Endocrinology and Metabolism*, 286(1): E8–13.

33. Lam YY, Janovska A, McAinch AJ, Belobrajdic DP, Hatzinikolas G, Game P, et al. (2011). The use of adipose tissue-conditioned media to demonstrate the differential effects of fat depots on insulin-stimulated glucose uptake in a skeletal muscle cell line. *Obesity Research and Clinical Practice*, 5: e43–e54.

34. Arkan MC, Hevener AL, Greten FR, Maeda S, Li ZW, Long JM, et al. (2005). IKK-beta links inflammation to obesity-induced insulin resistance. *Nature Medicine*, 11(2): 191–98.

35. Austin RL, Rune A, Bouzakri K, Zierath JR & Krook A (2008). siRNA-mediated reduction of inhibitor of nuclear factor-kappaB kinase prevents tumor necrosis factor-alpha-induced insulin resistance in human skeletal muscle. *Diabetes*, 57(8): 2066–73.

36. Fain JN (2006). Release of interleukins and other inflammatory cytokines by human adipose tissue is enhanced in obesity and primarily due to the nonfat cells. *Vitamins and Hormones*, 74: 443–77.

37. Weisberg SP, McCann D, Desai M, Rosenbaum M, Leibel RL & Ferrante AW Jr (2003). Obesity is associated with macrophage accumulation in adipose tissue. *The Journal of Clinical Investigation*, 112(12): 1796–808.

38. Harman-Boehm I, Bluher M, Redel H, Sion-Vardy N, Ovadia S, Avinoach E, et al. (2007). Macrophage infiltration into omental versus subcutaneous fat across different populations: effect

of regional adiposity and the comorbidities of obesity. *The Journal of Clinical Endocrinology and Metabolism*, 92(6): 2240–47.

39. Weisberg SP, Hunter D, Huber R, Lemieux J, Slaymaker S, Vaddi K, et al. (2006). CCR2 modulates inflammatory and metabolic effects of high-fat feeding. *The Journal of Clinical Investigation,* 116(1): 115–24.

40. Kanda H, Tateya S, Tamori Y, Kotani K, Hiasa K, Kitazawa R, et al. (2006). MCP-1 contributes to macrophage infiltration into adipose tissue, insulin resistance, and hepatic steatosis in obesity. *The Journal of Clinical Investigation*, 116(6):1494–1505.

41. Cinti S, Mitchell G, Barbatelli G, Murano I, Ceresi E, Faloia E, et al. (2005). Adipocyte death defines macrophage localization and function in adipose tissue of obese mice and humans. *The Journal of Lipid Research,* 46(11): 2347–55.

42. Strissel KJ, Stancheva Z, Miyoshi H, Perfield JW, 2nd, DeFuria J, Jick Z, et al. (2007). Adipocyte death, adipose tissue remodeling, and obesity complications. *Diabetes,* 56(12): 2910–18.

43. Murano I, Barbatelli G, Parisani V, Latini C, Muzzonigro G, Castellucci M, et al. (2008). Dead adipocytes, detected as crown-like structures, are prevalent in visceral fat depots of genetically obese mice. *The Journal of Lipid Research,* 49(7): 1562–68.

44. Spencer M, Yao-Borengasser A, Unal R, Rasouli N, Gurley CM, Zhu B, et al. (2010). Adipose tissue macrophages in insulin-resistant subjects are associated with collagen VI and fibrosis and demonstrate alternative activation. *American Journal of Physiology – Endocrinology and Metabolism*, 99(6): E1016–27.

45. Pasarica M, Gowronska-Kozak B, Burk D, Remedios I, Hymel D, Gimble J, et al. (2009). Adipose tissue collagen VI in obesity. *The Journal of Clinical Endocrinology and Metabolism,* 94(12): 5155–62.

46. Khan T, Muise ES, Iyengar P, Wang ZV, Chandalia M, Abate N, et al. (2009). Metabolic dysregulation and adipose tissue fibrosis: role of collagen VI. *Molecular and Cellular Biology,* 29(6): 1575–91.

47. Gregor MF & Hotamisligil GS (2007). Thematic review series: Adipocyte Biology. Adipocyte stress: the endoplasmic reticulum and metabolic disease. *The Journal of Lipid Research,* 48(9): 1905–14.

48. Zhang K & Kaufman RJ (2008). From endoplasmic-reticulum stress to the inflammatory response. *Nature,* 454(7203): 455–62.

49. de Ferranti S & Mozaffarian D (2008). The perfect storm: obesity, adipocyte dysfunction, and metabolic consequences. *Clinical Chemistry*, 54(6): 945–55.

50. Martinez FO, Sica A, Mantovani A & Locati M (2008). Macrophage activation and polarization. *Frontiers in Bioscience,* 13: 453–61.

51. Lumeng CN, DelProposto JB, Westcott DJ & Saltiel AR (2008). Phenotypic switching of adipose tissue macrophages with obesity is generated by spatiotemporal differences in macrophage subtypes. *Diabetes,* 57(12): 3239–46.

52. Aron-Wisnewsky J, Tordjman J, Poitou C, Darakhshan F, Hugol D, Basdevant A, et al. (2009). Human adipose tissue macrophages: m1 and m2 cell surface markers in subcutaneous and omental depots and after weight loss. *The Journal of Clinical Endocrinology and Metabolism,* 94(11): 4619–23.

53. Shaul ME, Bennett G, Strissel KJ, Greenberg AS & Obin MS (2010). Dynamic, M2-like remodeling phenotypes of CD11c+ adipose tissue macrophages during high-fat diet-induced obesity in mice. *Diabetes,* 59(5): 1171–81.

54. Porcheray F, Viaud S, Rimaniol AC, Leone C, Samah B, Dereuddre-Bosquet N, et al. (2005). Macrophage activation switching: an asset for the resolution of inflammation. *Clinical and Experimental Immunology,* 142(3): 481–89.

55. Desreumaux P, Ernst O, Geboes K, Gambiez L, Berrebi D, Muller-Alouf H, et al. (1999). Inflammatory alterations in mesenteric adipose tissue in Crohn's disease. *Gastroenterology,* 117(1): 73–81.

56. Maconi G, Greco S, Duca P, Ardizzone S, Massari A, Cassinotti A, et al. (2008). Prevalence and clinical significance of sonographic evidence of mesenteric fat alterations in Crohn's disease. *Inflammatory Bowel Diseases,* 14(11): 1555–61.

57. Bertin B, Desreumaux P & Dubuquoy L (2010). Obesity, visceral fat and Crohn's disease. *Current Opinion in Clinical Nutrition and Metabolic Care,* 13(5): 574–80.

58. Gambero A, Marostica M, Abdalla Saad MJ & Pedrazzoli J Jr (2007). Mesenteric adipose tissue alterations resulting from experimental reactivated colitis. *Inflammatory Bowel Diseases,* 13(11): 1357–64.

59. Thomaz MA, Acedo SC, de Oliveira CC, Pereira JA, Priolli DG, Saad MJ, et al. (2009). Methotrexate is effective in reactivated colitis and reduces inflammatory alterations in mesenteric adipose tissue during intestinal inflammation. *Pharmacological Research,* 60(4): 341–46.

60. Cereijido M, Contreras RG, Flores-Benitez D, Flores-Maldonado C, Larre I, Ruiz A, et al. (2007). New diseases derived or associated with the tight junction. *Archives of Medical Research,* 38(5): 465–78.

61. Muller CA, Autenrieth IB & Peschel A (2005). Innate defenses of the intestinal epithelial barrier. *Cellular and Molecular Life Sciences,* 62(12): 1297–307.

62. D'Inca R, Annese V, di Leo V, Latiano A, Quaino V, Abazia C, et al. (2006). Increased intestinal permeability and NOD2 variants in familial and sporadic Crohn's disease. *Alimentary Pharmacology and Therapeutics,* 23(10): 1455–61.

63. Cenac N, Coelho AM, Nguyen C, Compton S, Andrade-Gordon P, MacNaughton WK, et al. (2002). Induction of intestinal inflammation in mouse by activation of proteinase-activated receptor-2. *American Journal of Pathology,* 161(5): 1903–15.

64. Ye D, Ma I & Ma TY (2006). Molecular mechanism of tumor necrosis factor-alpha modulation of intestinal epithelial tight junction barrier. *American Journal of Physiology Gastrointestinal and Liver Physiology,* 290(3): G496–504.

65. Al-Sadi R, Ye D, Dokladny K & Ma TY (2008). Mechanism of IL-1beta-induced increase in intestinal epithelial tight junction permeability. *The Journal of Immunology,* 180(8): 5653–61.

66. Bumrungpert A, Kalpravidh RW, Chitchumroonchokchai C, Chuang CC, West T, Kennedy A, et al. (2009). Xanthones from mangosteen prevent lipopolysaccharide-mediated inflammation and insulin resistance in primary cultures of human adipocytes. *Journal of Nutrition,* 139(6): 1185–91.

67. Grisouard J, Bouillet E, Timper K, Radimerski T, Dembinski K, Frey DM, et al. (2010). Both inflammatory and classical lipolytic pathways are involved in lipopolysaccharides-induced lipolysis in human adipocytes. *Innate Immunity,* 18 November, DOI: 10.1177/1753425910386632 [Online]. Available: ini.sagepub.com/content/early/2010/10/14/1753425910386632.full.pdf [Accessed 12 January 2012].

68. Kopp A, Bala M, Buechler C, Falk W, Gross P, Neumeier M, et al. (2010). C1q/TNF-related protein-3 represents a novel and endogenous lipopolysaccharide antagonist of the adipose tissue. *Endocrinology,* 151(11): 5267–78.

69. Mantovani A, Sica A, Sozzani S, Allavena P, Vecchi A & Locati M (2004). The chemokine system in diverse forms of macrophage activation and polarization. *Trends in Immunology,* 25(12): 677–86.

70. Pond CM (2005). Adipose tissue and the immune system. *Prostaglandins, Leukotrienes, and Essential Fatty Acids,* 73(1): 17–30.

71. Peyrin-Biroulet L, Chamaillard M, Gonzalez F, Beclin E, Decourcelle C, Antunes L, et al. (2007). Mesenteric fat in Crohn's disease: a pathogenetic hallmark or an innocent bystander? *Gut,* 56(4): 577–83.

72. Tarantino G, Savastano S & Colao A (2010). Hepatic steatosis, low-grade chronic inflammation and hormone/growth factor/adipokine imbalance. *World Journal of Gastroenterology,* 16(38): 4773–83.

73. Postic C, Dentin R & Girard J (2004). Role of the liver in the control of carbohydrate and lipid homeostasis. *Diabetes and Metabolism,* 30(5): 398–408.

74. Szabo G & Bala S (2010). Alcoholic liver disease and the gut-liver axis. *World Journal of Gastroenterology,* 16(11): 1321–29.

75. Rao R (2009). Endotoxemia and gut barrier dysfunction in alcoholic liver disease. *Hepatology,* 50(2): 638–44.

76. Pastor Rojo O, Lopez San Roman A, Albeniz Arbizu E, de la Hera Martinez A, Ripoll Sevillano E & Albillos Martinez A (2007). Serum lipopolysaccharide-binding protein in endotoxemic patients with inflammatory bowel disease. *Inflammatory Bowel Diseases,* 13(3): 269–77.

77. Sun L, Yu Z, Ye X, Zou S, Li H, Yu D, et al. (2010). A marker of endotoxemia is associated with obesity and related metabolic disorders in apparently healthy Chinese. *Diabetes Care,* 8 June, 33(9):1925-32. DOI: 10.2337/dc10-0340 [Online]. Available: care.diabetesjournals.org/content/early/2010/06/03/dc10-0340.full.pdf+html [Accessed 12 January 2012].

78. Creely SJ, McTernan PG, Kusminski CM, Fisher M, Da Silva NF, Khanolkar M, et al. (2007). Lipopolysaccharide activates an innate immune system response in human adipose tissue in obesity and type 2 diabetes. *American Journal of Physiology – Endocrinology and Metabolism,* 292(3): E740–47.

79. Manco M, Putignani L & Bottazzo GF (2010). Gut microbiota, lipopolysaccharides, and innate immunity in the pathogenesis of obesity and cardiovascular risk. *Endocrine Reviews,* 31(6): 817–44.

80. Mehta NN, McGillicuddy FC, Anderson PD, Hinkle CC, Shah R, Pruscino L, et al. (2010). Experimental endotoxemia induces adipose inflammation and insulin resistance in humans. *Diabetes,* 59(1): 172–81.

81. Lu YC, Yeh WC & Ohashi PS (2008). LPS/TLR4 signal transduction pathway. *Cytokine,* 42(2): 145–51.

82. Kim JJ & Sears DD (2010). TLR4 and insulin resistance. *Gastroenterology Research and Practice,* 2010.

83. Savage DC (1977). Microbial ecology of the gastrointestinal tract. *Annual Review of Microbiology,* 31: 107–33.

84. Xu J & Gordon JI. (2003). Honor thy symbionts. *Proceedings of the National Academy of Sciences of the United States of America,* 100(18): 10452–59.

85. Camp JG, Kanther M, Semova I & Rawls JF (1989). Patterns and scales in gastrointestinal microbial ecology. *Gastroenterology,* 136(6): 1989–2002.

86. Bocci V (1992). The neglected organ: bacterial flora has a crucial immunostimulatory role. *Perspectives in Biology and Medicine,* 35(2): 251–60.

87. Macfarlane S, Woodmansey EJ & Macfarlane GT (2005). Colonization of mucin by human intestinal bacteria and establishment of biofilm communities in a two-stage continuous culture system. *Applied and Environmental Microbiology,* 71(11): 7483–92.

88. Anderson RC, Cookson AL, McNabb WC, Park Z, McCann MJ, Kelly WJ, et al. (2010). Lactobacillus plantarum MB452 enhances the function of the intestinal barrier by increasing the expression levels of genes involved in tight junction formation. *BMC Microbiology,* 10: 316.

89. Karczewski J, Troost FJ, Konings I, Dekker J, Kleerebezem M, Brummer RJ, et al. (2010). Regulation of human epithelial tight junction proteins by Lactobacillus plantarum in vivo and protective effects on the epithelial barrier. *American Journal of Physiology Gastrointestinal and Liver Physiology,* 298(6): G851–59.

90. Donohoe DR, Garge N, Zhang X, Sun W, O'Connell TM, Bunger MK, et al. (2011). The microbiome and butyrate regulate energy metabolism and autophagy in the mammalian colon. *Cell Metabolism,* 13(5): 517–26.

91. Bernet-Camard MF, Lievin V, Brassart D, Neeser JR, Servin AL & Hudault S (1997). The human Lactobacillus acidophilus strain LA1 secretes a nonbacteriocin antibacterial substance(s) active in vitro and in vivo. *Applied and Environmental Microbiology,* 63(7): 2747–53.

92. Ewaschuk JB, Diaz H, Meddings L, Diederichs B, Dmytrash A, Backer J, et al. (2008). Secreted bioactive factors from Bifidobacterium infantis enhance epithelial cell barrier function. *American Journal of Physiology Gastrointestinal and Liver Physiology,* 295(5): G1025–34.

93. Cani PD, Possemiers S, Van de Wiele T, Guiot Y, Everard A, Rottier O, et al. (2009). Changes in gut microbiota control inflammation in obese mice through a mechanism involving GLP-2-driven improvement of gut permeability. *Gut,* 58(8): 1091–103.

94. Frank DN, St Amand AL, Feldman RA, Boedeker EC, Harpaz N & Pace NR (2007). Molecular-phylogenetic characterization of microbial community imbalances in human inflammatory bowel diseases. *Proceedings of the National Academy of Sciences of the United States of America,* 104(34): 13780–85.

95. Smith PM & Garrett WS (2011). The gut microbiota and mucosal T cells. *Frontiers in Microbiology*, 2: 111.

96. Stappenbeck TS, Hooper LV & Gordon JI (2002). Developmental regulation of intestinal angiogenesis by indigenous microbes via Paneth cells. *Proceedings of the National Academy of Sciences of the United States of America*, 99(24): 15451–55.

97. Flint HJ, Duncan SH, Scott KP & Louis P (2007). Interactions and competition within the microbial community of the human colon: links between diet and health. *Environmental Microbiology*, 9(5): 1101–11.

98. Backhed F, Ding H, Wang T, Hooper LV, Koh GY, Nagy A, et al. (2004). The gut microbiota as an environmental factor that regulates fat storage. *Proceedings of the National Academy of Sciences of the United States of America*, 101(44): 15718–23.

99. Samuel BS, Shaito A, Motoike T, Rey FE, Backhed F, Manchester JK, et al. (2008). Effects of the gut microbiota on host adiposity are modulated by the short-chain fatty-acid binding G protein-coupled receptor, Gpr41. *Proceedings of the National Academy of Sciences of the United States of America*, 105(43): 16767–72.

100. Bjursell M, Admyre T, Goransson M, Marley AE, Smith DM, Oscarsson J, et al. (2011). Improved glucose control and reduced body fat mass in free fatty acid receptor 2-deficient mice fed a high-fat diet. *American Journal of Physiology – Endocrinology and Metabolism*, 300(1): E211–20.

101. Turnbaugh PJ, Backhed F, Fulton L & Gordon JI (2008). Diet-induced obesity is linked to marked but reversible alterations in the mouse distal gut microbiome. *Cell Host and Microbe*, 3(4): 213–23.

102. Turnbaugh PJ, Ley RE, Mahowald MA, Magrini V, Mardis ER & Gordon JI (2006). An obesity-associated gut microbiome with increased capacity for energy harvest. *Nature*, 444(7122): 1027–31.

103. Ley RE, Turnbaugh PJ, Klein S & Gordon JI. (2006). Microbial ecology: human gut microbes associated with obesity. *Nature*, 444(7122): 1022–23.

104. Ley RE, Backhed F, Turnbaugh P, Lozupone CA, Knight RD & Gordon JI (2005). Obesity alters gut microbial ecology. *Proceedings of the National Academy of Sciences of the United States of America*, 102(31): 11070–75.

105. Wu X, Ma C, Han L, Nawaz M, Gao F, Zhang X, et al. (2010). Molecular characterisation of the faecal microbiota in patients with type II diabetes. *Current Microbiology*, 61(1): 69–78.

106. Uddin M & Levy BD (2011). Resolvins: natural agonists for resolution of pulmonary inflammation. *Progress in Lipid Research*, 50(1): 75–88.

107. Ungaro R, Fukata M, Hsu D, Hernandez Y, Breglio K, Chen A, et al. (2009). A novel toll-like receptor 4 antagonist antibody ameliorates inflammation but impairs mucosal healing in murine colitis. *American Journal of Physiology Gastrointestinal and Liver Physiology*, 296(6): G1167–79.

108. Vijay-Kumar M, Sanders CJ, Taylor RT, Kumar A, Aitken JD, Sitaraman SV, et al. (2007). Deletion of TLR5 results in spontaneous colitis in mice. *The Journal of Clinical Investigation*, 117(12): 3909–21.

109. Vijay-Kumar M, Aitken JD, Carvalho FA, Cullender TC, Mwangi S, Srinivasan S, et al. (2010).

Metabolic syndrome and altered gut microbiota in mice lacking toll-like receptor 5. *Science*, 328(5975): 228–31.

110. Adkins Y & Kelley DS (2010). Mechanisms underlying the cardioprotective effects of omega-3 polyunsaturated fatty acids. *The Journal of Nutritional Biochemistry*, 21(9): 781–92.

111. Hellmann J, Tang Y, Kosuri M, Bhatnagar A & Spite M (2011). Resolvin D1 decreases adipose tissue macrophage accumulation and improves insulin sensitivity in obese-diabetic mice. *The FASEB Journal*, 25: 2399–407.

112. Vijay-Kumar M, Vanegas SM, Patel N, Aitken JD, Ziegler TR, Ganji V. (2011). Fish oil rich diet in comparison to saturated fat rich diet offered protection against lipopolysaccharide-induced inflammation and insulin resistance in mice. *Nutrition and Metabolism*, 8(1): 16.

113. Molin G (2001). Probiotics in foods not containing milk or milk constituents, with special reference to Lactobacillus plantarum 299v. *The American Journal of Clinical Nutrition*, 73(2): 380S–5S.

114. Trebichavsky I, Rada V, Splichalova A & Splichal I (2009). Cross-talk of human gut with bifidobacteria. *Nutrition Reviews*, 67(2): 77–82.

115. Cary VA & Boullata J (2010). What is the evidence for the use of probiotics in the treatment of inflammatory bowel disease? *Journal of Clinical Nursing*, 19(7–8): 904–16.

116. Lee BJ & Bak YT (2011). Irritable bowel syndrome, gut microbiota and probiotics. *Journal of Neurogastroenterology and Motility*, 17(3): 252–66.

117. Gourbeyre P, Denery S & Bodinier M (2011). Probiotics, prebiotics, and synbiotics: impact on the gut immune system and allergic reactions. *Journal of Leukocyte Biology*, 89(5): 685–95.

118. Topping DL, Fukushima M & Bird AR (2003). Resistant starch as a prebiotic and synbiotic: state of the art. *The Proceedings of the Nutrition Society*, 62(1): 171–76.

119. Clarke JM, Topping DL, Bird AR, Young GP & Cobiac L (2008). Effects of high-amylose maize starch and butyrylated high-amylose maize starch on azoxymethane-induced intestinal cancer in rats. *Carcinogenesis*, 29(11): 2190–94.

120. Kim YS & Ho SB (2010). Intestinal goblet cells and mucins in health and disease: recent insights and progress. *Current Gastroenterology Reports*, 12(5): 319–30.

121. An G, Wei B, Xia B, McDaniel JM, Ju T, Cummings RD, et al. (2007). Increased susceptibility to colitis and colorectal tumors in mice lacking core 3-derived O-glycans. *The Journal of Experimental Medicine*, 204(6): 1417–29.

122. Van der Sluis M, De Koning BA, De Bruijn AC, Velcich A, Meijerink JP, Van Goudoever JB, et al. (2006). Muc2-deficient mice spontaneously develop colitis, indicating that MUC2 is critical for colonic protection. *Gastroenterology*, 131(1): 117–29.

123. Mack DR, Michail S, Wei S, McDougall L & Hollingsworth MA (1999). Probiotics inhibit enteropathogenic E. coli adherence in vitro by inducing intestinal mucin gene expression. *American Journal of Physiology*, 276(4 Pt 1): G941–50.

124. Mattar AF, Teitelbaum DH, Drongowski RA, Yongyi F, Harmon CM & Coran AG (2002).

Probiotics up-regulate MUC-2 mucin gene expression in a Caco-2 cell-culture model. *Pediatric Surgery International,* 18(7): 586–90.

125. Amit-Romach E, Uni Z & Reifen R (2010). Multistep mechanism of probiotic bacterium, the effect on innate immune system. *Molecular Nutrition and Food Research,* 54(2): 277–84.

126. Faure M, Mettraux C, Moennoz D, Godin JP, Vuichoud J, Rochat F, et al. (2006). Specific amino acids increase mucin synthesis and microbiota in dextran sulfate sodium-treated rats. *Journal of Nutrition,* 136(6): 1558–64.

127. Sturm A & Dignass AU (2008). Epithelial restitution and wound healing in inflammatory bowel disease. *World Journal of Gastroenterology,* 14(3): 348–53.

128. Podolsky DK, Gerken G, Eyking A & Cario E (2009). Colitis-associated variant of TLR2 causes impaired mucosal repair because of TFF3 deficiency. *Gastroenterology,* 137(1): 209–20.

4

Pancreatic beta-cell failure in the pathogenesis of type 1 diabetes

Alexandra Sharland[1]

In essence, it is the failure of the cell known as the pancreatic beta cell to make and secrete adequate insulin, that leads to the development of all forms of diabetes mellitus. Type 1 diabetes is caused by immune destruction of pancreatic beta cells. While multiple pancreatic beta-cell autoantibody positivity is strongly associated with the progression to diabetes, it is not clear whether autoantibodies can cause initial beta-cell destruction, or whether antibody production is only triggered after episodes of beta-cell death have already occurred leading to clinical onset of type 1 diabetes. Indeed even though many of the major T cell autoantigens are derived from the same proteins recognised by the immune cells known as B cells, it is currently thought that type 1 diabetes is mainly mediated by subsets of effector T cells. Documented epidemiological data suggest environmental factors act upon a background of genetic susceptibility to establish pancreatic islet inflammation known as 'insulitis' and subsequent beta-cell dysfunction and loss. Understanding the nature of the environmental factors contributing to insulitis, beta-cell loss and the development of type 1 diabetes may provide the key to developing interventions to prevent or delay onset in at-risk individuals. To date, no clinical trials including immune-based approaches aimed at preventing type 1 diabetes onset in high-risk individuals have proven effective. This chapter will focus upon the evidence for genetic susceptibility, and some of the putative environmental triggers in type 1 diabetes which may ultimately lead to methods to protect beta cells, and to stimulate residual beta-cell function or regeneration without ongoing immune destruction.

Type 1 diabetes mellitus is an autoimmune disease with very well-defined genetic susceptibility. Individuals with a strong genetic predisposition to type 1 diabetes typically develop one or more autoantibodies against islet antigens, and grumbling islet inflammation or insulitis ensues, with slow destruction of the islets and attrition of the islet cell mass over a number of years. In most cases, clinical diabetes develops before the complete destruction of islet beta cells has occurred, whereas absence of functioning beta cells is the rule in longstanding type 1 diabetes.

---

1 Collaborative Transplantation Research Group, University of Sydney.

Although this pathway represents the characteristic pattern of disease progression, many aspects of the pathogenesis of type 1 diabetes are incompletely understood. Not all individuals with a genetic predisposition develop diabetes. Disease incidence can be influenced by additional genes inherited concurrently with the known high-susceptibility alleles, and by environmental factors. Insulitis can be difficult to detect, and when present, is often patchy. Whilst most patients with type 1 diabetes have one or more pancreatic islet autoantibodies detectable at the time of diagnosis, and the risk of developing diabetes increases with the number of autoantibodies an individual is producing, a small number of patients never have detectable islet autoantibodies. The progression from susceptibility to autoantibody production and beta cell loss is usually steady and inexorable, yet some elements of this process may be reversible. Animal studies have demonstrated the potential for islet beta cells to regenerate after the onset of clinical diabetes – such regeneration may be possible in humans as well, and offers a potential target for therapeutic intervention. These and other areas of current interest and controversy will be discussed further in the following sections.

Genetic susceptibility to type 1 diabetes

Over 40 gene loci have now been identified as being linked to the risk of developing type 1 diabetes [1]. Consistent with the notion of type 1 diabetes as an autoimmune disease, essentially all these genes influence the immune system at some level, thus affecting its ability to mount a response against islet autoantigens. The strongest predisposition to diabetes development is conferred by genes found in the Human Leucocyte Antigen complex on the short arm of chromosome 6, particularly the HLA class II loci, DR and DQ [2]. The highest-risk genotype includes some combination of HLA DR3 or DR4 with HLA DQ2 or DQ8. This genotype is present in around 2.4% of newborns, but its representation is much greater amongst individuals with diabetes [3]. Infants with this gene combination have a greater than 50% chance of developing type 1 diabetes by age 12, and this risk is increased further if an HLA-identical sibling is already affected by diabetes [3]. Conversely, other class II alleles such as DQ 0602, are associated with dominant protection from diabetes, even amongst autoantibody-positive first-degree relatives of patients with type 1 diabetes [4]. The function of HLA DR and DQ molecules is to present antigens to CD4-positive helper T cells, thus initiating a cognate immune response. Structural and computational studies of susceptibility and protective alleles have revealed a number of shared features which modify the ability of these class II molecules to present peptides derived from islet autoantigens to responding T cells [5]. Charged residues at critical positions within the peptide binding groove allow diabetogenic peptide epitopes to bind strongly with slow dissociation kinetics, promoting the priming of a range of autoreactive CD4+ T cells [5]. Consistent with these observations, possession of particular HLA DQ alleles is linked to antibody specificity, such that DQ8 is associated with the presence of insulin autoantibodies, and DQ2 is found in subjects with antibodies against glutamic acid decarboxylase (GAD65) [6]

HLA class I genes are also associated with diabetes susceptibility, and the presence of the common HLA A2 allele further increases the likelihood of developing diabetes in individuals with high-risk class II alleles [7, 8] Possession of HLA B39 increases overall risk, and is linked with earlier onset of disease [9]. HLA class I molecules present antigens to CD8+ T cells, the cell subset directly implicated in the final phase of islet destruction. A growing body of evidence supports a functional role for HLA-A2 in the display of antigenic peptides derived from insulin precursors and GAD on the beta-cell surface, thus triggering beta-cell killing by CD8+ T cells which recognise these antigens [10–12].

Autoimmunity arises from a failure of development or maintenance of self-tolerance, where either the deletion of potentially autoreactive T cells in the thymus, or the generation of regulatory T cells which can suppress autoreactivity in the periphery, is inadequate. Two rare single gene (or monogenic) disorders which affect these processes result in severe generalised autoimmunity, with diabetes as one manifestation. These conditions are known as IPEX (immune dysregulation, polyendocrinopathy, enteropathy, X-linked) in which regulatory T cells fail to develop appropriately due to a mutation in the FoxP3 transcription factor [13, 14] and APECED (autoimmune polyendocrinopathy – candidiasis – ectodermal dystrophy) where a defect in the protein AIRE prevents expression of otherwise tissue-specific genes (such as insulin) in the thymus, and blocks generation of self-tolerance to the proteins encoded by those genes [15]. Reminiscent of the mechanism underlying APECED, polymorphisms in the promoter of the insulin gene confer susceptibility to type 1 diabetes if they bind poorly to AIRE, and reduce insulin expression in the thymus [16, 17].

Recent advances in high-throughput sequencing technology have enabled genome-wide association studies (GWAS) to be performed in type 1 diabetes and other common disorders. These studies have confirmed that a number of other loci involved in the regulation of T cell function influence the likelihood of developing diabetes [18]. Such genes include PTPN 22, which encodes a tyrosine phosphatise which regulates T cell receptor signalling, and the genes encoding interleukin 2 receptor alpha chain and the co-inhibitory molecule CTLA4 [19]. Genes involved in innate immune responses to microorganisms have also been linked with diabetes susceptibility in recent studies, and intriguingly, these findings suggest one mechanism whereby genetic susceptibility can interact with environmental exposures to result in disease. IFIH1 is a gene which encodes the intracellular pathogen receptor MDA5 [19, 20]. MDA5 triggers immune responses to viral RNA derived from the enterovirus family, of which Coxsackie viruses are a member, and there is considerable circumstantial evidence linking Coxsackie infection with diabetes onset. Other intracellular nucleic acid receptors recently mapped in type 1 diabetes include the toll-like receptors TLR7 and TLR8 [21].

Environmental factors and type 1 diabetes

Whilst the growing epidemic of type 2 diabetes is common knowledge, it is less well appreciated that worldwide incidence of type 1 diabetes has been rising over the past few decades as well [22, 23]. Moreover, there has been a shift towards onset of clinical diabetes at an earlier age, such that the prevalence rate in individuals aged younger than 15 years is projected to increase by 70% between 2005 and 2020 [24]. These rapid changes in incidence and in age of onset, along with the lower than expected concordance between monozygotic twins, are characteristic of the operation of environmental factors upon a background susceptibility [25]. Consistent with the idea that the highest-risk genotypes require the least environmental pressure to result in overt diabetes, the changes in incidence have been most pronounced amongst those with moderate, rather than extreme genetic susceptibility [26]. In Australia, the incidence of type 1 diabetes in children with the highest risk alleles has remained stable over time, as has age at diagnosis. Conversely, a greater proportion of children with moderate-risk alleles is developing diabetes, and is doing so at a younger age [27]. Other hallmarks of environmental influence, such as seasonal variations in onset of clinical diabetes, are also largely confined to those at moderate genetic risk [28]. Understanding the nature of the environmental factors contributing to the development of overt diabetes may provide the key to developing interventions to prevent or delay onset in at-risk individuals, and there is considerable research concentration in this area. In this section, we will discuss the evidence for some of the putative environmental triggers of diabetes.

Viral infections

Infections with several viruses have been plausibly associated with the development of type 1 diabetes. 22% of children infected with rubella *in utero* later developed type 1 diabetes [29], and cross-reactivity between T cells recognising both rubella and GAD-derived peptides was demonstrated [30]. However, it now appears that impairment of islet development following pancreatic infection with rubella, rather than islet autoimmunity, may be the mechanism of rubella-associated type 1 diabetes [31].

Data linking infection with enterovirus or rotavirus to diabetes onset are tantalising, and evidence to support a potential pathogenetic role for these infections exists. Nevertheless, these findings have not been consistent across all groups studied, perhaps reflecting the complexity of the interactions between individual susceptibility and environmental factors as well as differences in study methodology.

In the longitudinal Diabetes Prediction and Prevention (DIPP) study from Finland, enterovirus infections were reported in the majority of subjects developing islet autoantibodies in the six months preceding initial antibody detection, whereas significantly fewer children without autoantibodies had been infected [32]. Other large longitudinal studies of genetically at-risk cohorts did not confirm these findings [33, 34]. Seemingly conflicting results may arise because different substrains of the same virus may not be differentiated by routinely available serological testing, and yet may have different diabetogenic potential. In addition, identical viruses could have different effects upon progression if encountered at different stages in the natural history of the disease [35].

Fulminant type 1 diabetes is an entity described in Japan, where direct infection of the islets and exocrine pancreas with enterovirus leads to upregulation of chemokine and cytokine secretion by islets, triggering infiltration with aggressive T cells and macrophages, and islet destruction within a matter of days [36]. However, pancreatic infection with enterovirus family members is also reported in diabetes cases with a less dramatic onset. Coxsackie virus is tropic for human beta cells, and virus-positive beta cells have been demonstrated in pancreas specimens from studies in children succumbing to severe metabolic complications of diabetes close to diagnosis, but not from control pancreata [37]. At symptom onset, multiple enterovirus nucleic acid sequences were identified in the peripheral blood cells of 50% of subjects, compared with 0% of age and sex-matched controls [38]. Moreover, T cells from a majority of recent-onset subjects proliferated in response to Coxsackie viral lysates [39]. One criticism of these data was that the controls were not matched with respect to diabetes risk, but recent reports from both the Diabetes Autoimmunity Study in the Young (DAISY) and DIPP studies have addressed these concerns. Amongst high-risk children with multiple islet autoantibodies, progression to clinical diabetes was significantly more frequent in those with evidence of a recent enterovirus infection than in those without [40, 41]. In addition to direct infection of the pancreas with enteroviruses such as Coxsackie, molecular mimicry between viral antigens and islet autoantigens has been postulated to trigger T cell reactivity against islets (discussed in [42]). The P2C non-structural protein of a diabetogenic strain of Coxsackie virus B4 shares extensive sequence similarity with GAD65, and virtually identical highly antigenic peptides can be derived from the two proteins [43].

Rotaviruses are double-stranded RNA viruses belonging to the Reovirus family. They are ubiquitous in the environment, and are the most frequent cause of gastroenteritis in young children [44]. The first indication that these agents may contribute to the development of type 1 diabetes came from studies demonstrating strong sequence homology between the rotavirus VP7 antigen and two epitopes recognised by islet-reactive T cells, one in GAD and one in IA-2 [45]. Longitudinal studies attempting to determine whether rotavirus exposure is associated with diabetes development have yielded varying results. The Australian BabyDiab study of at-risk children reported strong concordance between the appearance of islet autoantibodies and the detection of rotavirus-specific antibodies. Repeated rotavirus infection appeared to boost levels of anti-islet antibodies and coincided with epitope spreading and an increase in the number of autoantibody specificities present [46]. A later Finnish study failed to confirm these observations [47]. However, differences in the methodology used for determining rotavirus exposure may have contributed to this negative finding.

Lifestyle factors

Various other aspects of the modern lifestyle could be influencing the rise in incidence of type 1 diabetes (reviewed in [48]). Many of these (increased consumption of high-energy foods and foods containing trans-fatty acids, fructose or advanced glycation end-products, reduced energy expenditure due to declining levels of physical activity and maintenance of ambient temperatures within the thermoneutral zone for most of the time, reduced sleep duration) act through the mechanism of increasing insulin resistance, which will be discussed further below. In a seeming paradox, although exposure to some pathogenic viruses is linked to the development of type 1 diabetes, widespread adoption of clean living conditions with prevention or delay of exposure to environmental pathogens has also been implicated in the rise of autoimmune and allergic conditions, a theory termed the 'hygiene hypothesis' [49]. Changes in commensal gut bacteria, by increasing energy extraction from the diet, may also predispose to obesity and insulin resistance [50]. Finally, exposure to sunlight and consequent generation of vitamin D has progressively declined in many developed and developing countries over the past few decades. Several epidemiological studies have shown an inverse correlation between vitamin D intake and the incidence of type 1 diabetes [51, 52], and this link has been strengthened by the demonstration of protection against type 1 diabetes development by vitamin D administration in primary prevention studies in at-risk populations [53, 54].

Insulin resistance and type 1 diabetes

Insulin resistance in children and adults in the developed and developing world has been increasing in parallel with the rise in overweight and obesity, and could be making a significant contribution to the rising incidence of type 1 diabetes, in addition to its acknowledged role in type 2 diabetes. Analyses of a number of independent cohorts from Europe, the US and Australia have demonstrated that age at onset of type 1 diabetes was inversely proportional to body mass index (BMI) [55]. Not surprisingly, BMI was higher in subjects with moderate genetic risk, compared to those with high risk, and direct measurements of insulin sensitivity during metabolic testing confirmed that insulin resistance was an independent risk factor for progression to clinical type 1 diabetes in individuals with islet autoimmunity [56]. There are several ways in which insulin resistance could accelerate the development of type 1 diabetes in those with an underlying genetic predisposition. Insulin resistance means that the beta cells are obliged to increase insulin production in order to maintain blood glucose within the physiological range. Metabolic upregulation results in increased production of insulin precursor proteins as well as the cellular enzymes GAD and IA-2. Increased production results in increased presentation of peptides derived from these molecules on the surface of the beta cell, thereby increasing the chances of the beta cell being destroyed by a cytotoxic T cell which recognises these peptides. Insulin resistance per se 'accelerates the rate of beta-cell apoptosis through glucotoxicity and lipotoxicity' [57]. Furthermore, patients would be expected to cross the threshold at which remaining beta-cell function is no longer able to maintain glucose homeostasis at an earlier stage of beta-cell loss, in the presence of insulin resistance.

Pathogenesis and disease progression

Beta cells and autoantibodies in type 1 diabetes

The principal autoantibodies in type 1 diabetes recognise four islet autoantigens: insulinoma-associated antigen-2 (I–A2), insulin (micro IAA or mIAA), the 65 kD isoform of the enzyme glutamic acid decarboxylase (GAD65) and zinc transporter 8 (ZnT8) [58]. Whilst autoantibody positivity is strongly associated with the progression to diabetes, especially when antibodies against multiple islet determinants are present [59], it is not clear whether autoantibodies can cause beta-cell destruction, or whether antibody production is only triggered after episodes of beta-cell death have already occurred [60]. Antibody-producing B cells may also play a role in the pathogenesis of type 1 diabetes as professional antigen-presenting cells for T cells. In this regard, B cells can use their surface antibody to capture islet autoantigens before processing and presenting them to CD4+ T cells. B cells in turn receive help from the T cells which culminates in increased antibody secretion. This role of B cells is consistent with the observation that many of the major T cell autoantigens are derived from the same proteins recognised by B cells [61–63].

Insulitis

Infiltration of the pancreatic islets with lymphocytes ('insulitis') in patients who succumbed to diabetic complications close to the time of presentation was first noted in the 1960s [64] and has since been considered a hallmark of type 1 diabetes. Cross-sectional studies of tissues obtained close to diagnosis can yield important information about the final pre-clinical stages of the disease. Advances in the management of metabolic complications of diabetes mean that patients now rarely die with ketoacidosis, and most data are derived from historical collections of tissue [65]. Painstaking re-analysis of one such large cohort affirmed earlier observations that the degree of insulitis varied not only between patients but between regions of the pancreas and between individual islets [63, 65–67]. The investigators subdivided islets according to the percentage of remaining insulin-positive cells. The numbers of infiltrating cells increased as insulin-positive cell numbers declined, reaching a peak when less than 10% of insulin-containing cells remained. The density of infiltrate was then dramatically reduced in islets lacking insulin positivity. Although this was a cross-sectional study, the different categories of islets were interpreted as representing stages in the progression to beta-cell destruction, which was proceeding asynchronously [68]. At all stages, CD8+ T cells predominated in the infiltrate. B cells were preferentially found in more inflamed islets, whilst macrophages were a constant presence, albeit less frequent than CD8+ T cells. In this study, at least some degree of insulitis was found in all pancreas specimens, and overall, insulitis was detected in 12% of islets examined [68]. The observation that the density of the infiltrate increases substantially once beta-cell loss has reached a critical threshold is consistent with the idea that the drive to maintain glucose homeostasis upregulates the metabolic activity of the remaining beta cells, causing antigenic peptides to be produced and displayed on the cell surface in increasing amounts. This increases beta-cell susceptibility to CD8+ T cell-mediated killing and hastens the decline of the remaining beta-cell mass.

Much could be learned from the systematic histological study of the pancreas in at-risk and pre-diabetic individuals, as well as those with clinical diabetes of varying durations. However, obtaining tissue samples from these groups has previously been all but impossible. Recent initiatives have aimed to fill this void in our knowledge by screening organ donors for the presence of islet autoantibodies, and examining specimens of the pancreata of antibody-positive subjects. One such study of 62 antibody-positive donors found evidence of insulitis in only two individuals, a surprising result which led researchers to question the central role of islet inflammation in progression to diabetes [69]. Closer examination of the study cohort reveals that the two donors with insulitis were the only subjects with ≥3 autoantibodies, and also possessed high-risk HLA-DQ alleles. The increased age of this donor population compared with the usual age of onset of type 1 DM, single and low-titre antibody positive status of most of the subjects and relatively small number of islets examined per pancreas may all have contributed to the paucity of insulitis noted, and may mean that these findings do not reflect the general situation in prediabetes.

Efforts to gather pancreatic tissue from deceased organ donors of all ages have continued, largely under the auspices of the network for pancreatic organ donors with diabetes (nPOD), a program established by the Juvenile Diabetes Research Foundation. One of the first studies to be reported as a result of this initiative revealed that 30% of pancreata from donors with longstanding type 1 diabetes still contained numerous insulin positive cells in at least some islets [70]. Two distinct histological patterns were detected – one with patchy distribution of insulin-positive cells in a fraction of islets, co-incident with the upregulation of pro-survival signals in these islets. The second pattern was characterised by the presence of residual insulin-positive cells in 100% of islets. Subjects with this pattern were typically islet autoantibody-negative, and lacked high-risk HLA class II alleles, yet their disease displayed metabolic hallmarks of type 1 diabetes, including episodes of ketoacidisis [70]. These studies suggest that the pathogenesis of type 1 diabetes may be more heterogeneous than previously appreciated, and, at least a subset of patients have the potential to benefit from treatment approaches which stimulate residual beta-cell function or regeneration. More than 60 projects are currently underway using tissues collected through nPOD, and hopes are high that further new insights into diabetes pathogenesis will soon emerge from these.

Non-invasive imaging and monitoring of T cell function

Imaging of pancreatic islets and cells *in vivo* has to date proven very difficult in humans. The capacity to non-invasively screen for and sequentially monitor islet inflammation in at-risk, pre-diabetic, or type 1 diabetes patients would allow much greater refinement of risk stratification as well as enabling direct and timely assessment of the effect of interventions. In animal models of type 1 diabetes, the onset of insulitis is accompanied by increased 'leakiness' of the small blood vessels supplying the islets [71]. Magnetic Resonance Imaging (MRI) can be used to capture signals from injected magnetic nanoparticles, which exit the circulation through the leaky vessels and are engulfed by infiltrating macrophages in the pancreas. A recent report demonstrates that this imaging method can be adapted for use in humans, and is able to differentiate between subjects with recent-onset diabetes and controls [71]. Further development and more widespread adoption of this and other non-invasive imaging techniques, such as positron-emission tomography [72], have the potential to greatly increase our understanding of type 1 diabetes pathogenesis.

Efforts are being made to develop and validate assays of cell-mediated anti-islet reactivity which might be used to monitor changes in T cell function in those at risk for type 1 diabetes development, and subjects in prevention and early intervention trials of immunomodulation. A recent workshop sponsored by the Immune Tolerance Network evaluated two such assays for CD4+ T cells, a cellular immunoblot and a T cell proliferation assay [73]. Overall, these assays performed reasonably well in distinguishing patients with new-onset diabetes from normal controls with sensitivities of 94% and 58%, and specificities of 83% and 91%, respectively. Combination of the assays improved sensitivity, whilst maintaining specificity [73]. For CD8+ T cells, an islet-specific ELISPOT assay has been developed (ISL8SPOT, [74]). This assay measures interferon gamma-producing T cells in response to stimulation with a mixture of HLA-A2-restricted, beta cell-derived peptide epitopes. Beta cell-specific CD8+ T cells can thus be quantitated directly from unfractionated peripheral blood mononuclear cells. ISL8SPOT responses were clearly detectable in newly diagnosed patients with type 1 diabetes, but waned rapidly over the following six to 12 months as the rate of beta-cell destruction declined. Autoantibody levels remained constant over this period, suggesting that the T cell functional assays were more likely to reflect the patients' current immunological status than autoantibody titres [75]. HLA-A2 tetramers loaded with beta cell antigenic peptides are another tool which can be used to detect and quantitate islet-reactive CD8+ T cells [76]. These various assays are currently being evaluated for their suitability in monitoring responses to immunomodulatory treatments, and further information about these applications should soon become available.

On the opposite side of the T cell balance from the destructive effector cells are regulatory T cells, and attempts have also been made to assess regulatory T cell activity in type 1 diabetes. No consistent difference in the numbers of peripheral blood regulatory T cells have been identified between subjects with type 1 diabetes and normal individuals. Nonetheless, natural T regs isolated from type 1 diabetes patients are less potent suppressors than those isolated from control subjects, suggesting that function, rather than absolute number of these cells makes the paramount contribution to the disease state [77].

Interventions in at-risk individuals

The idea of being able to intervene in at risk or pre-diabetic individuals to prevent the onset of clinical diabetes is enormously appealing. Even with the most accurate predictive identification of high-risk groups, it should be remembered that not all members will develop diabetes. As a corollary, such trials must involve large numbers of subjects, and are very costly to conduct. Any interventions tested must be inherently very safe to maintain a balance between the risks and potential benefits to the participants. Interventions can be categorised as either non antigen-specific, or specific to various islet autoantigens. Dietary modifications are non antigen-specific interventions, and dietary substitutes and supplements studied in this way include hydrolysed cows' milk formula (Trial to Reduce IDDM in Genetically at Risk (TRIGR) study, [78]), vitamin D3 [79], Omega-3 fatty acids [80] and nicotinamide [81]. Another subgroup of prevention trials has aimed to induce specific tolerance to islet autoantigens by administering them via a route that is generally non-immunogenic. Accordingly, insulin has been given orally or intranasally to at-risk subjects. Whereas nicotinamide has been ineffective, early studies of vitamin D supplementation and of hydrolysed cow's milk formula have shown some benefit [82] and these interventions are now undergoing further evaluation. Results of insulin administration have been equivocal thus far [83].

The honeymoon phase and beta-cell regeneration

Up to 60% of patients newly diagnosed with type 1 diabetes achieve some improvement in functional beta-cell mass as measured by secretion of c-peptide and reduction in exogenous insulin requirement, after the initiation of insulin replacement therapy [84]. This period is often referred to as the 'honeymoon phase'. The mechanisms governing this short-lived improvement in function are incompletely understood, but probably involve restoration of function to insulin-depleted beta cells, perhaps accompanied by some true expansion of beta-cell mass [85].

A subset of patients with type 1 diabetes maintains small populations of functioning beta cells for many years after the onset of clinical type 1 diabetes [85], and these patients may be particularly amenable to therapies which aim to restore or improven glucose homeostasis via regeneration of existing beta-cell mass. In mouse models, three different mechanisms have been shown by different groups to result in the generation of new beta cells [87]. Replication of existing beta cells was responsible for beta-cell regeneration after subtotal ablation of beta cells in a transgenic mouse model [88], while recent reports have demonstrated that both beta-cell neogenesis from ductal precursors [89] and transdifferentiation from glucagon-secreting islet alpha cells [90, 91] can also occur under some circumstances. In the human pancreas, staining for the nuclear proliferation marker Ki-67 suggests that mature, differentiated beta cells can replicate, though the basal rate of replication is low (reviewed in [92]). Data supporting the existence of the other two mechanisms in humans are scant.

Arresting autoimmune islet destruction may allow beta-cell regeneration to emerge, but in adult humans, it is not clear whether this alone could be sufficient to reconstitute beta-cell mass and restore glucose homeostasis. In order to harness the potential of beta-cell regeneration, it is essential to understand how beta-cell turnover is controlled, and whether this could be manipulated in such a way as to produce a net accumulation of functional beta-cell mass. Murine studies indicate that a critical driver of beta-cell replication is glycolytic flux in the beta cell itself, reflected in the activity of the enzyme glucokinase [93]. Under physiological conditions, this is proportional to blood glucose levels, but glucokinase activity can be modified by a novel class of small-molecule drugs, the glucokinase activators, and thus represents a potential target for intervention [94]. Glucokinase activators are currently under development for the treatment of type 2 diabetes. They act by increasing the glucose affinity and maximum velocity of glucokinase [94]. Administration of glucokinase activators could eventually be used to enhance the low basal rate of beta-cell replication *in vivo*, thus permitting gradual regeneration of sufficient beta-cell mass from the remaining viable beta cells after the onset of clinical type 1 diabetes.

Gastrointestinal hormones (incretins) also play a role in regulation of beta-cell mass [95]. Glucagon-like peptide 1 (GLP-1) and glucose-dependent insulinotropic peptide (GIP) are produced and secreted by intestinal cells in response to dietary fat and carbohydrate. They increase insulin secretion by the beta cell via binding to G protein-coupled receptors (discussed in [96]). GLP-1 reduces beta-cell apoptosis [97], and may also stimulate beta-cell proliferation via the mitogen-activated protein (MAP) kinase [98] and Wnt [99] pathways, thus shifting the balance of beta-cell turnover towards accumulation. Treatment with currently available GLP-1 agonists such as exendin-4, or with inhibitors of the enzyme dipeptidyl peptidase 4 (DPP-IV), which degrades GLP-1 and GIP, increase beta-cell mass in diabetic rodents [100, 101]. These agents may have similar beneficial effects in humans if used in conjunction with treatments which target autoimmunity.

Conclusions

This is an exciting time for research in type 1 diabetes. Recent technological advances such as the ability to conduct genome-wide association studies or to undertake non-invasive imaging of the pancreas, coupled with initiatives such as nPOD, are greatly increasing our understanding of the aetiology and pathogenesis of type 1 diabetes. These insights will continue to suggest ways in which it might be possible to intervene in the course of the disease, both prior to and following the onset of clinical diabetes. Growing appreciation of the heterogeneity of type 1 diabetes will allow tailoring of treatment modalities to the particular subgroups of patients most likely to benefit from each type of intervention, while improved assays for monitoring anti-islet immune reactivity and response to treatment will inform clinical decisions and permit fine adjustment of immunomodulatory therapies.

References

1. Barrett JC, Clayton DG, Concannon P, Akolkar B, Cooper JD, Erlich HA, et al. (2009). Genome-wide association study and meta-analysis find that over 40 loci affect risk of type 1 diabetes. *Nature Genetics*, 41(6): 703–07.

2. Todd JA (1995). Genetic analysis of type 1 diabetes using whole genome approaches. *Proceedings of the National Academy of Sciences of the United States of America*, 92(19): 8560–65.

3. Aly TA, Ide A, Jahromi MM, Barker JM, Fernando MS, Babu SR, et al. (2006). Extreme genetic risk for type 1A diabetes. *Proceedings of the National Academy of Sciences of the United States of America*, 103(38): 14074–79.

4. Erlich H, Valdes AM, Noble J, Carlson JA, Varney M, Concannon P, et al. (2008). HLA DR–DQ haplotypes and genotypes and type 1 diabetes risk: analysis of the type 1 diabetes genetics consortium families. *Diabetes*, 57(4): 1084–92.

5. Parry CS & Brooks BR (2008). A new model defines the minimal set of polymorphism in HLA–DQ and –DR that determines susceptibility and resistance to autoimmune diabetes. *Biology Direct*, 3: 42.

6. Noorchashm H, Kwok W, Rabinovitch A & Harrison LC (1997). Immunology of IDDM. *Diabetologia*, 40 (Suppl. 3): B50–57.

7. Fennessy M, Metcalfe K, Hitman GA, Niven M, Biro PA, Tuomilehto J, et al. (1994). A gene in the HLA class I region contributes to susceptibility to IDDM in the Finnish population. Childhood Diabetes in Finland (DiMe) Study Group. *Diabetologia*, 37(9): 937–44.

8. Robles DT, Eisenbarth GS, Wang T, Erlich HA, Bugawan TL, Babu SR, et al. (2002). Millennium award recipient contribution. Identification of children with early onset and high incidence of anti-islet autoantibodies. *Clinical Immunology*, 102(3): 217–24.

9. Nejentsev S, Howson JM, Walker NM, Szeszko J, Field SF, Stevens HE, et al. (2007). Localization of type 1 diabetes susceptibility to the MHC class I genes HLA–B and HLA–A. *Nature*, 450(7171): 887–92.

10. Panagiotopoulos C, Qin H, Tan R & Verchere CB (2003). Identification of a beta-cell-specific HLA class I restricted epitope in type 1 diabetes. *Diabetes*, 52(11): 2647–51.

11. Panina-Bordignon P, Lang R, van Endert PM, Benazzi E, Felix AM, Pastore RM, et al. (1995). Cytotoxic T cells specific for glutamic acid decarboxylase in autoimmune diabetes. *Journal of Experimental Medicine*, 181(5): 1923–27.

12. Pinkse GG, Tysma OH, Bergen CA, Kester MG, Ossendorp F, van Veelen PA, et al. (2005). Autoreactive CD8 T cells associated with beta cell destruction in type 1 diabetes. *Proceedings of the National Academy of Sciences of the United States of America*, 102(51): 18425–30.

13. Bacchetta R, Passerini L, Gambineri E, Dai M, Allan SE, Perroni L, et al. (2006). Defective regulatory and effector T cell functions in patients with FOXP3 mutations. *The Journal of Clinical Investigation*, 116(6): 1713–22.

14. Wildin RS, Ramsdell F, Peake J, Faravelli F, Casanova JL, Buist N, et al. (2001). X-linked neonatal diabetes mellitus, enteropathy and endocrinopathy syndrome is the human equivalent of mouse scurfy. *Nature Genetics*, 27(1): 18–20.

15. Villasenor J, Benoist C & Mathis D (2005). AIRE and APECED: molecular insights into an autoimmune disease. *Immunology Reviews*, 204: 156–64.

16. Vafiadis P, Bennett ST, Todd JA, Nadeau J, Grabs R, Goodyer CG, et al. (1997). Insulin expression in human thymus is modulated by INS VNTR alleles at the IDDM2 locus. *Nature Genetics*, 15(3): 289–92.

17. Anderson MS, Venanzi ES, Klein L, Chen Z, Berzins SP, Turley SJ, et al. (2002). Projection of an immunological self shadow within the thymus by the aire protein. *Science*, 298(5597): 1395–401.

18. Todd JA, Walker NM, Cooper JD, Smyth DJ, Downes K, Plagnol V, et al. (2007). Robust associations of four new chromosome regions from genome-wide analyses of type 1 diabetes. *Nature Genetics*, 39(7): 857–64.

19. Todd JA (2010). Etiology of type 1 diabetes. *Immunity*, 32(4): 457–67.

20. Nejentsev S, Walker N, Riches D, Egholm M & Todd JA (2009). Rare variants of IFIH1, a gene implicated in antiviral responses, protect against type 1 diabetes. *Science*, 324(5925): 387–89.

21. Todd JA (2010). Etiology of type 1 diabetes. *Immunity*, 32(4): 457–67.

22. Diamond Study Group (2006). Incidence and trends of childhood type 1 diabetes worldwide 1990–1999. *Diabetic Medicine*, 23(8): 857–66.

23. Green A & Patterson CC (2001). Trends in the incidence of childhood-onset diabetes in Europe 1989–1998. *Diabetologia*, 44(Suppl. 3): B3–8.

24. Patterson CC, Dahlquist GG, Gyurus E, Green A & Soltesz G (2009). Incidence trends for childhood type 1 diabetes in Europe during 1989–2003 and predicted new cases 2005–20: a multicentre prospective registration study. *The Lancet*, 373(9680): 2027–33.

25. Ehehalt S, Dietz K, Willasch AM & Neu A (2009). Epidemiological perspectives on type 1 diabetes

in childhood and adolescence in Germany: 20 years of the Baden–Wurttemberg Diabetes Incidence Registry (DIARY). *Diabetes Care*, 33(2): 338–40.

26. Fourlanos S, Varney MD, Tait BD, Morahan G, Honeyman MC, Colman PG, et al. (2008). The rising incidence of type 1 diabetes is accounted for by cases with lower-risk human leukocyte antigen genotypes. *Diabetes Care*, 31(8): 1546–49.

27. Wentworth JM, Fourlanos S & Harrison LC (2009). Reappraising the stereotypes of diabetes in the modern diabetogenic environment. *Nature Reviews Endocrinology*, 5(9): 483–89.

28. Weets I, Kaufman L, Van der Auwera B, Crenier L, Rooman RP, De Block C, et al. (2004). Seasonality in clinical onset of type 1 diabetes in belgian patients above the age of 10 is restricted to HLA-DQ2/DQ8-negative males, which explains the male to female excess in incidence. *Diabetologia*, 47(4): 614–21.

29. Forrest JM, Turnbull FM, Sholler GF, Hawker RE, Martin FJ, Doran TT, et al. (2002). Gregg's congenital rubella patients 60 years later. *The Medical Journal of Australia*, 177(11–12): 664–67.

30. Ou D, Mitchell LA, Metzger DL, Gillam S & Tingle AJ (2000). Cross-reactive rubella virus and glutamic acid decarboxylase (65 and 67) protein determinants recognised by T cells of patients with type I diabetes mellitus. *Diabetologia,* 43(6): 750–62.

31. Bodansky HJ, Dean BM, Grant PJ, McNally J, Schweiger MS, Hambling MH, et al. (1990). Does exposure to rubella virus generate endocrine autoimmunity? *Diabetic Medicine*, 7(7): 611–14.

32. Salminen K, Sadeharju K, Lonnrot M, Vahasalo P, Kupila A, Korhonen S, et al. (2003). Enterovirus infections are associated with the induction of beta-cell autoimmunity in a prospective birth cohort study. *Journal of Medical Virology*, 69(1): 91–98.

33. Fuchtenbusch M, Irnstetter A, Jager G & Ziegler AG (2001). No evidence for an association of coxsackie virus infections during pregnancy and early childhood with development of islet autoantibodies in offspring of mothers or fathers with type 1 diabetes. *Journal of Autoimmunology*, 17(4): 333–40.

34. Graves PM, Rotbart HA, Nix WA, Pallansch MA, Erlich HA, Norris JM, et al. (2003). Prospective study of enteroviral infections and development of beta-cell autoimmunity: the Diabetes Autoimmunity Study in the Young (DAISY). *Diabetes Research and Clinical Practice*, 59(1): 51–61.

35. Honeyman M (2005). How robust is the evidence for viruses in the induction of type 1 diabetes? *Current Opinion in Immunology*, 17(6): 616–23.

36. Tanaka S, Nishida Y, Aida K, Maruyama T, Shimada A, Suzuki M, et al. (2009). Enterovirus infection, CXC chemokine ligand 10 (CXCL10), and CXCR3 circuit: a mechanism of accelerated beta-cell failure in fulminant type 1 diabetes. *Diabetes*, 58(10): 2285–91.

37. Ylipaasto P, Klingel K, Lindberg AM, Otonkoski T, Kandolf R, Hovi T, et al. (2004). Enterovirus infection in human pancreatic islet cells, islet tropism in vivo and receptor involvement in cultured islet beta cells. *Diabetologia*, 47(2): 225–39.

38. Yin H, Berg AK, Tuvemo T & Frisk G (2002). Enterovirus RNA is found in peripheral blood mononuclear cells in a majority of type 1 diabetic children at onset. *Diabetes*, 51(6): 1964–71.

39. Jones DB & Crosby I (1996). Proliferative lymphocyte responses to virus antigens homologous to GAD65 in IDDM. *Diabetologia*, 39(11): 1318–24.

40. Stene LC, Oikarinen S, Hyoty H, Barriga KJ, Norris JM, Klingensmith G, et al. (2010). Enterovirus infection and progression from islet autoimmunity to type 1 diabetes: the Diabetes and Autoimmunity Study in the Young (DAISY). *Diabetes*, 59(12): 3174–80.

41. Oikarinen S, Martiskainen M, Tauriainen S, Huhtala H, Ilonen J, Veijola R, et al. (2011). Enterovirus RNA in blood is linked to the development of type 1 diabetes. *Diabetes,* 60(1): 276–79.

42. Varela-Calvino R, Sgarbi G, Arif S & Peakman M (2000). T-Cell reactivity to the P2C nonstructural protein of a diabetogenic strain of coxsackievirus B4. *Virology*, 274(1): 56–64.

43. Kaufman DL, Erlander MG, Clare-Salzler M, Atkinson MA, Maclaren NK & Tobin AJ (1992). Autoimmunity to two forms of glutamate decarboxylase in insulin-dependent diabetes mellitus. *The Journal of Clinical Investigation*, 89(1): 283–92.

44. Honeyman M (2005). How robust is the evidence for viruses in the induction of type 1 diabetes? *Current Opinion in Immunology*, 17(6): 616–23.

45. Honeyman MC, Brusic V, Stone NL & Harrison LC (1998). Neural network-based prediction of candidate T-cell epitopes. *Nature Biotechnology*, 16(10): 966–69.

46. Honeyman MC, Coulson BS, Stone NL, Gellert SA, Goldwater PN, Steele CE, et al. (2000). Association between rotavirus infection and pancreatic islet autoimmunity in children at risk of developing type 1 diabetes. *Diabetes*, 49(8): 1319–24.

47. Blomqvist M, Juhela S, Erkkila S, Korhonen S, Simell T, Kupila A, et al. (2002). Rotavirus infections and development of diabetes-associated autoantibodies during the first 2 years of life. *Clinical & Experimental Immunology*, 128(3): 511–15.

48. Wentworth JM, Fourlanos S & Harrison LC (2009). Reappraising the stereotypes of diabetes in the modern diabetogenic environment. *Nature Reviews Endocrinology*, 5(9): 483–89.

49. Bach JF (2002). The effect of infections on susceptibility to autoimmune and allergic diseases. *The New England Journal of Medicine*, 347(12): 911–20.

50. Wentworth JM, Fourlanos S & Harrison LC (2009). Reappraising the stereotypes of diabetes in the modern diabetogenic environment. *Nature Reviews Endocrinology*, 5(9): 483–89.

51. Hypponen E, Laara E, Reunanen A, Jarvelin MR & Virtanen SM (2001). Intake of vitamin D and risk of type 1 diabetes: a birth-cohort study. *The Lancet*, 358(9292): 1500–03.

52. Scragg R, Sowers M & Bell C (2004). Serum 25-hydroxyvitamin D, diabetes, and ethnicity in the Third National Health and Nutrition Examination Survey. *Diabetes Care*, 27(12): 2813–18.

53. Stene LC & Joner G (2003). Use of cod liver oil during the first year of life is associated with lower risk of childhood-onset type 1 diabetes: a large, population-based, case-control study. *The American Journal of Clinical Nutrition*, 78(6): 1128–34.

54. Eurodiab Substudy 2 Study Group (1999). Vitamin D supplement in early childhood and risk for type I (insulin-dependent) diabetes mellitus: The EURODIAB Substudy 2 Study Group. *Diabetologia*, 42(1): 51–54.

55. Wilkin TJ (2009). The accelerator hypothesis: a review of the evidence for insulin resistance as the basis for type 1 as well as type 2 diabetes. *International Journal of Obesity (Lond)*, 33(7): 716–26.

56. Fourlanos S, Narendran P, Byrnes GB, Colman PG & Harrison LC (2004). Insulin resistance is a risk factor for progression to type 1 diabetes. *Diabetologia*, 47(10): 1661–67.

57. Wilkin TJ (2006). The accelerator hypothesis: a unifying explanation for type-1 and type-2 diabetes. *Nestle Nutrition Workshop Series: Clinical and Performance Programme*, 11: 139–50; discussion 150–53.

58. van Belle TL, Coppieters KT & von Herrath MG (2011). Type 1 diabetes: etiology, immunology, and therapeutic strategies. *Physiological Reviews*, 91(1): 79–118.

59. Eisenbarth GS & Jeffrey J (2008). The natural history of type 1A diabetes. *Arquivos Brasileiros de Endocrinologia Metabologia*, 52(2): 146–55.

60. van Belle TL, Coppieters KT & von Herrath MG (2011). Type 1 diabetes: etiology, immunology, and therapeutic strategies. *Physiological Reviews*, 91(1): 79–118.

61. Panagiotopoulos C, Qin H, Tan R & Verchere CB (2003). Identification of a beta-cell-specific HLA class I restricted epitope in type 1 diabetes. *Diabetes*, 52(11): 2647–51.

62. Panina-Bordignon P, Lang R, van Endert PM, Benazzi E, Felix AM, Pastore RM, et al. (1995). Cytotoxic T cells specific for glutamic acid decarboxylase in autoimmune diabetes. *The Journal of Experimental Medicine*, 181(5): 1923–27.

63. Skowera A, Ellis RJ, Varela-Calvino R, Arif S, Huang GC, Van-Krinks C, et al. (2008). CTLs are targeted to kill beta cells in patients with type 1 diabetes through recognition of a glucose-regulated preproinsulin epitope. *The Journal of Clinical Investigation*, 118(10): 3390–402.

64. Gepts W (1965). Pathologic anatomy of the pancreas in juvenile diabetes mellitus. *Diabetes*, 14(10): 619–33.

65. Coppieters KT & von Herrath MG (2009). Histopathology of type 1 diabetes: old paradigms and new insights. *The Review of Diabetic Studies*, 6(2): 85–96.

66. Gepts W (1976). Islet changes suggesting a possible immune aetiology of human diabetes mellitus. *Acta Endocrinologica Supplementum (Copenhagen)*, 205: 95–106.

67. Willcox A, Richardson SJ, Bone AJ, Foulis AK & Morgan NG (2009). Analysis of islet inflammation in human type 1 diabetes. *Clinical & Experimental Immunology*, 155(2): 173–81.

68. Foulis AK & Stewart JA (1984). The pancreas in recent-onset type 1 (insulin-dependent) diabetes mellitus: insulin content of islets, insulitis and associated changes in the exocrine acinar tissue. *Diabetologia*, 26(6): 456–61.

69. Willcox A, Richardson SJ, Bone AJ, Foulis AK & Morgan NG (2009). Analysis of islet inflammation in human type 1 diabetes. *Clinical & Experimental Immunology*, 155(2): 173–81.

70. In't Veld P, Lievens D, De Grijse J, Ling Z, Van der Auwera B, Pipeleers-Marichal M, et al. (2007). Screening for insulitis in adult autoantibody-positive organ donors. *Diabetes*, 56(9): 2400–04.

71. Gianani R, Campbell-Thompson M, Sarkar SA, Wasserfall C, Pugliese A, Solis JM, et al. (2010). Dimorphic histopathology of long-standing childhood-onset diabetes. *Diabetologia*, 53(4): 690–98.

72. Gaglia JL, Guimaraes AR, Harisinghani M, Turvey SE, Jackson R, Benoist C, et al. (2011). Noninvasive imaging of pancreatic islet inflammation in type 1A diabetes patients. *The Journal of Clinical Investigation*, 121(1): 442–45.

73. Martinic MM & von Herrath MG (2006). Control of graft-versus-host disease by regulatory T cells: which level of antigen specificity? *The European Journal of Immunology*, 36(9): 2299–303.

74. Seyfert-Margolis V, Gisler TD, Asare AL, Wang RS, Dosch HM, Brooks-Worrell B, et al. (2006). Analysis of T-cell assays to measure autoimmune responses in subjects with type 1 diabetes: results of a blinded controlled study. *Diabetes*, 55(9): 2588–94.

75. Mallone R, Martinuzzi E, Blancou P, Novelli G, Afonso G, Dolz M, et al. (2007). CD8+ T-cell responses identify beta-cell autoimmunity in human type 1 diabetes. *Diabetes*, 56(3): 613–21.

76. Martinuzzi E, Novelli G, Scotto M, Blancou P, Bach JM, Chaillous L, et al. (2008). The frequency and immunodominance of islet-specific CD8+ T-cell responses change after type 1 diabetes diagnosis and treatment. *Diabetes*, 57(5): 1312–20.

77. Cernea S & Herold KC (2010). Monitoring of antigen-specific CD8 T cells in patients with type 1 diabetes treated with antiCD3 monoclonal antibodies. *Clinical Immunology*, 134(2): 121–29.

78. Coppieters KT, Roep BO & von Herrath MG (2011). Beta cells under attack: toward a better understanding of type 1 diabetes immunopathology. *Seminars in Immunopathology*, 33(1): 1–7.

79. Akerblom HK, Krischer J, Virtanen SM, Berseth C, Becker D, Dupre J, et al. (2011). The Trial to Reduce IDDM in the Genetically at Risk (TRIGR) study: recruitment, intervention and follow-up. *Diabetologia*, 54(3): 627–33.

80. Eurodiab Sybstudy 2 Study Group (1999). Vitamin D supplement in early childhood and risk for type 1 (insulin-dependent0 diabetes mellitus. The EURODIAB Substudy 2 Study Group. *Diabetologia*, 42(1): 51–54.

81. Stene LC & Joner G (2003). Use of cod liver oil during the first year of life is associated with lower risk of childhood-onset type 1 diabetes: a large, population-based, case-control study. *The American Journal of Clinical Nutrition*, 78(6): 1128–34.

82. Gale EA, Bingley PJ, Emmett CL & Collier T (2004). European Nicotinamide Diabetes Intervention Trial (ENDIT): a randomised controlled trial of intervention before the onset of type 1 diabetes. *The Lancet*, 363(9413): 925–31.

83. Knip M, Virtanen SM, Becker D, Dupre J, Krischer JP & Akerblom HK (2010). Early feeding and risk of type 1 diabetes: experiences from the Trial to Reduce Insulin-dependent diabetes mellitus in the Genetically at Risk (TRIGR). *The American Journal of Clinical Nutrition*, in press.

84. van Belle TL, Coppieters KT & von Herrath MG (2011). Type 1 diabetes: etiology, immunology, and therapeutic strategies. *Physiological Reviews*, 91(1): 79–118.

85. Baker L, Kaye R & Root AW (1967). The early partial remission of juvenile diabetes mellitus: the roles of insulin and growth hormone. *Journal of Pediatrics*, 71(6): 825–31.

86. Weir GC & Bonner-Weir S (2010). Dreams for type 1 diabetes: shutting off autoimmunity and stimulating beta-cell regeneration. *Endocrinology*, 151(7): 2971–73.

87. Gianani R, Campbell-Thompson M, Sarkar SA, Wasserfall C, Pugliese A, Solis JM, et al. (2010). Dimorphic histopathology of long-standing childhood-onset diabetes. *Diabetologia*, 53(4): 690–98.

88. Gianani R (2011). Beta cell regeneration in human pancreas. *Seminars in Immunopathology*, 33(1): 23–27.

89. Nir T, Melton DA & Dor Y (2007). Recovery from diabetes in mice by beta cell regeneration. *The Journal of Clinical Investigation*, 117(9): 2553–61.

90. Bonner-Weir S, Li WC, Ouziel-Yahalom L, Guo L, Weir GC & Sharma A (2010). Beta-cell growth and regeneration: replication is only part of the story. *Diabetes*, 59(10): 2340–48.

91. Thorel F, Nepote V, Avril I, Kohno K, Desgraz R, Chera S, et al. (2010). Conversion of adult pancreatic alpha-cells to beta-cells after extreme beta-cell loss. *Nature*, 464(7292): 1149–54.

92. Chung CH, Hao E, Piran R, Keinan E & Levine F (2010). Pancreatic beta-cell neogenesis by direct conversion from mature alpha-cells. *Stem Cells*, 28(9): 1630–38.

93. Gianani R (2011). Beta cell regeneration in human pancreas. *Seminars in Immunopathology*, 33(1): 23–27.

94. Porat S, Weinberg-Corem N, Tornovsky-Babaey S, Schyr-Ben-Haroush R, Hija A, Stolovich-Rain M, et al. (2011). Control of pancreatic beta cell regeneration by glucose metabolism. *Cell Metabolism*, 13(4): 440–49.

95. Matschinsky FM (2009). Assessing the potential of glucokinase activators in diabetes therapy. *Nature Reviews Drug Discovery*, 8(5): 399–416.

96. Lavine JA & Attie AD (2010). Gastrointestinal hormones and the regulation of beta-cell mass. *Annals of the New York Academy of Sciences*, 1212: 41–58.

97. Baggio LL & Drucker DJ (2007). Biology of incretins: GLP-1 and GIP. *Gastroenterology*, 132(6): 2131–57.

98. Li Y, Cao X, Li LX, Brubaker PL, Edlund H & Drucker DJ (2005). Beta-Cell Pdx1 expression is essential for the glucoregulatory, proliferative, and cytoprotective actions of glucagon-like peptide-1. *Diabetes*, 54(2): 482–91.

99. Lavine JA & Attie AD (2010). Gastrointestinal hormones and the regulation of beta-cell mass. *Annals of the New York Academy of Sciences*, 1212: 41–58.

100. Liu Z & Habener JF (2008). Glucagon-like peptide-1 activation of TCF7L2-dependent Wnt signaling enhances pancreatic beta cell proliferation. *The Journal of Biological Chemistry*, 283(13): 8723–35.

101. Song WJ, Schreiber WE, Zhong E, Liu FF, Kornfeld BD, Wondisford FE, et al. (2008). Exendin-4 stimulation of cyclin A2 in beta-cell proliferation. *Diabetes*, 57(9): 2371–81.

102. Tian L, Gao J, Hao J, Zhang Y, Yi H, O'Brien TD, et al. (2010). Reversal of new-onset diabetes through modulating inflammation and stimulating beta-cell replication in nonobese diabetic mice by a dipeptidyl peptidase IV inhibitor. *Endocrinology*, 151(7): 3049–60.

5

Pancreatic beta-cell failure in the pathogenesis of type 2 diabetes

Jenny Gunton[1,2] and Christian M Girgis[1,2]

As the worldwide prevalence of type 2 diabetes continues to rise, there is mounting evidence that failure of the cells which make insulin – termed pancreatic beta (or β) cells, play a fundamental role at all stages in the pathogenesis. Beta-cell defects such as loss of the initial (first) phase of insulin secretion and inefficient insulin synthesis are seen years prior to the onset of type 2 diabetes. Later, it is the failure of beta cells to adequately respond to the demand for high insulin requirements that determines the onset of hyperglycaemia leading to the clinical diagnosis of type 2 diabetes. In this chapter, we will discuss the various proposed mechanisms of beta-cell failure in type 2 diabetes and address recent controversies in this field of research.

The prevalence of type 2 diabetes is rising at an alarming rate. In Australia alone, those affected by type 2 diabetes doubled from 3.4% in 1981 to 7.4% in a national sample of 11 247 adults in 1999 to 2002. An additional 16.4% of participants showed symptoms of prediabetes in this study, a sign of imminent trouble.

On a global scale, the International Diabetes Foundation projected that by 2030, up to 438 million people may be affected by this disease, accounting for more than 4.5% of the world's projected population [3]. China, the world's most populous nation, has not been spared as a recent survey reported a remarkably high diabetes prevalence of 9.7% (92.4 million adults) [4].

The burden of diabetes spans beyond the threat it poses to the individual sufferer and includes the greater effect on communities, the health economy and workforce. The estimated financial cost of type 2 diabetes in Australia is A$10.3 billion per annum which includes costs for carers (>A$4 billion), productivity losses (A$4.1 billion), direct costs to the healthcare system and the estimated direct costs of obesity (A$2.2 billion) [5].

Modern life is largely to blame for this surge in diabetes prevalence with the abundance of calorie-rich foods, the gross reduction in energy expenditure resulting from the use

---

1   Diabetes and Transcription Factors Group, Garvan Institute of Medical Research, Sydney.

2   Sydney Medical School, University of Sydney.

of cars and other labour-saving devices, the hours spent sitting in front of television or computer screens and the avoidance of outdoor activities. As described in earlier chapters, it is the collusion of such environmental factors with an individual's genetic predisposition that lead to pancreatic beta-cell failure that is characteristic of type 2 diabetes. However, the precise pathologic processes by which beta cells fail in their essential role in glucose homeostasis are incompletely understood and contentious.

This chapter will outline some of the proposed mechanisms of beta-cell failure in type 2 diabetes and touch on a couple of controversial issues that have characterised this field of research. However, it will first lay the groundwork with some basic principles in beta-cell physiology.

The beta cell

Since the initial description of the pancreatic islet by Paul Langerhans in 1869 as 'a network of small cells, almost perfect in homogeneity and structure, arranged in groups, scattered amongst the acinar cells of the pancreas' [6], understanding of this highly complex mini-organ has increased greatly. Five different endocrine cell types are found within the pancreatic islet, namely alpha cells that make glucagon, beta cells that make insulin, delta cells that make somatostatin, PP cells that make pancreatic polypeptide and epsilon cells that make ghrelin [7].

Although islets cells account for only 1%–2% of the pancreatic mass [8, 9], they receive 10% of the total pancreatic blood flow and are surrounded by a highly specialised system of fenestrated endothelial cells which provide critical signals for cell differentiation, development and function [10]. Other extracellular components, including extracellular matrix and neurons also play critical roles in influencing the behaviour of islet cells [11]. Beta cells are the dominant cell type of the human islet, accounting for 50% to 70% of islet cells [12]. Their main function, namely regulated insulin secretion, involves the integration of several stimuli which activate secretion when challenged and others that switch it off when the stimuli are no longer present. Whilst there is general agreement that the entry of glucose into the beta cell via specialised glucose transporters leads to a cascade of events including glucose phosphorylation by glucokinase and the closure of potassium-ion channels leading to membrane depolarisation and insulin secretion [13], the process is more complex. Following glucose entry into beta cells, insulin is secreted in two distinct phases and in an oscillatory, rather than a linear, pattern [14]. Further complexity can be found in the presence of secondary pathways of insulin secretion independent of ion channels [11], interactions between beta cells which influence behaviour [15] and the effect of gut-derived hormones, known as incretins, on beta-cell function [16]. The major steps in glucose-stimulated insulin secretion have been summarised in Figure 1.

However our understanding of beta-cell physiology is incomplete, with lack of understanding of the roles of a broad system of G-protein coupled receptors on the beta-cell surface [17], the effect of other nutrients such as amino acids and fatty acids on beta-cell function [18] and the role of vitamin D activating enzymes and receptors within the beta cell [19]. In seeking answers to these and many other questions, researchers in this field face a number of challenges. Significant inter-species differences in islet architecture [20] and responses to hyperglycaemia [21] pose a challenge that has made direct extrapolation of disease-related pathophysiology from rodents to humans tricky. Furthermore, the study of human pancreatic specimens, whilst insightful, does not always reflect *in vivo* beta-cell behaviour.

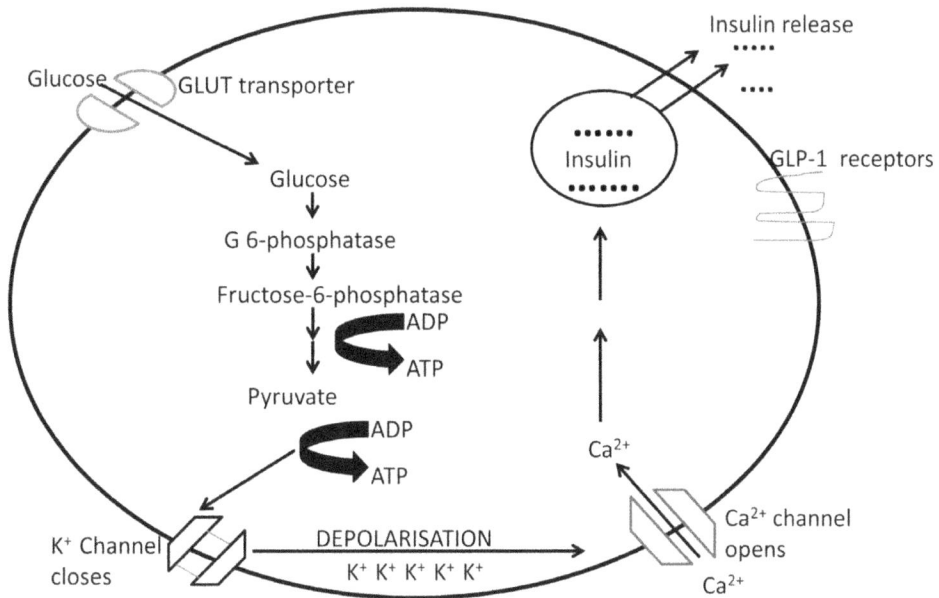

Figure 1. Steps involved in glucose-stimulated insulin secretion by the pancreatic beta cell. Following entry of glucose via GLUT transporters, phosphorylation by glucokinase occurs and pyruvate is formed via the process of glycolysis. This leads to increased activity of the TCA cycle within the mitochondria by which adenosine diphosphate (ADP) is converted to adenosine triphosphate (ATP). This causes closure of ATP-sensitive potassium channels, a wave of membrane depolarisation and the subsequent activation of voltage gated calcium channels. The entry of calcium into the cell is followed by vesicle docking and insulin granules are released into the circulation. Other factors play a role such as glucagon-like peptide 1 which has unique receptors in the beta-cell membrane.

There is no doubt that beta cells play an important role in the pathogenesis of type 2 diabetes but the complex nature of these cells and the difficulties encountered in 'unlocking' some of these complexities have inevitably led to some controversy in our understanding of the precise nature of this role.

Insulin resistance or defective beta cells?

A controversial issue for many years has been whether insulin resistance or impaired beta-cell function is the primary cause of type 2 diabetes. This controversy seems to have resulted from the complex interaction between both defects present early in the disease and the relative ease in measuring *in vivo* insulin resistance as compared to beta-cell function [22].

A 1992 study examining non-diabetic subjects at high risk of developing type 2 diabetes (ie women with prior gestational diabetes, high risk ethnic groups, people whose parents were both affected by type 2 diabetes) reported that insulin resistance was the predominant feature [23]. This was based on a glucose tolerance test which demonstrated supra-physiological insulin levels required to maintain normal glucose at two hours following a 75 gm oral glucose load. However, by only obtaining two-hour measurements, the high insulin levels were misinterpreted as representing normal beta-cell function compensating for a state of insulin resistance. As discussed above, insulin secretion is normally biphasic and the first phase of insulin secretion, maximal at 30 minutes following a meal, appears to be the first casualty of the beta cell in type 2 diabetes [12] Therefore, if values were measured at 30 minutes following the glucose load, different levels may have been found which would match the early rise in glucose, then followed by compensatory insulin hyper-secretion at two hours.

A prospective study of 200 non-diabetic Pima Indians, which is a group with a very high risk of type 2 diabetes, also reported that insulin resistance was the earliest feature in the 38 patients who went on to develop diabetes [24]. Lifestyle factors, such as obesity, sedentary lifestyle and high-fat diets correlated closely with this state of insulin resistance which was detected by the gold-standard technique, the hyperinsulinaemic-euglycaemic clamp. However, as the disease developed, the degree of insulin resistance did *not* change significantly but rather, a dynamic pattern of beta-cell activity emerged with early hyperinsulinaemia to maintain normoglycaemia being followed by a significant drop in insulin levels resulting in hyperglycaemia. It was therefore proposed that beta-cell failure was the final determinant in the development of hyperglycaemia in these patients.

For some time, 'beta-cell exhaustion' was the sole explanation for the failure in insulin secretion [20]. This is the concept that after a prolonged period of producing high amounts of insulin in order to overcome an insulin resistant state, otherwise normal beta cells eventually 'burn out' and permanently fail. Proponents of this hypothesis also describe distinct stages in the evolution of beta cells from a state of compensation to severe decompensation [25]. But the exhaustion concept has some limitations. Most patients with conditions characterised by insulin resistance – such as pregnancy, morbid obesity, Cushing's disease and acromegally – do not develop diabetes. Furthermore, studies in humans and rhesus monkeys suggest that the early hyperinsulinaemia may occur independently of insulin resistance and rather reflect 'beta-cell hyper-responsiveness' [26]. In addition, patients with mutations in the insulin receptor, who have severe insulin resistance from birth do not develop diabetes until their beta cells fail, usually in their teens or 20s [27]. Therefore, intrinsic defects in susceptible beta cells appear to be important both early in the development of diabetes and later when the cells undergo critical failure in their compensatory capacity.

Another five-year prospective study involving non-diabetic Pima Indians confirmed dual pathology involving both the beta cell and peripheral insulin sensitivity in the development of diabetes [28]. Amongst 48 non-diabetic subjects who were roughly equal for parameters of obesity and insulin resistance, the 17 who progressed to diabetes failed to increase their insulin secretion in response to progression of insulin resistance. Furthermore, they showed signs of defective beta-cell function even before the onset of impaired glucose tolerance. The 31 subjects who did not progress to diabetes demonstrated appropriate increases in insulin secretion as they gained weight and became more insulin resistant. Therefore, it was beta-cell function that determined the progression from insulin resistance to frank diabetes in this high-risk group.

A useful way to understand the interaction between insulin sensitivity and beta-cell function can be found in the disposition index [29]. In normal subjects, beta-cell function varies according to the degree of insulin sensitivity so that when non-diabetic individuals enter a phase of greater insulin resistance, such as in puberty, pregnancy or aging, beta cells 'rise to the occasion' and produce greater insulin as required. The relationship follows a hyperbolic pattern as seen in Figure 2, indicating a continuum of beta-cell responsiveness to variations in insulin sensitivity. The dotted, downward line in this figure represents the progression to diabetes as was displayed in the previous study [25] – while still glucose tolerant, susceptible individuals began to 'fall below the curve' with the inability of beta cells to respond appropriately to the degree of insulin resistance. The downward, rather than horizontal, trajectory of this dotted line indicates that deterioration in beta-cell function was of greater importance than the reduction in insulin sensitivity in the development of hyperglycaemia [20]. Therefore, in essence, type 2 diabetes may be considered a failure of beta-cell compensation.

Beta-cell failure and insulin resistance however need not be considered as separate entities. Pathways are emerging by which these otherwise disparate conditions may be linked. Striking examples exist in the insulin signalling pathway. For example, insulin receptor substrate-2 (IRS-2) promotes both cell growth, insulin secretion and plays a well-recognised role in insulin sensitivity [30]. Mice with IRS-2 mutations in their beta-cells develop diabetes. In addition, people with Akt2 mutations develop diabetes due to the combination of severe insulin resistance *and* impaired beta-cell dysfunction [31]. Insulin receptor mutations also associate with diabetes, both in people, and in mice. The transcription factor NF-kappaB plays an important role in both insulin resistance [32] and beta-cell behaviour [33]. Furthermore, complex processes which alter the behaviour of the mitochondria, the cell's own 'energy plant', are similar in insulin-resistant tissues and defective beta cells. Therefore, insulin resistance and beta-cell dysfunction may be aetiologically related and rather than predominating over the other, appear to conspire together in the development of diabetes.

Reduced beta-cell mass or function?

Currently, there is a debate concerning the relative roles of decreased beta-cell mass compared with decreased beta-cell function in diabetes pathogenesis [34].

Proponents of the reduced beta-cell mass argument refer to postmortem studies which demonstrate up to 40% reduction in the number of beta cells in subjects with prediabetes versus weight-matched non-diabetic individuals [35]. In addition, mutations of genes known to control beta-cell mass such as the pancreatic and duodenal homeobox 1 (Pdx-1) result in monogenic forms of diabetes, such as Maturity Onset Diabetes of the Young [36].

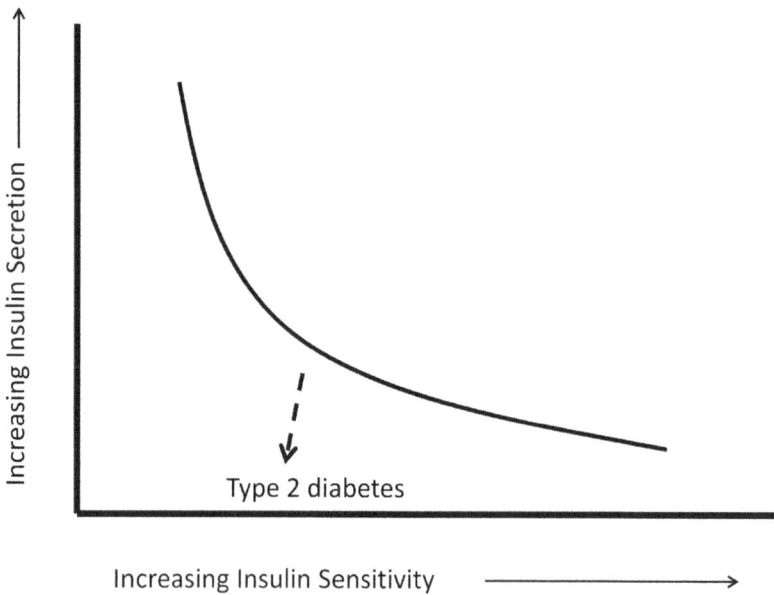

Figure 2. The 'disposition index' is a useful way to consider the relationship between insulin secretion and insulin sensitivity in both physiologic (ie curved line) and pathologic states (ie dotted line). This is based on data from a number of studies and has been adapted from Kahn et al. [26]. Individuals who develop type 2 diabetes head in a downward trajectory below the curve indicating that deterioration in beta-cell function (and thus less insulin secretion) is the main factor in the development of hyperglycaemia.

However, there are some limitations to this argument. Firstly, not all autopsy studies in diabetic subjects demonstrate relative reductions in beta-cell mass [37]. Secondly, beta-cell mass is highly variable even in normal individuals and may undergo substantial changes throughout a person's life [7]. Thirdly, it is difficult to see how a reduction of less than 50% of otherwise healthy beta cells could cause diabetes in the light of a recent *in vivo* islet donation from 50% of a healthy human pancreas which resulted in diabetes cure in the recipient and the absence of diabetes in the donor [38]. Furthermore, normal rats that underwent a 60% pancreatectomy remained normoglycaemic due to partial beta-cell regeneration and hyperfunction of remaining beta cells [39]. However, when these rats were challenged by the addition of 10% sugar to their water supply, impairment of the residual beta-cell mass and subsequent hyperglycaemia ensued. Therefore, in isolation, reduced beta-cell mass was insufficient to cause diabetes but rather required the presence of environmental factors to unmask the effect.

There are well-described functional defects in the beta cells of subjects with diabetes. As mentioned earlier, the loss of first phase insulin secretion is a particularly early defect [12]. Another is the loss of oscillations in insulin secretion, the importance of which relates to the regulation of hepatic glucose production under physiological conditions [40]. This may occur early in the disease, being found in non-diabetic relatives of people with type 2 diabetes [41]. Thirdly, inefficient conversion of the precursor peptide, pro-insulin, into insulin results in a four to fivefold increase in pro-insulin levels in the beta cells of patients with type 2 diabetes [42].

Defects within the incretin system may also result in early beta-cell dysfunction [14]. The incretins are a pair of gut hormones, namely glucagon-like peptide 1 and glucose-dependent insulinotropic polypeptide, which are released into the bloodstream after meal ingestion and stimulate insulin secretion in a glucose-dependent manner. The incretins increase the expression of genes important for insulin secretion, such as the GLUT2 and glucokinase genes, and beta-cell proliferation, such as PDX-1. Subjects with type 2 diabetes may display down-regulation of incretin receptors on the surface of beta cells [43], impaired incretin-induced insulin secretion [44] and increased degradation of incretin hormones [45]. Non-diabetic relatives of those with diabetes [46] and people with impaired glucose tolerance [47] may also display defects in the incretin system.

A whole range of gene expression defects are also associated with beta-cell dysfunction. My research group have previously demonstrated that proteins vital to beta-cell function and insulin secretion, known as the transcription factors HIF-1a [48] and ARNT [49], have significantly less expression in the pancreatic islets of diabetic versus non-diabetic subjects. Knockout mice lacking the genes for these proteins in insulin expressing cells develop glucose intolerance and impaired insulin secretion [44, 45]. In fact, the advent of genome-wide association studies (GWAS) in 2007 has led to an explosion of data on the possible genetic background of type 2 diabetes [20]. GWAS uses thousands of small nucleotide sequences throughout the genome to search for patterns linked to disease, using the human genome sequencing project as reference. The transcription factor 7-like 2 (TCF7L2) is to be most strongly linked to type 2 diabetes with important effects on beta-cell proliferation and function [50], incretin-related insulin secretion [39] and insulin secretion [51]. Polymorphisms in TCF7L2 are thought to account for ~20% of the population attributable risk of diabetes [52]. The important point here is that the genetic determinants of beta-cell function and mass appear closely linked.

Some investigators now refer to 'reduced functional beta-cell mass' rather than debating the predominance of reduced mass or defective function in diabetes causation [53]. The 'plasticity' of the functional beta-cell mass, that is, the concept that beta cells can undergo adaptive changes in both mass and function when challenged by insulin resistance has also received some attention.

Mechanisms of beta-cell failure

If defects in the functional beta-cell mass play such a critical role in diabetes pathogenesis, what are some of the mechanisms responsible for these defects? These have been summarised in Figure 3.

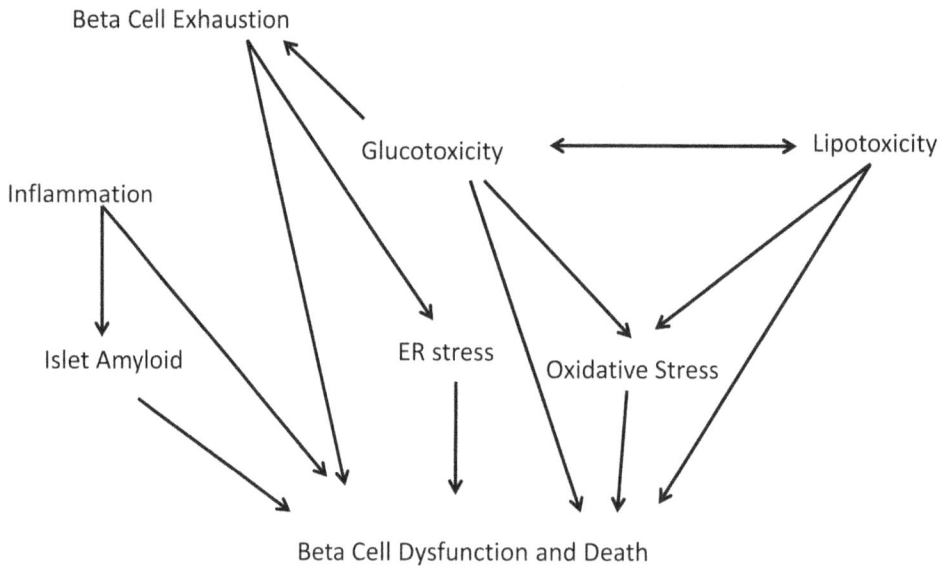

Figure 3. Proposed mechanisms of pancreatic beta (beta) cell dysfunction and death in type 2 diabetes. This flow-chart depicts the complex and multifactorial nature of cell dysfunction in this condition. For a description of the concepts and terms see the text.

Pancreatic islet inflammation

There is mounting evidence that chronic low-grade inflammation of the pancreatic islet can cause insulin secretory dysfunction and beta-cell apoptosis [54]. Most striking is the macrophage infiltration seen in the islets of mice and humans with type 2 diabetes prior to the onset of beta-cell death [55]. It is also known that islets and ductal cells respond to metabolic stress, such as hyperglycaemia [56] and exposure to fatty acids, by expressing cytokines particularly IL-1beta. While this may initially be protective, chronic expression of this cytokine may result in the production of reactive oxygen species, inflammation and eventual beta-cell death [49]. Furthermore, the use of anti-inflammatory therapies, such as an IL-1 receptor antagonists [57] or non-steroidal anti-inflammatory drugs [58] results in small improvements in beta-cell function independent of an effect on insulin resistance.

Inflammatory markers, such as the serum leukocyte count and c-reactive protein, are also elevated in patients with type 2 diabetes and in those at risk of diabetes [59].

There is emerging evidence linking obesity and beta-cell failure via an inflammatory pathway. Leptin, a hormone secreted by fat cells to control appetite, is often found in high levels in type 2 diabetes [60] and at such levels, has negative effects on insulin secretion [61] and may induce beta-cell apoptosis [62]. Conversely, adiponectin which has anti-inflammatory and insulin sensitising effects, appears to be down-regulated in diabetes [63]. In addition, fat-derived cytokines, fatty acids and lipoproteins may all have adverse effects on beta-cell function, suggesting a common inflammatory link between the various components of the metabolic syndrome.

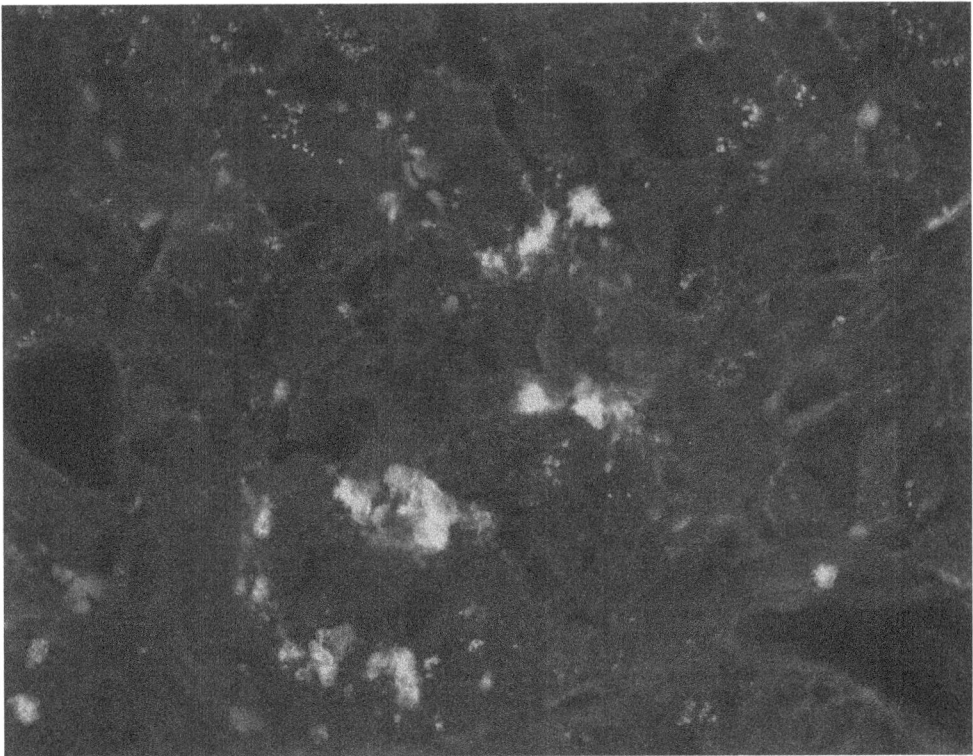

Figure 4. Islet amyloid deposition in a human with type 2 diabetes In the islet of this patient with diabetes, amyloid infiltration is seen as bright plaques in this grey scale image, thioflavin S stain.

Islet amyloid

Although islet amyloidosis has long been associated with beta-cell loss in type 2 diabetes [64], its precise role is uncertain. At postmortem, more than 90% of type 2 diabetic subjects have amyloid deposits in at least one islet compared to 12% of age-matched non-diabetic patients [65]. However, the number of islets affected is highly variable [66] and there is no relationship between duration of diabetes and the presence or severity of islet amyloid [67].

Islet amyloid fibrils are composed of amylin, a normally occurring peptide of the beta cell co-stored with insulin, which has folded abnormally and is initially deposited around islet capillaries but later within the islet space [30]. The increased production of pro-amylin accompanies the higher pro-insulin levels characteristic of type 2 diabetes and may be the first step to developing islet amyloid [68].

Although synthetic amyloid fibrils induce early beta-cell death *in vitro* [69], it is unclear whether amyloidosis is the direct cause of beta-cell failure *in vivo* or rather, the end-result of several distinct processes including inflammation, oxidative stress and mitochondrial damage. It is also currently debated whether the amyloid plaques per se are cytotoxic or rather small intracellular molecules that are precursors in the development of such plaques [70].

Endoplasmic reticulum stress

The endoplasmic reticulum (ER), a highly developed organelle that resides within the cell, is responsible for protein handling and packaging. Due to the high secretory demand placed on beta cells in type 2 diabetes, the endoplasmic reticulum may become overwhelmed by the production of high level of proteins [71]. A process called ER stress ensues whereby intracellular signals intending to protect the beta cells from the effects of inflammation [72] may eventually lead to the impairment of beta-cell function, the morphological appearance of ER swelling as proteins accumulate and subsequent beta-cell death.

ER stress may be mediated via genetic and environmental factors. Mice with mutations in proinsulin develop diabetes with morphological evidence of ER stress [20]. Exposure of islets to high glucose levels, cytokines and fatty acids may also lead to signs of ER stress [73].

Glucose toxicity

Glucose is the key physiological regulator of insulin secretion. Chronic hyperglycaemia is associated with impaired insulin secretion [74] and restoring normoglycaemia in subjects with diabetes has a clearly positive effect on beta-cell function [75].

There are several ways by which the exposure of beta cells to high glucose levels has toxic effects (glucotoxicity). The term 'beta-cell dedifferentiation' refers to an altered pattern of gene expression that results in substantial functional defects related to chronic hyperglycaemia [76]. Changes in beta-cell signalling and architecture are also possible effects of high glucose exposure [77]. The overproduction of reactive oxygen species, known as oxidative stress, is related to mitochondrial metabolism of high glucose levels and may result in beta-cell dysfunction or death [20].

Support for the oxidative stress hypothesis has come from a number of animal and human studies. The beta-cell over-expression of glutathione peroxidase, the enzyme that protects cells from oxidative damage, improved beta-cell mass and function in diabetic mice [78]. Higher concentrations of oxidative stress markers were found in islets from human subjects with type 2 diabetes and marked improvement in insulin secretion followed 24 hours of exposure to glutathione [79].

The failure of the beta cell's adaptive response to high glucose levels may precede dysfunction. The Fas-FLIP pathway involves a series of factors which are upregulated in response to high glucose levels and which result in greater beta-cell differentiation, proliferation and function [80]. However, in chronic hyperglycaemia, this adaptive pathway may eventually fail resulting in deterioration in beta-cell function and reduced survival [49].

Lipotoxicity

Whilst effective insulin secretion requires the presence of fatty acids [81], long-term exposure to excessive levels of this nutrient may also result in beta-cell toxicity [30]. The precise mechanism of so-called lipotoxicity is unclear but it may be due to genetic alterations in the expression of insulin and enzymes controlling insulin secretion [82], metabolic disturbances and ultimately, beta-cell death.

Studies in the Zucker diabetic fatty rat, considered a good model for obesity-related type 2 diabetes, have shown that the development of hyperlipidaemia parallels inadequate insulin secretion and the onset of diabetes [83]. However the lipid levels in this animal model are often extreme, so whether this reflects the human condition is debatable. Furthermore, fewer than 12% of obese hyperlipidaemic human subjects become diabetic [84], suggesting that lipotoxicity may be just one component in the development of beta-cell failure in type 2 diabetes.

Beta-cell exhaustion

It is speculated that after a prolonged period of insulin hypersecretion, depletion of readily available insulin granules may occur, thereby reducing the insulin secretory response [20]. Although we previously discussed the limitations of beta-cell exhaustion as the sole pathogenic mechanism, it may play a role in the wider, multifactorial setting of diabetes pathogenesis.

The strongest support for the exhaustion concept comes from studies examining the benefits of 'beta-cell rest' strategies. When inhibitors of insulin secretion, such as diazoxide or somatostatin, are given to animals or humans with diabetes, paradoxical increases in beta-cell function are observed following a period of 'rest' [85, 86]. Furthermore, human subjects with poorly controlled diabetes demonstrate a dramatic improvement in beta-cell function following a brief period of intensive glycaemic control [67]. A multicentre, randomised study of over 350 newly diagnosed patients confirmed that early intensive insulin therapy may facilitate recovery and maintenance of beta-cell function and protracted glycaemic remission better than oral hypoglycaemic agents for at least one year after diagnosis [87].

This leads to the discussion of the therapeutic implications of beta-cell failure and the possibility of reversing this complex process. Although a highly controversial and evolving area of research, the use of certain sulfonylureas such as glibenclamide has been linked to beta-cell death [88], while there is mounting evidence that incretin-based therapy and insulin replacement increase beta-cell mass in mice and have a positive effect on function [89]. However, a discussion on the nuances of beta-cell preservation in type 2 diabetes is beyond the scope of this chapter. For such a discussion, we refer the reader to a recent review on this topic [81].

Conclusion

Pancreatic beta-cell dysfunction plays a vital and complex role in the pathogenesis of type 2 diabetes. Ultimately, it is the failure of beta cells to respond to the insulin requirements posed by the prevailing level of insulin resistance that leads to the development of type 2 diabetes. We have discussed the evidence in support of various genetic and environmental factors that conspire together in this state of beta-cell susceptibility and 'decompensation'. The precise role of each and the search for a hypothesis which may unify these disparate concepts into a single paradigm is highly contentious and under active investigation. However, there is no doubt that beta-cell demise occurs in stages with early defects in beta-cell dysfunction, such as loss of first phase insulin secretion resulting in post-prandial hyperglycaemia following which progressive rises in glucose levels, fatty acids and insulin resistance place further stress on the beta cell, leading to eventual decline in its secretory capacity. Subtle components of the beta-cell stress mechanism, initially adaptive, such as changes to the endoplasmic reticulum and mitochondrium also eventually exacerbate the situation. Recent evidence suggests that early intervention to improve glycaemic control may improve beta-cell function and for at least a limited time period, may retard progression to beta-cell failure. Further research into the complex mechanisms of beta-cell failure may therefore offer hope in our collective fight against the global epidemic of type 2 diabetes.

References

1. Glatthaar C, Welborn TA, Stenhouse NS & Garcia-Webb P (1985). Diabetes and impaired glucose tolerance: a prevalence estimate based on the Busselton 1981 survey. *The Medical Journal of Australia,* 143(10): 436–40.

2. Dunstan DW, Zimmet PZ, Welborn TA, DeCourten MP, Cameron AJ & Sicree RA, et al. (2002). The rising prevalence of diabetes and impaired glucose tolerance: the Australian diabetes, obesity and lifestyle study (AusDiab). *Diabetes Care,* 25(5): 829–34.

3. Wild S, Roglic G, Green A, Sicree R & King H (2004). Global prevalence of diabetes: estimates for the year 2000 and projections for 2030. *Diabetes Care,* 27(5): 1047–53.

4. Yang W, Lu J, Weng J, Jia W, Ji L, Xiao J & Shan Z, et al. (2010). Prevalence of diabetes among men and women in China. *New English Journal of Medicine,* 362: 1090–101.

5.   Diabetes Australia (2010). Diabetes in Australia. [Online]. Available: www.diabetesaustralia.com.au/Understanding-Diabetes/Diabetes-in-Australia [Accessed 26 September 2011].

6.   Sakula A (1988). Paul Langerhans: a centenary tribute. *Journal of the Royal Society of Medicine,* 81(7): 414–15.

7.   Bonner-Weir S (1991). Anatomy of islet of Langerhans. In Samols E (Ed). *The endocrine pancreas* (pp15–27). New York: Raven.

8.   Rahier J, Guiot Y, Goebbels RM, Sempoux C & Henquin JC (2008). Pancreatic beta-cell mass in European subjects with type 2 diabetes. *Diabetes, Obesity and Metabolism,* 10(Suppl. 4): 32–42.

9.   Klöppel G, Löhr M, Habich K, Oberholzer M & Heitz PU (1985). Islet pathology and the pathogenesis of type 1 and type 2 diabetes mellitus revisited. *Survey and Synthesis of Pathology Research,* 4(2): 110–25.

10.   Lifson N, Lassa CV & Dixit PK (1985). Relation between blood flow and morphology in islet organ of rat pancreas. *American Journal of Physiology,* 249(1 Pt 1): E43–48.

11.   Kaido T, Yebra M, Cirulli V, Rhodes C, Diaferia G & Montgomery AM (2006). Impact of defined matrix interactions on insulin production by cultured human beta-cells: effect on insulin content, secretion and gene transcription. *Diabetes,* 55(10): 2723–29.

12.   Brissova M, Fowler MJ, Nicholson WE, Chu A, Hirshberg B & Harlan DM, et al. (2005). Assessment of human pancreatic islet architecture and composition by laser scanning confocal microscopy. *Journal of Histochemistry and Cytochemistry,* 53(2): 1087–97

13.   Straub SG, James RF, Dunne MJ & Sharp GW (1998). Glucose activates both K(ATP) channel-dependent and K(ATP) channel-independent signaling pathways in human islets. *Diabetes,* 47(5): 758–63.

14.   Perley MJ & Kipnis DM (1967). Plasma insulin responses to oral and intravenous glucose: studies in normal and diabetic subjects. *Journal of Clinical Investigation,* 46(12): 1954–62.

15.   Klee P, Bavamian S, Charollais A, Caille D, Cancela J, Peyrou M, et al. (2008). Gap junctions and insulin secretion. In Seino S & Bell GI (Eds). *Pancreatic beta cell in health and disease* (pp111–32). Japan: Springer.

16.   Ahren B (2006). Incretins and islet function. *Current Opinion in Endocrinology & Diabetes,* 13(2): 154–61.

17.   Ahren B (2009). Islet G protein-coupled receptors as potential targets for treatment of type 2 diabetes. *Nature Reviews Drug Discovery,* 8: 369–85.

18.   Nolan CJ & Prentki M (2008). The islet beta-cell: fuel responsive and vulnerable. *Trends in Endocrinology and Metabolism,* 19(8): 285–91.

19.   Lau SL, Clifton-Bligh R, Eismann J & Gunton JE (2008). A functional and regulated vitamin D system exists within Min-6 cells, an immortalized mouse-derived beta-cell line. *Australian Diabetes Society Annual Scientific Meeting.*

20.   Baetens D, Malaisse-Lagae F, Perrelet A & Orci L (1979). Endocrine pancreas: three-dimensional reconstruction shows two types of islets of Langerhans. *Science,* 206(4424): 1323–25.

21. Haataja L, Gurlo T, Huang CJ & Butler PC (2008). Islet amyloid in type 2 diabetes and the toxic oligomer hypothesis. *Endocrinology Review*, 29(3): 303–16.

22. Leahy JL & Pratley RE (2011). What is type 2 diabetes mellitus? Crucial role of maladaptive changes in beta cell and adipocyte biology In Robertson RP & Powers AC (Eds). *Translational endocrinology and metabolism: Type 2 Diabetes* (pp9–43). Maryland: The Endocrine Society.

23. Martin BC, Warram JH, Krolewski AS, Bergman RN, Soeldner JS & Kahn CR (1992). Role of glucose and insulin resistance in the development of type 2 diabetes mellitus: results of a 25-year follow-up study. *The Lancet,* 340(8825): 925–29.

24. Lillioja S, Mott DM, Howard BV, Bennett PH, Yki-Jarvinen H, Freymond D, et al. (1988). Impaired glucose tolerance as a disorder of insulin action. Longitudinal and cross-sectional studies in Pima Indians. *The New English Journal of Medicine,* 318(19): 1217–25.

25. Weir GC & Bonner-Weir S (2004). Five stages of evolving beta cell dysfunction during progression to diabetes. *Diabetes,* 53(S3): 16–21.

26. Hansen BC & Bodkin NL (1990). Beta-cell hyperresponsiveness: earliest event in the development of diabetes in monkeys. *The American Journal of Physiology,* 259(3): R612–17.

27. Krook, A & O'Rahilly S (1996). Mutant insulin receptors in syndromes of insulin resistance. *Baillieres Clinical Endocrinology and Metabolism,* 10(1): 97–122.

28. Weyer C, Bogardus C, Mott DM & Pratley RE (1999). The natural history of insulin secretory dysfunction and insulin resistance in the pathogenesis of type 2 diabetes mellitus. *Journal of Clinical Investigation,* 104(6): 787–94.

29. Kahn SE, Prigeon RL, McCulloch DK, Boyko EJ, Bergman RN, Schwartz MW, et al. (1993). Quantification of the relationship between insulin sensitivity and beta-cell function in human subjects: evidence for a hyperbolic function. *Diabetes,* 42(11): 1663–72.

30. Hennige AM, Burks DJ, Ozcan U, Kulkarni RN, Ye J, Park S, Schubert M, Fisher TL, et al. (2003). Upregulation of insulin receptor substrate-2 in pancreatic beta cells prevents diabetes. *Journal of Clinical Investigation,* 112(10): 1521–32.

31. George S, Rochford JJ, Wolfrum C, Gray SL, Schinner S & Wilson JC (2004). A family with severe insulin resistance and diabetes due to a mutation in *AKT2*. *Science,* 304(5675): 1325–28.

32. Shoelson SE, Lee J & Yuan M (2003). Inflammation and the IKK beta/I kappa B/NF kappa B axis in obesity- and diet-induced insulin resistance. *International Journal of Obesity and Related Metabolic Disorders,* 27(Suppl. 3): S49–52.

33. Donath MY, Storling J, Maedler K & Mandrup-Poulsen T (2003). Inflammatory mediators and islet beta cell failure: a link between type 1 and type 2 diabetes. *Journal of Molecular Medicine,* 81(8): 455–70.

34. Clark A (2008). Pancreatic islet pathology in type 2 diabetes. In Seino S & Bell GI (Eds). *Pancreatic beta cell in health and disease* (pp381–98). Japan: Springer.

35. Butler AE, Janson J, Bonner-Weir S, Ritzel R, Rizza RA & Butler PC (2003). Beta cell deficit and increased beta cell apoptosis in humans with type 2 diabetes. *Diabetes,* 52(1): 102–10.

36. Powers AC, Stein RW (2011). In Robertson RP & Powers AC (Eds). *Translational endocrinology and metabolism: type 2 diabetes* (pp95–116). Maryland: The Endocrine Society.

37. MacLean N & Ogilvie RF (1955). Quantitative estimation of pancreatic islet tissue in diabetic subjects. *Diabetes,* 4(5): 367–76.

38. Matsumoto S, Okitsu T, Iwanaga Y, Noguchi H, Nagata H, Yonekawa Y, et al. (2005). Insulin independence of unstable diabetic patient after single living donor islet transplantation. *Transplant Proceeding,* 37(8): 3427–29.

39. Leahy JL, Bonner-Weir S & Weir GC (1988). Minimal chronic hyperglycaemia is a critical determinant of impaired insulin secretion after an incomplete pancreatectomy. *Journal of Clinical Investigation,* 81(5): 1407–14.

40. Porkson N (2002). The in vivo regulation of pulsatile insulin secretion. *Diabetologia,* 45(1): 3–20.

41. O'Rahilly S, Turner RC & Matthews DR (1988). Impaired pulsatile secretion of insulin in relatives of patients with non-insulin-dependent diabetes. *The New England Journal of Medicine,* 318(19): 1225–30.

42. Kahn SE & Halban PA (1997). Release of incompletely processed pro-insulin is the cause of the disproportionate proinsulinemia of NIDDM. *Diabetes,* 46(1): 1725–32.

43. Shu L, Matveyenko AV, Kerr-Conte J, Cho JH, McIntosh CH & Maedler K (2009). Decreased TCF7L2 protein levels in type 2 diabetes mellitus correlate with downregulation of GIP- and GLP-1 receptors and impaired beta-cell function. *Human Molecular Genetics,* 18(13): 2388–99.

44. Meier JJ, Gallwitz B, Kask B, Deacon CF, Holst JJ, Schmidt WE, et al. (2004). Stimulation of insulin secretion by intravenous bolus injection and continuous infusion of gastric inhibitory polypeptide in patients with type 2 diabetes and healthy control subjects. *Diabetes,* 53(Suppl. 3): S220–24.

45. Mannucci E, Pala L, Ciani S, Bardini G, Pezzatini A, Sposato I, et al. (2005). Hyperglycaemia increases dipeptidyl peptidase IV activity in diabetes mellitus. *Diabetologia,* 48(6): 1168–72.

46. Meier JJ, Hucking K, Holst JJ, Deacon CF, Schmiegel WH & Nauck MA (2001). Reduced insulinotropic effect of gastric inhibitory polypeptide in first-degree relatives of patients with type 2 diabetes. *Diabetes,* 50(11): 2497–04.

47. Faerch K, Vaag A, Holst JJ, Glumer C, Pederson O & Borch-Johnsen K (2008). Impaired fasting glycaemia vs impaired glucose tolerance: similar impairment of pancreatic alpha and beta-cell function but differential roles of incretin hormones and insulin action. *Diabetologia,* 51(5): 853–61.

48. Cheng K, Ho K, Stokes R, Scott C, Lau SM, Hawthorne WJ et al. (2010). Hypoxia-inducible factor-1alpha regulates beta-cell function in mouse and human islets. *Journal of Clinical Investigation,* 120(6): 2171–83.

49. Gunton JE, Kulkarni RN, Yim S, Okada T, Hawthorne WJ, Tseng Y, et al. (2005). Loss of *ARNT/HIF1β* mediates altered gene expression and pancreatic-islet dysfunction in human type 2 diabetes cell. *Cell Metabolism,* 122: 337–49.

50. Liu Z & Habener JF (2010). Wnt signaling in pancreatic islets. *Advances in Experimental Medicine and Biology,* 654: 391–419.

51. da Silva Xavier G, Loder MK, McDonald A, Tarasov AI, Carzaniga R, Kronenberger K, et al. (2009). TCF7L2 regulates late events in insulin secretion from pancreatic islet beta cells. *Diabetes,* 58(4): 894–905.

52. Grant SFA, Thorleifsson G, Reynisdottir I, Benediktsson R, Manolescu A, Sainz J, et al. (2006). Variant of transcription factor 7-like 2 (*TCF7L2*) gene confers risk of type 2 diabetes. *Nature Genetics,* 38: 320–23.

53. Karaca M, Magnan C & Kargar C (2009). Functional pancreatic beta-cell mass: involvement in type 2 diabetes and therapeutic intervention. *Diabetes and Metabolism,* 35: 77–84.

54. Donath MY & Ehses JA (2008). Mechanisms of beta cell death in diabetes. In Seino S & Bell GI (Eds). *Pancreatic beta cell in health and disease* (pp75–89). Japan: Springer.

55. Ehses JA, Perren A, Eppler E, Ribaux P, Pospisilik JA, Maor-Cahn R, et al. (2007). Increased number of islet associated macrophages in type 2 diabetes. *Diabetes,* 56: 2356–70.

56. Maedler K, Sergeev P, Ris F, Oberholzer J, Joller-Jemelka HI, Spinas GA, et al. (2002). Glucose-induced beta-cell production of interleukin-1beta contributes to glucotoxicity in human pancreatic islets. *Journal of Clinical Investigation,* 110: 851–60.

57. Larsen CM, Faulenbach M, Vaag A, Volund A, Ehses JA, Seifert B, et al. (2007). Interleukin-1-receptor antagonist in type 2 diabetes mellitus. *The New England Journal of Medicine*, 356: 1517–26.

58. Zeender E, Maedler K, Bosco D, Berney T, Donath MY & Halban PA (2004). Pioglitazone and sodium salicylate protect human beta cells against apoptosis and impaired function induced by glucose and interleukin-1beta. *Journal of Clinical Endocrinology and Metabolism,* 89: 5059–66.

59. Pham MN, Hawa MI, Pfleger C, Roden M, Schernthaner G, Pozzilli P, et al. (2011). Pro- and anti-inflammatory cytokines in latent autoimmune diabetes in adults, type 1 and type 2 diabetes patients: action LADA 4. *Diabetologia,* 54(7): 1630–38 .

60. Weyer C, Funahashi T, Tanaka S, Hotta K, Matsuzawa Y, Pratley RE, et al. (2001). Hypoadiponectinaemia in obesity and type 2 diabetes: close association with insulin resistance and hyperinsulinaemia. *Journal of Clinical Endocrinology and Metabolism,* 86: 1930–35.

61. Kieffer TJ & Habener JF (2000). The adipoinsular axis: effects of leptin on pancreatic beta cells. *American Journal of Physiology: Endocrinology and Metabolism,* 278: E1–14.

62. Maedler K, Sergeev P, Ehses JA, Mathe Z, Bosco D, Berney T, et al. (2004). Leptin modulates beta cell expression of IL-1 receptor antagonist and release of IL-1beta in human islets. *Proceedings of the National Academy of Sciences USA,* 101: 8138–43.

63. Weyer C, Funahashi T, Tanaka S, Hotta K, Matsuzawa Y, Pratley RE et al. (2001). Hypoadiponectinaemia in obesity and type 2 diabetes: a close association with insulin resistance and hyperinsulinaemia. *Journal of Clinical Endocrinology and Metabolism,* 86: 1930–35.

64. Wright A (1927). Hyaline degeneration of the islets of Langerhans in non-diabetics. *American Journal of Pathology,* 3(5): 461–82.

65. Rocken C, Linke RP & Saeger W (1992). Immunohistology of islet amyloid polypeptide in diabetes mellitus: semi-quantitative studies in a post-mortem series. *Virchows Archive A: Pathological Anatomy and Histopathology,* 421: 339–44.

66. Clark A, Holman R, Matthews D, Hockaday T & Turner R (1984). Non-uniform distribution of islet amyloid in the pancreas of 'maturity-onset' diabetic patients. *Diabetologia*, 27: 527–28.

67. Westermark P (1984). Amyloid and polypeptide hormones: what is their interrelationship? *Amyloid: International Journal of Experimental and Clinical Investigation,* 1: 47–57.

68. Paulsson JF & Westermark GT (2005). Aberrant processing of human proislet amyloid polypeptide results in increased amyloid formation. *Diabetes,* 54: 2117–25.

69. Marzban L, Rhodes CJ, Steiner DF, Haataja L, Halban PA & Verchere CB (2006). Impaired NH2-terminal processing of human proislet amyloid polypeptide by the prohormone convertase PC2 leads to amyloid formation and cell death. *Diabetes*, 55: 2192–201.

70. Zraika S, Hull RL, Verchere CB, Clark A, Potter KJ, Fraser PE, et al. (2010). Toxic oligomers and islet beta cell death: guilty by association or convicted by circumstantial evidence? *Diabetologia,* 53: 1046–56.

71. Laybutt DR, Preston AM, Akerfeldt MC, Kench JG, Busch AK, Biankin AV, et al. (2007). Endoplasmic reticulum stress contributes to beta cell apoptosis in type 2 diabetes. *Diabetologia,* 50: 752–63.

72. Weber SM, Chambers KT, Bensch KG, Scarim AL & Corbett JA (2004). PPARgamma ligands induce ER stress in pancreatic beta cells: ER stress activation results in attenuation of cytokine signaling. *American Journal of Physiology: Endocrinology and Metabolism,* 287: E1171–77.

73. Marchetti P, Bugliani M Lupi R, Marselli l, Masini M, Boggi U, et al. (2007). The endoplasmic reticulum in pancreatic beta cell of type 2 diabetes patients. *Diabetologia*, 50: 2486–94.

74. Unger RH & Grundy S (1985). Hyperglycaemia as an inducer as well as a consequence of impaired islet cell function and insulin resistance: implications for the management of diabetes. *Diabetologia,* 28: 119–21.

75. Turner RC, McCarthy ST, Holman RR & Harris E (1976). Beta-cell function improved by supplementing basal insulin secretion in mild diabetes. *British Medical Journal,* 1: 1252–54.

76. Leahy JL, Cooper HE, Deal DA & Weir GC (1986). Chronic hyperglycaemia is associated with impaired glucose influence on insulin secretion: a study in normal rats using chronic in vivo glucose infusion. *Journal of Clinical Investigation,* 77: 908–15.

77. Leahy JL (2004). Detrimental effects of chronic hyperglycemia on the pancreatic β-cell. In LeRoith D, Olefsky JM & Taylor S (Eds). *Diabetes mellitus: a fundamental and clinical text* (pp115–27). Philadelphia: Lippincott.

78. Harmon JS, Bogdani M, Parazzoli SD, Mark SS, Oseid EA, Berghmans M, et al. (2009). Beta-cell specific overexpression of glutathione peroxidase preserves intranuclear MafA and reverses diabetes in db/db mice. *Endocrinology,* 150: 4855–62.

79. Del Guerra S, Lupi R, Marselli L, Masini M, Bugliani M, Sbrana S, et al. (2005). Functional and molecular defects of pancreatic islets in human type 2 diabetes. *Diabetes,* 54: 727–35.

80. Donath MY, Ehses JA, Maedler K, Schumann DM, Ellingsgaard H, Eppler E, et al. (2005). Mechanisms of beta cell death in type 2 diabetes. *Diabetes*, 54(Suppl. 2): S108–13.

81. Dobbins RL, Chester MW, Stevenson BE, Daniels MB, Stein DT & McGarry JDI (1998). A fatty acid – dependent step is critically important for both glucose- and non-glucose-stimulated insulin secretion. *Journal of Clinical Investigation,* 101: 2370–76.

82. Kebede M, Favaloro J, Gunton JE, Laybutt DR, Shaw M, Wong N, et al. (2008). Fructose-1,6-bisphosphatase overexpression in pancreatic beta-cells results in reduced insulin secretion: a new mechanism for fat-induced impairment of beta-cell function. *Diabetes,* 57: 1887–95.

83. Unger RH & Zhou YT (2001). Lipotoxicity of beta-cells in obesity and in other causes of fatty acid spillover. *Diabetes,* 50(Suppl. 1): S118–21.

84. Agren G, Narbro K, Naslund, Sjostrom L & Peltonen M (2002). Long-term effects of weight loss on pharmaceutical costs in obese subjects: a report from the SOS intervention study. *International Journal of Obesity Related Metabolism Disorders,* 26: 184–92.

85. Leahy JL, Bumbalo LM & Chen C (1994). Diazoxide causes recovery of beta-cell glucose responsiveness in 90% pancreatectomised diabetic rats. *Diabetes,* 44: 173–79.

86. Greenwood RH, Mahler RF & Hales CN (1976). Improvement in insulin secretion in diabetes after diazoxide. *The Lancet,* 1: 444–47.

87. Weng J, Li Y, Xu W, Shi L, Zhang Q, Zhu D, et al. (2008). Effect of intensive insulin therapy on beta-cell function and glycaemic control in patients with newly diagnosed type 2 diabetes: a multicentre randomised parallel-group trial. *The Lancet,* 371: 1753–60.

88. Efanova IB, Zaitsev SV, Zhivotovsky B, Kohler M, Efendic S, Orrenius S, et al. (1998). Glucose and tolbutamide induce apoptosis in pancreatic beta cells: a process dependent on intracellular xcalcium concentration. *The Journal of Biological Chemistry,* 273: 33501–07.

89. Leahy JL, Hirsch IB, Peterson KA & Schneider D (2010). Targeting beta-cell function early in the course of therapy for type 2 diabetes mellitus. *Journal of Clinical Endocrinology and Metabolism,* 95: 4206–16.

Specific risk groups and settings

6

Gender and obesity

Murray Fisher[1] and Natalie Chilko[1]

Multiple factors contribute to the development, maintenance and treatment of obesity. Viewing obesity through a gender relations approach helps to understand how an individual's interactions with others and society contributes to health opportunities and constraints, resulting in excess body weight. In gender relations theory, the body is viewed as both an agent and a product of social practice, whereby lifestyle behaviours influenced by an individual's context may impact on the physical body. This chapter presents life histories of two men in their 20s who have experience with obesity. Analysis of the production and power relations, relationships and symbolism reveal the marginalising effect of their obesity, and how gender interacts with other social structures including ethnicity and class. A holistic approach that considers how an individual configures their masculinity or femininity may assist in promoting and maintaining weight loss in obese individuals as it addresses the struggle in society experienced by many obese people.

Despite significant advances in nutrition, health and weight-loss treatments, there is a global epidemic of overweight and obesity [1]. Obesity is the result of significantly greater energy consumption than expenditure, and it is associated with long-term health problems including diabetes, cardiovascular disease, high-blood pressure, high cholesterol and some cancers [2]. Excess body weight has also been associated with depression, anxiety and low self-esteem [3]. Colagiuri and colleagues [4] estimate that the total direct cost of overweight and obesity in Australia was a substantial A\$21 billion in 2005. Obesity is a serious issue and current treatment strategies are modest at best with limited long-term success [5], making it critical to investigate new approaches to the prevention and treatment of obesity.

Gender research provides a new approach to understanding obesity. It is generally recognised that multiple factors contribute to excess weight, and medical, nursing and psychological literature have all considered this issue. The rapid increase in obesity rates worldwide suggests genetic causes alone are not sufficient to account for the epidemic and the importance of technology and sedentary lifestyles is well recognised [6]. Gender research has the potential to investigate the heterogeneity between and amongst men and women that may explain or give insight into why lifestyle behaviours are generally not altered by obese people. Consideration of an individual's experience of obesity will enable

---

1   Sydney Nursing School, University of Sydney.

the development of tailored weight-loss programs, rather than treatments that treat all men and all women as a collective group.

The gender relations approach

The contemporary theory of gender is gender relations, where gender is defined as 'a structure of social relations that centres on the reproductive arena, and the set of practices (governed by this structure) that bring reproductive distinctions between bodies into social processes' [7, p10]. Gender is an internally complex social structure that is actively constructed and comes into being as people (inter)act. An individual's gender is dynamic and constantly configured as it interacts with other social structures including ethnicity, sexuality and class. Multiple femininities and masculinities exist, and these are viewed as gender projects that can be challenged, reconstructed and contested [8, 9]. An individual's gender is considered relational to other's constructions of gender and thus people are positioned within a gender order. Hegemony, for example, is an idealised and dominant form of masculinity that is powerful, influential and strong. Other types of masculinity include complicit, marginalised and subordinated masculinities [6].

The body is a reproductive arena through which social practice occurs and gender is constructed. The body is both a recipient of social practice as well as an agent in social practice. As embodied beings we are recipients of emotions from others' actions, while simultaneously able to act in ways that create emotions in others. Social embodiment refers to the way bodies, as agencies, participate in society, and how in turn society affects bodies [10]. Some bodies for example encounter violence, accidents and sickness as a result of social practices, and this contributes to their configuration of gender [10]. To this end, obese bodies are constituted in social processes that are created in history and subject to change, and therefore could be explored as patterns of gendered social embodiment.

Gender, health and obesity

From the perspective of a gender relations approach, research on obesity demonstrates the validity of gender as a concept that manifests in social practice. For example, differences and inequalities between genders may help to explain general health differences among men and women. For example men are less likely to receive health screens, report symptoms and attend medical services than women [11, 12], and are more likely to engage in risky behaviour [13]. However not all men engage in risky behaviour and not all women have regular medical check-ups. Societal norms can influence the health of different genders beyond any biological sex differences, although there are differences in how people are affected. A gender relations approach focuses on how an individual's interactions with others and society significantly contribute both to opportunities for and constraints on health [14]. These, in turn, can give insight into the cause, maintenance and treatment of obesity.

The focus in the empirical literature on sex differences in obesity is a starting point for understanding the impact of gender on health behaviours. There are complex sex differences in the prevalence, effects and treatment of obesity. A growing number of studies for example suggest sex differences in rates of obesity exist in a dynamic relationship with ethnicity, age, geography and socioeconomic status worldwide [15–17]. Wang and Beydon's [15] systematic review and meta-regression analysis of obesity prevalence studies in the US reported large ethnic differences in obesity prevalence, especially among women. Minority groups, including non-Hispanic blacks and Mexican Americans, had a higher combined prevalence than non-Hispanic whites. Non-Hispanic blacks overall had the highest prevalence of obesity which, in women, was 20 percentage points higher than obesity prevalence among white women [15]. Prevalence was also affected by socioeconomic status (SES) and the effect differed by ethnic group. Less educated persons were more likely to be obese than their more educated counterparts, except amongst black women where higher education was associated with a higher rate of obesity [15].

The complex dynamic between sex, SES, ethnicity and obesity prevalence also exists in Australia. Obesity prevalence is higher among men and women from lower socioeconomic status, less educated people, Aboriginal and Torres Strait Islander peoples, and among migrants [18]. Data from the 2004 to 2005 National Health Survey indicate that people born overseas are more likely than people born in Australia to be overweight or obese, and within this group, men are more likely to be overweight or obese than women (58% compared to 43%). Indigenous Australians have nearly double the likelihood of non-Indigenous Australians to be obese, and are almost three times more likely to be morbidly obese [18].

The differences between males and females and the effects of obesity also appear to be complex. A recent meta-analysis of cross-sectional studies of depression and obesity (defined by BMI) in the community found a significant positive association for women but not men [19]. However another systematic review and meta-analysis of longitudinal studies revealed a reciprocal link between depression and obesity (n = 58 745) in both men and women [20]. This study also found a potential cultural influence as the risk of developing depression when obese was more pronounced in the American subjects compared to their European counterparts [20]. This complexity also exists in research on sex differences in obesity and anxiety, body image, quality of life [21–24], and weight loss. Considerable individual differences exist in the efficacy of weight-loss interventions, however this is often concealed by reporting mean differences [5]. Rates of dropout in weight-loss studies are also high (30%–60%) [5]. A range of behavioural, physiological and inherited factors have been put forward to explain the relative success of different individuals in losing weight through exercise [25].

Gender theory can help untangle the inconsistencies in the literature as it refrains from categorising men and women into groups, as gender is dependent on an individual's social and historical context. The failure to account for within-group and within-person variability has been suggested to be partially responsible for inconsistencies within the literature on sexual differences in other areas including healthcare utilisation [26]. Categorising by sex does not adequately explain why only some men and some women become obese, nor does it explain why only some obese men and some obese women lose a significant amount of weight. Biological and inherited characteristics are known to contribute to adipose profile

[6] and the propensity to lose weight [25]; however social factors of obesity are also strongly acknowledged. Gender relations theory focuses on how the body navigates through and how it is affected by society.

The study and its method

While there is growing research investigating sex differences in obesity, there is a paucity of studies investigating the role of gender. Gender as configurations of social practice may influence the lifestyle behaviours people engage in. It could be hypothesised that a person's positioning within the gender order will influence their ability to alter lifestyle behaviours (eating habits, smoking, diet and exercise), thus influencing their weight.

We conducted a study to examine, using a gender relations approach, the lived experience of men who are or have been obese. We investigated the impact obesity has on identity, social practice and gender relations in order to discover why individuals are successful (or not) in changing their lifestyles and behaviours. Life history methodology was used to collect personal narratives from obese men, two of which are presented here. The life history method is used to explain an individual's understanding of social events, movements and political causes, and how individual members of groups or institutions see, experience and interpret those events [27]. It is thus a useful way to gain a perspective on and understanding of the gendered experiences of obese men.

Data analysis consisted of the identification of patterns of social response to trace a historical dynamic of gender. A progressive-regressive method of analysis was employed where the life story provides the personal link to wider issues of history and culture [27]. In the first phase of analysis, a four-dimensional structural model of gender relations (production, power, emotion and symbolism) described by Connell [9, 10] was used to ascertain the informant's experience of gender and their position in the gender order. Each transcript was then analysed to map the informant's gender project – the construction and reconstruction of masculinity. Gender starting points and the trajectories of the gender projects are highlighted. These case studies were re-analysed to explore similarities and differences in the trajectories. These methods are consistent with those used in critical studies of men and masculinities [8, 28].

Group and context

Both men whose life stories are the subject of this study, have been significantly affected by their obesity throughout the course of their life and both are currently trying to lose weight. Lukman (24 years old) and Justin (25 years old) have similar starting points for their construction of masculinity and a strikingly similar gender project. They have a similar family history, both growing up in the middle class with relatively conservative parents. Both families were quite religious; Lukman's family was Coptic Christian and Justin's was Catholic. Lukman was born in Jordan and moved with his family when he was in Year 11 at school. Justin's background is Spanish (his mother) and Italian (his father). Both participants grew up in families with a conventional division of labour and a conventional power structure. They shared a closer relationship with their mothers than fathers. The mother was often quite involved in the participants' life while communication with the father was generally avoided and the relationship was tense. Lukman's father was obese and died two and a half years ago due to complications after surgery. Lukman has a family history of diabetes, cardiovascular disease, high-blood pressure and cancer. Both Justin's parents are alive and his mother struggles to lose weight. Both participants live at home and have been overweight since childhood.

Lukman and Justin appear to be at different points on the weight-loss trajectory. Although they currently weigh similar amounts, Justin, the heavier of the pair, became committed to weight loss at an earlier age. Lukman is 183 cm tall and weighs approximately 147 kg. Justin is 189 cm tall and weighs 136 kg. Their respective BMIs are 43.9 and 38.1. Lukman underwent gastric-sleeve banding two weeks prior to the interview and has so far lost 20 kg. His weight-loss efforts prior to surgery were minor, with his only significant attempt at the age of 13, when his family forced him to lose weight to make him more presentable for his sister's wedding. His father's health complications associated with the obesity have prompted Lukman's recent commitment to weight loss.

Justin has a longer weight-loss history, undergoing lap-band surgery after graduating high school at age 18. He weighed 250 kg at this point, and lost 40 kg in the following year. He comments that although he initially reduced his portion size and fat intake, no lifestyle changes were made and the weight-loss eventually plateaued at approximately 180 kg. Justin tried other methods of weight loss while at university, however these were largely unsuccessful. A significant change occurred when a friend introduced him to a weight-loss retreat, which he visited several times. This experience and access to information on nutrition, health and exercise inspired Justin to focus on his eating habits and caloric intake. He has been exercising regularly and closely monitoring his diet since then. He graduated from university in 2009 and spent the following year exercising and focusing on weight loss. He has a personal trainer, visits the gym regularly and has so far lost 114 kg. Although his BMI is still classified as obese, much of his weight is due to muscle mass and his latest visit to a physician reported that he was in good health.

Gender substructures analysis

The construction of masculinity of Lukman and Justin was analysed using Connell's [10] substructures of gender relations: a) *Gender production relations*: the gender division, allocation and organisation of labour; b) *Gender power relations*: the organisation of power, the way power is contested and the way groups mobilise to counteract power inequalities; c) *Cathexis or gender emotional relations*: a person's emotional attachment with another (or an object), including desire, sexuality and sexual relations; and d) *Symbolism*: the communication of gender ideologies.

Production

Lukman and Justin are situated in a similar subordinated position in production relations. They have an unimpressive work history, are currently unemployed, rely on other family members for financial support, and have limited qualifications and skills. They both experienced times at university that were difficult and resulted in failed subjects, and Justin partially attributes this to a low mood because of his weight. Both participants have a transient work history and no skills available to sell, resulting in a limited position in the labour market. Lukman has worked primarily in temporary jobs in the fast food industry, for the local council, in administrative roles, and for an IT company assembling computers for private use. Justin has worked at a call centre and recently in an IT sales job. They both lack any affection for these positions, and being relatively unskilled, they remain replaceable employees in the workplace.

Both Lukman and Justin have acknowledged a role of their weight in limiting their employment options. Lukman comments that for many jobs you 'need to look good in a shirt' and he believes he is not 'employable-looking'. Justin also indicates how his weight has affected his work: he resigned from his call centre position after believing staff perceived him as 'a grumpy person who couldn't talk to other people and couldn't relate and didn't have time for anybody', as he was struggling with severe back pain. His relationship with staff prior to the onset of back pain had been friendly and warm. Justin further indicates that working reduces time spent on weight loss,

> I found that the only way to lose weight is if you fully dedicate yourself to it, which means you can't have a job. (Justin)

He left his last job of three months because he was unhappy in the position and found this affected his eating habits and potential to gain weight.

Although Lukman and Justin have worked in abstract labour positions, they both express dissatisfaction with these roles and have a positive attitude to their future role in the labour market. They appear eager to support themselves. Justin is committed to 'find something I love doing and do it'. Lukman expresses feeling 'terrible' about having to rely on the financial support of his sister and her husband, and indicates his goals are to find work, finish uni, complete any postgraduate qualifications in psychology that may be necessary, and to eventually support himself and his mother. Justin intends to complete a personal training qualification and to pursue work in the fitness industry. Although these men are currently dispensable in the workplace, they express motivation to becoming a valuable contributor to the labour market.

Power

There have been significant issues of power in the lives of Lukman and Justin. They both cite an estranged relationship with their fathers from an early age. Both fathers were perceived as aggressive, with rare occasions of violence, and the mothers were the more approachable parent. They both believe however that their mothers also perceived them as powerless. Lukman labels his mother as the 'doting' mother, always involved and always enquiring about his wants and needs,

> I go to sleep and I wake up and all the clothes that are on my floor are gone and washed and waiting outside the room. (Lukman)

Justin acknowledges a more general perceived powerlessness because of his weight,

> I think that people saw that [the weight] and empathised and it just turned into a 'everyone has to take care of Justin' kind of thing … I was so overweight at one point that, you know, if I can't help myself, how can I help other people? (Justin)

They both believe their weight has significantly contributed to a powerlessness and marginalisation in society.

They also acknowledge their own role in power relations by recognising their chosen submissiveness in relationships. Justin comments that he was 'friendly to everyone so they would be friendly to me'. He used humour to be likeable and to avoid being the victim of bullying,

> Humour was a really big part of how I came to relate to people all through high school and further on. (Justin)

Lukman comments that he transformed from being 'a very social animal … a very involved person to more of an introvert.' He is unsure why this change occurred, but believes his obesity played a role in the transformation. He did experience some bullying during high school but nothing he couldn't really 'shrug off'. He believes his weight may have some role in it as 'first appearances mean a lot', but he says that the bullying disappeared when he was one-on-one with the perpetrators.

Importantly, both participants express a desire to increase their power. Lukman says that he wishes to 'survive without' the help of his doting mother and that he wishes to 'become more of an extrovert' so that he can advance in his career and in relationships. Justin is dedicated to training and eating nutritiously so that he can 'inspire people and eventually raise some money for some charities.' A key weight-loss trigger for both these men has been a desire to increase their power, and thus to improve their position in the gender order.

Cathexis: emotion and relationships

Relationships have been significantly affected by the obesity of these two men. Within the family unit, tension often arose because of weight,

> I felt like a lot of their fights started from arguments about me and my weight and how hard Dad was on me and how my Mum [was] giving me everything I want[ed]. (Justin)

Justin believes his dad may have felt 'helpless' and was unsure how to handle his increasing weight, resulting in their tense relationship. Obesity similarly affected Justin's ability to communicate with his father.

Obesity has also affected the friendships of the two men, however in a less overt way to relationships with their parents. Both men report having few sound friendships. Lukman believes he is more of 'a deep friendship kind of person' as he prefers close, intimate relationships over a 'legion of friends.' Obesity though has affected the activities that the men can participate in with friends. Justin comments that he 'wasn't really doing the same kind of things that other kids were' because he 'wasn't able to',

> I seemed to always be in a bit of a state of anxiousness or anxiety about … just about everyday things like if someone invited me out, would they be driving a sedan or a hatchback? Would I be able to fit in the passenger seat or the backseat? Would I be able to do the seatbelt up? (Justin)

He 'felt it was easier just to stay home than to be bothered with it because of all the things that I would have to encounter throughout the day.' Lukman also limits his social activities, avoiding going to the beach and places where he would have to take his shirt off. He feels more comfortable around people who are aware he is trying to lose weight; otherwise he becomes very self-conscious.

Obesity has also had a major role in the sexual relations of the two participants. Both participants reported having had a few, short-term relationships with a female partner that broke up primarily because of their low self-esteem.

> I don't feel confident enough to approach many people that I do find attractive and I do find that I'd like to get to know. And then, if I do get over that, if I do ask someone out, and then we do the relationship for a couple of months – I don't see myself as good enough, a lot of the time. (Lukman)

Justin also comments that he did not want to be seen with a girl because he was concerned about his appearance and he did not want to be an embarrassment. Despite losing a significant amount of weight, he still feels this way. His first girlfriend since the weight loss had also experienced a significant drop in weight and he comments that this made it easier to have a sexual relationship, as they felt less judgemental about the other's body. Justin however realises that he was insecure in the relationship,

> I was still really insecure about having a girlfriend. I had kind of come to the point in my life at one stage where I would be single for the rest of my life and I was fine with it. So I had thought. (Justin)

Lukman struggles with his sexuality and he believes his obesity has limited his sexual opportunities and ability to explore this. Although he believes he is a heterosexual, his first sexual encounter was with a gay man who he met through a friend. He is unsure if this was due to a 'lack of long-term success with females' or homosexual tendencies of his own:

> I figured what the hell, this might be the case. But I don't know if it's due to the lack of success, lack of long-term success, or is it just an individual thing? (Lukman)

He indicates that because of his obesity he has been prevented in investigating his sexuality further, noting this as one of the reasons for undergoing weight-loss surgery. He believes his attraction to men may be just sexual, and he thinks he may be 'bi-sexual with a heterosexual skew'.

Symbolism

The symbol of obesity in society has affected both participants and has had a role in triggering their weight loss. Lukman acknowledges that his decision to undergo gastric-sleeve surgery was partially due to a desire to 'fit in'. He comments that he wants to 'look normal'. Justin uses the train as an example,

> Getting on a train would always be difficult. Especially if it was busy or hot. I couldn't stand for too long so I'd need to find a seat but there's that whole thing where people don't really want you to sit next to them or don't want to sit next to you. There's that, there's the people watching you all the time, looking at what you do and making judgements. (Justin)

These men are aware of their marginalisation by others because of their weight. Justin believes many people judge obese people as selfish and lazy,

> I think people see overweight people like they only think about themselves. That they haven't got time for other people … It's like you think about feeding yourself before doing anything else. (Justin)

Both participants are aware of the symbolic meanings that subjugate the body and place stress on the construction of gender. The body is inextricably linked to gender, and as Parker [29] notes, a healthy looking physique is associated with a sense of respect for oneself and a commitment to health and fitness – the converse of the perception of obesity, as experienced by these men. The stigma associated with obesity is considerable [30].

Discussion

The two life histories presented here are valuable to the study of gender and health as they highlight the significant effect of the body on one's construction of masculinity. The weight of the participants has affected their position in the labour market, their power relations and their emotional and sexual relationships. This has resulted in their marginalisation and thus the construction of a marginalised masculinity.

The life-history methodology allows the dynamic of gender to be traced across the life course and the study of obesity serves as an interesting example of embodied masculinity developing over time. Both participants believed they would improve their position in the gender order by losing weight. Both men believe their weight loss will allow them to 'advance' in society, which is synonymous to being closer to achieving the hegemonic dividend, that is, being complicit with patriarchy and receiving its rewards. There is a sense that things will improve when they weigh less,

> I guess I keep thinking that if I lose weight or if I get to a certain point I'm going to be happy and everything is going to be fine. (Justin)

Weight loss is an embodied transformative process in these cases, essential for the reconfiguration of one's masculinity. Physicality is closely tied with gender and the desire to achieve a more powerful, athletic body is a trigger for weight loss.

One's position in the gender order, however, is not solely determined by the physical body. Social practices have a role in shaping an individual's body which exists in a reciprocal relationship with the individual's production, power, cathexis and symbolism. Justin, who is further along the weight-loss journey than Lukman, appears to be realising that his change in physical size is not matched with a change in positioning in the gender order,

> I still feel like a child. I don't feel like a man. I'm still living at home and my parents still see me the same way, as they always have. So they still treat me the same way with everything … I feel like I haven't grown up, I haven't been given responsibilities and I haven't learnt to do things for myself … I find myself 15 years old. If you were to look at me, you would see a man. But I don't feel that way … I don't feel like I've lived in the world. Until this point. (Justin)

Justin is struggling to reconfigure his masculinity despite weight loss. The marginalisation of obese people in terms of power, production and emotional and sexual relations has been well researched. A large study (n = 12 364) using telephone interviews found sexual behaviour differed for obese people compared to normal weight [31]. Obese women were less likely than women of normal weight to report having a sexual partner in the previous 12 months, and obese men were more likely to suffer from erectile dysfunction than normal weight men, and had fewer sexual partners [31]. Obesity has also been found to affect employment opportunities. A high BMI is associated with an increased likelihood of receiving a disability pension [32]. The evidence that obesity impacts negatively on job evaluations and hiring has also been rated as strong [30]. The stigma associated with obesity is considerable [30], comparable to racial discrimination [33], and this has a marginalising effect for many individuals.

Consideration of embodied masculinities and femininities in weight loss has the potential to contribute to individualising weight-loss plans. Justin commented that although surgery was necessary to lose the initial weight, he did not learn sustainable healthy behaviours from this process. His education in nutrition and lifestyle came from his time spent at a weight-loss retreat that focused on the personal experience in the weight-loss journey. Lukman, who has recently undergone gastric-sleeve surgery, recognises that his eating habits preceding surgery were unhealthy, but he did not indicate a desire to increase his exercise or engage in a healthy lifestyle now that he has had the surgery. Shah and colleagues' [34] review found weight-loss surgeries were associated with significant initial weight reduction, but that this was not maintained long term [34]. Douketis and colleagues' [5] systematic review of weight loss in obesity found weight loss of 25 kg to 75 kg in the two to four years following surgery, which was higher than the other interventions (eg diet therapy, pharmacologic therapy). Current weight-loss treatments overall for obese persons are modestly successful [35], however a focus on mean values may conceal individuals who do lose a significant amount of weight [5]. Justin comments:

> What I've started to realise is that there is no point that you can get to where things just change. It's what you do right now and what you do in your life as this weight loss is taking place that shapes how people react to you and how you react to others. So then it becomes

your life. Rather than wait till I weigh 100 kilos and then my life will be like this. As you go, your life starts to build and it incorporates all of this and it's not like you can put your life on hold, lose weight and then come back to it. (Justin)

It is an empirical question if an intervention involving a discussion about gender, personality and weight loss earlier in the weight-loss journey would facilitate quicker and sustained weight loss.

Conclusion

The life histories presented demonstrate the value of gender relations theory in analysing the obesity issue. Life-history methodology has the potential to shed light on the inconsistencies in data on the prevalence and effects of obesity by focusing on the individual experience. The cases presented highlight how the body is integral to constructing gender, but also how social aspects of ethnicity and class, as well as aspects of production, relationships and power, shape the body and contribute to the gender project. These preliminary results suggest that the construction of masculinity of an individual who is attempting to lose weight is closely tied with the body and that a trigger for weight loss may be a desire to improve one's position in the gender order. Challenges to maintaining this weight loss may however include the realisation that physical changes to the body are not the only obstacle to achieving a dominant form of masculinity or femininity. Weight-loss approaches that recognise the individual struggle with gender and the influence of other social structures may be an alternative to current, largely unsuccessful treatments of obesity.

References

1. International Obesity Task Force. Obesity prevalence worldwide [Online]. Available: www.iaso.org/iotf/obesity/ [Accessed 16 June 2011].

2. Stein CJ & Colditz GA (2004). The epidemic of obesity. *The Journal of Clinical Endocrinology & Metabolism*, 89(6): 2522–25.

3. Atlantis E & Ball K (2007). Association between weight perception and psychological distress. *International Journal of Obesity*, 32: 715–21.

4. Colagiuri S, Lee CMY, Colagiuri R, Magliano D, Shaw JE, Zimmet PZ, et al. (2010). The cost of overweight and obesity in Australia. *Medical Journal of Australia*, 192(5): 260–264.

5. Douketis JD, Macie C, Thabane L & Williamson DF (2005). Systematic review of long-term weight loss studies in obese adults: clinical significance and applicability to clinical practice. *International Journal of Obesity*, 29: 1153–67.

6. Power ML & Schulkin J (2008). Sex differences in fat storage, fat metabolism, and the health risks from obesity: possible evolutionary origins. *British Journal of Nutrition*, 99(5): 931–40.

7. Connell RW (2001). The social organization of masculinity. In SM Whithead & FJ Barrett (Eds). *The masculinities reader* (pp 30–50). Cambridge: Polity Press.

8. Connell RW (1995). *Masculinities*. Sydney: Allen & Unwin.

9. Connell RW (2000). *Men and the boys*. Sydney: Allen and Unwin.

10. Connell RW (2002). *Gender*. Cambridge: Polity Press.

11. Stoverinck MJ, Lagro-Janssen AL & Weel CV (1996). Sex differences in health problems, diagnostic testing, and referral in primary care. *Journal of Family Practice*, 43(6): 567–76.

12. Ladwig K-H, Mittag BM, Formanek B & Dammann G (2000). Gender differences of symptom reporting and medical healthcare utilization in the German population. *European Journal of Epidemiology*, 16(6): 511–18.

13. Lienard P (2011). Life stages and risk-avoidance: status- and context-sensitivity in precaution systems. *Neuroscience and Behavioural Reviews*, 35(4): 1067–74.

14. Schofield T, Connell RW, Walker L, Wood JF & Butland DL (2000). Understanding men's health and illness: a gender-relations approach to policy, research, and practice. *Journal of American College Health*, 48(6): 247–56.

15. Wang Y & Beydoun MA (2007). The obesity epidemic in the United States – gender, age, socioeconomic, racial/ethnic, and geographic characteristics: a systematic review and meta-regression analysis. *Epidemiologic Reviews*, 29(1): 6–28.

16. Paeratakul S, Lovejoy JC, Ryan DH & Bray GA (2002). The relation of gender, race and socioeconomic status to obesity and obesity comorbidities in a sample of US adults. *International Journal of Obesity*, 26(9): 1205–10.

17. Zhang Q & Wang Y (2004). Socioeconomic inequality of obesity in the United States: do gender, age, and ethnicity matter? *Social Science & Medicine*, 58(6): 1171–80.

18. National Preventative Health Taskforce (2009). *Australia: the healthiest country by 2020. The report of the National Preventative Health Strategy: the roadmap for action*. Including addendum for October 2008 to 2009. Canberra: National Preventative Health Taskforce.

19. de Wit L, Luppino F, van Straten A, Penninx B, Zitman F & Cuijpers P (2010). Depression and obesity: a meta-analysis of community-based studies. *Psychiatry Research*, 178(2): 230–35.

20. Luppino FS, de Wit LM, Bouvy PF, Stijnen T, Cuijpers P, Penninx BWJH et al. (2010). Overweight, obesity, and depression: a systematic review and meta-analysis of longitudinal studies. *Archives of General Psychiatry*, 67(3): 220–29.

21. Gariepy G, Nitka D & Schmitz N (2010). The association between obesity and anxiety disorders in the population: a systematic review and meta-analysis. *International Journal of Obesity*, 34(3): 407–19.

22. Barry D, Pietrzak RH & Petry NM (2008). Gender differences in associations between body mass index and DSM-IV Mood and Anxiety Disorders: results from the National Epidemiologic Survey on Alcohol and Related Conditions. *Annals of Epidemiology*, 18(6): 458–66.

23. Sorbara M & Geliebter A (2002). Body image disturbance in obese outpatients before and after weight loss in relation to race, gender, binge eating, and age of onset of obesity. *International Journal of Eating Disorders*, 31(4): 416–23.

24. White MA, O'Neil PM, Kolotkin RL & Byrne TK (2004). Gender, race, and obesity-related quality of life at extreme levels of obesity. *Obesity Research*, 12(6): 949–55.

25. Boutcher SH & Dunn SL (2009). Factors that may impede the weight loss response to exercise-based interventions. *Obesity Reviews*, 10(6): 671–80.

26. Addis ME & Mahalik JR (2003). Men, masculinity, and the contexts of help seeking. *American Psychologist*, 58(1): 5–14.

27. Plummer K (2001). *Documents of life: an invitation to a critical humanism*. London: Sage.

28. Messner MA (1992). *Power at play: sports and the problem of masculinity*. Boston: Beacon Press.

29. Parker A. (1996). Sporting masculinities: gender relations and the body. In M Mac an Ghaill (Ed). *Understanding masculinities: social relations and cultural arenas* (pp126–38). Buckingham: Open University Press

30. Puhl RM & Heuer CA (2009). The stigma of obesity: a review and update. *Obesity,* 17(5): 941–64.

31. Bajos N, Wellings K, Laborde C & Moreau C (2010). Sexuality and obesity, a gender perspective: results from French national random probability survey of sexual behaviours. *British Medical Journal*, 340: c2573.

32. Neovius K, Johansson K, Rössner S & Neovius M (2008). Disability pension, employment and obesity status: a systematic review. *Obesity Reviews*, 9(6): 572–81.

33. Puhl RM, Andreyeva T & Brownell KD (2008). Perceptions of weight discrimination: prevalence and comparison to race and gender discrimination in America. *International Journal of Obesity*, 32(6): 992–1000.

34. Shah M, Simha V & Garg A (2006). Long-term impact of bariatric surgery on body weight, comorbidities, and nutritional status. *The Journal of Clinical Endocrinology & Metabolism*, 91(11): 4223–31.

35. Franz MJ, VanWormer JJ, Crain L, Boucher JL, Histon T, Caplan W, et al. (2007). Weight-loss outcomes: a systematic review and meta-analysis of weight-loss clinical trials with a minimum 1-year follow-up. *Journal of the American Dietetic Association*, 107(10): 1755–67.

7

Preventing chronic disease to close the gap in life expectancy for Indigenous Australians

Alan Cass,[1,2] Paul Snelling[3] and Alex Brown[4]

Prevention of disease is a major aim of the Australian health system. Chronic diseases are responsible for approximately 80% of the burden of disease and injury in Australia, account for around 70% of total health expenditure, form part of 50% of GP consultations, and are associated with more than 500 000 person/years of lost full-time employment each year [1]. A small number of modifiable risk factors are responsible for the major share of the burden of preventable chronic disease. This chapter focuses on chronic kidney disease as an example of a preventable chronic disease that impacts heavily on the indigenous community, causing major morbidity and mortality. Key modifiable risk factors for chronic kidney disease include tobacco smoking, physical inactivity, poor nutrition, obesity and high blood pressure. Amongst Indigenous Australians, poor access to necessary preventative care, combined with the broader social determinants of health, acting across the life-course, contribute to the excess burden of chronic disease, including diabetes and chronic kidney disease. Improvements in maternal and early childhood health and development, educational attainment outcomes and access to safe and secure housing are critical 'building blocks' in national efforts to reduce the burden of chronic disease and to close the gap between the health status of Indigenous and non-indigenous Australians.

Burden of disease

The most recent estimates of the gap in life expectancy between Indigenous and non-Indigenous men and women are 12 and ten years respectively [2]. However, the true life expectancy of Indigenous Australians remains a matter of dispute. Research has shown a lower life expectancy in states or territories with more complete reporting of Indigenous deaths [3]. Amongst people aged 35 to 74 years, 80% of the mortality gap is attributable to chronic diseases. The inextricably related chronic diseases of blood vessels and metabolism – heart disease, diabetes, stroke and kidney disease – constitute half of this gap [2].

1   Sydney Medical School, University of Sydney.

2   George Institute for Global Health, Sydney.

3   Royal Prince Alfred Hospital, Sydney.

4   Baker IDI Heart and Diabetes Institute, Central Australia.

There are almost 20 000 Australians with severe or end-stage kidney disease (ESKD), who require ongoing dialysis or have received a kidney transplant. The incidence rate of ESKD among Indigenous Australians contrasts dramatically with that for non-Indigenous Australians. There is a steep gradient in the burden of kidney disease from urban areas, where rates are three to five times the national average, to rural areas where rates are ten to 15 times higher, to remote areas where rates are up to 30 times the national average [4, 5]. Between 2007 and 2008, there were almost 115 000 hospitalisations for regular dialysis for Indigenous Australians. This constitutes more than 40% of *all* hospital admissions for Indigenous Australians and dialysis hospitalisations occur at a rate 11 times that of non-Indigenous Australians [6]. While the burden of earlier stages of chronic kidney disease (CKD) amongst Indigenous Australians is less well documented, it is known to occur commonly. People with earlier stages of CKD are at high risk of death due to heart disease and at high risk of progression to ESKD.

Based on data from the AusDiab study, which surveyed the health of a large and representative sample of the adult population, about one in nine Australians aged 25 years and over have early CKD [7]. However, comprehensive population-based data for the national burden of CKD among Indigenous Australians are not available. Between 2004 and 2006 in Queensland, South Australia, Western Australia and the Northern Territory, CKD was recorded as the underlying cause of death in nearly 4% of all Indigenous deaths, a rate seven to 11 times higher than for non-Indigenous males and females respectively [8]. CKD was an associated cause in a further 12% of deaths [8]. Surveys in individual remote Aboriginal communities have documented high rates of early stages of CKD and its cardinal markers – reduced kidney function measured with a simple blood test and protein leakage into the urine from damaged kidneys. An audit of the screening and management of chronic disease in Aboriginal primary care, undertaken through the Kanyini Vascular Collaboration, has confirmed that more than 40% of regular adult attendees at Aboriginal primary care services who receive recommended screening tests have reduced kidney function or proteinuria [9]. This health service, rather than population-based data, underscores the burden of CKD which needs to be addressed.

Risk factors

Risk factors for CKD can be categorised as fixed and modifiable. Fixed-risk factors include a family history, genetic predisposition and increasing age [8]. Modifiable risk factors include low birthweight, socioeconomic disadvantage, diabetes, high-blood pressure, overweight and obesity, tobacco smoking, physical inactivity and poor nutrition [8, 10, 11]. Amongst Indigenous Australians, factors that arise early in the lifecourse, including poor maternal health and low birthweight and the burden of childhood infection and chronic inflammation, have been associated with increased risk of developing CKD [12, 13]. The associations between markers of socioeconomic disadvantage, including leaving school early, unemployment, low household income and house crowding, and ESKD rates, are particularly strong for Indigenous Australians [14].

Intervention across the life-course

Reducing the burden of CKD will require targeted interventions across the lifecourse, from before birth through childhood to adulthood (Figure 1). Whole of government interventions are required to address social disadvantage, and priority areas around housing, food supply and tobacco control can be directly related to CKD. Within the health sector, targeted screening, early intervention and evidence-based management to prevent the progression of kidney disease are required [15]. Although this chapter will focus on prevention, equitable access to necessary kidney disease treatment services must also be provided. Key service delivery issues that must be addressed by health providers and systems in order to better respond to the health, social and cultural needs of Indigenous Australians with kidney disease include:

1. Poor access to home- and community-based dialysis forcing the majority of patients from remote areas to relocate permanently to urban areas for treatment

2. Low kidney transplant rates

3. Making health services easier for Indigenous patients to navigate: key factors here include proximity to health services, availability of transport, minimal out-of-pocket costs for attendance and treatments, after-hours access, outreach services and mobile clinics, welcoming physical spaces and Indigenous staff as a critical point of contact

4. Inadequate provision of trained interpreters in Aboriginal languages

5. Pervasive miscommunication between Indigenous kidney patients and their healthcare providers (Figure 1) [16–19].

Primary prevention of kidney disease

Primary prevention initiatives are required from the antenatal period with the aim of preventing the development of CKD. High-quality evidence from controlled trials conducted within the Indigenous population, on the effectiveness of interventions to prevent the development of CKD is not currently available. Nevertheless, evidence indicates that the following initiatives would have a positive health impact generally and would affect intermediate outcomes known to be associated with the development of CKD:

1. Increased access to antenatal services to improve fetal and maternal health, and reduce the rates of low birthweight

2. Screening and intensive management of diabetes in pregnancy [20] and encouragement of breastfeeding [21] to help prevent the development of obesity and early onset of type 2 diabetes

3. Prevention of obesity in early childhood, particularly due to 'catch up growth' in those with low birthweight, as these people are at greatest risk of developing diabetes [22] and CKD [23]

4. Early childhood development initiatives to improve educational achievement and life-skills

5. Training community members to improve housing infrastructure and to maintain improvements [24]
6. Installing swimming pools in remote communities to reduce the prevalence of skin, middle ear and respiratory tract infections [25]
7. Community-based scabies control programs
8. Food supply initiatives to improve access to affordable healthy food [26]
9. Culturally appropriate healthy nutrition, physical activity and quit smoking programs and legislative initiatives to regulate tobacco advertising.

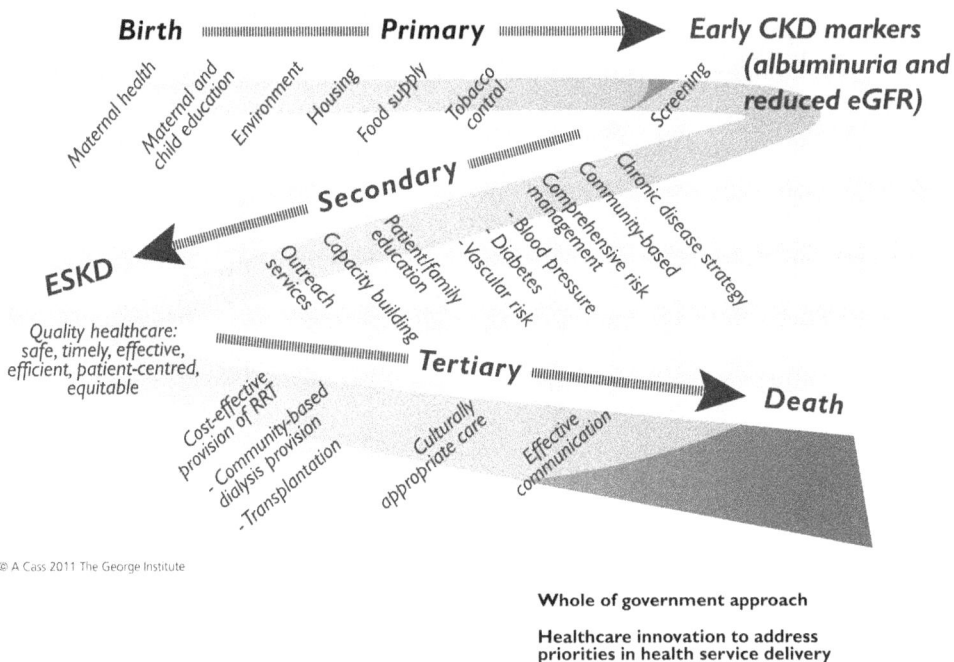

© A Cass 2011 The George Institute

Whole of government approach

Healthcare innovation to address priorities in health service delivery

Figure 1. A life-course approach to CKD prevention and management (Refer to the text for specific approaches as they relate to Indigenous Australians).

Primary care-based screening and early intervention to prevent disease progression

Screening tests for CKD in primary care should include:

1. A urine test for protein – specifically indicated is a first morning urine specimen tested for albumin. Albumin is an abundant protein in the blood. If detected in the urine, it indicates kidney damage. (If a first morning urine specimine cannot be obtained, a urine specimen obtained when a patient is attending primary care is acceptable.)
2. A blood test to measure serum creatinine – a breakdown product of muscle, usually produced in the body at a constant rate and filtered out of the body through the

kidneys. Where kidney function is reduced, the filtration rate falls and blood levels rise. The blood test result is used to estimate kidney function – commonly termed as estimated glomerular filtration rate or eGFR.

The Kanyini Vascular Collaboration (KVC), established in 2006, brings together Indigenous and non-Indigenous researchers, health providers and policy-makers in a research program aiming to improve the health outcomes of Indigenous Australians with heart disease, diabetes and kidney disease (www.kvc.org.au). The KVC Audit Study showed that approximately 40% of those people attending Aboriginal primary-care services, who are indicated for CKD screening, have the results of these tests entered into their medical record [9]. Primary care-based screening to facilitate early detection and evidence-based management of CKD has been shown to be cost-effective in the general population [27]. Evidence supports targeted screening of people at high risk of CKD – including Indigenous Australians aged 35 years and over; people with diabetes, high blood pressure or heart disease; smokers; people with a family history of CKD; and people who are overweight or obese. A comprehensive CKD screening program, if implemented as part of a coordinated chronic disease strategy, should have benefits both in terms of prevention of heart attacks, stroke and cardiac deaths as well as prevention of ESKD [27].

Modelled analyses utilising best Australian evidence regarding the population burden of diabetes and high-blood pressure, current practice patterns and randomised controlled trial-based evidence regarding the effectiveness of interventions, have demonstrated that primary care–based screening for CKD and its major risk factors, followed by evidence-based management of high blood pressure, diabetes and proteinuria, is likely to be highly cost-effective [27]. The KVC Audit Study has revealed evidence–practice gaps in the management of blood pressure and cholesterol in Aboriginal primary care, similar to gaps in mainstream primary care, which, if closed, would improve heart and kidney health outcomes for Indigenous Australians [9].

Substantial evidence underlines that lowering blood pressure is effective in reducing heart attacks, stroke and cardiac death [28] and favours the use of treatment regimens which include a particular class of drugs, ACE inhibitors, in slowing the progression of CKD [29]. Such evidence is most compelling for patients with kidney disease due to diabetes [30]. Diabetes is the leading cause of ESKD in many countries and is the primary cause or an associated condition for the vast majority of Indigenous Australians commencing dialysis for ESKD. As described in other sections of this book that address diabetes organ complications, large trials in people with diabetes have provided strong evidence that intensive control of blood glucose delays the onset or progression of diabetic kidney disease, particularly in its early stages [31]. Despite a lack of controlled trials indicating benefit within the Australian Indigenous population, chronic disease management programs in remote Aboriginal communities, which compared program results with disease rates for the population prior to the program, indicate the heart and kidney benefits from intensive management regimens [32].

The need for monitoring

Recent research has confirmed the lack of reliable, population-representative data for Indigenous Australians regarding the burden of CKD and related chronic conditions, risk factors for the development and progression of chronic disease, and utilisation of relevant preventative and treatment services. As concluded in the AIHW report on prevention of cardiovascular disease, diabetes and CKD [33]:

> There is clearly a need for ongoing monitoring in the area of prevention. However, better data are needed, in particular those based on measurement rather than self-reported data, as well as systematic data on population-level initiatives.

The Australian Health Survey (AHS), which commenced in 2011 and aims to involve around 50 000 Australians, will include an Aboriginal and Torres Strait Islander wave in 2012 [34]. This is a key step towards filling this data gap. Amongst its objectives, the AHS aims to estimate the prevalence of certain chronic conditions and selected biomedical and behavioural risk factors. Informed and consenting participants in the AHS, from a representative household-based sample of the population, will answer questions about their health; have their height, weight, waist circumference and blood pressure measured; and will be asked for separate consent to give blood and urine samples to measure markers of chronic disease including heart disease, diabetes and CKD. Such monitoring will form one necessary part of a coordinated prevention strategy aiming to reduce the burden of complex chronic disease amongst Indigenous Australians.

Conclusion

The National Indigenous Health Equality Summit, held in Canberra in March 2008, proposed a set of key targets to achieve the COAG commitment of closing the Aboriginal and Torres Strait Islander life expectancy gap within a generation. With the major contribution of premature death due to chronic diseases, we must comprehensively address chronic disease prevention and management using appropriate, sustainable and cost-effective strategies. The summit promulgated a prevention target relevant to CKD: 'Stabilize all-cause incidence of ESKD within five to ten years' [35]. Although ESKD directly affects fewer than 1500 Indigenous Australians [36], the impact of this chronic disease on families and communities is profound. Key findings of the recent Department of Health and Ageing Central Australia Renal Study [17] regarding the social and cultural impacts of ESKD include:

- For Aboriginal patients [in remote regions], uptake of treatment for ESKD has generally necessitated permanently moving away from kin and community. Consequences have included loss of social and cultural connectedness, loss of autonomy and control, and loss of status and authority.
- Key family and cultural leaders having to move away has profoundly affected communities.
- Patients moving to town for treatment are generally accompanied by immediate family carers and dependents. Research has estimated that as many as five people may follow

a person going for dialysis. This has implications for accommodation, social support services, employment and education.

These findings are relevant to the experiences of Indigenous Australians across remote Australia [37]. The devastating impact of ESKD was confirmed by many people interviewed for the Central Australia Renal Study. Their experiece underscores the imperative to prevent and optimise the management of CKD [17]:

> When my husband went onto dialysis, he got really angry and depressed … It was really hard. We had to move into town. There was no support to help us cope. He lost everything … he felt useless. (Wife of a dialysis patient, October 2010)

> I was born and bred on these lands. How on earth could I go all the way to the city, away from my family and country, knowing there was no possibility for them to come down and stay with me, no accommodation, no facilities … There's no way I could think about being so far away … I'd just be in total despair all the time. (Senior community member, September 2010)

References

1. National Preventative Health Strategy (2010). *Australia: the healthiest country by 2020. The report of the National Preventative Health Strategy: the roadmap for action*. Canberra: National Preventative Health Strategy.

2. Australian Institute of Health and Welfare (2011). *Contribution of chronic disease to the gap in adult mortality between Aboriginal and Torres Strait Islander and other Australians*. Canberrra: Australian Institute of Health and Welfare.

3. Australian Institute of Health and Welfare (2011). *Comparing life expectancy of indigenous people in Australia, New Zealand, Canada and the United States: conceptual, methodological and data issues*. Canberra: AIHW.

4. Cass A, Cunningham J, Wang Z & Hoy W (2001). Regional variation in the incidence of end-stage renal disease in Indigenous Australians. *Medical Journal of Australia*, 175(1): 24–27.

5. Preston-Thomas A, Cass A & O'Rourke P (2007). Trends in the incidence of treated end-stage kidney disease among Indigenous Australians and access to treatment. *The Australian and New Zealand Journal of Public Health*, 31(5): 419–21.

6. Australian Institute of Health and Welfare (2010). *Chronic kidney disease hospitalisations in Australia 2000–01 to 2007–08*. Canberra: Australian Institute of Health and Welfare.

7. White SL, Polkinghorne KR, Atkins RC & Chadban SJ (2010). Comparison of the prevalence and mortality risk of CKD in Australia using the CKD Epidemiology Collaboration (CKD-EPI) and Modification of Diet in Renal Disease (MDRD) Study GFR estimating equations: the AusDiab (Australian Diabetes, Obesity and Lifestyle) Study. *American Journal of Kidney Disease*, 55(4): 660–70.

8. Australian Institute of Health and Welfare (2009). *An overview of chronic kidney disease in Australia 2009*. Canberra: Australian Institute of Health and Welfare.

9.   Peiris DP, Patel AA, Cass A, Howard MP, Tchan ML, Brady JP, et al. (2009). Cardiovascular disease risk management for Aboriginal and Torres Strait Islander peoples in primary healthcare settings: findings from the Kanyini Audit. *Medical Journal of Australia*, 191(6): 304–09.

10.   Cass A, Cunningham J, Wang Z & Hoy W (2001). Social disadvantage and variation in the incidence of end-stage renal disease in Australian capital cities. *The Australian and New Zealand Journal of Public Health*, 25(4): 322–26.

11.   White SL, Perkovic V, Cass A, Chang CL, Poulter NR, Spector T, et al. (2009). Is low birth weight an antecedent of CKD in later life? A systematic review of observational studies. *American Journal of Kidney Disease*, 54(2): 248–61.

12.   Hoy WE, Hughson MD, Singh GR, Douglas-Denton R & Bertram JF (2006). Reduced nephron number and glomerulomegaly in Australian Aborigines: a group at high risk for renal disease and hypertension. *Kidney International*, 70(1): 104–10.

13.   White AV, Hoy WE & McCredie DA (2001). Childhood post-streptococcal glomerulonephritis as a risk factor for chronic renal disease in later life. *Medical Journal of Australia*, 174(10): 492–96.

14.   Cass A, Cunningham J, Snelling P, Wang Z & Hoy W (2002). End-stage renal disease in Indigenous Australians: a disease of disadvantage. *Ethnicity and Disease*, 12(3): 373–78.

15.   Cass A, Cunningham J, Snelling P, Wang Z & Hoy W (2004). Exploring the pathways leading from disadvantage to end-stage renal disease for Indigenous Australians. *Social Science & Medicine,* 58(4): 767–85.

16.   Cass A, Lowell A, Christie M, Snelling PL, Flack M, Marrnganyin B, et al. (2002). Sharing the true stories: improving communication between Aboriginal patients and healthcare workers. *Medical Journal of Australia*, 176(10): 466–70.

17.   Department of Health and Ageing (2011). *Central Australia renal study June 2011*. Part 3: Technical Report. Canberra: Department of Health and Ageing.

18.   Yeates KE, Cass A, Sequist TD, McDonald SP, Jardine MJ, Trpeski L, et al. (2009). Indigenous people in Australia, Canada, New Zealand and the United States are less likely to receive renal transplantation. *Kidney International*, 76(6): 659–64.

19.   Australian Institute of Health and Welfare (2011). *Chronic kidney disease in Aboriginal and Torres Strait Islander people 2011*. Canberra: Australian Institute of Health and Welfare.

20.   Dabelea D & Pettitt DJ (2001). Intrauterine diabetic environment confers risks for type 2 diabetes mellitus and obesity in the offspring, in addition to genetic susceptibility. *Journal of Pediatric Endocrinology & Metabolism,* 14(8): 1085–91.

21.   Pettitt DJ, Forman MR, Hanson RL, Knowler WC & Bennett PH (1997). Breastfeeding and incidence of non-insulin-dependent diabetes mellitus in Pima Indians. *The Lancet*, 350(9072): 166–68.

22.   Yajnik CS (2002). The lifecycle effects of nutrition and body size on adult adiposity, diabetes and cardiovascular disease. *Obesity Review*, 3(3): 217–24.

23.   Hoy WE, Rees M, Kile E, Mathews JD & Wang Z (1999). A new dimension to the Barker hypothesis: low birthweight and susceptibility to renal disease. *Kidney International*, 56(3): 1072–77.

24. Pholeros P, Rainow S & Torzillo PJ (1994). *Housing for health: towards a healthier living environment for Aborigines*. Sydney: HealthHabitat.

25. Silva DT, Lehmann D, Tennant MT, Jacoby P, Wright H & Stanley FJ (2008). Effect of swimming pools on antibiotic use and clinic attendance for infections in two Aboriginal communities in Western Australia. *Medical Journal of Australia*, 188(10): 594–98.

26. Rowley KG, Daniel M, Skinner K, Skinner M, White GA & O'Dea K (2000). Effectiveness of a community-directed 'healthy lifestyle' program in a remote Australian Aboriginal community. *The Australian and New Zealand Journal of Public Health*, 24(2): 136–44.

27. Howard K, White S, Salkeld G, McDonald S, Craig JC, Chadban S, et al. (2010). Cost-effectiveness of screening and optimal management for diabetes, hypertension, and chronic kidney disease: a modeled analysis. *Value in Health*, 13: 196–208.

28. Turnbull F (2003). Effects of different blood-pressure-lowering regimens on major cardiovascular events: results of prospectively designed overviews of randomised trials. *The Lancet*, 362(9395): 1527–35.

29. Jafar TH, Schmid CH, Landa M, Giatras I, Toto R, Remuzzi G, et al. (2001). Angiotensin-converting enzyme inhibitors and progression of nondiabetic renal disease. A meta-analysis of patient-level data. *Annals of Internal Medicine,* 135(2): 73–87.

30. Jafar TH, Stark PC, Schmid CH, Landa M, Maschio G, de Jong PE, et al. (2003). Progression of chronic kidney disease: the role of blood pressure control, proteinuria, and angiotensin-converting enzyme inhibition: a patient-level meta-analysis. *Annals of Internal Medicine*, 139(4): 244–52.

31. Jun M, Perkovic V & Cass A (2011). Intensive glycemic control and renal outcome. In Lai KN & Tang SCW (Eds). *Diabetes and the kidney* (pp196–208). Basel: Karger.

32. Hoy W, Baker PR, Kelly AM & Wang Z (2000). Reducing premature death and renal failure in Australian Aboriginals: a community-based cardiovascular and renal protective program. *Medical Journal of Australia*, 172(10): 473–78.

33. Australian Institute of Health and Welfare (2009). *Prevention of cardiovascular disease, diabetes and chronic kidney disease: targeting risk factors*. Canberra: Australian Institute of Health and Welfare.

34. Australian Bureau of Statistics (2011). Australian Health Survey [Online]. Available: http://www.abs.gov.au/websitedbs/D3310114.nsf/home/australian+health+survey [Accessed: 21 September 2011]

35. Aboriginal and Torres Strait Islander Social Justice Commissioner and the Steering Committee for Indigenous Health Equality (2008). Close the Gap – National Indigenous health equality targets: outcomes from the National Indigenous Health Equality Summit Canberra, 18–20 March 2008. Sydney: Human Rights and Equal Opportunity Commission.

36. Australia and New Zealand Dialysis and Transplant Registry (2011). *ANZDATA Registry 2010 report*. Adelaide: Australia and New Zealand Dialysis and Transplant Registry.

37. Anderson K, Devitt J, Cunningham J, Preece C & Cass A (2008). 'All they said was my kidneys were dead': Indigenous Australian patients' understanding of their chronic kidney disease. *Medical Journal of Australia*, 189(9): 499–503.

8

The case for and against the regulation of food marketing directed towards children

Bridget Kelly,[1] Rohan Miller[2] and Lesley King[1]

Authoritative and comprehensive reviews of studies on the nature and extent of food marketing to children indicate that children are exposed to high levels of food marketing and that the 'marketed diet' typically comprises energy-dense, micronutrient-poor foods. However, the implication of causality between marketing, product exposures and childhood obesity is not universally accepted. A vigorous discussion rages about appropriate policy responses to children's exposure to food marketing. The advocacy by many health and consumer groups for tighter government restrictions on food marketing is juxtaposed to the views held by many in the food and advertising industries. Pivotal in this debate is the role of evidence in policy decisions and the appropriateness of industry self-regulation versus government intervention in food marketing. This chapter will explore the dietary and health implications of children's exposure to unhealthy food marketing and present arguments for and against regulations to restrict this marketing.

Unhealthy food marketing to children has become a highly politicised debate in Australia and internationally. Health and consumer groups cite substantial bodies of research that children's exposure to unhealthy food marketing is a contributing factor in the development of children's food preferences and purchases, and hence plays a role in rising rates of childhood obesity. As such, these groups have called on government to restrict marketing as an obesity prevention initiative. At the same time, the food and advertising industries rebut these claims, and promulgate the relative benefits of industry self-regulatory mechanisms. This chapter presents both public health and marketing perspectives, in the form of a 'head to head' debate presenting arguments for and against regulation of food marketing.

A key driver in this debate comes from psychological research that children are highly vulnerable to advertising promotions and consequently require protection from this form of marketing. One reason for this is because young children, especially those less than five years of age, are unable to distinguish commercial content from non-commercial content [1]. For example, when viewing television, very young children are unable to differentiate

---

1 Prevention Research Collaboration, Sydney School of Public Health, University of Sydney.

2 University of Sydney Business School.

between a program and an advertisement break. For older children, despite being able to identify advertising, these children still have an impaired ability to interpret marketing messages critically as they lack the necessary cognitive skills and experience. Up until the age of eight years, most children are unable to recognise the persuasive nature of advertising effectively, and tend to accept advertising as truthful, accurate and unbiased [1].

While children's vulnerability to some forms of marketing has been recognised, the effect of marketing and the most appropriate approach to limit children's marketing exposure is contested by health and industry groups. The key points of debate covered in this chapter concern the quality and sufficiency of evidence which underpins any regulatory initiative, the range of media that would need to be covered by any regulation, and the quality and type of foods that are advertised and potentially subject to regulation.

The case FOR regulating food marketing directed towards children

The effect of marketing on children's food choices and habits

There is a large and accumulating body of research to support the association between the marketing of energy-dense nutrient-poor ('unhealthy') foods and beverages, and childhood obesity. This includes at least seven major systematic reviews synthesising the scientific evidence on the impact of food marketing to children [2–8]. Most of these systematic reviews have been commissioned by key health organisations, such as the Institute of Medicine in the US and the World Health Organization, and have been updated regularly to include new evidence. Such reviews take into account the quality of evidence, by considering methodological limitations and consistency between studies.

The most recent systematic review, commissioned by the World Health Organization in 2008, found that food advertising has a modest impact on children's nutrition knowledge, their food preferences and their consumption patterns, with subsequent implications for weight gain and obesity [8]. In particular, research indicated that children are able to recall a high number of food advertisements and that these advertisements were enjoyed and discussed amongst their peers [9–11]. Further, advertisements created a desire in children to purchase food products, and the majority of children either purchased these products themselves or asked their parents to buy these products for them [12–14].

Importantly, food marketing is thought to operate at both the brand and the food category level [8], thereby influencing not only the particular product brands that children choose but also their broader consumption patterns. For example, advertisements for a particular brand of confectionery will not only generate a desire for that brand but also for confectionery in general [8].

Contribution of food marketing to childhood obesity

The causes of obesity are many and complex, comprising an array of sociological, environmental and genetic influences. Unhealthy food marketing is only one such environmental factor that contributes to the obesity-promoting environment. Other factors, such as family and peer networks, engagement in physical activity, and socioeconomic status also influence children's food choices and risk of weight gain and obesity [5].

In the context of the full range of contributing factors, the specific contribution that television food advertising makes to childhood obesity is estimated to be small to moderate in size, with some studies estimating that 2% of the variation in food choice and obesity is attributed to this advertising [15]. However, even small effects in statistical terms can have an appreciable effect when they influence a large population and are ongoing. These estimated effects are based on the contribution of television food advertising alone, and may be increased when marketing from other forms of media are included [5]. Given that the majority of advertised foods are energy dense and nutrient poor, this advertising encourages additional consumption of these food types that are already consumed in excess by Australian children [16]. Data from the 1995 National Nutrition Survey identified that energy-dense, nutrient-poor foods contribute 41% of children's daily energy intake, while dietary recommendations allow for between 5%–20% of energy from these discretionary foods [16]. In addition, the act of television viewing itself contributes to sedentary lifestyles and obesity, independent of the effects of food advertising [17].

Researchers have predicted that the magnitude of the specific effect of food advertising on food behaviours and weight is at least the same as that of many other determinants of obesity, including family and parents, peers and socioeconomic status [8]. Therefore, food marketing has as much impact on obesity as these other factors and is amenable to intervention, making it one of a number of potential levers for change.

Nature and scope of food marketing to children

Evidence on the effect of food marketing on children's food preferences and consumption is concerning as the majority of advertised foods are high in fat, sugar and/or salt. Indeed, the top products that are advertised to children internationally on television are sugar-sweetened breakfast cereals, soft drinks, confectionery and high-fat savoury snacks, while the promotion of healthy food choices, including fruit, vegetables, whole grains and milk is virtually non-existent [8]. The frequency of advertisements for fast food restaurants is also increasing [8]. One study from Australia identified that even during a A$5 million government campaign promoting fruit and vegetable consumption, television advertisements for healthy foods only contributed to 5% of all food advertisements across the whole study period, while 82% were for high-fat/high-sugar foods [18]. The heavy and ubiquitous marketing of these unhealthy food and beverage products assists in promoting these products as normal and desirable.

Most of the research and attention on children's exposure to food marketing has been directed to television food advertising. However, it is widely acknowledged that food marketing encompasses a range of different media platforms and food marketing campaigns are increasingly integrating these different marketing channels to more widely promote their messages [19].

These marketing channels include: *broadcast media* (eg television, cinema and radio); *new technology* (eg the internet and SMS/text messaging); *print media* (eg magazines and newspapers); *promotions* (eg premium offers, celebrity endorsements, cartoon characters, health and nutrient claims and product placements); *places* (eg school canteens and vending machines, sporting events and supermarkets); *price* where products are sold at cheaper prices to make them more available and appealing to children; *packaging* that is appealing to children; *product expansion* by selling multiple variations of a product; and *public relations* by sponsoring television programs, sporting events, fundraising and establishing or donating money to charity.

Data on industry marketing expenditure can be used to assess the spread of media used by food marketers. While available Australian information is limited, data from the UK indicate that between 2003 and 2007 there was a 19% increase in industry expenditure on food and beverage advertising, from £704m to £838m [20]. Over the same time period, expenditure on print advertising increased the most, with an increase of 159% or £107m. By comparison, expenditure on television food advertising increased by only 6% or £34m [20]. From this expenditure information, it appears that food marketers are shifting away from traditionally used advertising modes, such as television. Of concern is that these other forms of media are often used by children without parental supervision, making them more difficult for parents to monitor and control.

Some examples of integrated marketing campaigns by food companies promoting products high in fat, sugar, and/or salt have included the Nestle Smarties 8 Colours of Fun campaign (www.smarties-australia.com.au, accessed 20 June 2011). This campaign involved the creation of multi-media clips featuring eight young children teamed up with musicians, sculptors, dancers, photographers and installation artists to create an artwork inspired by each of the eight different Smarties colours. These clips were then broadcast through the Smarties website and online social networking sites, including YouTube and Facebook, as well as through television, press and in-store promotions. The Streets Paddle Pop Elemagika Lick-a-Prize campaign is a further example of integrated marketing (www. paddlepop.com.au, accessed 20 June 2011). This campaign incorporated a short film starring the Paddle Pop Lion, a website featuring branded games, a Facebook page, and a competition requiring the purchase of Paddle Pop ice-creams to uncover prize codes listed on ice-cream sticks. Additional codes for prizes could be found in television and magazine advertisements.

The power of pestering

The raison d'être of marketing is to create a desire for advertised products. In the case of children, marketing can influence their own food purchases, as well as the purchase behaviour of parents [21]. Children's purchase requests, often referred to as 'pester power' or 'purchase influence attempts', can create tension in child–parent relationships and result in the purchase of these products despite parents' awareness of their poor nutritional quality [22]. As such, advertising commentators have claimed that 'by advertising to children, companies are encouraging the child to nag their parents into buying something that is not good for them, they don't need or the parent cannot afford' [23]. This phenomenon of children 'nagging' for advertised products has been repeatedly reported by parents [8].

In the supermarket setting, children employ various techniques to encourage parents to purchase food items. For example, in a qualitative study from the UK, children reported that they kept on requesting products until their parents conceded. This is typified in the response from one child, who was reported as saying 'you just keep saying please mum, please mum, please mum, and then she gets it' [24].

Research also indicates that children's purchase requests often result in actual product purchases. In a review of studies on the effect of children's purchase requests on parents' purchasing responses, children were found to request products an average of 15 times per supermarket visit (around one request for every two minutes spent in the supermarket), and around half of all children's requests were successful [22]. Further, children's exposure to food marketing increased their purchase requests for advertised foods [22].

Parents' responses to children's purchase requests are also likely to be influenced by their socioeconomic status. In interviews conducted with over 1000 parents and their children in the UK, the most socially disadvantaged parents were more open to persuasion by children and were more likely to agree to the statement 'I buy what the children want', compared to less disadvantaged parents [25].

As such, the marketing of unhealthy food to children impedes the ability of parents to promote and support healthy eating. This appears to be particularly the case for socially disadvantaged families, who are also the most vulnerable to excessive weight gain and obesity [26]. In the face of exceedingly sophisticated and integrated food marketing campaigns, spanning multiple media platforms, parents' ability to subjugate children's purchase requests are likely to be further diminished.

The role of industry self-regulation in minimising harm to children from unhealthy food marketing

In recent times, there has been vigorous discussion regarding appropriate policy responses to the issue of children's high and diversifying exposure to the marketing of unhealthy food and beverages. In particular, there has been significant advocacy from health and consumer groups calling for government restrictions to protect children from these promotional messages. Meanwhile, the food and advertising industries have been actively involved in promoting self-regulatory approaches to limit this marketing. These may be seen as good corporate responsibility, or more likely, as a means of diverting criticism and impeding government regulations.

In an analysis of available regulations to restrict unhealthy food marketing to children across 73 countries between 2004 and 2006, most new regulations came from the food and advertising industries [27]. The number of countries with industry self-regulations increased from 11 in 2004 to 23 by the end of 2006, including the revision and extension of industry codes in Australia, Canada and the US [27]. These regulatory codes are typically overseen by an industry body and participation by individual food companies is voluntary.

In Australia, the Australian Food and Grocery Council, the national body representing food and grocery manufacturers, introduced the Responsible Children's Marketing Initiative in 2009, which aims to 'provide a framework for food and beverage companies to promote healthy dietary choices and lifestyles to Australian children' [28]. As well, the Australian Association of National Advertisers introduced a similar initiative in 2009 relating to the quick service (fast food) industry [29].

Independently conducted evaluations of the Australian Food and Grocery Council code have compared the amount of television advertising from companies participating in this self-regulatory initiative before and after its introduction [30]. These evaluations show that overall unhealthy food advertising did not decrease following the introduction of the codes, despite a reduction in television advertisements for unhealthy food items by participating companies. The main reason for the ineffectiveness of this self-regulation was the limited participation in these codes by food companies [30]. As at May 2011, only 17 food companies had signed up to this initiative.

As well, in an analysis of the nutrition criteria used to define foods as appropriate to be marketed to children, industry-developed nutrition criteria vary between companies and tended to be more permissive than independently developed standards [31]. Of the 52 food products that were assessed, only 38% were considered healthy by independent criteria, although 83% were deemed appropriate using industry standards including items such as chocolate, confectionery, sugary drinks and ice-cream [31].

The findings of these evaluations indicate that self-regulatory initiatives, in their current form, are insufficient to curb the amount of unhealthy food marketing that children are exposed to and the effect of this marketing. By comparing successful and less successful self-regulatory initiatives across a range of industries, including tobacco, alcohol, fisheries and forestry industries, Sharma and colleagues proposed eight standards that should be met if self-regulation is to be effective [32]. These included input from all stakeholders, transparency, meaningful objectives, objective evaluation and public reporting, and oversight [32]. In the case of food and beverage marketing, self-regulatory initiatives would require: the input of health and consumer groups as well as government and the food and advertising industries; transparency in developing standards on how breaches can be reported; be targeted towards reducing children's exposure to unhealthy food marketing and the persuasiveness of this marketing; be regularly evaluated for their effectiveness; involve public reporting on industry's adherence to regulations; and be overseen by an appropriate regulatory or health body.

The role of government in creating real and sustainable change in children's exposure to unhealthy food marketing

Governments have a clear leadership role, particularly in relation to the protection of children, protecting public health, overseeing broadcast and non-broadcast information environments and balancing the operation of free markets in the public interest. In the case of food marketing to children, government can provide leadership through statutory regulation or through co-regulation with industry. Statutory regulation has been most commonly called for by health and consumer advocates, as this has the benefit of being independent, having greater accountability, ensuring unilateral compliance across all industry groups and of operating within the public interest.

In 2010, the World Health Organization released a set of recommendations for limiting the marketing of foods and non-alcoholic beverages to children [33]. One recommendation was that government should play a lead role in developing, monitoring and evaluating regulations to limit children's exposure to unhealthy food marketing.

Evidence of the effectiveness of statutory regulations to reduce children's exposure to unhealthy food marketing

Government restriction on television advertising to children has been a longstanding policy in Sweden (since 1991), Norway (since 1992), and across all media in Quebec, Canada (since 1980). While no systematic evaluations of the effectiveness of these regulations have been conducted, there is a small amount of research to indicate that these regulations have been effective in reducing children's exposure to unhealthy food advertising and the effect of this marketing.

One study from Quebec examined household purchases of breakfast cereals between English-speaking children, exposed to American television, and French-speaking children who tended to watch more French-language television. At the time of this research, French-language television channels banned advertisements targeting children whereas television broadcast from the US was not subject to these restrictions. Findings from this study indicate that English-speaking children, who had a higher exposure to advertisements for children's cereals, had significantly higher household purchases of advertised cereals compared to French-speaking children [34]. Research also indicates that children in Quebec have the lowest prevalence of obesity across all Canadian provinces, and the second lowest prevalence of overweight [35].

Additionally, in 2008 the Office of Communications in the UK introduced restrictions on the scheduling of television advertising of food and drink products to children. Under these regulations, advertisements for unhealthy food and beverage products were precluded from being shown in or around programs specifically designed for children or of appeal to children less than 16 years of age, and on dedicated children's channels. An evaluation of the impact of these regulations on children's exposure to unhealthy food advertising found that, compared to 2005, children saw around 34% fewer unhealthy food advertisements in the year following the introduction of regulations [36]. As such, these government regulations have been effective in reducing children's exposure to unhealthy food and beverage advertising and reducing the effect of this marketing on food purchases.

The case AGAINST regulating food marketing directed towards children

A complex array of rules and regulations already exists governing food marketing across multiple tiers of government. Social contract theory has long acknowledged the need for common rules in order for people to protect themselves and one another from harm. That food marketing should be regulated is not an issue; however, questions need to be asked about the veracity and standard of evidence that justify changes to the existing legislation and self-regulation frameworks, how the outcomes of the new laws will be measured, what will happen if the new laws don't have the desired effect, and what other implications will additional regulations present to our market economy. Any proposed change to the regulation of food marketing should be realistic and likely to be effective in behavioural change. Considerable doubt exists that even the most extreme restrictions to the existing level of Australia's commercial speech will render the desired behavioural change.

What is marketing: now and in the immediate future?

The overwhelming body of academic literature discussing food marketing is embedded in the era of television dominated mass marketing characterised by the *Mad Men* television series (see www.amctv.com/shows/mad-men). However, television advertising is no longer omnipotent; marketing professionals, regulators and consumers face increasingly fragmented media. Experience is king. Companies seek to engage with consumers by offering elements of emotions, logic and general thought processes to connect with the consumer. Pushing a message is passé: consumers are the recipients of thousands of commercial marketing messages, each day. There is no way that consumers can react to all of the advertising or marketing communications they receive and they have become expert at filtering out unwanted messages.

In the *Mad Men* era of mass media primacy it was commonly assumed there was a linear relationship called a purchase funnel that was also encapsulated in hierarchical advertising models. These simple advertising models generalised that brand awareness led to familiarity with the brand, then to consideration for purchase, the act of purchase, and thereafter, repeated purchase. However, as categories and brands matured, new empirically based behavioural models of consumer behaviour were proposed suggesting habits were a major consideration in stable markets [37].

Consistent with the behavioural models, streetwise marketers sought to influence purchase decisions at or immediately before the point of purchase; in effect, to encourage brand switching. This shift largely explains the ascent of marketing techniques such as sampling, premiums, coupons, discounts, in-store radio, signs, and shelf space (slotting) in the marketing mix in order to influence short-term purchase behaviour, and ideally leading to repeat purchase or habit. It also provides historical context to the contemporary view that consumers undertake an increasingly sophisticated and technologically driven journey along many brand touch-points rather than being causally influenced by single or multiple forms of media. These marketing tactics, however, are not always successful, nor do they typically deliver long-term behavioural change [38].

Causality: silver or rusting bullet?

The case for regulating food marketing to children is based on assumptions that food advertising has a causal influence on children's food choices and that this contributes to rising rates of childhood obesity. It is also assumed that regulatory restrictions or bans on food advertising will reduce rates of obesity and associated health problems. These assumptions appear to be unwarranted due to a lack of evidence and the continued evolution of communications practice. Holland et al. comment that the perceived threat of obesity is deemed to be so great that efforts to contain it may be subjected to less scrutiny than they warrant [39]. Suggested remedies based on incorrect assumptions are likely to be ineffective [40].

There are a number of possible causal relationships between television viewing and obesity. Critics of food advertising assume that more television viewing leads to more exposure to food advertising which in turn leads to purchase requests and hence increased consumption of unhealthy advertised foods. Television viewing might also lead to increased snacking and reduced family meal times. Increased television viewing may also be associated with a more sedentary lifestyle and hence reduced physical activity. Research linking television viewing with obesity and health outcomes generally do not attempt to distinguish between these three possible explanations of the relationship [5].

Correlational studies do not show causation

It is a fallacy of logic that correlational studies can show a causal relationship between marketing or advertising and obesity. Most of the reviews alleging that food advertising causes obesity have been largely based on correlational studies examining television viewing. For example, the US Institute of Medicine Committee on Food Marketing and the Diets of Children and Youth published a report cited by Livingstone [5] concluding, on the basis of 123 studies, that television advertising influences the food and drink preferences, purchase requests, and short-term consumption of children aged two to 11 years.

Livingstone [5] noted that the typical research designs linking marketing to behaviour/ diet and to health outcomes were mostly surveys with low quality measures and low causal inference validity. Ecological validity was mostly high as these surveys considered real world behaviour. Most of these studies assessed exposure to advertisements through assessing general television viewing. Livingstone noted that only five findings from four published studies combined high causal inference validity and high ecological validity. None of these four studies demonstrated that exposure to advertising causes obesity. One study using a quasi-experimental design found that advertising exposure produced more favourable evaluations of products compared to non-exposure, but this did not affect purchasing decisions [41].

Much recent research on the link between advertising and obesity has largely been correlational in design because researchers have assumed that there is sufficient evidence of a causal link between the two [5]. However, this assumption seems inappropriate as research has not been able to disentangle confounding factors, such as lack of physical activity, or parental factors, that could plausibly have much larger effects on obesity. For example, there is research suggesting that higher levels of television watching are associated with permissive parenting styles that may be associated with less parental control over children's dietary behaviours [42]. The relevance of this causal assumption must also be questioned with the decline in television viewing and the proliferation of other 'screens' increasingly used by children, adolescents and adults.

Mass media impact: going down

Technology evolves constantly, and rapidly. Moore's law predicts technological changes will occur at an exponential rate (approximately). Marketing communications are at the cutting edge of the technological development, often underpinning the commercial business model for change. Moreover, internet-based communications are increasingly integrated with other media, other forms of promotion, and even product offerings. From a research perspective, the rapid evolution of technologically based innovations in marketing makes their impact hard to assess, especially in a timely way, and also suggests evidence-based regulations will lag considerably behind marketing practice.

If advertising causes obesity through its influence on consumption of unhealthy foods then it would be reasonable to assume that rising rates of obesity would be accompanied by a rise in children's exposure to advertising and an increase in consumption of advertised foods [42]. Conclusions that advertising leads to obesity have been based largely on studies of television advertising [1–8]. However, children's television viewing has declined rather than increased over the last two decades [42]. Furthermore, due to the widespread diffusion of cable television, an increasing number of children spend more time watching channels with little or no outside product advertising than watching broadcast television programs.

Expenditure on television advertising for food is only one indicator of possible advertising influence and should not be assumed a measure of behavioural change. Moreover, advertising expenditure needs to be considered against changes in the cost for advertising, real dollar changes and declining audience levels (implying higher costs for a consistent level of reach and frequency). This means it costs considerably more in real dollars to have the same reach and frequency in 2012 than in 1992. Data from the UK suggest that food advertising on television declined from 34% of advertising in 1982 to 18% in 2002 [43].

Technological innovations have also reduced how much attention children pay to advertising. For example, the use of remote controls encourage channel surfing, and the introduction of video recorders, themselves largely rendered obsolete by the digital innovations TiVo and Foxtel, mean that viewers can record then zip (fast forward) or zap (switch to another channel) with minimal advertising exposure. In fairness, however, television ratings in Australia suggest only a very small percentage of viewers presently do this. As digital television broadcasting increases, the percentage of viewers who pre-record shows for later watching will likely increase, further leading to declining levels of advertising impact.

Technology is shifting traditional free-to-air television from omnipotence to a background media (similar to the audience shift from radio following the introduction of television). Accompanying the decline in television viewing led by younger demographics, there appears to be an increase in non-television 'screen time', such as computer use, videos, DVDS and video games [42]. Time playing video games is positively associated with risk of obesity [42] as is computer usage time [44], and yet video games are largely advertisement free and what advertising they have is not usually food related. There has also been an increase in media multi-tasking (such as computer, iPad, SMS or Facebook use) during television viewing times, meaning that children pay less attention to commercials [42]. Additionally, studies of television suggest viewing might also conflate time spent watching videos and DVDs with time watching commercial television [7]. These factors together suggest that children's exposure and susceptibility to food advertising, and particularly televised advertising, has significantly decreased while obesity rates are claimed to be increasing. None of these moderating developments have been factored into research based in the *Mad Men* era.

It is also largely unexplained why television is claimed to lead to a causal relationship when other media do not. For example, a study on magazine advertisements for healthy and less-healthy foods found no effects on hunger or food preferences in pre-adolescent children [45]. Clearly more research on non-television food marketing is required in order to make informed decisions as to why regulation should occur primarily in one form of media rather than all media, and why advertisements on television are assumed to be problematic yet those in other media are ignored.

The advertising–obesity causality argument also ignores culturally based consumption habits. For example, in New Zealand, demand for fish and chips, an unadvertised product, is substantially larger than demand for heavily advertised fast foods such as hamburgers [40]. It is also argued that demand for a product can be primarily influenced by price and consumer wealth [40]. Reductions in advertising may lead to cost-based competition that could be passed on to consumers through price reductions and can have the effect of increasing consumption. Therefore, restricting food advertising could actually increase consumption of unhealthy foods, unless measures to increase the price, such as a 'sin tax' were introduced.

Obesity: evolving, but not necessarily growing

Research from the UK suggests that dietary energy intake has declined between 1983 and 1999 [43]. Similarly, US data show that Americans decreased their consumption of fat between 1965 and 1995 [40]. If advertising caused obesity due to increased consumption of unhealthy foods there would logically only be evidence of increased energy consumption. The findings that energy consumption has decreased while obesity has risen suggest the cause of obesity is not necessarily increased energy input. Rather, there may be an under-addressed issue related to decreasing energy output, that is, decreased physical activity and lifestyle.

The importance of decreased physical activity needs to be considered when interpreting findings that exposure to television advertising is modestly correlated with obesity. Cross-sectional studies have found that children's television viewing is positively associated with increased consumption of fat, sweet and salty snacks and carbonated beverages. Researchers assume that television exposure affects food consumption via advertising and consequent purchase requests to parents [46]. Studies finding a correlation between television watching and obesity/health outcomes often understate other potential explanatory variables, including the nature of any assumed causal relationship [5]. Excess television watching might be a symptom, rather than a cause, of a sedentary lifestyle leading to obesity [45]. Obesity might cause a sedentary lifestyle in a reciprocal manner. Most studies do not distinguish between whether it is hours of watching television, or amount of advertising seen, that leads to unhealthy eating behaviour [5], although the 1983 study by Bolton [15] is a notable exception. Bolton found that exposure to food advertising had a significant although small effect on snacking (explaining 2% of the variance) but did not have a significant direct effect on energy intake. Bolton found that the influence of parental snacking frequency was stronger than that of food advertising. Food advertising did not have a significant effect on nutrient balance (deviation from percentage of Recommended Daily Intake) for specific nutrients. Parent nutrient balance explained 9% of the variance in nutrient balance.

Interestingly, an intervention to reduce time spent viewing television and playing video games was successful in reducing these behaviours and participants did have a reduction in body mass index (BMI) compared to a control group [47]. However, there was no reduction in high-fat foods or daily servings of highly advertised foods in the diet of the experimental group. Therefore, reducing exposure to television advertising did not appear to have an impact on diet. The authors suggested that decreases in BMI associated with reduced television viewing were due to increases in low-intensity physical activity. One of these studies did find that advertising affected consumption of orange juice (but not of unhealthy foods), but another of these studies found no effect of advertising on purchasing behaviour. Furthermore, reducing television viewing, and presumably exposure to food advertising, did not produce dietary changes but may have increased physical activity. Therefore, the apparent link between food advertising and obesity might be due largely to the associated sedentary lifestyle, a finding supported by Wong et al. [48]. Additionally, the correlation between television viewing and obesity might also be due to unobserved confounding factors [40]. For example, parents who restrict children's hours of television viewing might also encourage healthier diets and lifestyles.

Additional support for the role of lifestyle factors relating to lack of physical activity on obesity is drawn from findings from New Zealand that television viewing was inversely correlated with parental socioeconomic status (SES) [40]. The authors suggested that higher SES families could afford more after-school activities, such as sports electives to keep children occupied. Low SES families often left children unsupervised during after-school hours as it was common for both parents to be working. Children might therefore have tended to occupy their time watching television rather than engaging in outdoor activities. Fear of 'stranger danger' for children playing with little or no supervision, and other possible physical harm through participation in sports, reinforces the view that a sedentary lifestyle may be safer than a more physical lifestyle.

Critics of food advertising have argued that even though the amount of variance in BMI explained by exposure to food advertising appears to be small, the cumulative effects are sufficiently important to warrant restricting or banning food advertising aimed at children. Implementing such restrictive policies might be misguided. Sweden introduced a comprehensive ban on all television advertising aimed at children in 1991 and childhood obesity rates in that country continued to rise [49].

Is the problem too much food, or only the wrong food?

It has been argued that imposing restrictions on advertising of unhealthy foods would be unfair because unhealthy foods have not been clearly defined [50]. Critics of food advertising complain that advertised foods do not match 'recommended diets' [7], yet there is a lack of expert consensus about what constitutes a healthy diet [49]. Proponents of the traditional 'food pyramid' recommend that people derive most of their energy from carbohydrates, yet an increasingly popular alternative view is that energy should be obtained mostly from protein and fat [49].

Developing guidelines for 'acceptable' foods to be advertised would appear to be highly complicated. It is clear that research is continually evolving: perfect knowledge about the perfect diet does not yet exist. Therefore a simpler alternative would be to ban all food advertising altogether. However, banning all food advertising would make it impossible to use television and other media to promote healthy food choices. An experimental study comparing the effects of advertisements for either healthy or junk foods found that, contrary to expectations, advertisements for junk foods did not enhance attitudes or intentions to these foods. On the other hand, advertisements for healthy foods actually did enhance attitudes and intentions to these foods in children who had seen these ads compared to children not exposed to them. This experiment suggests that advertising of healthy foods could actually have a beneficial impact on children's dietary habits [51].

Evidence that advertising of healthy foods can have a beneficial impact on diet was shown by research into the advertising of high-fibre cereals. Advertising containing information that high-fibre foods can reduce the risk of cancer was followed by an increase in market share for these products [42]. Regulations may prohibit certain truthful claims about foods that might be useful to consumers, eg calorie reductions can only be advertised if they are greater than 25% compared to a reference food. Producers might therefore lack incentives to reduce calorie content if they cannot meet this threshold.

Conclusion

The debate about the appropriateness and efficacy of any additional regulation of advertising of unhealthy foods to children centres around key themes: the definition of 'unhealthy' foods, the range of media that would be encompassed by any regulation, and importantly, the interpretation of available evidence. Public health, and food and marketing industries draw from overlapping bodies of evidence regarding the impact of food marketing on children's food consumption and obesity patterns, but draw different conclusions. The complexities of defining both the unhealthy foods and range of media (including new social media) to be covered by any regulation are widely recognised.

The potential of regulatory initiatives to reduce children's exposure to food marketing to some extent is also widely recognised, with debate focused on who should control such regulations. The further impact of this on children's diets and obesity levels is more uncertain, given the broader obesity-promoting environment in which we live. There is scope for the debate to broaden, for example, to introduce regulation to encourage the marketing of healthier foods and improve food product formulation. Or to foster a new approach to self-regulation which has full industry participation and consistent standards for defining unhealthy foods. Future work in this area should focus on estimating the actual impact of food marketing on children's food consumption patterns and obesity, and the development of transparent and meaningful regulations (either statutory or self-regulatory) which truly seek to improve the healthiness of the marketing environment for children.

References

1. American Psychological Association (2004). Report of the APA taskforce on advertising and children. [Online]. Available: www.apa.org/pi/families/resources/advertising-children.pdf [Accessed 16 January 2012].

2. Dalmeny K, Hanna E & Lobstein T (2003). Broadcasting Bad Health: Why food advertising needs to be controlled: International Association of Consumer Food Organisations.

3. Escelante de Cruz A. The junk food generation. A multi-country survey of the influence of television advertisements on children. Consumers International 2004 [22 July 2011]. [Online]. Available: epsl.asu.edu/ceru/Articles/CERU-0407-227-OWI.pdf [Accessed 16 January 2012].

4. Hastings G, McDermott L, Angus K, Stead M & Thomson S (2006). *The extent, nature and effects of food promotion to children: a review of the evidence.* Technical Paper Prepared for The World Health Organization; Geneva.

5. Livingstone S (2006). *New research on advertising foods to children: an updated review of the literature.* Published as Annex 9 to Ofcom Television Advertising of Food and Drink Products to Children consultation. London: Office of Communications (Ofcom).

6. McGinnis MJ, Gootman JA & Kraak VI (2006). *Food Marketing to Children and Youth: threat or Opportunity?* Food and Nutrition Board, Board on Children, Youth and Families, Institute of Medicine of the National Academies. [Online]. Available: books.nap.edu/catalog/11514.html [Accessed 16 January 2012].

7. Hastings G, Stead M, McDermott L, Forsyth A, MacKintosh AM, Rayner M, et al. (2003). Review of research on the effects of food promotion to children. Prepared for the Food Standard Agency. Glasgow: Centre for Social Marketing.

8. Cairns G, Angus K & Hastings G (2009). The extent nature and effects of food promotion to children: a review of the evidence to December 2008. Prepared for the World Health Organization. United Kingdom: Institute for Social Marketing, University of Stirling.

9. Hitchings E, Moynihan P & Moynihan P (1998). The relationship between television food advertisements recalled and actual foods consumed by children. *Journal of Human Nutrition and Dietetics*, 11(6): 511–17.

10. Barry TE & Hansen RW (1973). How race affects children's TV commercials. *Journal of Advertising Research*, 13(5):63–67.

11. Batada A & Borzekowsk D (2008). Snap! Crackle! What? Recognition of cereal advertisements and understanding of commercials' persuasive intent among urban, minority children in the US. *Journal of Children and Media*, 2(1): 19–36.

12. Carruth BR, Goldberg DL & Skinner JD (1991). Do parents and peers mediate the influence of television advertising on food-related purchases? *Journal of Adolescent Research*, 6(2): 253–71.

13. Marshall D, O'Donohoe S & Kline S (2007). Families, food, and pester power: beyond the blame game? *Journal of Consumer Behaviour*, 6(4): 164–81.

14. Maryam A, Mehdi MR, Masood K, Mosoomeh G, Nasrin O & Yadollah M (2005). Food advertising on Iranian children's television: A content analysis and an experimental study with junior high school students. *Ecology of Food and Nutrition*, 44(2): 123–33.

15. Bolton RN (1983). Modeling the impact of television food advertising on children's diets. In JH Leigh & JCR Martin (Eds). *Current issues and research in advertising* (pp173–99). Ann Arbor: University of Michigan

16. Rangan AM, Randall D, Hector DJ, Gill TP & Webb KL (2008). Consumption of 'extra' foods by Australian children: types, quantities and contribution to energy and nutrient intakes. *European Journal of Clinical Nutrition*, 62(3): 356–64.

17. Landhuis CE, Poulton R, Welch D & Hancox RJ (2008). Programming obesity and poor fitness: the long-term impact of childhood television. *Obesity*, 16(6): 1457–59.

18. Chapman K, Kelly B, King L & Flood V (2007). Fat chance for Mr Vegie TV ads. *Australian and New Zealand Journal of Public Health*, 31(2): 190.

19. Dalmeny K, Hanna E & Lobstein T (2003). Broadcasting bad health: why food advertising needs to be controlled. London: The International Association of Consumer Food Organizations.

20. United Kingdom Department of Health (2008). Changes in food and drink advertising and promotion to children: a report outlining the changes in the nature and balance of food and drink advertising and promotion to children, from January 2003 to December 2007. [Online]. Available: www.dh.gov.uk/prod_consum_dh/groups/dh_digitalassets/@dh/@en/documents/digitalasset/dh_089123.pdf [Accessed 16 January 2012].

21. Story M & French S (2004). Food advertising and Marketing Directed at Children and Adolescents in the US. *International Journal of Behavioral Nutrition and Physical Activity*, 1(3).

22. McDermott L, O'Sullivan T, Stead M & Hastings G (2006). International food advertising, pester power and its effects. *International Journal of Advertising*, 25(4): 513–39.

23. Spungin P (2004). Parent power, not pester power. *International Journal of Advertising and Marketing to Children*, 5(3): 37–40.

24. Wilson G & Wood K (2004). The influence of children on parental purchases during supermarket shopping. *International Journal of Consumer Studies*, 28(4): 329–36.

25. Ofcom (2004). Childhood Obesity – Food Advertising in Context. Children's Food Choices, Parents' Understanding and Influence, and the Role of Food Promotion. Office of Communication. [Online]. Available: www.ofcom.org.uk/research/tv/reports/food_ads/report.pdf [Accessed 16 January 2012].

26. King T, Kavanagh AM, Jolley D, Turrell G & Crawford D (2006). Weight and place: a multilevel cross-sectional survey of area-level social disadvantage and overweight/obesity in Australia. *International Journal of Obesity*, 30(2): 281–87.

27. Hawkes C (2007). Regulating and litigating in the public interest: regulating food marketing to young people worldwide: trends and policy drivers. *American Journal of Public Health*, 97(11): 1962–73.

28. Australian Food and Grocery Council (2010). The Responsible Children's Marketing Initiative. [Online]. Available: www.afgc.org.au/industry-codes/advertising-kids.html [Accessed 25 August 2010].

29. Australian Association of National Advertisers. Australian Quick Service Restaurant Industry Initiative for Responsible Advertising and Marketing to Children (2009). [19 January 2010]; Available from: www.aana.com.au/documents/QSRAInitiativeforResponsibleAdvertisingandMarketingtoChildren June2009.pdf.

30. King L, Hebden L, Grunseit A, Kelly B, Chapman K & Venugopal K (2010). Industry self regulation of television food advertising: responsible or responsive? *International Journal of Pediatric Obesity*. DOI: 10.3109/17477166.2010.51731.

31. Hebden L, King L, Kelly B, Chapman K, Innes-Hughes C & Gunatillaka N (2010). Regulating the types of foods and beverages marketed to children: how useful are food industry commitments. *Nutrition & Dietetics* 67(4):258–66.

32. Sharma LL, Teret SP & Brownell KD (2010). The food industry and self-regulation: standards to promote success and to avoid public health failures. *American Journal of Public Health*, 100(2):240–46.

33. World Health Organization. Set of recommendations on the marketing of foods and non-alcoholic beverages to children. Geneva 2010.

34. Goldberg M (1990). A quasi-experiment assessing the effectiveness of TV advertising directed to children. *Journal of Marketing Research*, 27:445–54.

35. GPI Atlantic. Cost of obesity in Quebec. 2000 [23 March 2011]; Available from: www.gpiatlantic.org/pdf/health/obesity/que-obesity.pdf.

36. Ofcom. Changes in the nature and balance of television food advertising to children. 2008 [23 March 2011]; Available from: stakeholders.ofcom.org.uk/market-data-research/tv-research/hfssdec08/.

37. Ehrenberg ASC & Ehrenberg A (1988). *Repeat-buying: facts, theory and applications.* London: Oxford University Press.

38. Lawson M, McGuinness D & Esslemont D (1990). The effect of in-store sampling on the sale of food products. *Marketing Bulletin*, 1: 1–6.

39. Holland KE, Blood RW, Thomas I, Lewis S, Komesaroff PA & Castle DJ (2011). Our girth is plain

to see: an analysis of newspaper coverage of *Australia's Future 'Fat Bomb'*. *Health, Risk & Society*, 13(1): 31–46.

40. Eagle L, Bulmer S, De Bruin A & Kitchen KJ (2004). Exploring the link between obesity and advertising in New Zealand. *Journal of Marketing Communications*, 10: 49–67.

41. Greenberg BS & Brand JE (1993). Television news and advertising in schools: the Channel One controversy. *Journal of Communication*, 43(1): 143–51.

42. Zywicki TJ, Holt D & Ohlhausen, MK (n.d.). Obesity and advertising policy. George Mason School of Law Working Paper Series. Working Paper 3 [Online]. Available: law.bepress.com/gmulwps/gmule/art3/ [Accessed 17 April 2011].

43. Ambler T (2004). Does the UK promotion of food and drink to children contribute to their obesity? Centre for marketing working paper, No. 4–901. London Business School, Centre for Marketing.

44. Russ SA, Larson K, Franke TM & Halfon N (2009). Associations between media use and health in US children. *Academic Paediatrics*, 9(5): 300–06.

45. King L & Hill AJ (2008). Magazine adverts for healthy and less healthy foods: effects on recall but not hunger or food choice by pre-adolescent children. *Appetite*, 51(1): 194–97.

46. Carter OBJ (2006). The weighty issue. *Health Promotion Journal of Australia,* 17: 5–11.

47. Robinson TN (1999). Reducing children's television viewing to prevent obesity: a randomised controlled trial. *Journal of the American Medical Association*, 282(16): 1561–67.

48. Wong ND, Hei TK, Qaqundah PY, Davidson DM, Bassin SL & Gold KV (1992). Television viewing and pediatric hypercholesterolemia. *Pediatrics*, 90: 75–79.

49. Harker D, Harker M & Svensen S (2007). Attributing blame. *Journal of Food Products Marketing*, 13: 33–46.

50. Australian Association of National Advertisers (2009). Letter to Nicola Roxon, Minister for Health and Aging. 23 October 2009.

51. Dixon HG, Scully ML, Wakefield MA, White VM & Crawford DA (2007). The effects of television advertisements for junk food versus nutritious food on children's food attitudes and preferences. *Social Science and Medicine*, 65: 1311–23.

9

Benefits of developing a whole-school approach to health promotion

Jenny O'Dea[1]

This chapter examines the school experience as a determinant of future health, including discussion of how broad dimensions such as physical health, emotional wellbeing, cultural identity and psychosocial development, may be developed and enhanced within a whole-school health-promoting context. Healthy behaviours can be established in young people, and these behaviours tend to translate into healthy habits in adulthood, which are subsequently modelled and passed on to the following generations. In this chapter, the salience of health promotion in schools is presented in terms of preventing obesity and type 2 diabetes by promoting a healthy body image, establishing positive food habits and encouraging involvement in sport and physical activity. The potential 'ripple effect' that school health promotion can have via families and communities is also addressed as an additional avenue which can be utilised and embraced by teachers, health professionals and communities.

Links between health and education outcomes

One way to promote health in schools is to highlight the important links between a child's health status and their academic achievement. As recently as 2010, the United Nations' 2010 Human Development Report clearly reiterated the predictive nature of health and education variables by stating that 'education, health, nutrition and sanitation complement each other, with investments in any one contributing to better outcomes in the others' [39]. Other researchers agree and demonstrate how literacy and numeracy are inextricably interwoven with education, and education is concurrently a key predictor of life opportunities, including economic development, psychological wellbeing, health status and social spheres [4, 33]. It is recognised that healthy students are more able and ready to learn [25], and that improving the health of students and the school environment has positive outcomes for learning and academic results.

An example of this important association is given in some recent studies which clearly demonstrate the predictive relationships between physical activity and educational performance and achievement, and show that physical activity is positively related to

---

1   Faculty of Education and Social Work, University of Sydney.

brain function and cognitive performance [14, 37]. Positive relationships have also been documented between academic achievement and both physical activity [5, 20] and sports participation [10, 11]. Field and colleagues [11] found that students who reported having high physical activity and exercise participation also reported having higher grade point averages (GPAs), better family relationships, lower levels of drug use and better mental health, than those who reported participating in physical activity and exercise less often. Vigorous levels of physical activity are also positively associated with overall grade score [6, 7, 12, 16, 35].

Similarly, recent studies of nutrition and cognitive function also reinforce earlier reports that dietary components favourably influence cognitive function and academic achievement in children and adolescents. For example, comparisons of studies among school-aged children indicate that breakfast consumption is more beneficial to cognitive function and academic performance than skipping breakfast, particularly in those whose nutritional status is already compromised by social disadvantage and poverty [3, 15, 23]. Recent reviews and experimental studies present a working hypothesis that a breakfast of low-glycaemic index is beneficial to the blood glucose supply to the brain, and that this effect is likely to explain the positive relationship between breakfast consumption and the cognitive and academic performance of schoolchildren [24, 36].

Other studies provide ongoing evidence for the link between the academic achievement and health status of children, with a recent report also proposing clear pathways between socioeconomic position, physical activity, mental health and educational performance in adolescents [19].

A whole-school, health-promoting schools framework

Whilst the links between child health and academic achievement become more cemented in the recent international research literature, governments, schools and local communities have become increasingly perceived as having the major responsibility for child health promotion, childhood obesity and type 2 diabetes prevention. Much of the resultant pressure placed on governments has been in the area of providing procedures and resources for health promotion.

One way of ensuring a collaborative and developmental process on which to base health promotion is the World Health Organization (WHO) health-promoting schools framework [43]. This framework outlines a holistic approach to foster health within a school and its local community by engaging health and education officials, teachers, students, parents, health professionals and community leaders in making common, coordinated and sustained efforts to promote health. A 'whole-school' or health-promoting school approach is one which has an organised set of policies, procedures, activities, and structures designed to protect and promote the overall health and wellbeing of students, staff, and wider school and community members.

The health-promoting schools concept is based on the previously outlined premise that education and health are inseparable and that health supports successful learning, and successful learning supports health [39, 43]. The ideology of the health-promoting schools framework states that the whole school and its surrounding community must implement policies, practices, and other measures that respect individual self-esteem, are culturally appropriate, provide multiple opportunities for success, and acknowledge group efforts and intentions as well as personal achievements. A health-promoting school also strives to improve the health of school personnel, families, and community members as well as students, and it works with community leaders to help them understand how the community and environment is influential in affecting health and education.

The WHO guiding principles for developing health-promoting schools include the holistic nature of health, gender equity, involvement and ownership of the whole-school community, participatory decision-making, sustainability, cultural appropriateness, and inclusion of measures to increase health literacy. WHO defines health literacy as the cognitive and social skills that determine the motivation and ability of individuals to gain access to, understand, and use information in ways that promote and maintain health [43]. Thus, the health-promoting school promotes empowerment of students, teachers, parents, school staff, and community members because they learn to obtain and use health information.

The framework focuses on three areas of intervention within the school and its local community: 1) School curriculum, teaching, and learning; 2) School ethos, environment, and organisation; 3) School–community partnerships and services.

The overall guiding principles for the development of health-promoting schools include the following:

- Good health supports lifelong learning, living and wellbeing.
- Students grow and learn in a safe, caring, responsive and empowering environment.
- Health-promoting schools view health holistically, addressing the physical, social, cultural, mental, intellectual and spiritual dimensions of health comprehensive programs.
- Equal access by male and female students from all population groups to educational opportunities is essential for promoting quality of life.
- Health-promoting schools ensure a coordinated, comprehensive approach to health and learning by linking curriculum with the school ethos/environment and the community.
- Health-promoting schools are inclusive – the whole community of students, parents, staff and local agencies are engaged in school activities.
- Active participation is based on respecting skills, values and experiences of parents, students and staff.
- Collaborative, participatory decision-making and personal action provide the conditions for the empowerment of individuals and the school community.
- Staff and parent wellbeing is an integral part of health-promoting school activity.
- Partnerships result in action which is more effective, efficient and sustainable.

- Addressing health literacy is an important component of a health-promoting school.
- The contribution of diverse cultures and groups is supported and valued.

In a recent report of a health-promoting schools project in Africa, MacNab and colleagues [21] demonstrate how these basic principles can have wide relevance and application in multiple international settings. In this oral health and nutrition project, the researchers demonstrate how health-promoting schools provide information and support systems that can be catalysts for behavioural changes to improve health globally and reduce healthcare costs [21].

Unfortunately, school-based health education programs face many challenges such as inconsistent health messages in the child's home or community environment, coupled with communication barriers between the health and education communities [25]. Health-promoting schools practitioners can overcome these issues by collaborating with community representatives, opening the lines of communication, distributing clear messages to the community and engaging students, parents, teachers, and health and education professionals. Health-promoting schools can empower students to make positive decisions about their health and allow them to take such knowledge home to their families.

Inchley and colleagues [17] expressed concern that a common approach toward health promotion and education in a school setting had been a focus on specific, short-term interventions that produce observable change in students' health related behaviours. Such short-term initiatives neglect to fully embrace the philosophy behind health-promoting schools, which states that long-term gains will only follow if initiatives are integrated into a more diverse, multifaceted health-promotion strategy that supports sustained change [17]. This is in accordance with the concept of a whole-school and community approach that encompasses a combined and collaborative effort.

A successful whole-school approach to health promotion must also provide opportunities to utilise broader social, economic and environmental factors as catalysts for positive behavioural change [34]. Further successes can be attributed to drawing connections between curriculum and learning imperatives within the school environment as well as placing value on the partnerships between the school and community [34].

Factors that affect health promotion in a positive and negative way

The delivery of health education and promotion is a very important factor to be considered, as there are many components that can impact the way health education is received by its target recipients.

Potential resistance to the messages presented in health interventions is often reported among adolescents [40]. School students often do not respond well to the paternalistic nature of health-education interventions and can have an oppositional response if they see the intervention as a threat to, or removal of, their freedom to determine their own health status [41]. Whitehead [40], however, explains a continuum to counter this, whereby the less educating a health intervention is, and the more health promoting it becomes, the less likely the strategy is to be rejected by its target group.

Alternatively, a program that is properly planned, implemented and delivered can have a profoundly positive impact, as recently demonstrated in the Brighter Smiles Africa oral health program which generated more positive attitudes towards health-related practices for the wider community [21].

A recent study conducted by Xin-Wei and colleagues [44] discusses the development of an overall health-promoting school program in a province of China. It was reported that with community collaboration, it was feasible to implement the health-promoting schools concept in rural and urban schools in both resource-poor and adequately resourced schools. This study subsequently reported enhanced student educational outcomes as well as improvement in the emotional and social wellbeing of students and the broader school community [44].

Development of health-promoting schools

The long-term planning and partnerships required to produce health-promoting schools do not develop overnight and it is unrealistic to assume that such initiatives will lead to immediate change. Inchley and colleagues [17] suggest that there are four themes that should be given the major focus in planning and development of school health promotion programs. These include: 1) recognition – ownership and empowerment, 2) leadership and management, 3) collaboration, and 4) integration [17]. Deliberately utilising these major themes in health-promotion activities reduces barriers to implementation, promotes ease of access beyond narrow individual behavioural outcomes, and aims instead to improve the school as a whole organisation, whilst supporting teachers and facilitating sustainable long-term health improvement.

Rowe and colleagues [34] also recognise the importance of school leadership and management naturally forming from within the school environment, rather than being imposed from outside of the school or the local community. The role of such leadership is critical in engaging others in the program implementation.

There are many factors that influence whether a school will be able to adopt and implement a health-promoting schools approach. A recent Canadian study found that there were four predictors relating to school organisational characteristics that carried great weight in determining the adoption of a health-promoting schools approach: 1) the presence of leaders within schools, 2) perceived school contextual barriers, 3) school investment in healthy lifestyles, and 4) belief in collective efficacy [8]. These findings imply that emphasis should not be placed solely on strategies designed to 'sell' the health-promoting schools concept to schools, but also on strategies that support the organisational change required to incorporate it within schools [8].

The health-promoting schools framework involves shifting from practices that rely predominantly on classroom-based health education to a more integrated construct of health promotion that encompasses both children's attitudes and behaviours as well as their environment [8]. The framework outlines requirements for a planned and sequential health-education curriculum across all age groups and the need for inter-sectoral and cross-curricular approaches.

An example of this concept in regard to obesity prevention, would be a coordinated, cross-curricular approach using a deliberate focus on promotion of healthy eating habits and prevention of fad dieting and subsequent weight-gain cycles in health-education classes (skill development to reduce the influence of peer-group pressure), English classes (the impact of persuasive advertising), and science (normal composition and nutritional needs of the human body). The cross-curricular approach ensures health messages remain balanced and consistent across subject areas. In addition, the utilisation of a health-promoting schools framework emphasises teacher training in specific areas and the opportunity for teachers to reflect on their own values, beliefs, prejudices and life experiences in order to be effective role models. In regard to the long-term prevention of body image problems, promotion of lifelong physical activity, healthy eating, and obesity and diabetes prevention, teachers and other school and community personnel are likely to require training to better understand these problems, training in effective and safe preventive strategies, and access to counselling and referral services.

First, do no harm

Before governments and other agencies leap into actions that they assume to be beneficial in the promotion of child and adolescent health and the prevention of childhood obesity and type 2 diabetes, we must remember to employ one of the most important principles of modern medicine and prevention science, 'First, do no harm'.

Programs aimed at healthy eating or increased physical activity that are not adequately planned, pre-tested or inappropriately delivered, have the potential to do more harm than good [28]. Those who work with young people in any health-promoting capacity need to recognise the vulnerability of children and adolescents of both genders to body image and eating concerns and that weight-focused programs are already known to result in further feelings of shame, guilt and hopelessness and a subsequent low participation in physical activity [31].

The 'First, do no harm' approach is not just salient for obesity, diabetes and other disease prevention, but rather an imperative that should be actively considered for all health-education and promotion campaigns. The potential to cause inadvertent and undesirable outcomes when delivering obesity or type 2 diabetes prevention activities should be a serious consideration for all health professionals, teachers and educators. Such risk can be summarised in the following four major points:

- Implementation of 'treatment' rather than 'prevention': for example, measuring and diagnosing student overweight or obesity based only on a one-off BMI measure that does not take into account many factors such as pubertal stage, ethnicity, muscularity or adiposity; or providing weight-loss advice.

- Inadvertent suggestion of fad dieting and other weight-loss techniques that are likely to be unsupervised and thereby fail: for example, discussing weight loss and inadvertent promotion of dieting rather than promoting weight maintenance or a healthy lifestyle; inadvertently encouraging disordered eating or suggestion that dieting behaviour is normal and/or desirable.

- Creation of stigmatisation, prejudice and discrimination: for example, suggesting that health is exclusively associated with slimness, weighing students and having them plot their BMI on a chart, inadvertently encouraging weight and BMI comparisons, focusing on weight rather than growth as evidenced by height, fitness and overall health markers, labelling and shaming overweight and obese students. This can also stigmatise overweight or obese students as having a 'problem', being a 'failure' and promote the idea that in order to be 'healthy', students must lose weight.

- Undesirable outcomes of unplanned approaches. Inadvertently creating weight concerns can lead to weight-loss attempts that are particularly unhealthy and harmful such as smoking for weight control, vomiting, laxatives, excessive exercise or avoidance of exercise, shame of body, social isolation and depression. In some recent literature, researchers have identified the link between eating disorders and obesity, particularly in young women seeking bariatric surgery [13]. In these research reports the obesity is the likely result of a binge-eating disorder which ought to be treated by psychiatric and psychological interventions, rather than by simplistic surgical intervention or health promotion. The obvious link between eating disorders and weight gain require further recognition and research.

Nutrition promotion in schools

It has long been recognised that schools have the potential to make significant and long-lasting contributions to promoting healthy eating habits in children and adolescents [34]. Sound child nutrition offers many varied benefits, including growth, brain function, intelligence, immunity to infections, energy regulation, better concentration and behaviour, dental health, prevention of lifestyle diseases and the development of good eating habits, many of which are likely to continue into late adolescence and adulthood. School students who are properly nourished tend to demonstrate better classroom learning behaviours, fewer disciplinary problems, better attention and increased attendance [26].

Normal growth and weight control are other benefits of a nutritious diet, but these factors are often not considered most important to parents. Hence, the focus on other important positive benefits as outlined above which are crucial in the engagement of families in health promotion. An interesting point related to child and adolescent nutrition is that the food habits learned at theses stages of life are often carried on and taught to future generations of children. This can ensure healthy food habits for the next generation of children or, conversely, the continuation of poor eating habits and the risk of adult ill-health.

Food and nutrition are very interesting and relevant topics for children and adolescents of all ages, but all too often this material is taught in a very negative way. Teachers and other health educators often focus on telling students what NOT to eat rather than encouraging them to enjoy healthy options. This approach is negative and unnecessarily narrow because the key components of human nutrition are balance, variety, enjoyment and moderation. In this regard, there is no one food that cannot be included in a balanced diet. School personnel and health professionals need to approach the topic of nutrition education using the 'balance, variety, moderation' messages in a consistent manner.

While nutrition has long been included in health-education curricula in Westernised nations, there has been a recent increase in the recognition of the social and environmental factors that influence food choice, which has extended the focus to include the whole-school community, rather than narrowly approaching nutrition education from just one avenue [34].

As an example of a health-promoting schools approach, a primary school in the UK developed an approach called Kids Café which empowered the students to prepare, sell and serve nutritious food to staff and students. This initiative is an example of how the health-promoting schools approach can be utilised to instigate changes in the school environment that support and encourage healthy eating habits among children [34]. Further, the Kids Café initiative provides an example of how to promote the availability, affordability and accessibility of nutritious foods in the school environment.

Other examples of positive, health-promoting schools nutrition activities include the following:

- School gardens – students grow fresh vegetables; examine environmental factors in food production; demonstrate the affordability of and accessibility to nutritious foods; learn about nature, nutrition and health; create recipes for vegetables; develop a sense of ownership of the health promotion initiative; become empowered to make choices regarding their project; raise funds. This kind of mutual support where the students are contributing to the public community and the local shops are supporting their schools is a good example of a whole-school approach having a positive impact beyond the school environment.

- Cookery sessions – students learn about an array of foods from multicultural origins; develop recipe-modification skills; enjoy healthy eating in a social situation; develop budgeting and consumerism skills; master cooking skills.

- Healthy school canteen – students learn to choose healthy options; teachers model healthy eating; pricing policies demonstrate influences on food choices.

- Shopping/supermarket tours – students learn consumerism skills, value for money, budgeting, how to interpret food packaging and labels, food law, food safety, how to decipher advertising messages, the food supply and the food distribution chain.

- Classroom food tasting activities – students have a set class break for fruit and vegetable snack; school programs provide milk, breakfast, fruit, water bottles or water fountains/dispensers; local vendors provide food products.

- Environmental initiatives – soft-drink machines removed, water fountains installed and regularly maintained; marketing initiatives scrutinised; canteens implement healthy food and drink policy, canteens provide healthy choices, sponsorship by food companies should be scrutinised, local food producers and media are utilised to reinforce program aims.

For further reading on this topic please see the book by Worsley [47].

Promotion of a healthy body image

The promotion of a healthy body image is desirable because it impacts on many aspects of adolescent health including self-image, psychological health [31], participation in physical activity [9], avoidance of dangerous dieting and it is part of the array of self-concept factors that promote and protect general child health status [22].

The evidence presented by Canadian researcher Niva Piran and her colleagues [32] recognises that teachers are on the 'frontline' with students and in a position of power to convey critical information, values, norms and other culturally encumbered material. This position of intensive interaction allows teachers great potential to become involved in the prevention and treatment of eating disorders and childhood obesity, and should be geared towards health education and promotion [32]. School-based health-promotion programs can have a positive and lasting impact on body image, eating behaviours, attitudes, and the self-image of adolescents [30]. There is also great potential to address the surrounding issues of body dissatisfaction, self-esteem and self-efficacy in a safe and health-promoting environment.

The environment in which issues such as obesity, eating disorders and unhealthy weight-loss practices, are didactically taught via classroom 'lessons', is considered to be a 'toxic' environment which has the potential to cultivate these problems [18]. Such programs, like the information-giving approach, can glamourise and normalise eating disorders and disturbances, as well as introduce young people to methods of fad dieting and weight control that are dangerous and health harming, such as laxative abuse and starvation. Unintentional harmful effects have been reported when teachers and school staff inadvertently transfer their own poor body image, lack of interest in sport or physical activity or weight prejudices to the impressionable young people in their care. Piran [32, p4] discussed teachers being role models and the importance of examining their own past body-anchored experiences and attitudes, including 'weightism'. This critical consciousness could reduce the potential for inadvertent transference of misinformation, prejudices and inappropriate advice from teacher to student.

Suggestions for body image improvement initiatives in schools include the following:

- Design of school uniforms and sports uniforms in which students feel comfortable, fashionable, culturally appropriate and less concerned about their body image. An example of this is a sport/swim uniform that is designed for use by Muslim girls.
- Implementation of a 'free' physical education uniform so that students can be active in their own choice of clothing or swimwear. For example, students are allowed to wear board shorts and rash vests to swimming.

- Implementation of a policy that allows students to wear their sports uniform to school on the day of sport or physical education to avoid having to change in school changing rooms.
- Addressing privacy/modesty issues such as placing doors on school change cubicles and covering school showers with curtains.
- Implementing body image promotion activities for both girls and boys.

Promoting physical activity

The health benefits of regular physical activity in children and adolescents have been well established in the research literature for many decades [26, 47] as have the health risks of physical inactivity or a sedentary lifestyle [1, 2, 27]. Promoting physical activity is a clear public health policy objective [42] and one which lends itself to school-based promotion.

Physical activity among children and adolescents can be basically divided into organised and non-organised activities and the promotion of both is important for children's health and wellbeing.

The promotion of physical activity within a health-promoting schools framework would incorporate some of the following strategies:

- Promoting opportunities for children and adolescents to be physically active as part of daily life eg walking or riding bikes to school, providing play time at school, providing play time before and after school, planning specifically targeted physical activity programs that are supervised before and after school
- Assisting school teachers in the delivery and resourcing of school sport and physical activity
- Promoting non-competitive, cooperative games and physical activity environments
- Offering non-structured options such as walking, martial arts, free play or gardening in school physical activity programs
- Providing structural enablers at school such as safe bike routes, secure bike racks or lock-up areas for bicycles
- Restructure playgrounds by using colorful markings and providing different types of game equipment
- Avoid or reduce the time required for uniform changing and showering at school sport or physical education classes. Allow sports uniforms to be worn to school on the day of sport or physical education
- Avoid activities in which students wait for their turn in a queue – find an activity to keep all students active during the whole class
- Produce innovative activity areas including climbing equipment, rock walls, skate areas and free play materials
- Designing modest and/or self-selected sports uniforms and swimwear to encourage participation and reduce body consciousness

- Providing same gender physical activities as an option in order to reduce competitive behaviours and self/body consciousness

- Implementing environmental changes to enable more physical activity and to address barriers to physical activity eg providing safe public spaces for physical activity, providing seasonally appropriate activities in the community, such as indoor heated swimming pools, providing play areas and equipment in high-rise housing areas

- Involve parents in monitoring sedentary time and promoting adequate sleep and daily physical activity of their children

- Provide teacher training to update skills, knowledge and resources.

Conclusions

Research reinforces the suggestion that educators need preventive strategies that encompass objectives of holistic health promotion including healthy eating, improved body image, increased physical activity as well as prevention of obesity and type 2 diabetes. School-based programs may provide an efficient and effective way to approach these problems utilising a health-promoting schools framework which encompasses a range of influences internal and external to the school environment. The holistic focus of the framework targets numerous aspects of promoting a healthy lifestyle including school curricula, policies and attitudes as well as the local environment and community activities, services and resources. Collaboration among school, home and community, which is central to implementing the framework, enables a shared language and a shared way of working and understanding each other [43].

The school environment is crucial in determining future health as it complements the classroom learning and provides a basis for knowledge, beliefs, attitudes and behaviours that will almost certainly be carried into the young persons' future life.

References

1. Aires L, Andersen LB, Mendonça D, Martins C, Silva G & Mota J (2010). A 3-year longitudinal analysis of changes in fitness, physical activity, fatness and screen time. *Acta Paediatrica*, 99(1): 140–44.

2. Andersen LB, Harro M, Sardinha LB, Froberg K, Ekelund U, Brage S & Anderssen SA (2006). Physical activity and clustered cardiovascular risk in children: a cross-sectional study (The European Youth Heart Study). *The Lancet*, 368(9532): 299–304.

3. Benton D (2008). The influence of children's diets on their cognition and behaviour. *European Journal Nutrition*, 47(Suppl. 3): 25–37.

4. Buchmann C, DiPrete T & McDaniel A (2008). Gender inequalities in education. *Annual Review of Sociology*, 34(1): 319–37.

5. Caterino M & Polak E (1999). Effects of two types of activity on the performance of second-, third-, and fourth-grade students on a test of concentration. *Perceptual and motor skills*, 89: 245–48.

6. Coe D, Pivarnik J, Wormack C, Reeves M & Malina R (2006). Effect of physical education and activity levels on academic achievment in children. *Medicine & Science in Sports & Exercise*, 39(8): 1515–19.

7. Daley A & Ryan J (2000). Academic performance and participation in physical activity by secondary school adolescents. *Perceptual and motor skills,* 91(2): 531–34.

8. Deschesnes M, Trudeau F & Kebe M (2010). Factors influencing the adoption of a health promoting school approach in the province of Quebec, Canada. *Health Education Research*, 25(3): 438–50.

9. Dounchis JZ, Hayden HA & Wilfley DE (2001). Obesity, body image, and eating disorders in ethnically diverse children and adolescents. In Thomspon JK & Smolak L (Ed). *Body image, eating disorders, and obesity in youth: assessment, prevention and treatment* (pp67–98). Washington DC: American Psychological Association.

10. Dwyer T, Sallis J, Blizzard L, Lazarys R & Dean K (2001). Relationship of academic performance to physcial activity and fitness in children. *Pediatric Exercise Science,* 13: 225–37.

11. Field T, Diego M & Sanders CE (2001). Exercise is postively related to adolescents' relationships and academics. *Adolescence*, 36(141): 105.

12. Fisher M, Juszczak L & Friedman S (1996). Sports participation in an urban high school: academic and psychologic correlates. *Journal of Adolescent Health*, 18(5): 329–34.

13. Grilo C, Masheb R, Brody M, Burke-Martindale C & Rothschild B (2005). Binge eating and self-esteem predict body image dissatisfaction among obese men and women seeking bariatric surgery. *International Journal of Eating Disorders*, 37(4): 347–51.

14. Hillman C, Erickson K & Kramer A (2008). Be smart, exercise your heart: exercise effects on brain and cognition. *Nature Reviews Neuroscience*, 9(1): 58–65.

15. Hoyland A, Dye L & Lawton C (2009). A systematic review of the effect of breakfast on the cognitive performance of children and adolescents. *Nutrition Research Reviews*, 22: 220–43.

16. Huang T, Goran M & Spruijt-Metz D (2006). Associations of adiposity with measured and self-reported academic performance in early adolescence. *Obesity*, 14(10): 1839–45.

17. Inchley J, Muldoon J & Currie C (2006). Becoming a health promoting school: evaluating the process of effective implementation in Scotland. *Health Promotion International*, 22(1): 65–71.

18. Irving LM & Neumark-Sztainer D (2002). Integrating the prevention of eating disorders and obesity: feasible or futile? *Preventative Medicine*, 34: 299–309.

19. Kantomaa M, Tammelin T, Demakakos P, Ebeling H & Taanila A (2010). Physical activity, emotional and behavioural problems, maternal education and self-reported educational performance of adolescents. *Health Education Research*, 25(2): 368–79.

20. Keays J & Allison K (1995). The effects of regular moderate to vigorous physcial activity on student outcomes: a review. *Canadian Journal of Public Health*, 86(1): 62–65.

21. MacNab AJ, Radziminiski N, Budden H, Kasangaki A, Zavuga R, Gagnon FA & Mbabali M (2010). Brighter Smiles Africa: translation of a Canadian community-based health-promoting school program to Uganda. *Education for Health*, 23(2): 1–8.

22. Mann M, Hosman CMH, Schaalma HPS & DeVries NK (2004). Self-esteem in a broad spectrum approach for mental health promotion. *Health Education Research*, 19(4): 357–72.

23. McBean L & Miller G (1999). Enhancing the nutrition of America's youth. *Journal of the American College of Nutrition*, 18(6): 563–71.

24. Micha R, Rogers P & Nelson M (2010). The glycaemic potency of breakfast and cognitive function in school children. *European Journal of Clinical Nutrition*, 64(9): 948–57.

25. Moag-Stahlberg A (2004). Action for healthy kids: focus on state teams–current initiatives for sound nutrition and physical activity programs in schools. *Topics in Clinical Nutrition*, 19(1): 41–44.

26. Mota J, Ribeiro JC, Carvalho J, Santos MP & Martins J (2010). Television viewing and changes in body mass index and cardiorespiratory fitness over a two-year period in schoolchildren. *Pediatric Exercise Science*, 22(2): 245–53.

27. Must A & Strauss RS (1999). Risks and consequences of childhood and adolescent obesity. *International Journal of Obesity and Related Metabolic Disorders*, 23(Suppl. 2): S2–11.

28. O'Dea J (2002). Can body image education programs be harmful to adolescent females? *Eating Disorders*, 10: 1–13.

29. O'Dea J (2005). School-based health education strategies for the improvement of body image and prevention of eating problems: an overview of safe and successful interventions. *Health Education*, 105(1):11–33.

30. O'Dea J & Maloney D (2000). Preventing eating and body image problems in children and adolescents using the health promoting schools framework. *Journal of School Health*, 70(1): 18–21.

31. O'Dea J (2006). Self-concept, self-esteem and body weight in adolescent females: a three-year longitudinal study. *Journal of Health Psychology*, 11(4): 599–611.

32. Piran N (2004). Teachers: on 'being' (rather than 'doing') prevention. *Eating Disorders*, 12: 1–9.

33. Ross C & Willigen M (1997). Education and the subjective quality of life. *Journal of Health and Social Behavior*, 38(3): 275–97.

34. Rowe F, Stewart D & Somerset S (2010). Nutrition education: towards a whole-school approach. *Health Education*, 110(3): 197–208.

35. Sanders C, Field T, Diego M & Kaplan M (2000). Moderate involvement in sports is related to depression levels among adolescents. *Adolescence*, 35(140): 793–97.

36. Taki Y, Hashizume H, Sassa Y, Takeuchi H, Asano M, Asano K & Kawashima R (2010). Breakfast staple types affect brain gray matter volume and cognitive function in healthy children. *PLoS ONE*, 5(11): e15213.

37. Tomporowski P, Davis C, Miller P & Naglieri J (2008). Exercise and children's intelligence, cognition, and academic achievement. *Educational Psychology Review*, 20(2): 111–31.

38. United Nations. Human Development Report (2003). *Millennium development goals: a compact among nations to end human poverty*. Oxford: United Nations Development Programme.

39. United Nations. Human development report (2010). *The real wealth of nations: pathways of human development*. New York: United Nations Development Programme.

40. Whitehead D (2006). The health-promoting school: what role for nursing? *Clinical Nursing Roles*, 15: 264–71.

41. Whitehead D & Russell G (2004). How effective are health education programmes: resistance, reactance, rationality and risk? Recommendations for effective practice. *International Journal of Nursing Studies*, 41: 163–72.

42. World Health Organization (2002). *The world health report 2002: reducing risks, promoting healthy life*. Geneva: World Health Organization.

43. World Health Organization (1998). *Health promoting schools: a healthy start for living, learning and working*. Geneva: World Health Organization.

44. Zhang XW, Liu LQ, Zhang XH, Guo JX, Pan XD, Aldinger C, Yu SH & Jones J (2008). Health-promoting school development in Zhejiang Province, China. *Health Promotion International*, 23(3): 220–30.

45. Yager Z & O'Dea JA (2005). The role of teachers and other educators in the prevention of eating disorders and child obesity: what are the issues? *Eating Disorders*, 13:261–78.

46. Yang X, Telama R, Hirvensalo M, Viikari JS & Raitakari OT (2009). Sustained participation in youth sport decreases metabolic syndrome in adulthood. *International Journal of Obesity*, 33(11): 1219–26.

47. Worsley T (2008). *Nutrition promotion: theories and methods, systems and settings*. Crows Nest: Allen & Unwin.

10

Health implications of overweight and obesity in children and adolescents

Shirley Alexander[1,2]

Overweight and obesity has been associated with a wide range of health and psychosocial problems that impact negatively on quality and length of life. The exact relationship between obesity and premature mortality is controvertible but there are strong and clear associations between increasing weight and risk of most major chronic diseases. Obesity is now the most common chronic disorder of childhood, and may adversely affect a child's health with immediate medical and psychosocial consequences. However the more significant risk in children and adolescents who are obese is the tendency for obesity to persist in adulthood leading to greater potential for the early development of chronic disease and reduced life expectancy.

The validity of adverse health implications in relation to excessive body fat in childhood and adolescence has come into question in recent years, with warnings that exaggeration of risk may lead to potential increases in eating disorders or body image problems [1, 2]. However, a substantial body of research exists demonstrating that both overweight and obesity can have profound effects on the health of a child or adolescent [3, 4].

Childhood obesity is a multisystem disease with significant immediate and long-term medical and psychosocial complications, which were previously associated with onset in adulthood. Ethnic origin, cultural background, genetic susceptibility, environmental factors and socioeconomic status contribute to the risk of developing obesity-related complications. Furthermore, childhood overweight and obesity tracks into adolescence and adulthood. A recent systematic review found that persistence of overweight and obesity was greater with increasing weight status and age [5]. For overweight children (under 12 years of age), the risk of becoming an overweight adult ranged from two- to tenfold compared with normal weight children. For obese children the relative risk for becoming an obese adult was in the higher range. Similarly, for overweight/obese adolescents (aged 12 to 18 years), the risks of becoming overweight/obese as an adult was higher than in younger children, with between 24%–90% of overweight adolescents becoming overweight/obese adults. Risk of

1 Discipline of Paediatrics and Child Health, Sydney Medical School, University of Sydney.

2 Weight Management Services, Children's Hospital, Westmead.

persistence of obesity is also greater if at least one parent of the child or adolescent is obese [6]. Obesity early on in life is a predictor of later morbidity and mortality [6]. Given that obesity during adolescence increases the risk for chronic disease and premature death in adulthood, independently of adult obesity, forecasts of potential decline in life expectancy of current and future generations are perturbing and plausible [7, 8].

The following gives an overview of clinically important medical and psychosocial complications associated with childhood and adolescent overweight and obesity. Table 1 provides a summary of these complications.

Table 1. Potential obesity-associated complications among children and adolescents

System	Health problems
Psychosocial	Social isolation and discrimination, decreased self-esteem, learning difficulties, body image disorder, bulimia
	Medium and long term: poorer social and economic 'success', bulimia
Respiratory	Obstructive sleep apnoea, asthma, poor exercise tolerance
Orthopaedic	Back pain, slipped femoral capital epiphyses, tibia vara, ankle sprains, flat feet
Hepatobiliary	Non-alcoholic fatty liver disease, gallstones, gastro-oesophageal reflux
Reproductive	Polycystic ovary syndrome, menstrual abnormalities
Cardiovascular	Hypertension, adverse lipid profile (low HDL cholesterol, high triglycerides, high LDL cholesterol), raised inflammatory markers
	Medium and long term: increased risk of hypertension and adverse lipid profile in adulthood, increased risk of coronary artery disease in adulthood, left ventricular hypertrophy
Endocrine	Hyperinsulinaemia, insulin resistance, impaired glucose tolerance, impaired fasting glucose, type 2 diabetes mellitus
	Medium and long term: increased risk of type 2 diabetes mellitus and metabolic syndrome in adulthood
Neurological	Benign intracranial hypertension
Skin	Acanthosis nigricans, striae, intertrigo

Psychosocial impact

The most prevalent of obesity-related complications are related to psychosocial consequences, with risk being greater in girls compared to boys, and increasing with age [6]. Childhood obesity is highly stigmatised, with affected children being seen by other children as young as four years, as lazy, unhygienic and socially incompetent [9]. Peer-relationship problems are more prevalent in overweight and obese children, adolescents and even preschool-aged children [10]. Low self-esteem, anxiety and depression, and social isolation are more common in overweight and obese children and adolescents who may also suffer high levels of teasing and bullying [9]. Weight-based teasing may further contribute to negative psychosocial behaviour, including disordered eating, depression and suicidal ideation [11]. Overweight school-aged children are more likely to be bullied than normal-weight peers with obese children even more so [12, 13]. Bullying may take the form of physical aggression (overt bully) or what is termed relational bullying (eg withdrawing friendship or spreading lies). Bullying reportedly reduces throughout adolescence but whether this also occurs in relation to overweight/obesity is undetermined, though Janssen and colleagues report an association between weight status and peer victimisation in 11 to 14 year olds but not in 15 to 16 year olds [13]. Differentiation in relation to bullying, gender and weight is also unclear. There is a suggestion however that overweight/obese boys tend to suffer overt bullying whereas overweight/obese girls are victims of relational bullying [14]. Furthermore, presumably because of increased size in relation to peers thus enabling physical dominance, obese boys are more likely to be overt bullies [12].

Overweight and obese children tend to have reduced athletic ability, potentially leading to exclusion from physical activities and contributing to a vicious cycle of reduced opportunity to improve gross motor skills, further exclusion and inactivity [15]. Similarly, weight status may have a negative influence on academic achievement. Poorer school performance may result from a combination of factors. An increase in absenteeism has been noted in overweight and obese children compared with normal-weight peers, and reduced school attendance is associated with negative academic outcomes [16]. Absenteeism may be as a result of obesity-related ill-health or from school avoidance, which may be secondary to victimisation. Furthermore, difficulties with concentration secondary to sleep deprivation from obstructive sleep apnoea (see below) may also contribute to poor academic performance.

Many obese children have good self-esteem with few or no psychological issues. However, a systematic review of cross-sectional, longitudinal and intervention studies found strong evidence of a negative impact on global self-esteem and quality of life in obese children and adolescents compared with healthy-weight peers, with no clear differences in age groups [17]. Moreover, in the severely obese treatment-seeking child, the psychosocial impact of obesity can be profound, with studies indicating a significant reduction in health-related quality of life, with impairment equating to that of a child diagnosed with cancer [15, 17]. In addition, the psychosocial problems may persist into adulthood, particularly for obese adolescent girls. Longitudinal data indicate young obese women are less likely to marry, have fewer years of higher education, and have higher rates of poverty with lower levels of income compared with normal weight peers [18].

Obstructive sleep aponea (OSA)

Obesity is a major risk factor for sleep-disordered breathing, particularly obstructive sleep apnoea (OSA), a condition characterised by recurrent prolonged episodes of partial and/

or complete upper-airway obstruction resulting in disruption of normal breathing and sleep patterns. The prevalence of OSA in the normal paediatric population is around 2%; however in children and adolescents with obesity the prevalence is significantly higher, ranging from 13% to 59%, depending on diagnostic criteria, age, ethnicity and pubertal status [19, 20]. For every 1 kg/m^2 increment in body mass index beyond the mean for age and sex, the risk of OSA appears to increase by 12% [21]. The underlying mechanisms for this increased risk are unknown. It is not simply related to enlargement (hypertrophy) of the tonsils, as, even after adeno-tonsillectomy (first line treatment in OSA in children and adolescents), residual OSA persists in around 50% of obese children compared with only 10%–20% of non-obese children [22].

Untreated OSA is associated with attention and behavioural problems (found in up to 58% of obese children, compared with 10% of the general paediatric population [23]), cognitive impairment and poor school performance, in part as a result of disturbed sleep and even recurrent low level hypoxia. Furthermore, OSA has been associated with cardio-metabolic complications, such as hypertension, ventricular hypertrophy, insulin resistance and abnormal blood lipid profile. The common pathway appears to be induction of chronic inflammation, the process beginning in childhood and persisting into adulthood, particularly if the OSA is left untreated [24].

Insulin resistance and type 2 diabetes mellitus

Childhood obesity is associated with a number of metabolic complications, including insulin resistance (IR), a pre-diabetic state. The presence of insulin resistance increases the risk of developing type 2 diabetes mellitus and cardiovascular disease, and also appears to predict future cardiovascular risk [25]. The prevalence of insulin resistance is difficult to ascertain as there is no single simple reliable marker to determine a universal cut-point. Furthermore ethnicity and age (in particular pubertal status) influence insulin levels. However, studies using a simple blood marker of insulin resistance (homeostasis model of insulin resistance) have found a prevalence of IR ranging from 45%–80% in obese children, 10%–60% in overweight children and 2%–20% in normal-weight children [26]. Similarly, in the 2004 New South Wales Schools Physical Activity and Nutrition Study, in which fasting blood from randomly sampled 15-year-old school students was analysed, raised levels of fasting insulin (another marker of insulin resistance) were found in 68%, 30% and 7%, of obese, overweight and healthy-weight boys respectively, and in 44%, 42% and 11% of obese, overweight and healthy-weight girls respectively [27]. Increasing body mass index and deep abdominal fat are associated with increasing insulin resistance and there is a degree of heritability with an increased risk of developing insulin resistance in those with a strong family history of type 2 diabetes.

The number of cases of type 2 diabetes has been increasing in the paediatric population over the past couple of decades in parallel with the rise in paediatric obesity. The overall prevalence of children and adolescents with type 2 diabetes is 1%–4%, with rates being much higher in certain racial and ethnic groups, including Native American, African American, Hispanic, Indian sub-continent and Indigenous Australian populations, and lower in northern European countries [28]. Type 2 diabetes in childhood can present with life-threatening ketoacidosis (around 10% of cases) or hyperglycaemic hyperosmolar non-ketotic syndrome (3.7% of cases) [29, 30]. The consequences of type 2 diabetes in young people may be more marked than in adults. Disease progression is normally related to decline in beta-cell function and altered insulin sensitivity. The decline in glycaemic control following initial diagnosis of type 2 diabetes tends to occur over a period of ten to 12 years in adults, but appears to evolve more rapidly in children, within two to four years of diagnosis, with those presenting in diabetic ketoacidosis manifesting greater and more rapid decline [31]. In addition, cardiovascular fitness is significantly impaired in comparison with obese youth who do not have type 2 diabetes.

Hypertension, cardiovascular disease and the metabolic syndrome

Obesity in childhood, and especially adolescence, is associated with the development of cardiovascular abnormalities, including atherosclerotic changes in the aorta and cardiac vasculature, and decreased arterial distensibility. Furthermore, obese children are more likely to develop such changes at an earlier age than normal-weight children [32, 33]. Both left ventricular hypertrophy and arterial hypertension are significantly more prevalent in obese children and adolescents, with the prevalence of hypertension increasing progressively with body mass index. Adolescents with obesity are three times more likely to be hypertensive than those in lower weight ranges [34, 35]. Arterial hypertension is a highly prevalent cardiovascular risk factor in young obese individuals and is predictive of sustained hypertension and end-organ damage in early adulthood [36]. In the previously mentioned 2004 NSW Schools Physical Activity and Nutrition Survey, high blood pressure was found in 37%, 36% and 14% of obese, overweight and healthy-weight boys, respectively, and in 22%, 7% and 5% of obese, overweight and healthly-weight girls, respectively [27].

The clustering of cardiovascular risk factors (insulin resistance, hypertension, abdominal obesity and dyslipidaemia – also termed the metabolic syndrome) are predictors of adult cardiovascular disease. Clustering of two or more cardiovascular risk factors is more prevalent in obese children and adolescents, and, depending on the definition used, 1.2%– 22.6% of children and adolescents have the metabolic syndrome, with rates ranging from 30% up to 60% observed in those who are overweight or obese [36–38]. Moreover, mid-childhood obesity is associated with a sevenfold increased chance of developing cardiovascular disease risk factors in adolescence [39].

Dyslipidaemia

Dyslipidaemia, most commonly raised serum concentrations of low-density lipoprotein (LDL) cholesterol and triglycerides and reduced concentrations of high-density lipoprotein (HDL) cholesterol, occurs in overweight and obese children and adolescents, particularly those who have abdominal obesity. Up to 50 % of obese adolescents may have some degree of dyslipidaemia [40, 41].

Fatty liver disease

Paediatric obesity is associated with a spectrum of liver abnormalities known as non-alcoholic fatty liver disease (NAFLD). The disease ranges from simple fatty infiltration of the liver (hepatic steatosis), to fatty liver with inflammation and fibrosis (non-alcoholic steatohepatitis). NAFLD is the most common paediatric liver abnormality, related to the increasing childhood obesity epidemic and is associated with the metabolic syndrome (central obesity, hypertension, dyslipidemia and insulin resistance). The true prevalence and severity of NAFLD is unknown because of problems with standardisation of disease definition, diagnostic modalities and variations by ethnicity. However, prevalence ranges from 3%–77% in obese children and adolescents have been quoted [42]. Additionally, the natural history of paediatric NAFLD is not established as long-term studies are lacking. Current evidence suggests that a minority of adolescents with NAFLD develop progressive liver disease, leading to liver failure or transplantation, and this is most likely in patients with advanced fibrosis at baseline [43].

Musculoskeletal complications

There is increased awareness that child and adolescent obesity may not only lead to major orthopaedic complications, such as slipped capital femoral epiphyses (where the developing head of the femur shifts backwards resulting in a weakened hip joint) and tibia vara (Blount disease, progressive bowing of the legs), but also a number of other issues involving the whole of the musculoskeletal system. Compared with normal-weight peers, obese children and adolescents have a higher incidence of musculoskeletal pain (eg back pain, lower limb pain especially knees and feet), and genu valgum (knocked knees), greater hinderance to lower limb functioning and gait, and increased risk of fractures (as obese children generally have reduced bone mass after adjusting for size and often vitamin D deficiency as well) [44]. Slipped capital femoral epiphyses, a debilitating condition of the hip joint requiring surgical intervention, is significantly associated with obesity: up to 80% of cases of slipped capital femoral epiphyses are associated with obesity. Unfortunately, weight loss does not resolve the condition, although it helps alleviate the severity and potential for developing bilateral disease. Likewise Blounts disease is strongly associated with increased weight whereby weight loss alleviates but does not resolve the condition [44].

Polycystic ovary syndrome

Obese adolescent girls are at risk of polycystic ovary syndrome (PCOS), a syndrome of elevated androgen levels and ovulatory dysfunction. The prevalence appears to be increasing. It is associated with obesity, insulin resistance, and other elements of the metabolic syndrome. It should be suspected in girls, with hirsutism or severe acne and/or menstrual irregularity, especially if they have obesity and insulin resistance [45]. There is mounting evidence that females with PCOS are at increased long-term risk of endometrial cancer (if PCOS is untreated), cardiovascular and metabolic complications later in adulthood. PCOS is also the most common cause for infertility.

Idiopathic intracranial hypertension

Idiopathic intracranial hypertension (also known as pseudotumour cerebri), is more prevalent in obese children and adolescents, although more so in obese adolescents rather than younger children [46]. It is a rare condition which can cause severe visual impairment or blindness and presents with headaches and a range of potential symptoms.

Skin problems

Obesity is associated with a number of skin manifestations, including acanthosis nigricans, in association with insulin resistance. Acanthosis nigricans appears as hyperpigmented, velvety-thickened skin most often seen on the neck, in the axillae, groin, knuckles or knees. It may be mistaken for a dirty neck and may be a cause of embarrassment in more marked cases. Treatment of the insulin resistance, either by weight loss or pharmacologically, results in reduction or resolution of the manifestation. Other skin complications associated with obesity include striae (stretch marks) and a tendency for fungal infections (intertrigo) in areas where moisture is trapped, such as in skin folds.

Other medical complications

The above list of obesity-associated complications is not exhaustive. Additional complications such as gastro-oesophageal reflux disease, constipation, daytime wetting and nocturnal enuresis (bedwetting), nutritional deficiencies, gallstone formation and bulimia are all problems that are either exacerbated by the association of obesity or have an increased prevalence in overweight and obese children and adolescents. Moreover, seemingly less major difficulties, such as an inability to attend to personal hygiene or reach to tie one's shoelaces, can result from being obese and have a major impact on quality of life.

Conclusion

Childhood and adolescent obesity is a multifactorial, multisystem disease, the prevalence of which has been rising exponentially in recent decades. A considerable body of evidence exists highlighting the significant adverse health-related impacts of childhood and adolescent obesity. Recognised obesity-related complications range from psychosocial issues, these being the most prevalent, to medical ailments such as insulin resistance, hypertension and non-alcoholic fatty liver disease. Importantly, the adverse effects may not only have immediate implications but also can affect health in the longer term, independent of adult obesity. As childhood obesity tends to persist into adulthood, the risk of obesity-related morbidity and mortality is further increased. However, a reduction in total body fat has the potential to alleviate or resolve the adverse health outcomes, thus appropriate assessment and management of such children and adolescents is warranted.

References

1. O'Dea JA (2008). Gender, ethnicity, culture and social class influences on childhood obesity among Australian schoolchildren: implications for treatment, prevention and community education. *Health and Social Care in the Community,* 16(3): 282–90.

2. *The Telegraph* (April 2008). 'Obesity crusade' drives children to anorexia [Online]. Available: www.telegraph.co.uk/news/uknews/1896136/Obesity-crusade-drives-children-to-anorexia.html [Accessed September 2011].

3. Bell LM, Byrne S, Thompson A, Ratnam N, Blair E, Bulsara M, Jones TW & Davis EA (2007). Increasing body mass index z-score is continuously associated with complications of overweight in children, even in the healthy weight range. *The Journal of Clinical Endocrinology and Metabolism*, 92(2): 517–22.

4. Denney-Wilson E, Hardy LL, Dobbins T, Okely AD & Baur LA (2008). Body mass index, waist circumference, and chronic disease risk factors in Australian adolescents. *Archives of Pediatrics & Adolescent Medicine*, 162(6): 566–73.

5. Singh SA, Mulder C, Twisk JWR, van Mechelen W & Chinapaw MJM (2008). Tracking of childhood overweight into adulthood: a systematic review of the literature. *Obesity Reviews*, 9(5): 474–88.

6. Reilly JJ, Methven E, McDowell ZC, Hacking B, Alexander D, Stewart L & Kelnar CJH (2003). Health consequences of obesity. *Archives of Disease in Childhood*, 88: 748–52.

7. Bjorge T, Engeland A, Tverdal A & Smith GD (2008). Body mass index in adolescence in relation to cause-specific mortality: a follow-up of 23,000 Norwegian adolescents. *American Journal of Epidemiology*, 168: 30–37.

8. Olshansky SJ, Passaro DJ, Hershow RC, Layden J, Carnes BA, Brody J, Hayflick L, Butler RN, Allison DB & Ludwig DS (2005). A potential decline in life expectancy in the United States in the 21st century. *The New England Journal of Medicine*, 352(11): 1138–45.

9. Rees R, Oliver K, Woodman J & Thomas J (2011). The views of young children in the UK about obesity, body size, shape and weight: a systematic review. *BMC Public Health*, 11: 188.

10. Boneberger A, von Kries R, Milde-Busch A, Bolte G, Rochat MK & Ruckinger S for the GME study group (2009). Association between peer relationship problems and childhood overweight/obesity. *Acta Paediatrica*, 98(12): 1950–55.

11. Eisenberg ME, Neumark-Stanzer D & Story M (2003). Associations of weight-based teasing and emotional wellbeing among adolescents. *Archives of Pediatrics & Adolescent Medicine*, 157(8): 733–38.

12. Griffiths LJ, Wolke D, Page AS & Horwood JP, for the ALSPAC Study (2006). Obesity and bullying: different effects for boys and girls. *Archives of Disease in Childhood*, 91(2): 121–25.

13. Janssen I, Craig WM, Boyce WF & Pickett W (2004). Associations between overweight and obesity with bullying in school-aged children. *Pediatrics*, 113(5): 1187–94.

14. Pearce MJ, Boergers J & Prinstein MJ (2002). Adolescent obesity, overt and relational peer victimization, and romantic relationships. *Obesity Research*, 10: 386–93.

15. Schwimmer JB, Burwinkle TM & Varni JW (2003). Health-related quality of life of severely obese children and adolescents. *Journal of the American Medical Association*, 289(14): 1813–19.

16. Geier AB, Foster GD, Womble LG, McLauglin J, Borradaile KE, Nachmani J, Sherman S, Kumanyika S & Shults J (2007). The relationship between relative weight and school attendance among elementary schoolchildren. *Obesity*, 15: 2157–61.

17. Griffiths LJ, Parsons TJ & Hill AJ (2010). Self-esteem and quality of life in obese children and adolescents: a systematice review. *International Journal of Pediatric Obesity*, 5(4): 282–304.

18. Viner RM & Cole TJ (2005). Adult socioeconomic, educational, social and psychological outcomes of childhood obesity: a national birth cohort study. *British Medical Journal*, 330(7504): 1354–57.

19. Arens R, Muzumdar H (2010). Childhood obesity and obstructive sleep apnea syndrome. *Journal of Applied Physiology*, 108(2): 436–44.

20. Verhulst SL, Van Gaal L, De Backer W & Desager K (2008).The prevalence, anatomical correlates and treatment of sleep-disordered breathing in obese children and adolescents. *Sleep Medicine Reviews*, 12(5): 339–46.

21. Redline S, Tishler PV, Schluchter M, Aylor J, Clark K & Graham G (1999). Risk factors for sleep-disordered breathing in children: associations with obesity, race, and respiratory problems. *American Journal of Respiratory and Critical Care Medicine*, 159(5): 1527–32.

22. Bhattacharjee R, Kheirandish-Gozal L, Spruyt K, Mitchell RB,Promchiarak J, Simakajornboon N, Kaditis AG, Splaingard D, Splaingard M, Brooks LJ, Marcus CL, Sin S, Arens R, Verhulst SL & Gozal D (2010). Adenotonsillectomy outcomes in treatment of OSA in children: a multicenter retrospective study. *American Journal of Respiratory and Critical Care Medicine*, 182(5): 676–83.

23. Agranat-Meged AN, Deitcher C, Goldzweig G, Leibson L, Stein M & Galili-Weisstub E (2005). Childhood obesity and attention deficit/hyperactivity disorder: a newly described comorbidity in obese hospitalized children. *International Journal of Eating Disorders*, 37(4): 357–59.

24. Bhattacharjee R, Kim J, Kheirandish-Gozal L & Gozal D (2011). Obesity and obstructive sleep apnea syndrome in children: a tale of inflammatory cascades. *Pediatric Pulmonology*, 46(4): 313–23.

25. Sinaiko AR, Steinberger J, Moran A, Hong CP, Pineas RJ & Jacobs DR (2006). Influence of insulin resistance and body mass index at age 13 on systolic blood pressure, triglycerides, and high-density lipoprotein cholesterol at age 19. *Hypertension*, 48(4): 730–36.

26. Nelson RA & Bremer AA (2010). Insulin resistance and metabolic syndrome in the pediatric population. *Metabolic Syndrome and Related Disorders*, 8: 1–14.

27. Booth M, Okely AD, Denney-Wilson E, Hardy L, Yang B & Dobbins T (2006). *NSW Schools Physical Activity and Nutrition Survey (SPANS) 2004*. Full report. Sydney: NSW Department of Health.

28. L'Allemand-Jander D (2010). Clinical diagnosis of metabolic and cardiovascular risks in overweight children: early development of chronic diseases in the obese child. *International Journal of Obesity*, 34: S32–36.

29. Rewers A, Klingensmith G, Davis C, Petitti DB, Pihoker C, Rodriguez B, Schwartz ID, Imperatore G, Williams D, Dolan LM & Dabelea D (2008). Presence of diabetic ketoacidosis at diagnosis of diabetes mellitus in youth: the Search for Diabetes in Youth Study. *Pediatrics*, 121(5): e1258–66.

30. Fourtner SH, Weinzimer SA & Levitt Katz LE (2005). Hyperglycemic hyperosmolar non-ketotic syndrome in children with type 2 diabetes. *Pediatric Diabetes*, 6(3): 129–35.

31. Levitt Katz LE, Magge SN, Hernandez ML, Murphy KM, McKnight HM & Lipman T (2011). Glycemic control in youth with type 2 diabetes declines as early as two years after diagnosis. *The Journal of Pediatrics*, 158(1): 106–11.

32. Whincup PH, Gilg JA, Donald AE, Katterhorn M, Oliver C, Cook DG & Deanfield JE (2005). Arterial distensibility in adolescents: the influence of adiposity, the metabolic syndrome, and classic risk factors. *Circulation*, 112(12): 178–97.

33. Mittelman SD, Gilsanz P, Mo AO, Wood J, Dorey F & Gilsanz V (2010). Adiposity predicts carotid intima-media thickness in healthy children and adolescents. *The Journal of Pediatrics*, 156(4): 592–97.

34. Maggio AB, Aggoun Y, Marchand LM, Martin XE, Hermann F, Beghetti M & Farpour-Lambert NJ (2008). Associations among obesity, blood pressure, and left ventricular mass. *The Journal of Pediatrics*, 152(4): 489–93.

35. Movahed M, Bates S, Strootman D & Sattur S (2011). Obesity in adolescence is associated with left ventricular hypertrophy and hypertension. *Echocardiography*, 28(2): 150–53.

36. L'Allemand D, Wiegand S, Reinehr T, Müller J, Wabitsch M, Widhalm K & Holl R on behalf of the APV-Study Group (2008). Cardiovascular risk in 26,008 European overweight children as established by a multicenter database. *Obesity*, 16(7): 1672–79.

37. de Ferranti SD, Gauvreau K, Ludwig DS, Neufeld EJ, Newburger JW & Rafai N (2004). Prevalence of the metabolic syndrome in American adolescents: findings from the Third National Health and Nutrition Examination Survey. *Circulation*, 110: 2494–97.

38. Tailor AM, Peeters PHM, Norat T, Paolo Vineis & Romaguera D (2010). An update on the prevalence of the metabolic syndrome in children and adolescents. *International Journal of Pediatric Obesity*ity, 5(3): 202–13.

39. Garnett SP, Baur LA, Srinivasan S, Lee JW & Cowell CT (2007). Body mass index and waist circumference in midchildhood and adverse cardiovascular disease risk clustering in adolescence. *The American Journal of Clinical Nutrition*, 86(3): 549–55.

40. Harel Z, Riggs S, Vaz R, Flanagan P & Harel D (2010). Isolated low HDL cholesterol emerges as the most common lipid abnormality among obese adolescents. *Clinical Pediatrics (Phila)*, 49(1): 29–34.

41. NSW Centre for Overweight and Obesity. NSW Schools Physical Activity and Nutrition Survey (SPANS) (2004). [Online]. Available: www.health.nsw.gov.au/pubs/2006/pdf/spans_full.pdf [Accessed 19 October 2011].

42. Widhalm K & Ghods E (2010). Nonalcoholic fatty liver disease: a challenge for paediatricians. *International Journal of Obesity*, 34: 1451–67.

43. Feldstein AE, Charatcharoenwitthaya P, Treeprasertsuk S, Benson JT, Enders FB & Angulo P (2009). The natural history of non-alcoholic fatty liver disease in children: a follow-up study for up to 20 years. *Gut*, 58(11): 1538–44.

44. Chan G & Chen CT (2009). Musculoskeletal effects of obesity. *Current Opinion in Pediatrics*, 21(1): 65–70.

45. Hassan A & Gordon CM (2007). Polycystic ovary syndrome update in adolescence. *Current Opinion in Pediatrics*, 19(4): 389–97.

46. Genizi J, Lahat E, Zelnik N Mahajnah M, Ravid S & Shahar E (2007). Childhood-onset idiopathic intracranial hypertension: relation of sex and obesity. *Pediatric Neurology*, 36(4): 247–49.

11

Child and adolescent obesity in Asia

Mu Li[1] and Michael J Dibley[1]

Childhood obesity is a rapidly growing public health problem in developing countries. World Health Organization estimated that in 2010, of 43 million overweight/obese children worldwide, about 35 million of them were living in developing countries. In this chapter we will present case studies on what is happening in Vietnam, Indonesia, Thailand and China, the developing countries in the Southeast and East Asia that are undergoing rapid socioeconomic development and urbanisation. We will also explore the possibilities of what the governments and communities can do to address the emerging childhood obesity epidemic in these countries.

Although high rates of childhood obesity have been evident for some time across North America, Europe, and parts of the Western Pacific, including Australia [1], in recent years lower- and middle-income countries have joined the trend. As a result, the absolute number of children who are overweight or obese is now much higher in developing than developed countries [2]. At the end of 2010, 43 million preschool-aged children were overweight or obese – a prevalence of 6.7%, up from 4.2% in 1990 globally [3]. The World Health Organization (WHO) has declared childhood obesity 'one of the most serious public health challenges of the 21st century' [4]. Overweight and obesity in childhood are not simply 'shrugged off' in adulthood. Longitudinal studies show that when acquired early, overweight and obesity can have serious adverse effects in later life, such as metabolic and cardiovascular risks [5–7]. Importantly, obese children have a 25%–50% risk of progressing to obesity in adulthood, and this risk may be as high as 78% in obese adolescents [5].

This chapter reports on the background of a Regional Collaboration for Childhood Obesity Prevention Research program, funded by AusAID (the Australian Government's Overseas Aid Program), with participants from China, Vietnam, Indonesia and Thailand. These countries have enjoyed rapid economic growth in recent decades (Table 1), with increased gross national income and family disposable income which are accompanied by a shift from under- to over-nutrition [8–12]. Childhood obesity has become a major public concern in these countries. In this chapter we will review prevalence and trend data from these four countries, discuss the similarities and differences, and highlight social, behavioural and environmental factors associated with the rapid growth of childhood obesity. We will also explore intervention strategies for the East and Southeast Asia region.

---

1   Sydney School of Public Health, University of Sydney.

Table 1. Income (GNI per capita) and level of urbanisation by country*

	Thailand	China	Indonesia	Vietnam
Income level	Upper Middle	Upper Middle	Lower Middle	Lower Middle
GNI per capita	4210 US$	4260 US$	2580 US$	1100 US$
2009 Urban population (%)	34	44	53	28

* Based on World Bank 2010 data

Definitions of child and adolescent overweight and obesity

Unlike the situation in adulthood, body mass index (BMI; weight/height^2) differs, physiologically, by age, sex and development stage in children and adolescents. Thus, BMI rises in the first year, falls during preschool years, reaching its lowest point between four to seven years, before rising once more into adolescence and adulthood. Because of this, the standard definition of overweight and obesity in adulthood cannot be used when describing the paediatric population. Several different ways of defining child and adolescent overweight and obesity are commonly used (Table 2), with no one universal consensus definition having been agreed upon. Some of the currently used international definitions are described below. They are mainly based upon BMI, but have used somewhat different approaches for defining the cut-off points for healthy weight, overweight and obesity.

Table 2 Different definitions of child and adolescent overweight and obesity

	International Obesity Task Force IOTF reference (Cole et al, 2000)	World Health Organization WHO reference (WHO 1995)	World Health Organization WHO reference (WHO 2006)	World Health Organization WHO reference (WHO 2007)
Age	2-18 y	6-19 y	0-5 y	5-19 y
Data and reference populations	Survey data from the US, Brazil, Britain, Hong Kong, Singapore and the Netherlands	US NHANES I data based on NCHS 1977 reference	Data from Brazil, Ghana, India, Norway, Oman, and the US	US NHANES I data based on NCHS 1977 reference + < 5 child growth standards samples
Overweight	BMI-for-age cut-offs derived from BMI – age curves passed BMI of 25 at age 18	BMI 85th percentile	BMI > =+ 2SD	BMI > =+ 1SD
Obesity	BMI-for-age cut-offs derived from BMI – age curves passed BMI of 30 at age 18	BMI 95th percentile	BMI > =+ 3SD	BMI > =+ 2SD

The International Obesity Task Force definition

The International Obesity Task Force (IOTF) has recommended BMI cut offs-based on the centile curves that at age 18 pass through the adult cut-off points of 25 kg/m^2 and 30 kg/m^2 to define overweight and obesity among children and adolescents. In 2000, Cole and his colleagues, on behalf of the IOTF, published a table of age- and sex-specific cut-off points based upon a compilation of nationally representative cross-sectional growth studies from six countries – Brazil, UK, Hong Kong, the Netherlands, Singapore, and the US [13]. These cut-off points are useful in epidemiological research to classify overweight and obesity and for international comparison of trends in overweight and obesity. This IOTF definition also provides continuity between the childhood and adulthood definitions of overweight and obesity.

The World Health Organization reference

In 1995 a WHO Expert Committee recommended that the sex- and age-specific BMI 85th and 95th percentiles in the BMI for age reference charts developed by Must et al. [14] be used to define overweight and obesity for adolescents aged ten to 19 years, and that obesity in children aged less than ten years be defined as weight-for-height z-score >2 [15]. This definition has now been superseded, although published papers may refer to it.

The WHO Child Growth Standard and the WHO growth reference for school-aged children and adolescents

The WHO has subsequently recommended two other approaches to defining overweight and obesity in the paediatric population, depending upon the age of the child. For children aged from birth to 59 months, the new WHO Child Growth Standard for children [16] is based on the WHO Multicentre Growth Reference Study which looked at the growth of healthy children from Brazil, Ghana, India, Norway, Oman, and the US. Overweight and obesity are defined as the proportion of children with BMI-for-age values >2 standard deviations (SDs) and greater than 3 SDs, respectively, from the WHO Child Growth Standard median [17].

For five- to 19-year-olds, the WHO growth reference (2007) is a reconstruction of the 1977 National Center for Health Statistics/WHO reference [18, 19]. Overweight, obesity and severe obesity are defined as the proportion of children with BMI-for-age values >1 SDs, >2 SDs and >3 SDs respectively, from the World Health Organization Growth Reference median [19].

Thus, there remains considerable variation in the approaches to defining overweight and obesity in the paediatric age group. And, as you will see below, other definitions are also being used in individual countries. This highlights the importance of knowing what definition is being used, especially if comparisons are made between different countries or different studies. Importantly, when looking at trends over time, then it is important to use the same definition at the different time points.

What's happening? Childhood obesity situation by country

Thailand: childhood obesity prevalence and trends

There have been two nationally representative surveys for obesity in children aged two to 12 years in Thailand, the Second National Health Examination Survey in 1997 and the National Child Health Survey in 2001 [20]. Over these four years, there was a substantial rise in obesity prevalence, as defined using the Thai growth reference (developed in 1995 and based on weight-for-height percentile) [21]. Obesity prevalence in preschool-aged children (two to five years) increased from 5.8% in 1997 to 7.9% in 2001. It increased to a lesser degree in children aged six to 12 years: from 5.8% to 6.7% [20]. Obesity was much more prevalent in children living in urban areas.

A recent nationwide survey involving 47 389 grade six primary school children in urban settings found that 16.7% children were overweight or obese [21]. The results were echoed by a study of preschool-aged children (four to six years) in central Thailand. Using the Thai growth reference, the prevalence of overweight (defined as BMI between the 90th and 97th percentile) was 16.1% in the urban group and 8.7% in rural group, and the prevalence of obesity (BMI greater than the 97th percentile) was 22.7% in the urban group compared with 7.4% in the rural group [22].

The prevalence of childhood obesity appears to be relative to the level of development of the region. For example, the prevalence of childhood overweight (defined this time as weight-for-height z-score greater than 2 SDs) in seven- to nine-year-old school children in Knon Kaen Municipality, in northeast Thailand, was 10.8% [23], compared with 15.6% in children (six to 12 years old; this time defined as BMI >85th percentile for age and sex) from Hat Yai, in southern Thailand, an economically advanced metropolitan region [24]. It is noticeable, however, that different references were applied in these studies, and hence direct comparisons cannot be made.

In a five-year follow-up study tracking overweight from childhood to adolescence in Hat Yai, Mo-Suwan et al. [25] found that children who were overweight in childhood were more likely to be overweight as adolescents. Overall 11.8% children remained overweight, with a higher proportion of boys (13.9%) than girls (10.1%).

Social, behavioural and environmental factors associated with childhood obesity

Several studies have examined the social determinants of childhood obesity in Thailand. Socioeconomic status (SES), as measured by parents' education levels and monthly household income levels, are positively associated with increased risk [22, 25, 26]. Thus, children of parents with high education levels or high household incomes are more likely to have a high BMI. Other factors such as a high BMI for father or mother, a family history of obesity and physically inactivity are also associated with increased child BMI [25].

China: childhood obesity prevalence and trends

School-aged children and adolescents

In China, there are two nationally representative data collection systems. The China National Survey on Students' Constitution and Health (CNSSCH) is a national initiative by the Ministries of Education, Health, Science and Technology, State National Affairs and State Sports Administration. It started in 1985 and is repeated every five years for school-aged children and adolescents (aged seven to 18 years). The available data from the 1985, 1995, 2000 and 2005 surveys show that the prevalence of overweight and obesity (using the Group of China Obesity Task Force definition, BMI 85th to 95th and BMI greater than 95th percentile) [27] has steadily increased from 1985. The changes were particularly remarkable in seven- to 12-year-old boys from urban settings, with the prevalence of overweight increasing dramatically from 1.7% to 25%, and that of obesity from 0.1% to 11.7%, between 1985 and 2005 [28]. A geographic gradient has also emerged from the CNSSCH data. The prevalence of overweight and obesity is highest in children from the most advanced metropolitan centres such as Beijing and Shanghai and other coastal large cities, followed by the medium/small coastal cities, then the inland big cities, and finally the medium/small inland cities [29]. This suggests that the childhood obesity epidemic in China is largely driven by economic and social development, and it is still at its early stage. The China National Nutrition and Health Surveys (CNNHS) have been carried out every ten years since 1982. The 1982, 1992 and 2002 data (analysed using the IOTF definition for obesity) for school-aged children (aged seven to 17 years) revealed very similar results to the CNSSCH. The prevalence of childhood obesity was low in early 1980, but there was a threefold increase over the subsequent 20 years [30].

The China Health and Nutrition Survey (CHNS) is a longitudinal subnational study carried out in nine provinces in the eastern part of China since 1991 with the most recent data being from 2006. The trend data show that the mean BMI of seven- to 17-year-old Chinese children and adolescents has increased steadily from 17.4 kg/m^2 (95% CI: 17.3, 17.5) in 1991 to 18.3 kg/m^2 (95% CI: 18.1, 18.5) in 2006, after adjusting for age, sex and urban/rural residence. There was a corresponding increase in overweight and obesity prevalence (IOTF definition) during the same period, from 5.2% to 13.2% [31]. The results from this dataset were higher than those obtained from the CNNHS, despite the same reference cut-off points being used. One of the explanations is that this is not a nationally representative sample, and that the economic development in the provinces in the eastern part of China sampled is relatively advanced.

A number of provincial and municipal levels studies have also shown similar patterns. Based on analysis of the CNSSCH data, the overall prevalence of overweight and obesity in seven- to 18-year-olds from Shandong Province, in eastern China, increased from 2.2% in 1985 to 31.2% in 2010 for boys and from 2.3% to 19.1% for girls, using the Chinese weight-for-height criteria [32]. In a cross-sectional survey conducted in 2004 [33] among 1800 junior high school students (aged 11 to 17 years) in Xi'an Metropolitan area, in northwest China, the overall overweight and obesity prevalence (using the IOTF definition) was

16.3%, with a significant sex difference: 19.4% for boys and 13.2% for girls. The prevalence was higher in children living in urban area and from rich families.

Preschool-aged children (under seven years)

Although there are no national representative data for assessing childhood obesity in younger children, the nine cities epidemiological surveys, carried out by the Coordinating Group of Nine Cities Study on the Physical Growth and Development of Children in 1986, 1996 and 2006, provide trend data on children under seven years of age [34].The nine cities are Beijing, Harbin and Xi'an in the north, Shanghai, Nanjing and Wuhan in the central region and Guangzhou, Fuzhou and Kunming in the south. The 2006 survey included 112 945 children. Using the National Centre for Health Statistics/WHO reference (weight-for-height >10% and >20%), the overall prevalence of overweight and obesity was 6.3% (6.6% for boys and 5.9% for girls) and 3.2% (3.8% for boys and 2.5% for girls) respectively [34]. Compared with the 1986 results, the prevalence of overweight nearly tripled in 20 years, with an average annual increase of 6.9% [34].

Another subnational survey began in 1986 in children aged zero to six years covering 11 cities in the east, central and southern regions. There have been two subsequent surveys with a ten-year interval. The most recent survey was in 2006, with total sample size of 84 766 [35]. The prevalence of overweight and obesity (WHO Child Growth Standard; BMI greater than 1 SD and greater than 2 SD) was 19.8% (22.2% for boys and 17% for girls) and 7.2% (9.9% for boys and 5.3% for girls), respectively. Due to the different definitions used, the data for similar age groups in the two 2006 surveys are not comparable. In fact, there was a threefold difference for the overweight prevalence and more than twofold difference for obesity prevalence. Nevertheless, both surveys have consistently shown that overweight and obesity prevalence is higher in boys than in girls.

A similar sex difference was found in Shanghai; the obesity rate (National Centre for Health Statistics /WHO reference, with weight-for-height greater than 20%) in 5188 kindergarten children (aged from three to six years) was 8.3%, with 10.3% for boys and 7.1% for girls [36].

In a large sample study involving 262 738 preschool children (aged from 3.5 to 6.4 years) in three provinces (Hebei in the north, Zhejiang and Jiangsu in the south), the overall prevalence of overweight and obesity (IOTF definition) was 7.4% [37]. However, unlike the findings in the two large scale subnational surveys described above, the prevalence of overweight/obesity was higher for girls (7.8%, 95% CI: 7.1, 8.0) than for boys (6.9%, 95% CI: 6.8, 7.1). An interesting finding from this survey is that the children residing in rural areas, both north and south, had a relatively higher risk of being overweight/obese compared with children from urban settings in the south (adjusted relative risk = 2.58, 95% CI: 2.43, 2.73; and relative risk = 1.15, 95% CI: 1.09, 1.21; respectively). The possible explanations of the difference of the prevalence of overweight/obesity between children from rural areas of north and south include differences in genetic factors and dietary habits. Furthermore, Zhejiang and Jiangsu are two of the most developed coastal provinces. The small difference in overweight/obese prevalence between rural and urban children from the south may be attributed to the narrowing gap of living standards and lifestyle between rural and urban population in the more economically advanced areas in China.

Social, behavioural and environmental factors associated with childhood obesity

In general, due to the disparities in economic and social development, childhood obesity prevalence is higher in urban than rural settings [28, 29, 38]. A study from Xi'an reported that adolescents from wealthier families, or whose parents were overweight or obese, or those who had permission to purchase snacks with pocket money, were 1.7, 1.8 and 1.5 times more likely to be overweight/obese, respectively, than their counterparts [38]. Risk factors identified in boys included consuming sweetened soft drink four or more times/ week (odds ratio [OR] = 1.6) or more than 1100 ml/day (OR = 1.9) and higher levels of energy consumption (medium to high-energy intake OR = 1.5 and 1.9, respectively) [38, 39]. Interestingly, having a mother with tertiary education was associated with a higher prevalence of overweight/obesity in boys (OR = 2.2) but not in girls [38]. Having breakfast outside the family home was a stronger dietary risk factor in girls only (OR = 1.7, 95% CI 1.1–2.3) [39].

In the 2004 study on obesity and metabolic syndrome among 21 198 children (two to 18-year-old) in Beijing [40], obesity (after adjustment for age, sex, puberty and residential area) was significantly associated with a range of factors. These include: being physically inactive (less than one hour/day physical activity, including physical education class, physical activities after school, walking or bike riding to and from school), spending two or more hours per day watching TV, on the computer or playing video games, snacking frequently (three or more times/week), consuming Western fast foods or having reduced hours of sleep (<10 hours for six- to 12-year-olds and <8.5 hours for 13- to 18-year-olds). However, there was no significant association between obesity and consumption of sweetened beverage [40].

The reported risk factors from the nine cities epidemiological survey and other studies for obesity in preschool-aged children (birth to seven years) included having a good appetite and fast eating [34], high parental BMI or parental overweight [34, 41], maternal overweight [41], watching more than two hours a day of TV [34, 41], lower maternal education level [41, 42] and a lower paternal education level [42]. In infants and young children (aged one to 35 months), a higher total energy intake, formula feeding in the first four months and introduction to semi-solids before four months of age were significantly associated with overweight [42]. Other factors such as caesarean section birth [34], birth weight more than 3000 grams [43], sleeping less than 11 hours/night [44] were associated with overweight or obesity in children in this age group.

Indonesia: childhood obesity prevalence and trends

Data from the National Basic Health Research in 2007 showed that overnutrition existed among all age groups in Indonesia [12]. In children under five years, 12% were overweight (WHO Child Growth Standard BMI >2 SD), which was very close to the prevalence of undernutrition in the same age group (14 %, WHO weight-for-height less than –2 SD). In six to 14-year-olds, the prevalence of obesity (WHO Growth Reference BMI greater than 2 SD) was 10% and 6% for boys and girls, respectively. In the 15 years and above age group, the combined overweight and obesity (defined as BMI between 25 to 27 kg/m² and >27 kg/m² respectively) was 19%. As found in other countries, in the six- to 14-year-old age group, the prevalence of overweight was higher in children living in urban areas than in their rural counterparts: 11% for urban boys vs 9% for rural boys, and 7% for urban girls vs 6% for rural girls [12].

Although these nationally representative data were only collected recently, overweight and obesity among primary school-aged children have been documented earlier [12, 45]. In a cross-sectional study involving 3000 pre-pubertal school-aged children from Central Java, the overall prevalence of overweight was 2.7% (IOTF definition). The prevalence of overweight in the non-poor urban group was 4.9%, which was five times higher than the rural group [46]. Obesity prevalence was higher for boys than for girls, but no sex difference for overweight prevalence was found. The Yogyakarta five-year (1999 to 2004) tracking study from pre-pubertal children to adolescents found that the prevalence of overweight (US Centers for Disease Prevention and Control reference BMI 85th to 95th percentile) and obesity (BMI ≥95th percentile) increased from 4.2% and 1.9%, to 8.8% and 3.2% respectively, over this time [47]. Moreover, all obese children stayed obese over the five-year period, and 85% of the overweight children remained overweight [47].

Social, behavioural and environmental factors associated with childhood obesity

The reported factors associated with overweight and obesity from Indonesia include urban (versus rural) residence and higher family income levels, as seen in Thailand and China. Children from non-poor urban families had a higher risk of becoming overweight or obese [46].

Vietnam: childhood obesity prevalence and trends

Adolescents

Systematic national data on the prevalence of child and adolescent obesity are not available in Vietnam. The reported studies are from Ho Chi Min City (HCMC), in adolescents as well as preschool-aged children. Two recent epidemiological surveys conducted in 2002 and 2004, in junior high school students (aged from 11 to 16 years) that revealed a rapid decline in the prevalence of underweight (US Centers for Disease Prevention and Control growth reference BMI Z-score less than −2 SD) halved in just these two years. At the same time, the overall prevalence of overweight and obesity (IOTF definition) more than doubled, from 5.9% to 11.7% and from 0.7% to 2.1%, respectively [48]. The increase in prevalence of overweight and obesity was particularly marked in boys, from 7.8% (95 CI: 3.2, 17.9) and 1.2 (95% CI: 0.3, 4.0) in 2002 to 16.2% (95% CI: 13.3, 19.5) and 3.1 (95% CI: 2.2, 4.4) in 2006, especially in the younger age groups. Furthermore, the largest increase was seen in boys from wealthiest families. These findings are similar to results from the study in Xi'an, China [33].

Preschool-aged children

The 2005 cross-sectional survey of a representative sample of 670 preschool-aged children (aged from 48 to 65 months) in urban areas of HCMC [11] found a remarkably high prevalence (IOTF definition) of overweight (20.5%, 95% CI: 17.5, 24.3) and obesity (16.3%, 95% CI: 13.2, 20.4). The prevalence trend between 2002 and 2005 in preschool-aged children in HCMC are consistent with the findings for adolescents [48]. The total prevalence of overweight/obesity in preschoolers almost doubled from 2002 to 2005 (21.4%, 95% CI: 17.5, 25.8 and 36.8% 95% CI: 32.0, 41.8 respectively). The increase was greater for boys (from 22.6% to 40.8%) than for girls (from 20.4% to 32.8%) and of particular interest was the increase in the less wealthy districts: from 16.9% (95% CI: 13.3, 21.2) to 35.9% (95% CI: 29.4, 42.9) in three years [49]. However, unlike the findings reported by Hong et al. [48] for adolescents, there was no significant difference in the level of overweight/obesity for children from poor and rich families.

Social, behavioural and environmental factors associated with childhood obesity

Significant associations have been demonstrated between childhood overweight/obesity and family social status (fathers having secondary school or above education, fathers working as professionals, and mothers having government employment), both parents having a BMI ≥23 kg/m^2 [50], one or both parents being overweight [49], children being from wealthy families and having a birth weight ≥4000 grams [11]. Prolonged breastfeeding and longer duration of sleeping at night have a protective effect [11]. Many of these factors have also been identified in studies from Thailand and China.

Common characteristics of childhood obesity among the four Asian countries and differences from the West

The common characteristics of childhood overweight and obesity in Thailand, China, Indonesia and Vietnam include the:

• rapid increase in prevalence, especially in younger age groups
• sex difference in prevalence, highest in younger boys
• rural/urban residence differences in prevalence of overweight/obesity
• higher prevalence of overweight and obesity amongst children from households with higher economic status.

However, since the definitions used to define overweight and obesity vary from country to country, and from study to study, direct comparison of epidemiological data across countries is extremely difficult.

In contrast to what has been shown in these four Asian countries, the prevalence of childhood obesity appears to be plateauing in a number of developed countries, including Australia [51–53]. No sex differences in the prevalence of overweight/obesity in children and adolescents have been found in the UK [54], US [52] and Sweden [55]. It has been suggested that the higher prevalence in boys in Asia is at least partially related to a societal view that favours boys over girls [48] and the traditional cultural belief that a fat child symbolise the prosperity of the family [31]. The socioeconomic gradient in relation to prevalence, including the urban/rural disparity, suggests that the childhood obesity epidemic in countries undergoing economic transition is driven by the environment and lifestyle to which the children are exposed. For instance, in urban areas of Asian countries it is common for both parents to work fulltime, having little time to prepare nutritious foods. In particular, children from higher income families tend to eat out more, including Western-style fast food, and often have pocket money to buy snacks [38]. This is a different pattern from developed countries where childhood obesity is more prevalent in lower socioeconomic status families [54, 56].

Disease consequences of childhood obesity

In adults, the cut-off values defining overweight or obesity are based on the related disease risk. There are no risk-based BMI values for children and adolescents, largely due to the time span between childhood obesity and when the adverse outcomes may occur [57]. Nevertheless, a body of evidence has shown a strong association between childhood obesity and major cardiovascular disease risk factors, such as diabetes, hypertension and metabolic syndrome (MetS) in children and adolescents. The tracking studies from Thailand and Indonesia clearly demonstrate that there is a strong tendency for overweight and obese children to remain overweight or obese into adolescence. This tendency, of course, is not confined to Asian countries [58, 59].

In a study that reviewed medical records of diabetic patients in the Division of Paediatric Endocrinology, Faculty of Medicine, Siriraj Hospital in Hat Yai, south Thailand, children and adolescents diagnosed with type 2 diabetes increased from 5% in the mid 1980 to mid 1990s to 17.9% in the late 1990s [60]. This coincided with the increase of obesity prevalence from 5.8% to 13.3% [60]. The mean age of diabetic children was 11.6 years with a mean BMI of 27.8 kg/m^2 [60]. In the 2006 nine cities epidemiological survey conducted in China, both the systolic (SBP) and diastolic (DBP) blood pressure of children aged three to six years were higher in obese children than in children of normal bodyweight [35]. Based on data analysis from the 2002 Chinese National Health Survey, overweight and obese adolescents (aged 15 to 17.9 years, the Group of China Obesity Task Force definition) were 3.3 and 3.9 times more likely, respectively, to have high blood pressure than their normal-weight peers, with systolic and diastolic blood pressure being about ten and five mmHg higher than in those of normal weight [61, 62]. Type 2 diabetes was found in 0.2% of seven-to 12-year-olds and 0.4% of 12-to 18-year-olds. As many as 62% of children and adolescents had dyslipidaemia or other lipid profile abnormalities [62]. Overweight was a risk factor for hyperglycaemia (OR = 2.3, 95% CI: 1.0, 5.4). More alarmingly, overweight and obesity were associated with high dyslipidaemia (OR = 1.5, 95% CI: 1.2, 1.9 and OR = 1.8, 95% CI: 1.3, 2.5 respectively), high triglyceride (OR = 1.9, 95% CI: 1.5, 2.4 and OR = 3.3, 95% CI: 2.4, 4.5 respectively), high SBP (OR = 3.4, 95% CI: 1.5. 7.5 and OR = 5.0, 95% CI: 1.5, 16.4 respectively), high DBP (OR = 2.7, 95% CI: 1.5. 4.8 and OR = 3.1, 95% CI: 1.2, 8.1 respectively) and MetS (OR = 15.4, 95% CI: 6.8. 34.8 and OR = 47.9, 95% CI: 16.0, 143.1 respectively) [62].

Two recent publications reported on survey results of MetS, using the International Diabetes Foundation definition [63], in children and adolescents from Guangzhou, China [64] and HCMC, Vietnam [65]. The overall prevalence of the metabolic syndrome in seven- to 14-year-olds from Guangzhou was 6.6%, and much higher in overweight (20.5%) and obese (33.1%) children [64]. Similarly, the metabolic syndrome was more prevalent in overweight/obese children from HCMC. Being physically active was associated with a lower odds of developing the metabolic syndrome [65]. These findings illustrate that childhood obesity poses immediate consequences to child and adolescent health.

The possibility for intervention: where to start?

Childhood obesity is a complex problem with no easy solution. The results of many intervention studies aimed at preventing obesity in school-aged children remain inconclusive due to lack of long-term follow-up [66]. Indeed, Li et al. [67] conducted a systematic review of school-based intervention studies for the prevention or reduction of excess weight gain among Chinese children and adolescents and found that most of the published studies (lasting between ten weeks to three years) were uni-dimensional, mostly focusing on improving knowledge, physical activity levels and/or diet. None of the trials demonstrated convincing efficacy. In 2009 WHO published a systematic review, 'Interventions on diet and physical activity: what works?' [68], which examined close to 400 publications between 1995 and 2005. The authors showed that multi-component interventions involving the family, school, community and government, and interventions that are adapted to the local context were the most successful [68–70]. Unfortunately, the representation of studies from low-middle income countries in the WHO review was extremely low (less than 13%). This highlights the urgent need for well-designed intervention programs to be implemented in low and middle-income countries. In the meantime, the extent to which examples of successful programs for reducing childhood obesity in developed countries could be adapted to the context of low- and middle-income countries, should be explored.

At the national level, Singapore's experience can provide some insight into national intervention programs within an Asian country that shares a similar social and cultural background and dietary patterns. Although the prevalence of childhood obesity in Singapore was not as high as in the countries described in this chapter, concerns about obesity-related morbidities had prompted the government to introduce national health promotion and disease prevention policies and programs from the early 1990s [71]. Specific policies and programs were developed for populations in different settings, including schools, communities and workplaces. Several programs were targeted at school-aged children. The Trim and Fit program was one of the longest running programs (1992 to 2006), and aimed to reduce obesity prevalence and to increase children's fitness level. Although the program achieved its overall goals, it also raised concerns about the extra pressure that overweight and obese students were subjected to, as well as stigmatisation towards them, as a result of the way in which that particular program was implemented. The program was terminated in 2006 and replaced by the Holistic Health Framework program [72]. The important point here is that nationwide programs in Singapore were implemented by government in order to prevent and control overweight and obesity in the population, in a similar manner to national strategies for controlling communicable diseases [71]. The Thai government has recently endorsed its national obesity prevention plan. This nationwide approach to the problem is a step in the right direction.

At the community level, one successful Australian example of an obesity prevention program is the Romp & Chomp project. This four-year obesity demonstration program was targeted towards preschool children aged less than five years, and their families, in two communities in Victoria [69]. It was designed, planned and implemented as a partnership by a range of government and non-government organisations [73].The intervention led to a significantly lower intake, by children, of packed snacks and sweet drinks, as well as a significantly higher frequency of vegetable intake. An evaluation of early childhood environments undertaken as part of this study found that no sweet drinks were being offered in any of the early childhood settings. Healthy eating policies and healthy food guidelines were implemented, and there was an increase in the availability of nutrition and physical activity resources [73]. This project demonstrated that a whole-community and settings-based approach can create environments for young children that are less obesogenic and that promote healthy weight from early age. More importantly, it shows that actions can be taken to prevent childhood obesity.

Challenges and opportunities

There are a number of challenges and opportunities in addressing the rising prevalence of overweight and obesity among children and adolescents in Asia.

1. There is an important need to gather quality nationally representative epidemiological data in all countries in order to monitor trends over time and to inform decision-making in policy development and intervention programs. Currently, China has national data collection systems in place; while Thailand and Indonesia have collected nationally representative data through the Thai National Child Health Survey (2001) and the Indonesian Basic Health Research (2007); Vietnam has the national child nutrition surveillance program, which is still orientated towards the surveillance of under-nutrition in children aged <5 years. The challenge is to achieve a robust national data collection system that can monitor the trends regularly and consistently.

2. It is important to determine the applicability of the international definitions of overweight and obesity for Asian children and adolescents. Work is under way to collate and analyse childhood obesity epidemiological data from the four countries. The data and the national growth references (Thailand and China) will be evaluated against the WHO Child Growth Standards and the WHO Growth Reference for five to 19-year-olds, as well as the IOTF definition.

3. One of the biggest challenges is to determine the value of the current definitions of childhood overweight and obesity in predicting disease risks. This will need a monitoring system to track the development of non-communicable diseases from childhood right into adolescence and adulthood.

4. Because countries in the region are facing similar issues, a regional approach to prevention may be warranted. One of the opportunities for reseach collaboration is

to gain a better understanding of the causative factors of childhood obesity in Asian countries. We have already identified the role of food and beverage marketing targeted at children as a research priority.

5. Evidence of effective intervention strategies and programs in countries undergoing economic and nutrition transition is urgently needed. Further research is needed to evaluate obesity prevention interventions in different age groups and settings in transition countries. These interventions will need to address the risk factors found in these countries.

Conclusion

As illustrated by data from Thailand, China, Indonesia and Vietnam, the childhood obesity epidemic in transition nations shows no signs of slowing down. Although undergoing rapid economic growth these countries share with more developed countries some common social, behavioural and environmental factors that are associated with a higher prevalence of childhood overweight and obesity. There are also characteristics that are unique to the region, such as higher rates of obesity in boys from wealthier families. It is important, therefore, to develop policies and intervention programs that are culturally appropriate to prevent and reduce rates of childhood obesity for the region.

References

1. Wang Y & Lobstein T (2006). Worldwide trends in childhood overweight and obesity. *International Journal of Pediatric Obesity*, 1: 11–25.

2. World Health Organization (2009). *Population-based prevention strategies for childhood obesity: report of a WHO forum and technical meeting*. Geneva: World Health Organization.

3. de Onis M, Blossner M & Borghi E (2010). Global prevalence and trends of overweight and obesity among preschool children. *The American Journal of Clinical Nutrition*, 92(5): 1257–64.

4. World Health Organization (2011). Childhood overweight and obesity [Online]. Available: www.who.int/dietphysicalactivity/childhood/en/ [Accessed 8 February 2011].

5. Deitz W (1994). Critical periods in childhood for the development of obesity. *The American Journal of Clinical Nutrition*, 59: 955–59.

6. Leunissen R, Kerkhof G, Stijnen T & Hokken-Koelega A (2009). Timing and tempo of first-year rapid growth in relation to cardiovascular and metabolic risk profile in early adulthood. *Journal of the American Medical Association*, 301(21): 2234–42.

7. Monteiro P & Victora C (2005). Rapid growth in infancy and childhood and obesity in later life: a systematic review. *Obesity Review*, 6(2): 143–54.

8. Kosulwat V (2002). The nutrition and health transition in Thailand. *Public Health Nutrition*, 5(1A): 183–89.

9. National Bureau of Statistics of China (2010). China Statistical Yearbook 2010 [Online]. Available: www.stats.gov.cn/tjsj/ndsj/2010/indexch.htm. [Accessed 9 September 2011].

10. Zhai F, Wang H, Du S, He Y, Wang Z, Ge K, et al. (2009). Prospective study on nutrition transition in China. *Nutrition Reviews*, 67(Suppl. 1): S56–61.

11. Dieu H, Dibley M, Sibbritt D & Hanh T (2007). Prevalence of overweight and obesity in preschool children and associated socio-demographic factors in Ho Chi Minh City, Vietnam. *International Journal of Pediatric Obesity*, 2(1): 40–50.

12. Usfar A, Lebenthal E, Atmarita, Achadi E, Soekirman & Hadi H (2010). Obesity as a poverty-related emerging nutrition problems: the case of Indonesia. *Obesity Review*, 11(12): 924–28.

13. Cole T, Bellizzi M, Flegal K & Dietz W. (2000). Establishing a standard definition for child overweight and obesity worldwide: international survey. *British Medical Journal*, 320(7244): 1240–43.

14. Must A, Dallal G & Dietz W. (1991). Reference data for obesity: 85th and 95th percentiles of body mass index (wt/ht2) and triceps skinfold thickness. *The American Journal of Clinical Nutrition*, 53(4): 839–46.

15. World Health Organization (1995). *Physical status: the use and interpretation of anthropometry*. Report of a WHO Expert Committee. Technical Report Series No. 854. Geneva: World Health Organization.

16. World Health Organization (2006). *WHO child growth standards: methods and development: length/ height-for-age, weight-for-age, weight-for-length, weight-for-height and body mass index-for-age*. Geneva: World Health Organization.

17. World Health Organization (2008). *Training course on child growth assessment*. Geneva: World Health Organization.

18. de Onis M, Onyango A, Borghi E, Siyam A, Nishida C & Siekmann J (2007). Development of a WHO growth reference for school-aged children and adolescents. *Bulletin of the World Health Organization*, 85: 660–67.

19. de Onis M, Onyango A, Borghi E, Siyam A, Nishida C & Siekmann J (2007). Development of a WHO growth reference for school-aged children and adolescents. *Bulletin of the World Health Organization*, 85: 649–732.

20. Aekplakorn W & Mo-suwan L (2009). Prevalence of obesity in Thailand. *Obesity Reviews*, 10(6): 589–92.

21. Mo-suwan L (2008). Childhood obesity: an overview. *Siriraj Medical Journal*, 60(1): 37–40.

22. Sakamoto N, Wansorn S, Tontisirin K & Marui E (2001). A social epidemiologic study of obesity among preschool children in Thailand. *International Journal of Obesity Related Metabolic Disorders*, 25(3): 389–94.

23. Langendijk G, Wellings S, van Wyk M, Thompson S, McComb J & Chusilp K (2003). The prevalence of childhood obesity in primary school children in urban Khon Kaen, northeast Thailand. *Asia Pacific Journal of Clinical Nutrition*, 12(1): 66–72.

24. Mo-suwan L, Junjana C & Puetpaiboon A (1993). Increasing obesity in school children in a transitional society and the effect of the weight control program. *Southeast Asian Journal of Tropical Medicine and Public Health*, 24(3): 590–94.

25. Mo-suwan L, Tongkumchum P & Puetpaiboon A (2000). Determinants of overweight tracking from childhood to adolescence: a 5 y follow-up study of Hat Yai schoolchildren. *International Journal of Obesity Related Metabolic Disorders*, 24(12): 1642–47.

26. Mo-suwan L & Geater A (1996). Risk factors for childhood obesity in a transitional society in Thailand. *International Journal of Obesity Related Metabolic Disorders*, 20(8): 697–703.

27. Group of China Obesity Task Force (2004). Body mass index reference norm for screening overweight and obesity in Chinese children and adolescents. *Zhonghua Liu Xing Bing Xue Za Zhi*, 25(2): 97–102.

28. Cui Z & Dibley M. (2010). Secular treand in childhood obesity and associated risk factors in China from 1982 to 2006. In J O'Dea & M Eriksen (Eds). *Childhood obesity prevention: international research, controversies, and interventions* (pp104–16). New York: Oxford University Press.

29. Ji C & Cooperative Study on Childhood Obesity: Working Group on Obesity in China (WGOC) (2008). The prevalence of childhood overweight/obesity and the epidemic changes in 1985–2000 for Chinese school-age children and adolescents. *Obesity Review*, 9(Suppl. 1): 78–81.

30. Li Y, Schouten E, Hu X, Cui Z, Luan D & Ma G (2008). Obesity prevalence and time trend among youngsters in China, 1982–2002. *Asia Pacific Journal of Clinical Nutrition*, 17(1): 131–37.

31. Cui Z, Dibley MJ, Huxley R & Wu Y (2010). Temporal trends in overweight and obesity of children and adolescents from nine provinces in China from 1991–2006. *International Journal of Pediatric Obesity*, 5(5): 365–74.

32. Zang Y & Wang S (2011). Secular trends in body mass index and the prevalence of overweight and obesity among children and adolescents in Shandong, China, from 1985 to 2010. *Journal of Public Health (Oxf)*, 1–7.

33. Li M, Dibley M, Sibbritt D & Yan H (2006). An assessment of adolescent overweight and obesity in Xi'an City, China. *International Journal of Pediatric Obesity*, 1(1): 50–58.

34. Li H & Collaboration Group of Nine Cities Study on the Physical Growth and Development of Children (2008). A national epidemiological survey on obesity of children under 7 years of age in nine cities of China, 2006. *Zhonghua Er Ke Za Zhi*, 46(3): 174–78.

35. Ding Z & Collaboration Group of Nine Cities Study on the Physical Growth and Development of Children (2008). A national epidemiological survey on obesity of children under 7 years of age in nine cities of China, 2006. *Zhonghua Er Ke Za Zhi*, 46(3): 174–78.

36. Zhang J, Yuan L & Wei M (2002). The current status of obesity epidemiology and prevention in preschooler. *Maternal and Child Health Care of China*, 17: 376–78.

37. Liu J, Ye R, Li S, Ren A, Li Z, Liu Y, et al. (2007). Prevalence of overweight/obesity in Chinese children. *Archives of Medical Research*, 38(3): 882–86.

38. Li M, Dibley M, Sibbritt D & Yan H (2008). Factors associated with adolescents' overweight and obesity at community, school and household levels in Xi'an City, China: results of hierarchical analysis. *European Journal of Clinical Nutrition*, 62(5): 635–43.

39. Li M, Dibley M, Sibbritt D & Yan H (2010). Dietary habits and overweight/obesity in adolescents in Xi'an City, China. *Asia Pacific Journal of Clinical Nutrition*, 19(1): 76–82.

40. Shan X, Xi B, Cheng H, Hou D, Wang Y & Mi J (2010). Prevalence and behavioral risk factors of overweight and obesity among children aged 2–18 in Beijing, China. *International Journal of Pediatric Obesity*, 5(5): 383–89.

41. Jiang J, Rosenqvist U, Wang H, Greiner T, Ma Y & Toschke A (2006). Risk factors for overweight in 2- to 6-year-old children in Beijing, China. *International Journal of Pediatric Obesity*, 1(2): 103–08.

42. Jiang J, Rosenqvist U & Wang H (2009). Relationship of parental characteristics and feeding practices to overweight in infants and young children in Beijing, China. *Public Health Nutrition*, 12(7): 973–78.

43. Zhang X, Liu E, Tian Z, Wang W, Ye T, Liu G, et al. (2009). High birth weight and overweight or obesity among Chinese children 3–6 years old. *Preventative Medicine*, 49(2–3): 172–78.

44. Jiang F, Zhu S, Yan C, X J, Bandla H & Shen X. (2009). Sleep and obesity in preschool children. *The Journal of Pediatrics,* 154(6): 814–18.

45. Soekirman, Hardinsyah, Jus'at I & Jahari A (2002). Regional study of nutritional status of urban primary schoolchildren. 2. West Jakarta and Bogor, Indonesia. *Food and Nutrition Bulletin*, 23(1): 31–40.

46. Julia M, van Weissenbruch M, de Waal H & Surjono A (2004). Influence of socioeconomic status on the prevalence of stunted growth and obesity in prepubertal Indonesian children. *Food and Nutrition Bulletin*, 25(4): 354–60.

47. Julia M, van Weissenbruch M, Prawirohartono E, Surjono A & Delemarre–van de Waal H (2008). Tracking for underweight, overweight and obesity from childhood to adolescence: a 5-year follow-up study in urban Indonesian children. *Horm Res*, 69(5): 301–06.

48. Hong T, Dibley M, Sibbritt D, Binh P, Trang N & Hanh T (2007). Overweight and obesity are rapidly emerging among adolescents in Ho Chi Minh City, Vietnam, 2002–2004. *International Journal of Pediatric Obesity*, 2(4): 194–201.

49. Dieu H, Dibley M, Sibbritt D & Hanh T. (2009). Trends in overweight and obesity in pre-school children in urban areas of Ho Chi Minh City, Vietnam, from 2002 to 2005. *Public Health Nutrition*, 12(5): 702–09.

50. WHO Expert Consultation (2004). Appropriate body-mass index for Asian populations and its implications for policy and intervention strategies. *The Lancet*, 363(9403): 157–63.

51. Popkin B (2010). Recent dynamics suggest selected countries catching up to US obesity. *The American Journal of Clinical Nutrition,* 91(1): 284S–8S.

52. C, Carroll M, Curtin L, Lamb M & Flegal K (2010). Prevalence of high body mass index in US children and adolescents, 2007–2008. *Journal of the American Medical Association*, 303(3): 242–49.

53. Olds T, Tomkinson G, Ferrar K & Maher C (2010). Trends in the prevalence of childhood overweight and obesity in Australia between 1985 and 2008. *International Journal of Obesity*, 34(1): 57–66.

54. Jebb S, Rennie K & Cole T (2004). Prevalence of overweight and obesity among young people in Great Britain. *Public Health Nutrition*, 7(3): 461–65.

55. Sundblom E, Sjoberg A, Blank J & Lissner L (2010). Childhood obesity: recent trends in Sweden including socioeconomic differences. In J O'Dea & M Eriksen (Eds). *Childhood obesity prevention: international research, controversies, and interventions* (pp164–73). New York: Oxford University Press.

56. O'Dea J (2003). Differences in overweight and obesity among Australian schoolchildren of low and middle/high socioeconomic status. *Medical Journal of Australia*, 179(1): 63.

57. Lloyd L, Langley-Evans S & McMullen S (2010). Childhood obesity and adult cardiovascular disease risk: a systematic review. *International Journal of Obesity*, 34(1): 18–28.

58. Singh A, Mulder C, Twisk J, van Mechelen W & Chinapaw M (2008). Tracking of childhood overweight into adulthood: a systematic review of the literature. *Obesity Review*, 9: 474–88.

59. Suchiindran C, North K, Popkin B & Gordon-Larsen P (2010). Association of adolescent obesity with risk of severe obesity in adulthood. *Journal of the American Medical Association*, 304: 2042–47.

60. Likitmaskul S, Kiattisathavee P, Chaichanwatanakul K, Punnakanta L, Angsusingha K & Tuchinda C (2003). Increasing prevalence of type 2 diabetes mellitus in Thai children and adolescents associated with increasing prevalence of obesity. *Journal of Pediatric Endocrinology & Metabolism* 16(1): 71–77.

61. Chen C (2008). Overview of obesity in mainland China. *Obesity Review*, 9(Suppl. 1): 14–21.

62. Li Y, Yang X, Zhai F, Piao J, Zhao W, Zhang J, et al. (2008). Childhood obesity and its health consequence in China. *Obesity Review*, 9(Suppl. 1): 82–86.

63. Zimmet P, Alberti K, Kaufman F, Tajima N, Silink M, Arslanian S, et al. (2007). The metabolic syndrome in children and adolescents: an IDF consensus report. *Pediatric Diabetes*, 8(5): 299–306.

64. Liu W, Lin R, Liu A, Du L & Chen Q (2010). Prevalence and association between obesity and metabolic syndrome among Chinese elementary school children: a school-based survey. *BMC Public Health*, 10: 780.

65. Nguyen T, Tang H, Kelly P, van der Ploeg H & Dibley M (2010). Association between physical activity and metabolic syndrome: a cross-sectional survey in adolescents in Ho Chi Minh City, Vietnam. *BMC Public Health*, 17(10): 141.

66. Summerbell C, Waters E, Edmunds L, Kelly S, Brown T & Campbell K (2005). Interventions for preventing obesity in children. *Cochrane Database of Systematic Reviews*, 3: CD001871.

67. Li M, Li S, Baur L & Huxley R (2008). A systematic review of school-based intervention studies for the prevention or reduction of excess weight among Chinese children and adolescents. *Obesity Review*, 9(6): 548–59.

68. World Health Organization (2009). Interventions on diet and physical activity: what works [Online]. Available: www.who.int/dietphysicalactivity/whatworks/en/ [Accessed 9 July 2011].

69. de Silva-Sanigorski A, Bell A, Kremer P, Nichols M, Crellin M, Smith M, et al. (2010). Reducing obesity in early childhood: results from Romp & Chomp, an Australian community-wide intervention program. *The American Journal of Clinical Nutrition*, 91(4): 831–40.

70. Bautista-Castano I & Doreste J (2004). Effectiveness of interventions in the prevention of childhood obesity. *European Journal of Epidemiology*, 19: 617–22.

71. Ho T (2010). Prevention and management of obesity in children and adolescents-the Singapore experience. In J O'Dea & M Eriksen (Eds). *Childhood obesity prevention: international research, controversies, and interventions* (pp240–49). New York: Oxford University Press.

72. Soon G, Koh Y, Wong M & Lam P (2008). *Obesity prevention and control efforts in Singapore: 2008 case study*. The National Bureau of Asian Research, USA.

73. WHO Collaboration Centre for Obesity Prevention & Deakin University (2009). Outcome and impact evaluation of Romp & Chomp: preliminary report. Deakin University.

Ethics, policy and regulation

12

The ethical implications of intervening in bodyweight

Stacy M Carter,[1,2] Ian Kerridge,[1] Lucie Rychetnik[1,2] and Lesley King[3]

This chapter is about the ethical implications of health sector actions intended to change individuals' or communities' weight. We consider these implications using two hypothetical cases. The first is Megan, a 15-year-old girl whose BMI is in the range defined as obese. She has been unable to lose weight and her parents are considering seeking clinical help. The second case is the population of the state where Megan lives, in which 35% of adults and 15% of children are reportedly overweight, and 17% of adults and 5% of children obese. The minister for health, prompted by these statistics, is determined to take action. What ethical issues are relevant for Megan, her parents, and the health professionals they may consult? What ethical issues are relevant for the citizens of the state, their minister for health and their bureaucrats? How does a focus on the care of individuals impact on public health, and how might community-level interventions affect people like Megan? Interventions designed to treat and prevent obesity in individuals and in communities raise important ethical issues. These issues are both distinct and overlapping; because the interventions have different goals, risks and benefits, moral compromise is always necessary. The central task is to think through the ethical and philosophical issues before action is taken: whether in clinical medicine or in public health. We present ethical approaches that can assist in such reasoning.

In this chapter we examine the ethical implications of intervening in weight, and the ethical difference between intervening in the weight of individuals and the weight of populations. We discuss these issues via two cases: Megan, a hypothetical 15-year-old girl, and Australia, the country where Megan lives. We conclude that there are distinct and overlapping ethical concerns at individual and population levels, and that at both levels moral compromise is necessary. Both clinicians and public health professionals need to consider the ethical issues and implications before action is taken. Using our two cases, this chapter provides examples of such reasoning.

---

1   Centre for Values, Ethics and the Law in Medicine, University of Sydney.

2   Sydney School of Public Health, University of Sydney.

3   Prevention Research Collaboration, Sydney School of Public Health, University of Sydney.

Megan

Megan is 15 and a high-school student. She is technically 'overweight': 165 cm tall and 76 kg, with a body mass index of 27.9 kg/m². Megan has always been larger than many of her peers. As a young child Megan wasn't aware of her weight, but began to be self-conscious in primary school after being teased by a fellow student for being fat. Since then she has become increasingly fearful of bullying. Megan has two close friends, but other students often tease her during breaks at school. In physical education classes she is often overlooked in team selections and teased by fellow pupils.

Megan's parents became worried about her weight when she was six. They enrolled Megan in several team sports over the years, but she begged to be allowed to discontinue each one: she felt uncoordinated and awkward and was resented by teammates, who saw her as a liability. When she was ten, her parents began putting her on diets. In the last four years she has tried a meal replacement product, Weight Watchers, a grapefruit diet and the Atkins diet: each time Megan lost weight but regained it. Friends, family members, teachers, or even complete strangers frequently comment about Megan's weight. When this happens, she thinks: 'Don't they realise? I already know I'm fat and I'm trying to fix it!' Megan's parents worry about her future; they hear constant media reports about health risks, depression and other problems associated with higher weights.

Someone suggests Dr Jim Spright – a general practitioner experienced in managing overweight in adolescence – as a good starting point to 'do something' about Megan's weight, and Megan's parents decide to seek his professional advice.

The population in which Megan lives

Megan lives in a metropolitan city in Australia, where approximately 21% of adults are considered obese and 35% overweight, and 25% of children aged five to 17 overweight or obese [1]. The hypothetical health minister, prompted by these statistics, public health officials and academics, decides that she wants a formal overweight and obesity strategy. An Obesity Summit is convened to discuss policy options. Academics, public servants, public health officials, commercial weight-loss service providers, exercise industry representatives, food industry manufacturing and retail representatives, surgeons, endocrinologists and general practitioners – including Dr Spright – are all invited.

Over the course of the summit, participants discuss many options. How should food be labelled and marketed? Should marketing for some foods be banned? Should healthy behaviours be mandated? Should health department money be spent on projects with departments of public transport and urban planning? Should spending be focused on kids or on adults? What should be done in schools? Should bariatric surgery be publicly funded, how and for whom? How should social marketing be used, and what can it achieve? Their goal is to produce feasible, acceptable recommendations for actions that will reduce the population prevalence of overweight and obesity significantly by 2020.

Individuals and populations as a focus for action

A distinction between intervening in the lives of individuals – like Megan – and intervening in populations – like Australia – is fundamental to public health practice. An iconic statement of this was made by Geoffrey Rose in his 1985 paper 'Sick individuals and sick populations' [2]. Rose noted that within our population, we tend to treat average states as 'normal', and deviation from such states as 'abnormal' [2]. We present to doctors as patients because we perceive ourselves to be 'abnormal'. The goal of clinicians is to determine whether we are 'abnormal', and if so, explain why. Rose argued that this is an investigation of why variation occurs *within* a population [2]; in the case of weight, for example, a doctor tries to determine why a patient is fatter than the rest of the population. This is done through direct clinical interaction – a relatively intimate and proximal exchange. The clinician's problem-solving is based on examination of the patient and listening to the patient's story, and can take into account many aspects of their lives. The clinician attempts to determine causes for that individual, and achieve the best outcome for them. This might require advocacy for that person against systems designed to ration services.

Rose argued that this important clinical process provides only partial understanding of health problems. If a causal factor is distributed evenly throughout a population, everyone in that population is equally exposed to it. Thus a clinician is unlikely to 'see' it as a causal factor for a patient like Megan, because, within the doctor's population of patients, it does not explain why some patients are thin and others fat. The only way we can 'see' the effect of such an omnipresent factor is to compare a whole population that is heavier on average – say Australia – with one that is leaner on average – say Japan [3]. To make such a comparison changes the key question from 'Why do some Australian individuals weigh more than their peers?' to 'Why is overweight more common in Australia and less common in Japan?' These two explanations, Rose argued, may rest on different causal factors [2]. This led Rose to distinguish between two kinds of intervention: the 'high-risk' strategy, in which individual cases in the high-risk 'tail' of a distribution were identified and treated, and the 'population strategy' where root causes were identified and altered to potentially shift the entire distribution slightly towards lower risk [2]. Although Rose noted strengths and weaknesses of each, he proposed that the 'population strategy' could lead to a greater average improvement in health because of its radical intervention in root causes for whole populations.

Clinicians must act in the best interests of a patient, within a health system inevitably constrained by resource limitations. In contrast, population health interventions focus on whole populations, and public health policy-makers on allocating resources to maximise efficiency; this means such policy-makers may need to be less sensitive to the complexities of individuals' lives, and more conscious of equity and opportunity cost across whole populations. In the clinical case, the patient presents to the clinician and asks for treatment. In the case of public health, the population is unlikely to have asked to have its 'incidence' reduced, making the rights and responsibilities of all involved less clear.

Clinical ethics and public health ethics

Ethics is the study of *what should be done*: a prescriptive, systematic analysis of what is required for human wellbeing [4]. The descriptions above reveal the potential for incompatibility between the ethics of clinical medicine and the ethics of public health. They occur in a different milieu, take different objects, seek different objectives, and work from different information. It is perhaps unsurprising then that the development of clinical ethics has been reasonably distinct from the development of public health ethics.

Ethics has been a concern of the medical profession for over two millennia: in this sense, medical ethics is not new. However the focus on ethical analysis and reform of clinical medicine and biotechnology has intensified since the development of bioethics in the 1960s [5]. Clinical ethics grew and developed during the second half of the 20th century but during this period public health ethics was relatively neglected [6–8]. Systematic attempts to establish an ethic for public health began in earnest in the 21st century producing, for example, a specialist journal [9], full-length books [10] and technical reports [11, 12].

Approaches to clinical ethics

A number of moral frameworks have been proposed to guide clinical decision-making, including casuistry (case-based reasoning), narrative ethics and the ethics of care [4]. The most dominant framework, however, has been principle-based ethics (sometimes referred to as 'principlism' [12]. Much-criticised, much-revised and extremely influential, it focuses on four central and two derived principles for ethical conduct (hence the name): respect for the autonomy of the patient, beneficence (doing good for the patient), non-maleficence (not doing harm to the patient), ensuring justice, veracity (practicing honestly) and respect for the patient's privacy and confidentiality. While each of these principles is important, they are, in themselves, not action-guiding and must always be specified and balanced and supported by rules that describe their scope, authority and relevant processes. Respect for autonomy, therefore, requires that a patient's consent is sought before commencing treatment, but does not demand that a patient's decisions always be respected, irrespective of the cost. Likewise, rules for consent must be clearly articulated to outline who can consent, what capacities are required before one can consent, and what should be done where a person is unable, because of illness, to consent. While this approach is deceptively simple, and may obscure considered ethical critique, the fact that it provides a moral framework that appears consistent with clinical practice has led to its widespread adoption by the health professions.

Approaches to public health ethics

In contrast to clinical ethics, there is little consensus on the best approach to ethics in public health, except for a general agreement that public health ethics requires its own framework [7, 13]. To date the literature has suggested five key issues in evaluating public health actions: benefits and harms of intervention (or non-intervention), problem definition and telos (ultimate purpose), fairness and distributive justice, process and procedural justice, and rights [5, 11, 14–20].

Maximising benefit, minimising harm

The framework most commonly associated with public health is utilitarianism, a consequentialist and welfarist philosophical position that emphasises achieving the greatest good for the greatest number of people. Utilitarians are firstly concerned with the effectiveness or benefit of an intervention [5, 14, 17, 19, 21] and the balance of any benefits to the attendant burdens [5, 14]. Possible concerns here include coercion, infringement, intrusion or undermining of human rights (see below) [11, 14, 16, 17] whether the response is proportional to the problem [14], whether the action is necessary [14, 19], and the cost of the intervention, including the opportunity cost [17, 19]. It is also important here to consider the quality of evidence on matters of ethical concern [15, 19, 20].

Problem definition and telos

Some writers emphasise the severity of the problem or risk addressed [17] and the goals of intervention as key issues for ethical evaluation. More ethical interventions are thought to relate to severe problems, fundamental causes, conditions and environments, and/or to address the ill-health that people impose on each other rather than the ill-health people impose upon themselves, because this is more respectful of the autonomy of individuals [5, 15].

Increasing fairness or distributive justice

Other writers have argued that social justice, community, common good and/or recognition of mutual vulnerability are the best basis for public health ethics [6, 22, 23]. These writers suggest that it is most important to evaluate the fairness of goals and interventions, and the distribution of benefits and burdens, especially with regard to vulnerable groups and health inequalities [5, 11, 14, 15, 17, 19, 21]. For these writers, goods in public health may be more valuable if they can be obtained only, or more efficiently, through collective action or if benefits pertain to whole communities [5, 14, 17, 19, 21], such as through provision of supportive environments or assisting communities to act [11, 16].

Process and procedural justice

Another approach is less concerned with principles, values or justifications, and more with processes and procedural justice. This approach values collaboration and participation [14, 15], transparency and accountability (including informing or disclosing, speaking truthfully, and providing public justification) [14–16, 19, 20] acknowledging and accommodating diversity, applying fair process when consensus cannot be reached [14, 15], obtaining consent, determining community acceptance or ensuring adequate mandate for intervention [11, 15, 19], and building and maintaining trust [14, 15].

Rights as a basis for public health

The final domain argues – broadly – that human rights provide the most coherent, egalitarian, universalisable and critical framework for public health [7, 17]. These rights generally include protection of privacy and confidentiality [15] and respecting the 'right to health' enshrined in some international agreements, which entails a 'positive right' to health improvement [7, 17, 24]. Limiting an individual's freedoms is justified only to prevent harm to others, that is, respecting their 'negative right' to non-interference – sometimes called the Millian harm principle, after John Stuart Mill [7, 16, 21, 24].

A central problem for all approaches to public health ethics

Consideration of each of these domains is necessary for a comprehensive account of any public health intervention. All approaches, arguably, can inform decisions regarding a key problem in public health ethics: the degree to which coercion – forcing someone to act against their own will – or paternalism – interfering with someone's liberty or autonomy without their consent to make them better off – are ethically permissible in public health [25, 26]. This is a central issue because degrees of coercion and paternalism have been key to the successes of public health [7, 11, 21] – think of seatbelt laws, gun control, fluoridation, sanitation and food hygiene regulations. A central challenge for public health is thus to define exactly when paternalism and/or coercion are permissible, and under what conditions, and what responsibilities this may entail for governments and individuals [18].

Some public health actions are justified by qualifying the paternalism involved. Three justificatory qualifications are made. The first is that the paternalism is 'soft' – that is, that it restricts only ill-informed and involuntarily actions. The second is that the paternalism is 'weak' – that is, that it interferes only when a person's actions are inconsistent with their own goals. The final justification is that the paternalism is 'welfare oriented' – that is, that those intervening are concerned only for a person's physical and psychological condition, as opposed to preventing them from being 'morally corrupted' [11, 18, 21]. These distinctions are a matter of degree and need to be argued on a case-by-case basis.

Some, particularly those concerned with rights and with procedural justice, argue that a simplistic opposition – paternalism or coercion versus freedom – obscures the complex relationship between these concepts, and de-emphasises the positive freedoms that public health interventions can promote [21]. Although voluntarism is not always effective [6], freedoms can decrease the need for coercion. If states engage communities, earning trust that negative freedoms will be respected, individuals may be more likely to seek help; conversely coercive interventions may be less effective or drive epidemics underground [7, 14, 17]. In addition, even strongly paternalistic actions could be moderated by democratic oversight or a community-level mandate [27]. These scholars would argue that by engaging communities paternalism can be lessened and better justified.

We have now considered both clinical and public health ethics. In clinical ethics, a clinician engages directly with a patient and the problem she presents. The clinician attempts to act in the patient's best interests and to advocate on her behalf. The clinician seeks to determine what has made that individual patient atypical – 'high risk' – in the distribution of her peers. More ethical clinical conduct, broadly speaking, will be that which respects the patients' autonomy, does her good, does not harm her, treats her justly and honestly, and respects her privacy and confidentiality. In public health, the situation is different. A decision-maker engages with 'problems' that are most likely to be defined statistically by the state, and may not be priorities for the community. The public health professional – if applying a 'population' strategy – will seek to determine what makes this population different from other populations in regard to that problem, and to intervene in these 'root causes', ideally in a way that maximises benefit, minimises harm, seeks justice, is procedurally transparent, minimises violation of the rights of individuals, and can justify any coercion or paternalism entailed.

What ethical issues are relevant for Megan, her parents and Dr Spright?

Megan and her parents attend Dr Spright's office for a long appointment. Spright's training, as Rose would say [2], is to find the 'causes of Megan's case', that is to find a causal explanation for why Megan, as an individual, deviates from the average or desired weight for her age. During the appointment he asks many questions about Megan – about her development, diet, exercise, other illnesses, symptoms, schooling, friends and family. He takes measurements and samples. He discusses the evidence for, and his experience with, a variety of approaches and services – dietary regimes, weight-loss clubs, specialist physicians and centres and exercise programs.

Dr Spright – Jim – has done continuing education courses in clinical ethics. He is keenly aware that his interactions with Megan and her mother are ethically charged, and that bioethical principles are expressed daily through the actions of doctors like him. Jim tries to conduct himself ethically, as he would with any other patient. In the interests of non-maleficence, he recommends actively against some programs and services that he thinks are non-evidence based and exploitive. His beneficence is expressed through offering evidence-based options that he thinks will help. He tries to respect the autonomy of both Megan and her parents in their conversation. Jim knows that Megan has her own opinions and goals and tries to draw her out whenever he can. He tries to inform but not over-inform, pulling back when they seem to be overwhelmed. He offers his own opinion – with clear reasons – when Megan and her mother ask for it. He is careful not to act in ways that could undermine Megan's self-esteem, and he gently asks questions about the role of her family in her daily habits, not assuming that she is completely independent in her choices [28]. Apart from being sensitive to whether or not Megan's family can afford private services, and whether they are insured, Jim doesn't consider the cost of different treatments when making his recommendations – he considers only whether or not he thinks they are best for Megan.

In this sense, Megan is like any one of Jim's patients. However Megan is also unlike many of Jim's patients. Megan is apparently well. If she suffers from any current condition, it is the psychological effects of the stigma commonly experienced by fat people [29]. Jim is not being asked to treat a current, urgent medical condition like a broken finger or an acute infection. Instead he is being asked to 'treat' two problems: a future risk (that Megan will experience future weight-related health problems), and a socially produced psychological condition (the product of her stigmatisation). Jim does not think about Megan in this way, however. Because of his expertise and training, because he has read many reports showing that obesity is potentially damaging for health, and because Megan and her mother are asking him for assistance he defines Megan's weight as 'a problem'. He sets about explaining why she is fatter than other 15-year-olds, and seeks to provide an individually tailored solution in the most ethical way possible. This individualism is a natural product of case analysis, attention to ethical principles and clinical problem-solving. It is, however, very different from what happens at the Obesity Summit.

What ethical issues are relevant for Australian citizens, their minister for health and their bureaucrats?

The week after Jim sees Megan, he attends the Obesity Summit. Before he goes he reads some of the preparatory material, but it doesn't seem clear to him which strategies are evidence based and which are not. A lot of evidence is presented for the prevalence of overweight and obesity, but not much about the effectiveness or implementation of programs. Megan is on his mind as he travels to the meeting in Canberra. What good will this do her, he wonders? In fact, what difference will this make for anyone?

There are several hundred people at the summit. Jim notices that not many of the participants seem to be obese themselves. After the Welcome to Country ceremony the health minister is introduced. She stands amid the applause, walks to the microphone and begins her opening speech.

> We face a crisis in this country. Two-thirds of Australian men are overweight. Half of Australian women are overweight. A quarter of our children are overweight. Many of us are dying of the diseases that are complications of obesity, such as diabetes and cardiovascular disease.
>
> The question is what we do about it. Answering that question is what we are here for.
>
> Australians are simply eating more kilojoules than they are burning. Everyday foods that have become part of our daily diet are laden with kilojoules. Most ordinary snacks – ice-creams, chocolate bars, soft drinks – would require an hour of fast walking to burn off. We are adding these snacks to our diets and simultaneously doing less and less exercise.
>
> Somehow, we have to find a way to eat less and move around more. We need to lose some weight. I don't think the answer is banning things. We don't want to shut down industries, or gag their right to advertise. We don't want to tell people that they can't have treats, that they can't celebrate with their families. We need to find ways to make people feel responsible for their own actions. We need to encourage industries to self-regulate. We need to encourage people to make better choices. We need to give people better information.
>
> Your job is to work out how best we can do that. It's the most important health challenge facing this country today. I will look forward to receiving the recommendations from the meeting. Thank you for agreeing to be a part of it.

Over the next few days, health bureaucrats, consumer advocates, representatives of industry, and experts from public health, epidemiology, nutrition, health economics, exercise physiology, health education and law rise to the minister's challenge – presenting sometimes conflicting data regarding the costs to the community, and to individuals, of the 'obesity epidemic' and calling for support for a range of interventions to meet it.

The summit concludes with a resolution calling upon the federal and state governments to prioritise two strategies: 1) a large, persuasive social marketing campaign aimed at raising awareness of the problem and motivating individuals to do something about their diet and sedentary behaviours; and 2) greater funding for obesity-related medical consultations and for bariatric surgery, including for adolescents. These recommendations are broadly acceptable to most political interests at the summit. They give something to both public health professionals and clinicians. They locate the problem and its solution with individual citizens; they permit egalitarian rhetoric via statistics showing equal 'reach' and 'access'; they appear to be minimally restrictive on people's freedoms; and they provide new income streams for some interests while not limiting the income streams of commercial interests. And, perhaps most persuasively, they are framed as being 'evidence based' – although in reality they are no more or less evidence based than other possibilities considered at the summit.

In many ways the Obesity Summit is a success. It stimulates passing media interest in obesity, it brings together a range of disciplinary and sectional interests into open dialogue about obesity, and it generates clear recommendations for action. But closer examination of the summit reveals many of the assumptions that underpin policy-making around obesity, the limitations of this model of analysis and decision-making, and the potential value of a framework for explicit consideration of issues of ethics and evidence in public health.

The minister's opening speech is familiar to anyone who has been audience to such occasions. It begins – as such speeches often do – by conflating overweight and obesity, associating overweight or obesity with death, and suggesting a need for weight loss, or at least behaviour change. Although the rhetorical power of this is clear, the evidence suggests that it is somewhat misleading. Many systematic reviews distinguish between the health effects of obesity versus overweight (showing overweight to be significantly less risky or even, at some ages, and in some situations, protective) and there are contradictory findings about the benefits of weight loss [eg 30–34]. The speech also frames individual actions as the key problem to be solved, and implicitly advocates a purpose for intervention: encouraging individuals to change their actions. Indeed, the minister explicitly guards the audience against restriction of trade and commerce, makes no mention of environmental contributors to obesity and (implicitly) restricts the critique of government. It is easy to argue that this fails to address the fundamental root causes, conditions and environments that might stimulate such behaviours, ignores the ill-health that people impose on each other, and in fact focuses on preventing people from harming themselves.

The speech also emphasises that obesity is harmful and suggests that public health action will be beneficial. Throughout the summit, experts present competing accounts of the benefits and harms of various interventions, and many of the small group discussions focus on these evaluations. Such evaluative practices are fundamental in both public health planning and utilitarianism. Inasmuch as there is a positive right to health improvement, or responsibility for public health practitioners to improve health, then advocacy for action – including advocacy of its benefits – is reasonable and required. Yet while there is much optimistic talk of benefits, there is often very little focus on potential harms. Jim might well think about Megan – an overweight but not obese adolescent coping with teasing, anxiety and reduced self-esteem – and wonder how some of the interventions proposed at the summit might affect her. Interventions such as the withdrawn Singaporean school-based program Trim and Fit have been empirically associated with negative outcomes such as bullying and eating disorders for young people [35], often while producing the desired reductions in weight. This demonstrates the importance of going beyond 'effectiveness' – for example, measures of desired behaviour change – by employing ethical reasoning. It also suggests the need for better measurement of potential harms, including stigmatisation [20].

Public health decisions should rely on evaluations of harm and benefit [5, 11, 14, 16, 17, 19]. But the utilitarian ideal of balancing all relevant benefits and harms based on evidence is unlikely to be achieved [36]. Evidence is consumed in the context of political, social, media and lobbying pressures. Our hypothetical Obesity Summit is a conglomeration of interest groups jostling for prime position, and threatening harms such as job losses, restrictions on commercial freedom of speech, or damage to economic productivity. Little wonder then that public health professionals, with the best intentions, feel a responsibility to provide the most compelling evidence they can about the health benefits of interventions! Even the purest utilitarian decision-making requires weighing up of non-equivalent, and perhaps non-comparable, benefits and harms. Simple utilitarianism can also be limited by inattention to egalitarian ideals. Fairness is rarely measured [23] or addressed in mainstream public health strategies [eg 37], despite its rhetorical prominence in public health documents [38]. Although recent commentaries have asserted Rose's deep concern for egalitarianism [39], the idea of shifting an entire population towards slightly lower risk is sometimes used to justify prioritising utilitarian average benefit over greater fairness in distribution of benefit. This is a values-based rather than an empirically based commitment [6, 22, 23]. Regarding weight, empirical evidence suggests that – for example – higher weight is associated with lower educational achievement [40], that the poorest Australian neighbourhoods have 2.5 times as many fast-food outlets as the richest neighbourhoods [41], and that the objective weight and subjective perception of the acceptability of weight in adolescents varies according to their socioeconomic status [42]. Thus, fair distribution may be at least as ethically important as average benefit.

And what of rights, freedoms, coercion and paternalism? Although many scholars interested in these areas have focused on pandemic contagious disease [16, 43], the issues are also critical in chronic states such as overweight, for which the threat of harm is less immediate and less certain. Tobacco and alcohol provide examples of risk factors for which an argument can perhaps be made that behaviour constitutes a threat to others (environmental tobacco smoke and violence, respectively). At the Obesity Summit, economists attempt to provide arguments about such other-regarding harms, including costs to the taxpayer, caring burdens on families and work absenteeism. But while each of these issues seem relevant, for the most part they fail to gain traction in discussions regarding how the government should intervene in response to obesity, in part, because these are; a) non-health costs; b) based on highly abstracted models; and c) vulnerable to the way in which overweight versus obese individuals are classified. Any empirical uncertainties regarding differential risks between these groups become highly ethically relevant to these debates, raising questions about the basis for justification of intervention.

One group of scholars has answered this question with procedural justice. If, they argue, decision-makers make themselves accountable to communities, or can demonstrate a community mandate for action, they are justified in acting. Models for such mandates can range from the most broad (eg democratic election of a government) to the most specific (eg deliberative processes that actively inform and engage a representative sample of citizens and seek consensus on a course of action for a specific problem such as overweight). Summits – like our hypothetical one – can help to meet the more limited requirements of transparency in decision-making. However, they also raise questions about the circumstances under which mandate can be said to have been achieved. If summits are populated entirely by 'experts' – even if that includes 'expert' consumer advocates – can they be said to provide a real mandate? Who should legitimately make decisions about public health priorities? [44] Is it realistic to expect ordinary citizens to engage in public health decision-making? Could such engagement be achieved under the right conditions? These questions are yet to be answered; they bring us to the relationship between individual and community-level intervention.

Individual and community-level intervention: thinking across boundaries

Jim Spright feels strangely unsatisfied with the whole process. It felt to him like a 'political exercise', and he is not convinced by the outcome. He thinks about what these strategies might do for Megan, and for Australia. The campaign may increase the stigma that Megan experiences at school. Greater funding for surgery and consultations may increase healthcare costs, expectations of services and distribution of services across the population. Spright is conservative with referrals for surgery, as he's concerned about potential, as yet unknown, future harms of the procedure. He's also concerned that the increased healthcare costs may have only a marginal impact on the weight or health of the population. In fact, he muses, the campaign might inspire Megan to assent to more radical interventions, like surgery, whether or not that is in her best interests. He also thinks about his poorer patients, because he knows that they are less likely to respond to this campaign, and have less access to surgery. And he wonders whether these strategies might prove to be of most benefit to those who are already receptive to health messages, who already think about their health, and who already have reasonable access to healthcare.

Jim then thinks about how health fits into the lives of his patients. He has been reading lately about 'healthism' [45], the accusation that public health prioritises health outcomes over other outcomes regardless of the goals of the individuals and populations they serve. People clearly value their 'health', he thinks, but what does this mean? 'Health' and 'public health' can be defined very narrowly or very broadly [44, 46, 47]. Jim can see that these strategies serve narrow definitions of health as physical health, but he wonders whether they are good for people's health more broadly: for their wellbeing. In his consultations with a patient like Megan, he can carefully explore life goals, values, what her weight means and how this relates to her emotional wellbeing, fulfilment and happiness. This is difficult, and time consuming, but it can be done. However Jim knows that weight is not simply an individual matter [48]. If we're going to intervene in weight in communities, how can we think about the relationship between community and individual goals and freedoms?

We suggest that the best way of thinking about the ethics of intervening in individuals' weight and communities' or populations' weight is to think about both at once, and to consider the relationship between them. This is surprisingly rare, perhaps because few individuals work across the clinical–population health boundary. However, as is clear from the summit recommendations to support both an extensive social marketing campaign and the medical and surgical management of obesity, it is readily apparent that individuals and communities mutually interact.

This suggests that it is a mistake to understand issues like obesity, and the public health responses to them, as simply a contest between respect for individual liberty (or autonomy) and our responsibilities as citizens, and that there is merit in exploring some of the various 'third way' positions between individualism and collectivism that have been suggested in public health ethics [6, 7, 14, 17, 21, 27, 36, 49–52]. This work suggests several answers for Jim's concerns that might help public health strategies to be more ethically justifiable. Respect for individual autonomy is, largely, a concern with freedom – with the freedom to be and to do as one wishes. However, as relational approaches to autonomy have shown us, these freedoms are not a purely individual matter: they are constituted in relationships. The communities that we belong to produce goods: things that we value. It been proposed that these goods are of two kinds: aggregative and corporate [52]. Aggregative goods are simply the aggregation of individual goods. Corporate goods, however, are an 'emergent social property' of communities: they can only be obtained through community collaboration or cooperation [52]. Corporate goods of public health interventions might include, for example, the creation of conditions that support sustainable future improvements in health, the development of new shared and valued cultural practices, or community attributes like solidarity or diversity. Corporate goods have a future orientation – rather than simply providing a present benefit, they provide a benefit available to future communities. This distinction resonates with Munthe's call for public health interventions that both 1) promote population health, and 2) promote 'equal (and real) opportunities for everyone to be more healthy' [50]. For Munthe, this required providing the freedom to be healthy or unhealthy (including by preventing others from constraining our health opportunities), but the means only to be healthy [50].

To take such a 'third way' position on intervention in weight would assist decision-making for both individual and population-level interventions. It provides an ethical rationale that resonates with Rose's concern for intervention in 'root causes'. Changing the price structure and composition of the food sold in supermarkets, providing usable public transport, or designing a local community to provide healthier food outlets and better opportunities for walking would be recognisable interventions in root causes – of health, not just of weight. Critically, they are also corporate goods – the kind that can only be achieved through collective effort and which provide sustainable future benefit. They provide opportunities for health and prevent others – like food producers – from constraining our health opportunities; however they do not constrain individuals' freedoms to live unhealthily if that is what they desire. Mulvaney-Day has shown, on the basis of social network analyses, that the people one cares about – that is, one's affective network – may be a more important influence on weight than the people who live nearby [53]. They suggest that ethical interventions engage at a meso-level – the level of community – leveraging existing relationship networks to change the opportunities available to people. This may, at least in part, explain the popularity of programs such as School Kitchen Gardens [54] which provide opportunities for existing affective networks to make changes together. Such programs also potentially provide both opportunities and corporate goods by changing the norms and practices in a social group, allowing those to be handed down through generations.

The solutions chosen by the summit provide none of these collective community-level goods. Instead, the summit used a collective process to support individualistic solutions, with little evidence of engagement with the important ethical issues raised for clinical or public health practice. This does not, of course, suggest that participants were ignorant of, or insensitive to, many of the ethical issues that underpin medicine and public health, but rather, that these issues were not explicitly addressed, that the limitations of 'evidence' were not made clear, that the complex relationships between individuals and the communities in which they live were not fully exposed and that the socio-moral goals of healthcare were not made explicit. These are important failings, because the values, focus, scope and goals of clinical medicine and public health are both distinct and overlapping; because interventions to address problems affecting individuals and communities may have different goals, risks and benefits, and because moral compromise in the design and delivery of healthcare is always necessary. For both clinicians and public health decision-makers, the central task is to think through the ethical and philosophical basis for actions before they are taken.

References

1. Australian Institute of Health and Welfare (2010). *Australia's health 2010*. Australia's health series no. 12. Cat. no. AUS 122. Canberra: Australian Institute of Health and Welfare.

2. Rose G (1985). Sick individuals and sick populations. *International Journal of Epidemiology*, 14(1): 32–38.

3. World Health Organization (2006). *Global database on body mass index*. Geneva: World Health Organization.

4. Kerridge I, Lowe M & Stewart C (2009). *Ethics and law for the health professions*. 3rd edn. Annandale, NSW: The Federation Press.

5. Kass NE (2001). An ethics framework for public health. *American Journal of Public Health*, 91(11): 1776–82.

6. Kass NE (2004). Public health ethics: from foundations and frameworks to justice and global public health. *Journal of Law Medicine & Ethics*, 32(2): 232–42.

7. Bayer R & Fairchild AL (2004). The genesis of public health ethics. *Bioethics*, 18(6): 473–92.

8. Callahan D & Jennings B (2002). Ethics and public health: forging a strong relationship. *American Journal of Public Health*, 92(2): 169–76.

9. Dawson A & Verweij M (2009). *Public health ethics*. Oxford, UK: Oxford University Press.

10. Holland S (2007). *Public health ethics*. Cambridge: Polity.

11. Nuffield Council on Bioethics (2007). *Public health: ethical issues*. London: Nuffield Council on Bioethics.

12. Beauchamp TL & Childress JF (2001). *Principles of biomedical ethics*. 5th edn. New York: Oxford University Press.

13. Beauchamp DE (1976). Exploring new ethics for public health: developing a fair alcohol policy. *Journal of Health Politics Policy and Law*, 1(3): 338–54.

14. Childress JF, Faden RR, Gaare RD, Gostin LO, Kahn J, Bonnie RJ, et al. (2002). Public health ethics: mapping the terrain. *Journal of Law Medicine and Ethics*, 30(2): 170–78.

15. Center for Health Leadership and Practice, Public Health Institute, Public Health Leadership Society Ethics Work Group and Public Health Leadership Society Standing Committee on Public Health Ethics (2002). *Principles of the ethical practice of public health*. New Orleans, LA: Public Health Leadership Society.

16. Upshur RE (2002). Principles for the justification of public health intervention. *Canadian Journal of Public Health–Revue Canadienne De Sante Publique*, 93(2): 101–03.

17. Gostin KG (2003). Public health ethics: tradition, profession, and values. *Acta Bioethica*, 9(2): 177–88.

18. Jennings B, Kahn J, Mastroianni A & Parker LS (2003). *Ethics and public health: model curriculum*. Washington: Health Resources and Services Administration, Association of Schools of Public Health and Hastings Centre.

19. Baum NM, Gollust SE, Goold SD & Jacobson PD (2007). Looking ahead: addressing ethical challenges in public health practice. *Journal of Law Medicine & Ethics*, 35(4): 657–67.

20. Carter SM, L, Lloyd B, Kerridge IH, Baur L, Bauman A, Hooker C & Zask A (2011). Evidence, ethics, and values: a framework for health promotion. *American Journal of Public Health*, 101(3): 465–72.

21. Faden R & Shebaya S (2010). Public health ethics. In EN Zalta (Ed). *The Stanford encyclopedia of philosophy* [Online]. Available: plato.stanford.edu/entries/publichealth-ethics/ [Accessed 5 September 2011].

22. Baylis F, Kenny NP & Sherwin S (2008). A relational account of public health ethics. *Public Health Ethics*, 1(3): 196–209.

23. Daniels N (2008). *Just health*. Cambridge: Cambridge University Press.

24. Thomas JC, Sage M, Dillenberg J & Guillory VJ (2002). A code of ethics for public health. *American Journal of Public Health*, 92(7): 1057–59.

25. Anderson S (2008). Coercion. In EN Zalta (Ed). *The Stanford encyclopedia of philosophy* [Online]. Available: plato.stanford.edu/archives/fall2008/entries/coercion/ [Accessed 2 September 2011].

26. Dworkin G (2010). Paternalism. In EN Zalta (Ed). *The Stanford encyclopedia of philosophy* [Online]. Available: plato.stanford.edu/archives/sum2010/entries/paternalism/ [Accessed 2 September 2011].

27. Dawson A & Verweij M (2008). The steward of the Millian state. *Public Health Ethics*, 1(3): 193–95.

28. Entwistle VA, Carter SM, Cribb A & McCaffery K (2010). Supporting patient autonomy: the importance of clinician–patient relationships. *Journal of General Internal Medicine*, 25(7): 741–45.

29. Puhl RM & Heuer CA (2009). The stigma of obesity: a review and update. *Obesity*, 17(5): 941–64.

30. Janssen I & Mark AE (2007). Elevated body mass index and mortality risk in the elderly. *Obesity Reviews*, 8(1): 41–59.

31. Lenz M, Richter T, Muhlhauser I, Lenz M, Richter T & Muhlhauser I (2009). The morbidity and mortality associated with overweight and obesity in adulthood: a systematic review. *Deutsches Arzteblatt International*, 106(40): 641–48.

32. McGee DL & Diverse Populations Collaboration (2005). Body mass index and mortality: a meta-analysis based on person-level data from twenty-six observational studies. *Annals of Epidemiology*, 15(2): 87–97.

33. Oreopoulos A, Padwal R, Kalantar-Zadeh K, Fonarow GC, Norris CM & McAlister FA (2008). Body mass index and mortality in heart failure: a meta-analysis. *American Heart Journal*, 156(1): 13–22.

34. Romero-Corral A, Montori VM, Somers VK, Korinek J, Thomas RJ, Allison TG, Mookadam F & Lopez-Jimenez F (2006). Association of bodyweight with total mortality and with cardiovascular events in coronary artery disease: a systematic review of cohort studies. *The Lancet*, 368(9536): 666–78.

35. Lee HY, Lee EL, Pathy P & Chan YH (2005). Anorexia nervosa in Singapore: an eight-year retrospective study. *Singapore Medical Journal*, 46(6): 275–81.

36. Wyniaa MK (2005). Oversimplifications I: physicians don't do public health. *The American Journal of Bioethics*, 5(4): 4–5.

37. Carter SM, Hooker LC & Davey HM (2009). Writing social determinants into and out of cancer control: an assessment of policy practice. *Social Science & Medicine*, 68(8): 1448–55.

38. First International Conference on Health Promotion (1986). Ottawa Charter for Health Promotion, WHO/HPR/HEP/95.1. Ottawa: World Health Organization, 21 November.

39. Rose G, Khaw K-T & Marmot M (2008). *Rose's strategy of preventive medicine: updated edition*. Oxford: Oxford University Press.

40. Cameron AJ, Welborn TA, Zimmet PZ, Dunstan DW, Owen N, Salmon J, Dalton M, Jolley D & Shaw JE (2003). Overweight and obesity in Australia: the 1999–2000 Australian diabetes, obesity and lifestyle study (AusDiab). *Medical Journal of Australia*, 178(9): 427–32.

41. Reidpath DD, Burns C, Garrard J, Mahoney M & Townsend M (2002). An ecological study of the relationship between social and environmental determinants of obesity. *Health & Place*, 8(2): 141–45.

42. O'Dea JA & Caputi P (2001). Association between socioeconomic status, weight, age and gender, and the body image and weight control practices of 6- to 19-year-old children and adolescents. *Health Education Research*, 16(5): 521–32.

43. Bayer R (1988). AIDS and the ethics of public-health: challenges posed by a maturing epidemic. *Aids*, 2: S217–S221.

44. Ruger JP (2010). *Health and social justice*. New York: Oxford University Press.

45. Skrabanek P (1994). *The death of humane medicine and the rise of coercive healthism*. Suffolk: The Social Affairs Unit.

46. Rothstein MA (2002). Rethinking the meaning of public health. *Journal of Law Medicine & Ethics*, 30(2): 144–49.

47. Buchanan DR (2000). *An ethic for health promotion: rethinking the sources of human wellbeing*. New York: Oxford University Press.

48. Holm S (2008). Parental responsibility and obesity in children. *Public Health Ethics*, 1(1): 21–29.

49. EuroPHEN (European Public Health Ethics Network) (2006). Public policies, law and bioethics: a framework for producing public health policy across the European Union. European Union Member States: Funded by the European Commission, DG Research, under FP5, Quality of Life Programme QLG6–CT–2002–02320, www.europhen.net.

50. Munthe C (2008). The goals of public health: an integrated, multidimensional model. *Public Health Ethics*, 1(1): 39–52.

51. Jennings B (2009). Public health and liberty: beyond the Millian paradigm. *Public Health Ethics*, 2(2): 123–34.

52. Widdows H & Cordell S (2011). Why communities and their goods matter: illustrated with the example of biobanks. *Public Health Ethics*, 4(1): 14–25.

53. Mulvaney-Day N & Womack CA (2009). Obesity, identity and community: leveraging social networks for behavior change in public health. *Public Health Ethics*, 2(3): 250–60.

54. Gibbs L, Staiger P, Townsend M, Macfarlane S, Block K, Gold L, Johnson B, Long C, Kulas J, Ukoumunne OC & Waters E (2009). *Evaluation of the Stephanie Alexander Kitchen Garden Program*. Melbourne: The Stephanie Alexander Kitchen Garden Foundation [Online]. Available: www.kitchengardenfoundation.org.au/about–the–program/proving–it–works [Accessed 2 September 2011].

13

How law and regulation can add value to prevention strategies for obesity and diabetes

Roger S Magnusson[1]

Steadily rising rates of overweight and obesity among adults and children in Australia and elsewhere are fuelling debate about the most effective and appropriate strategies for obesity prevention. This chapter defends a role for law in policy efforts to prevent obesity and to improve nutrition at the population level. Rather than targeting individuals and seeking to directly influence their dietary choices and patterns of physical activity, I argue that the best opportunities for law lie in improving the environment in order to support healthier choices and to reduce exposure to the wide range of factors that have made weight gain increasingly common. Secondly, this chapter presents four Australian case studies, with comparisons from the US and the UK, to illustrate the variety of priority interventions that could take legal form.

On my first day of law school, I was introduced to the law of contracts and the law of torts. In five years of lectures, however, never once did I come across the 'law of obesity prevention'. Hitherto, preventing obesity has never been considered part of the role of law or lawyers. Lawyers have never been called on to defend the role of law in obesity prevention, or to identify the content of a package of legal interventions having that goal. The same might be said about the law of cardiovascular disease, or diabetes prevention.

Historically, public health law in Australia, Britain and the United States has been the law of unsanitary premises, abatement, and quarantine. Later, it evolved to include notifiable diseases, HIV/AIDS, tobacco control, and more recently – certainly in the United States – the law of public health emergencies and 'pandemic preparedness'. In other respects, public health laws in all three countries have developed in a reactive and haphazard manner, reflecting successive health crises, fears and political priorities that vary between jurisdictions. Writing about English public health legislation, Robyn Martin argues that it neither has the promotion of health as its primary focus, 'nor does it particularly address the causes of ill-health'. Instead, its focus is on inadequate premises, 'on an understanding that ill-health results from identifiable bodies escaping from a physical source' [1]. Only more recently, as Australian public health acts have undergone a process of renewal, has

---

1   Sydney Law School, University of Sydney.

legislation become more proactive, and less issue-specific. South Australia's new *Public Health Act* is the first such act in Australia to include specific provisions for the prevention of non-communicable conditions [2].

Quite apart from this, rising rates of overweight and obesity among adults and children have been fuelling debate about the most effective and appropriate strategies for prevention. Legal scholarship on obesity prevention, although relatively recent, is increasing in popularity, although with substantial differences that reflect the constitutional structure and political traditions of each country [3–9]. Suggested legal strategies are wide-ranging and extend far beyond the boundaries of the health sector and the traditional 'turf' of public health Acts.

This chapter defends a role for law in policy efforts to prevent obesity and to improve nutrition at the population level. Rather than targeting individuals directly and seeking to coerce dietary changes, or greater levels of physical activity, I argue firstly that the best opportunities for law lie in improving the environment in order to support healthier choices and to reduce exposure to the wide range of factors that have made weight gain increasingly common. This emphasis is significant: by focusing on policy, systems and environmental changes, rather than behavioural change directly, law can address the factors that shape patterns of behaviour at a population level, while avoiding the coercive and discriminatory laws to which an excessive emphasis on 'personal responsibility' could lead [10–13].

Secondly, having set out a philosophy or framework for how law can contribute to obesity prevention, this chapter presents four case studies to illustrate the variety of legal interventions in this area. Each case study will be argued through in sufficient detail to illustrate the contested nature of legal interventions, with comparisons between regulatory developments in Australia, the US and the UK.

The trend towards population weight gain: why does it matter?

The prevalence of overweight and obesity is based on measurements of body mass index (BMI), which divides weight in kilograms by height squared (m²). In Australia, results from the 2007–2008 National Health Survey showed that 68% of men, and 55% of women were either overweight (BMI 25.0–29.9 kg/m²) or obese (BMI ≥30 kg/m²), based on measured BMI [14]. Among children aged seven to 15, almost 25% were overweight or obese, rising from 20.7% in 1995, and 11.5% in 1985 [15]. According to a Victorian government study, if current trends continue, 83% of males and 67% of females will be overweight or obese by 2025, as well as over one-third of children [16].

In Australia in 2003, cardiovascular disease (CVD) and cancer accounted for some 37% of the total burden of disease [17].[2] Table 1 illustrates the extraordinary impact of *modifiable risk factors* on disability-adjusted life years (DALYs) from all causes in Australia, and on the leading causes of disease burden, including CVD and cancer. In 2003, overweight and obesity accounted for 7.5% of the burden of disease: almost as much as smoking (7.8%).

---

2 The term 'burden of disease' refers to a combination of years of life lost through premature mortality, combined with the years of *healthy life lost*, due to disease. Typically, the burden of disease is measured in disability-adjusted life years, or DALYs.

Table 1. The contribution of behavioural risk factors to the burden of disease in Australia, 2003*

Determinant	% of DALYS (all causes)#	% of DALYS (specific causes)^
Tobacco	7.8%	20.1% of cancer
High blood pressure	7.6%	42.1% of CVD
Overweight & obesity	7.5%	19.5% of CVD
Physical inactivity	6.6%	23.7% of CVD
High blood cholesterol	6.2%	34.5% of CVD
Alcohol harm	3.3%	3.1% of cancer
Alcohol benefit	−1.0%	−4.7% net benefit on CVD
Lack of adequate fruit, vegetable intake	2.1%	9.6% of CVD

* Begg S, Vos T, Barker B, Stevenson C, Stanley L & Lopez A (2007). *The burden of disease and injury in Australia, 2003.* Canberra: AIHW. PHE 82 (p74).
# Disability-adjusted life years
^ Contribution of each risk factor is independent of other risk factors (analysis is not additive)

Overweight and obesity are risk factors for high blood pressure, raised cholesterol, impaired glucose tolerance, a range of chronic conditions including CVD (coronary heart disease and stroke), type 2 diabetes, a variety of cancers (including colon, breast and ovarian cancer), as well as gallbladder disease, osteoarthritis, gout, and sleep apnoea [18]. Many of these conditions are exacerbated by high blood pressure (for which excess salt consumption is a risk factor), high blood cholesterol (for which excess consumption of saturated fat is a risk factor), and inadequate intake of fresh fruit and vegetables. According to one estimate, in 2007, around 24% of type 2 diabetes, 21% of cardiovascular disease, 25% of osteoarthritis, and 21% of colorectal, breast, uterine and kidney cancer were attributable to obesity [19].

In the US, the prevalence of obesity (defined as BMI >30 kg/m^2) remained relatively stable from 1960 to 1980 but climbed sharply thereafter, from 15% in 1976 to 1980, to 34% in 2007–2008 [20, 21]. Over the same period, obesity in children and adolescents (aged two to 19 years) tripled from over 5% to 17% [22]. Overall calorie intake, mean intake from carbohydrates, and absolute fat intake also increased over this period [23, 24]. Some epidemiologists warn that increases in BMI in the US, and its impact on diabetes, CVD and other conditions, will increasingly outweigh the positive impact on life expectancy of declining smoking rates, and could cause a decline in life expectancy at birth and at older ages during the first half of this century [25–27]. In Australia, D'Arcy, Holman and Smith have warned that, based on recent trends in population weight gain, by the time they are 20, the life expectancy of Australian children will fall two years, pulling them back to 2001 and 1997 levels for males and females, respectively [28].

In 2010, Colagiuri and colleagues estimated the total direct costs of overweight and obesity in Australia in 2005 at A$21 billion, with an additional A$35.6 billion spent by government on pensions and subsidies [29]. Between 2003 and 2033, treatment costs for type 2 diabetes are estimated to increase by 520%, from A$1.3 billion to A$8 billion, largely driven by the impact of rising obesity rates on diabetes prevalence [30]. In the US, by 2008, annual medical costs attributable to obesity are estimated to have reached US$147 billion [31]. In 2007, RAND Corporation estimated that if current trends continue, by 2020 up to one-fifth of all healthcare expenditures could be obesity related [32].

Debates about the right policy approach to population weight gain

The susceptibility of *individuals* to weight gain is influenced both by non-modifiable factors such as age, sex and genetics, and by modifiable dietary and physical activity patterns. Modifiable factors contributing to energy oversupply include the frequency and energy value of the food eaten (fat and alcohol contain more calories per gram than protein and carbohydrates), and the duration and intensity of physical activity. On the other hand, obesity is also a *population issue*: the weight distribution of the population as a whole has drifted steadily to the right over the past two decades.

The rapid changes in national obesity rates over the past few decades suggest that it is environmental influences upon average eating and physical activity patterns within the population that explain the epidemic, rather than individual or genetic factors [33, p118]. Previous generations shared our genes and physiology, but rates of obesity were lower. Explaining the trend towards weight gain solely in terms of people eating too much and exercising too little is self-evident, but ignores the impact of environmental and policy factors on changes in *average behaviour*, and hence the causes of the trend itself. The temptation to explain an emerging epidemic, such as obesity, purely in terms of the private choices of individuals also obscures the contribution of corporate behaviour (such as the food industry) to population health trends, as well as the responsibility of governments to create the conditions for a healthy lifestyle. Understanding this is critical if we are to develop an effective response.

If Australians, as a population, were to adopt a healthier lifestyle, there is little doubt that life expectancy, and healthy life expectancy, could dramatically increase. For example, the INTERHEART study found that over 90% of the risk of heart attack in men and women, young and old, across all geographical regions and ethnic groups, could be predicted by eight risk factors, several of which are certainly modifiable [34]. These are: smoking, physical inactivity, obesity, high blood pressure, high blood cholesterol, diabetes, inadequate fruit and vegetable intake, and psychosocial stressors.

Knowing this, however, is not enough. As the trend towards weight gain illustrates, people find it difficult to eat healthily and to maintain energy balance. In a survey of over 150 000 Americans, 76% were non-smokers, 40% had a healthy weight, 23% had the appropriate intake of fruit and vegetables, and 22% exercised regularly. But only 3% of the sample were following all four of these healthy lifestyle factors [35]. One of the authors of the study said: 'The effect of following these [lifestyle guidelines] is greater than anything else medicine has to offer. I don't know anything a doctor's office can do that would reduce your risk of diabetes or cardiovascular disease by 80% or 90%' [36]. In Australia, Atlantis and colleagues found that while 55% of Australians are eating enough fruit, less than one in four were meeting national guidelines for physical activity (a minimum of 2.5 hours per week of moderate-intensity physical activity, including walking, spread across five or more days per week). Less than 15% were meeting eating enough vegetables, and less than 5% were doing all three [37].

Faced with policy challenges as complex and contested as obesity, there is a temptation for governments in liberal, market-oriented societies – facing coordinated pressure from food and beverage manufacturers and retailers – to frame the problem as one that *individuals* face. The answer seems blindingly obvious: every individual should exercise more 'personal responsibility'. In well-quoted comment, Australia's former health minister, the Hon. Tony Abbott MHR said:

> It is estimated that obesity adds about a billion dollars a year currently to the nation's health bill. Obviously I would rather that we didn't have to spend that money … but in the end if people are obese it's because they're eating too much or they're exercising too little, and the answer is in the hands of those individuals [38].

This is wise counsel – *for individuals*. However, as a conceptual framework for reducing national healthcare costs and the burden of disease caused by obesity and diabetes, it will continue to fail.

Unless motivational strategies and health promotion can magically unlock new personal resources for healthy living that are not already being tapped by the weight-loss industry, or neutralised by the variety of influences in modern societies that make healthy living difficult (such as time poverty, long commutes, loss of cooking skills, food marketing and the ubiquity of cheap, unhealthy food), then this is a counsel of despair. Governments are often attracted to health promotion campaigns using mass media, which were an effective tool in tobacco control strategies. As Wakefield and colleagues point out, however, media campaigns are likely to be more successful when the behaviour that needs to be changed is 'one-off or episodic'. This is not the case with healthy eating and physical activity, which requires sustained discipline and daily effort, well after the campaigns have ended (39). Furthermore, the norms about 'normal weight' are changing. Surveys indicate that males and females in the US [40] and the UK [41], and Australian males [42] do not perceive their (over)weight accurately. Unless individuals recognise when they are overweight, they may have little reason to alter their lifestyles.

To summarise so far: taking responsibility for health is an excellent idea for individuals. However, populations cannot necessarily be expected to 'take responsibility' or to 'shape up' in the way that individuals (sometimes) can. Mass media campaigns are part of a comprehensive policy response, but governments need to be realistic about what they can achieve. To arrest the population-wide trend towards weight gain, we need to address factors to which the population as a whole is exposed: the social forces that shape the way people live [43].

Where does law and regulation fit with obesity prevention strategies?

Most models for understanding the causes of health and disease recognise that health outcomes are the result of a complex interplay of environmental, socioeconomic, biological and individual behavioural factors, partially modified by interactions with the healthcare system (Figure 1) [44]. Strategies for obesity prevention tend to reflect different assumptions about the relative importance of the policy, systems and environmental factors that lie *outside* of the individual, the behavioural factors that *are* the individual, and the biological and genetic influences that lie *within* the individual. The discussion above has already pointed out the limitations of strategies that focus narrowly on the behavioural domain, relying on mass marketing to encourage personal responsibility and motivationally led, self-directed changes in behaviour. As discussed below, each of the strategic domains set out in Figure 1 – the *environment* (from global to local level), *individual behaviours*, and the *health system* – provide opportunities for regulatory interventions that could contribute to healthier eating and improvements in physical activity at a population level. The challenge for public health lawyers is to identify law reform priorities and to make the case for those interventions which are best implemented through legal and regulatory processes.

(i) Regulating the healthcare system

Population growth and the ageing of the population mean that Australia's healthcare system will face a higher burden of chronic disease in future. In 2008, for example, over one million Australians had type 2 diabetes, and over 242 000 of them had it as a result of being obese (an increase of 137% over 2005 figures) [19]. Law plays a crucial role in improving the effectiveness of clinical care; for example, by creating stable rules for the sharing of patient data within an electronic health records system that enjoys public trust, yet permits optimal access to a patient's data at all points of care. In Australia, important elements towards achieving this include the development of a personally controlled electronic health records service [45], which builds on the Healthcare Identifiers Service that uniquely identifies individuals and healthcare providers [46, 47].

In a bold experiment, New York City extended notifiable disease reporting to chronic disease risk factors, through the mandatory reporting of haemoglobin A1c (glycated haemoglobin, a measure of blood glucose control). By making diabetes a notifiable disease, the New York City Department of Health and Mental Hygiene is creating a registry that will map the epidemiology of hyperglycaemia and help to facilitate care for the estimated one-third of diabetics who are unaware of their condition [48–50].[3] Although controversial

---

3 Following a pilot project in the Bronx, patients in New York City with blood glucose levels above a certain level receive information (on an opt-out basis) about the lifestyle changes required to reduce health risks. Treating physicians are given a report which enables them to identify patients whose diabetes is not well controlled, and a summary of glycaemic control among patients in the practice which can be compared with a NYC benchmark.

[51], this initiative deserves careful study elsewhere. Due to the frequent co-location or clustering of chronic disease risk factors in the same individual [52–54], the New York City law could assist in identifying other risk factors for chronic disease in individuals who – not coincidentally – tend to be of lower socioeconomic status [55–57]. Ironically, it is this capacity for chronic disease risk surveillance to potentially contribute to reducing health inequalities that also enables this strategy to be framed as discrimination against poor people of colour.

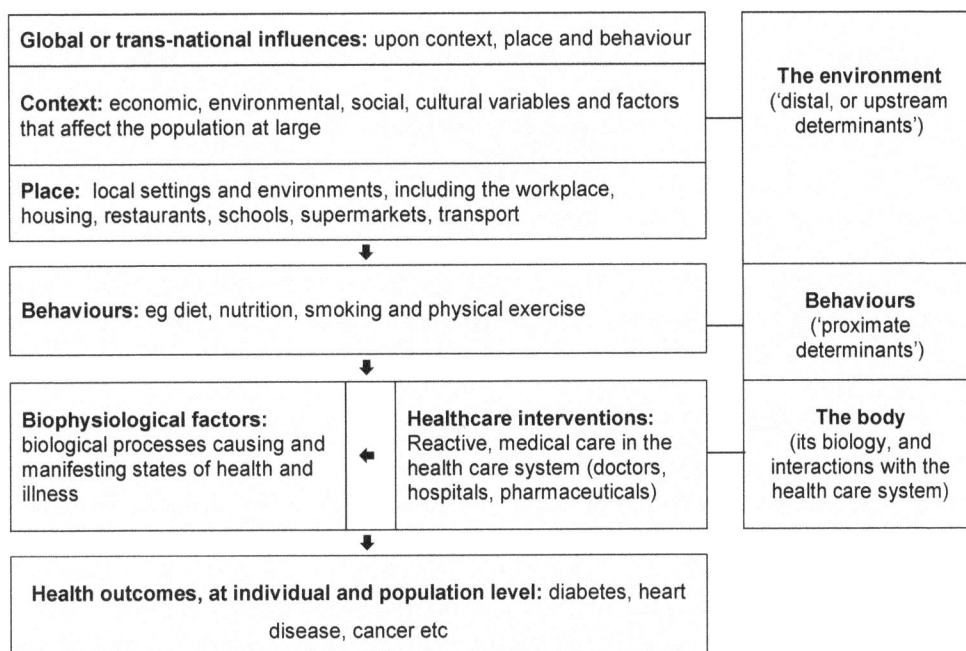

Global or trans-national influences: upon context, place and behaviour	**The environment** ('distal, or upstream determinants')
Context: economic, environmental, social, cultural variables and factors that affect the population at large	
Place: local settings and environments, including the workplace, housing, restaurants, schools, supermarkets, transport	
⬇	
Behaviours: eg diet, nutrition, smoking and physical exercise	**Behaviours** ('proximate determinants')
⬇	
Biophysiological factors: biological processes causing and manifesting states of health and illness ⬅ **Healthcare interventions:** Reactive, medical care in the health care system (doctors, hospitals, pharmaceuticals)	**The body** (its biology, and interactions with the health care system)
⬇	
Health outcomes, at individual and population level: diabetes, heart disease, cancer etc	

Figure 1. A simplified, hierarchical model of the determinants of health and disease

In addition to improving diagnosis and treatment, regulation can enhance the process of integrating secondary prevention within primary healthcare systems. The Australian Government has taken several initiatives in this direction, including the introduction of new Medicare item numbers providing reimbursement for general practitioners to carry out medical check-ups on patients aged from 45 to 49 who present with identifiable risk factors for chronic disease, and patients aged from 40 to 49 whose risk factors (including excess weight) put them at risk of developing type 2 diabetes [58].[4] In its comprehensive review of strategies for chronic disease prevention, the National Preventative Health Taskforce recommended that the Medical Benefits Schedule should support prevention through practice-level incentive payments or payments to individual medical practitioners to support brief interventions and a followup consultation directed to tobacco, alcohol,

---

4 For patients with diagnosed chronic or complex health conditions, Medicare rebates are payable for a limited number of consultations with allied health professional services, as part of an Enhanced Primary Care plan coordinated by a general practitioner: Australian Government Department of Health and Ageing. Enhanced Primary Care Program, at: www.health.gov.au/epc.

obesity, or other risk factors for chronic disease [59, p260]. In the UK, pay-for-performance contracts have been a feature of general practice reform; a substantial proportion of GP income depends upon 'quality points' that are earned when practice targets are met, including those for the assessment and management of risk factors for heart disease, asthma and diabetes [60, 61]. Unlike Australia, patient registration with local NHS practices facilitates continuity of care and a stable patient group for measuring performance.

In Australia, the Practice Incentive Program currently supports performance-based incentive payments to general practices for the successful management of diabetes patients, amongst other areas [62, 63]. The Australian Primary Care Collaboratives program also supports primary practices to improve their capacity to manage and reduce risk factors in the patient group, and to improve management of chronic and complex conditions [64, 65].

From July 2011, the Australian Government began to roll out a network of independent, primary healthcare organisations, known as Medicare Locals [66]. Building on the existing Divisions of General Practice, Medicare Locals identify service gaps and develop formal and informal linkages to integrate the care provided by different service providers. Their role also includes the delivery of health promotion and risk prevention programs targeted to the risk profiles of local communities [67, pp8, 48].

(ii) Targeting the behaviours of individuals

Many people would intuitively understand legal strategies for obesity prevention as crude attempts at behaviour modification, whether through education, financial incentives and disincentives, or more direct forms of control. More benign interventions include evaluative food labelling initiatives which, quite apart from encouraging reformulation by food manufacturers, aim to alter purchasing patterns by educating consumers about the nutrient qualities of foods. Less benign interventions that might be seen as 'targeting' the behaviour or weight status of individuals include restrictions on taxpayer-funded medical procedures for obese patients and smokers [68–70], or the elimination of community rating resulting in differential premiums for private health insurance, and other restrictions in coverage, based on one's obesity or health status.

In April 2008, Japan introduced a legal requirement on companies and local governments to measure the waistlines of Japanese people aged from 40 to 74 as part of their annual check-up. Japan has adopted official limits for waistlines – 33.5 inches for men, and 35.4 inches for women, based on International Diabetes Federation estimates for identifying health risks. Companies and local governments that fail to meet targets for measuring waistlines will be fined [71]. These policies raise the question of who should bear responsibility for the rising prevalence of lifestyle risk factors, including obesity, not to mention the ethics of intruding into the lives of individuals and discriminating against them based on weight [10–12].

Imposing an additional tax on high-fat or high-salt foods, or eliminating tax concessions for novated vehicle leases, illustrate policies that aim to 'nudge' behaviour in a healthier direction by increasing the costs of unhealthy choices and regulating in order to make the healthy choice the 'default option' [12, 72]. These policies are defended on the basis that people find it difficult to make choices that are consistent with their longer-term preferences and welfare, for reasons that include limited willpower, inadequate information and cognitive constraints, and social and cultural influences, including advertising [12, 73]. People are also *overoptimistic*, preferring current consumption while discounting its future, adverse impacts on them *personally* [74].[5] On the other hand, policies can subtly shape patterns of choice within populations in ways that are not necessarily mediated through the *conscious* deliberations of individuals. Interventions of this kind are best understood as being directed at the broader environment, rather than at individuals.

(iii) Improving the quality of the economic, social, physical and policy environment

Although debate persists about the underlying drivers of energy imbalance and weight gain, economic factors are crucial [75, 76]. Relevant factors include the reduced cost of food (particularly energy-dense carbohydrates), and the growth of a commercial food sector marketing processed snack foods (leading to an increase in snacking). Pre-prepared and pre-packaged foods are ubiquitous and heavily marketed, and manufacturers compete for market share by satisfying human preferences for energy-dense, fatty, salty, and sweet foods. Boyd Swinburn points out that the trend towards population weight gain is evidence of commercial success [77], although weight gain brings longer-term costs that the industry externalises. In addition to the changing food culture, technological change has resulted in high levels of car use, and less need for both incidental physical activity and arduous work. Entertainment is frequently passive; not surprisingly, there is a correlation between overweight and hours spent watching television [78].

Scholars point out that population weight gain is, in fact, a normal response to these environmental influences upon diet and physical activity patterns [76]. Two factors follow. Firstly, if the causes of population weight gain lie in the environmental domain, then mitigation 'require[s] socioeconomic, not health sector reforms' [76, p12]. A feature of so-called population health approaches to obesity prevention is the emphasis on interventions that address these 'upstream' environmental and socioeconomic determinants. As Geoffrey Rose stated, a population health approach 'attempts to remove the underlying causes that make the disease common' [79]. To the extent that this can be done successfully, a population health approach has the capacity to shift 'entire risk factor distributions at the population level, not simply the causes of cases at the individual level' [80].

On the other hand, this does not mean that obesity prevention is the process of identifying and seeking to reverse the factors that plausibly explain the population trend. Not only would it be impossible to reverse the processes of economic development and globalisation that have given us higher incomes, labour-saving devices, television, pre-prepared food, and a higher proportion of women in the paid workforce, it would also be highly undesirable. Rather than return society to the Stone Age, the policy priority is to identify

---

5   As Marteau, Oliver and Ashcroft [74] point out, 'Unfortunately, the health costs of many behaviours occur in the future, whereas their benefits are enjoyed in the present. The so-called obesogenic environment reflects the operation of these two principles – that is, an environment that contains a plethora of readily realized options that offer immediate gratification but that cause and sustain obesity'.

feasible, evidence-informed and culturally acceptable ways of counteracting the impacts of an 'obesogenic' environment. Necessarily, this involves finding ways of effectively achieving population nutrient intake goals: reducing salt, fat and free sugars, improving intake of fibre and fresh fruit and vegetables, and increasing levels of physical activity [81].

I would argue that the best opportunities for law lie in addressing the socioeconomic and environmental factors that are driving the increase in average weight gain. 'Privatising' the obesity epidemic – confining it to the healthcare setting, or emphasising personal responsibility to the exclusion of everything else – is unlikely to reverse the trend. Until policy-makers focus on the influences to which *populations are exposed*, there will be nothing to prevent the occurrence of new cases [33, p178]. On the other hand, to the extent that societies are successful in creating supportive environments that encourage healthier lifestyles, it will be 'less necessary to keep on persuading individuals' [79]. By using legal and policy levers to alter the obesogenic environment, the goal is to 'outweigh' those environmental contributors to energy imbalance that it is not feasible to change. An environment that better supports healthier choices and lifestyles will also be a more fertile ground for education strategies and health promotion, and for targeted strategies pursuing behaviour change and significant weight reduction among high-risk groups [82–85].

A final point to make is that where the absolute risk of the population is too high – because, for example, average weight, salt or saturated fat intake is too high – it is not the case that the only ones to benefit from prevention policies are those who have the highest *relative risk* by virtue of being on the far right hand tail of the distribution. The risk of diabetes, for example, rises modestly with BMI within the normal range, and exponentially at higher levels [86]. Although interventions may benefit the smaller number of people at highest risk, the greatest benefit may be among the much larger number of people in the middle part of the disease distribution who are exposed to a relatively low risk [33, pp176–78, 87].

The importance of a 'plausible policy basket'

Before suggesting some law reform priorities for obesity prevention, a dose of realism is needed. No society has yet succeeded in reversing the future reservoir of disease and healthcare expenditure that population weight gain will produce [88]. Given the tenacity of many of the conditions that currently contribute to poor diet and sedentary lifestyle – from long working hours and lack of time, to geographically dispersed suburbs – multiple policy changes will be needed. Implementing a sufficiently broad basket of policies through the political process will be extremely challenging, and incremental progress is the most likely scenario. Nevertheless, serious action on obesity prevention is needed now, before things get worse, relying on the best available evidence, monitoring the entire basket of policies, and adding promising new ones as they become feasible. Insisting on cast-iron evidence of effectiveness for each new policy is an invitation to policy paralysis. Sensibly, the National Preventative Health Taskforce called for a 'trialling of a package of interventions' accompanied by monitoring and evaluation: a 'learning by doing' approach [67, p92].

Scholars including Anjali Jain have pointed out that since there are multiple determinants of population weight gain, 'solutions are also likely to be multifactorial, with no single intervention providing widespread success. Thus it is less important to isolate why an approach is successful, than it is to find interventions that work' [89, p1388]. It is the combined impact of a basket of 'plausible interventions' that is likely to make a difference: no single policy is likely to deliver a 'king hit'. At the same time, it is the complex and multi-factorial nature of population weight gain that makes law reform a constant struggle. In so far as policy-makers seek to regulate individual behaviours in ways that move beyond education and advice-giving, they run the risk of offending civil libertarians. In so far as they adopt a population health perspective and move upstream, seeking to influence the social and economic determinants of obesity and chronic disease, they risk offending the free marketeers. Since a population-wide approach necessarily seeks to achieve changes in the behaviours of large number of people, policies will inevitably have an impact on those who do not perceive themselves to be at risk and who may resent the 'interference'. Selling temperance is difficult at the best of times, and becomes even harder when the food industry unites in opposition to a proposed policy initiative, decrying the lack of evidence, in circumstances when the scale of the benefit to public health is unknown, despite its likely value as part of a package of interventions. Critics fume that public health should stick to what it knows best: communicable diseases control, and keeping bugs out of the food supply. They resent public health becoming a smokescreen for interference in the market economy, or for policies to redress health inequalities by re-shaping the political economy [90–93].

Obesity prevention and the struggle for regulatory control

Ultimately, law's role in chronic disease and obesity prevention boils down to the exercise of raw political power. As Stephen Leeder points out, 'It's war' [94]. Underlying reasons for opposing the use of law and regulation as tools for obesity prevention are not difficult to uncover. Firstly, obesity is neither contagious, nor *readily* transmitted to others (notwithstanding evidence that obesity – probably through its behavioural antecedents – spreads through social ties over significant periods of time) [95]. It follows that the justification for interfering with individual preferences in order to protect the population from health risks to which it has not consented, is absent.

Secondly, the goal that underlies at least some interventions for obesity prevention involves *reducing consumption*, whether it be total calories, the amount of saturated fat in the diet, or the habit of snacking. The interests of the food and beverage industry, on the other hand, lie in avoiding policies that could de-stabilise revenue flows based on consumer preferences and markets – as shaped by industry.

Thirdly, obesity prevention strategies are often vulnerable to attack by economic conservatives and libertarians who frame the prospect of any regulation – even controls on advertising and clearer nutrition labelling – as evidence of 'nanny state' interference with the personal autonomy of consumers and parents [90–93, 96, 97].⁶ The Hon. Tony Abbott MHR stated in 2006:

> I don't think we can put people in cotton wool. I don't think we can cover our population in cling-wrap. I think people need to retain substantial authority over how they live their lives … I think the role of the Government, in this instance at least, is not so much to regulate, let alone to ban. I think its role is to encourage, to inform and to give good example [98].

An alternative view would acknowledge that governments are stewards of the health of the population, and have a responsibility to invest in policies that support healthier lifestyles in ways that do not unduly burden individual freedom. To the extent that governments acknowledge this responsibility, a population health approach offers important advantages. By targeting the influences upon – and *influencers* of – behaviour, rather than the behaviour itself, regulatory interventions can contribute to health improvement without stigmatising individuals, or micro-managing their lifestyles [99]. Success in tobacco control, for example, came about while substantially preserving the liberty of adults to smoke where this does not jeopardise the health of others [100].

The obstacles to effective obesity prevention *law reform* are not only ideological. Effective structures for facilitating a comprehensive, inter-sectoral approach do not even exist. Government agencies have their own entrenched cultures: it can be difficult to collaborate with them, difficult to usurp their turf, and difficult to route around them. Political leadership is required from the top, and federalism complicates everything [101, 102]. With this in mind, the remainder of this chapter reviews four case studies for legal and regulatory interventions to support obesity prevention.

Priorities for law and regulation in the prevention of population weight gain

So far, I have argued that a sustainable approach to reversing the trend towards population weight gain calls for a 'plausible policy basket' that focuses significantly – not necessarily exclusively – on creating environments that better support physical activity and healthy eating. Piecemeal, ad hoc responses are unlikely to have a major impact, due to the combined force of the many factors that subtly encourage excess energy intake and a sedentary lifestyle.

The strategies that law can deploy as a tool to prevent obesity and to encourage an active lifestyle can be described in different ways [5–8]. Gostin's well-known model [103] includes:

- laws that shape the informational environment, for example, mandatory front-of-pack nutrition labelling [104], restaurant calorie labelling of 'standard food items' [105–107], and laws restricting the advertising of energy-poor, nutrient-poor foods to children;
- economic policies that alter the costs of behaviour, such as taxes on sugary, fizzy drinks [108, 109];

---

6 As Joseph Sullum (90) writes, 'The war on fat … reflects an anti-capitalist perspective that views people as helpless automatons manipulated into consuming whatever big corporations choose to produce. The anti-fat crusaders want to manipulate us too, but for our own good' (p23).

- laws that shape the physical environment, for example, through infrastructure investment, planning controls on the density of fast food outlets [110], or New York City's 'green cart' permit scheme to increase the availability of fresh fruit and vegetables [111, 112];

- social policies to address social disparities, for example, subsidising the freight costs of fresh fruit and vegetables to remote indigenous locations [67, pp134–35]; and

- prescriptive controls on business; for example, bans on the use of trans fats [113].

Each of these examples illustrates ways in which regulation can change the 'external' environment. In addition, however, regulation has an 'internal aspect', which refers to governance initiatives whose focus is institutional reform, and structures for improving the strategic and organisational capacity of government to respond to health challenges. This is the focus of the first of four case studies, below.

(1) Improving governance structures for cross-sectoral collaboration and policy leadership

> Goal: To deliver an inter-sectoral, whole-of-government approach to policy development for obesity prevention

In 2008 to 2009, Australia's federal government spent A$112.8 billion on health, but only 2% of this (A$2.3 billion) was spent on public health [114]. At present, public health functions compete for funding within health departments that are focused on treating the sick. In addition to the difficulty of achieving more adequate investment, however, lies the challenge of achieving a voice in policy development in sectors *beyond health*. In the context of obesity prevention, this means a voice in policies relating to transport and urban development, local government, agriculture and food (production, manufacture, retail, catering, advertising), education, and taxation [115]. Achieving an inter-sectoral, all-of-government approach to strategy, policy and program development is perhaps the most important priority for taking innovative and incremental steps that could reduce the burden of disease, and healthcare expenditures, in Australia's ageing population.

Developing architecture to support an inter-sectoral approach to policy development requires strategic choices, including between an essentially government-focused, and a community-focused structure. One model is a 'politically owned' governance structure with a mandate – secured through high-level (preferably cabinet-level) leadership and support – to forge cross-departmental links and to develop an integrated response that is consistent with the government's commitment to act. This model might include inter-departmental taskforces or standing committees that provide the opportunity for relevant ministries to consider the negative impact of their policies and programs on shared health goals, as well as opportunities for a more coherent, all-of-government approach.

The National Obesity Prevention Act of 2008, a federal bill introduced into the 110th US Congress, illustrates the first kind of structure [116]. This bill would have established an inter-Departmental Task Force, supported by an Advisory Committee on Obesity, with a mandate to develop a government-wide strategy for obesity prevention, supported by goals for each agency, with a requirement for each agency to review its budgets and programs and to determine their impact on physical activity, nutrition and obesity rates. The bill would also have required each agency to report annually on its implementation of the national strategy and its impact on obesity rates.

Although this bill was never passed, its essential structure is reflected in President Obama's more recent National Prevention, Health Promotion and Public Health Council [117], which recently published the National Prevention Strategy [118] and is tasked with monitoring the policies of a dozen federal agencies, reporting annually on progress towards the goals in the strategy, and suggesting corrective actions to agencies to assist them to achieve the goals. In the UK, the Blair government adopted a multi-sectoral approach to health inequalities, setting out the commitments, key actions and spending required for each department as part of the all-of-government strategy. Importantly, the strategy was overseen by a Cabinet sub-committee chaired by the deputy prime minister [119].

An alternative model for supporting an inter-sectoral approach is an independent-of-government structure that is less constrained by party politics, but nevertheless has a clear mandate to advise on policy options. On the one hand, the benefits of this second model include its independence from the entrenched cultures and agendas of existing departments, its likely capacity to engage more effectively with consumers, business, and the NGO sector, and its ability to perform functions governments might wish to avoid, such as evaluating industry practices. On the other hand, this remoteness and lack of political power could limit the effectiveness of such a body in genuinely influencing the policy agenda of departments and in raising the profile of possible solutions.

A third model of particular relevance to Australia is a 'portfolio agency' with a statutory mandate that lies outside the health department, but within the health portfolio, with executive leadership reporting directly to the minister.[7] With adequate resources and a statutory mandate, such an agency may be able to move more effectively between departments and to assume the role of 'honest broker', while engaging effectively with business and community groups. The functions of the CEO of the recently established Australian National Preventive Health Agency include encouraging partnerships with industry, non-government organisations, and the community sector; developing standards and codes of practice relating to preventive health matters; advising the minister, and publishing a biannual report on the state of preventive health in Australia. If requested to do so, the CEO can also make recommendations about preventive health to the federal health minister, to the Australian Health Ministers' Conference, to state and territory governments and the Australian Local Government Association [120]. It seems clear, however, that the functions of the new agency have been designed to prevent it from interfering in departmental policies or in the political sphere, as distinct from engaging in health promotion and on non-legislative and voluntary actions by business and within the community sector.

---

7   Examples of portfolio agencies, each with their establishing acts, include the National Health and Medical Research Council (NHMRC), Cancer Australia, and the National Blood Authority (NBA).

In 2009, the National Preventative Health Taskforce proposed a Prime Minister's Council for Active Living driving the development and implementation of a National Framework for Active Living encompassing transport, the built environment, and social engagement [67, pp99–100]. The aim was that the Prime Minister's Council would develop a business case for consideration by the Council of Australian Governments for a new funding partnership that would link future infrastructure funding in these areas to the agreed outcomes for active living. This recommendation was rejected on the grounds that the National Preventive Health Agency, and other existing mechanisms including Medicare Locals and the national Partnership Agreement on Preventive Health, could deliver appropriate outcomes [59, pp34–35].

Chronic disease prevention competes with many other issues for the attention and resources of cabinet, ministers and departments. The easier option, as reflected in the National Preventive Health Agency, is to create agencies to lead efforts to encourage behavioural change by individuals through mass media campaigns and voluntary actions. Important as they are, these investments need to be matched by governance structures that facilitate serious consideration of how all ministries and sectors can shape their policies in order to encourage and even privilege healthier food choices and a more physically active lifestyle.

(2) Reducing or eliminating advertising of high-sugar, high-salt, high-saturated-fat (HSSF) foods to children

> Goal: To reduce or eliminate diet-distorting commercial influences on children's diets due to the relentless marketing of energy-dense, nutrient-poor foods; to reduce 'pester power' and to support parents in exercising personal responsibility to provide a healthy diet for children

The exposure of children to television advertising of energy-dense, nutrient-poor foods has become a litmus test for the willingness of governments to use regulation to create a healthier food environment for children [121]. Evidence suggests that Australian parents are concerned about food advertising to children and support stronger regulation [122]. On the other hand, due to assumptions about personal responsibility and commercial freedom, reducing food advertising to adults is not seriously on anyone's agenda, even where constitutional constraints do not preclude it. Overweight and obese children are more likely to remain so in adulthood [123], and to the extent that unhealthy food advertising could be reduced, it would not only assist parents to exercise parental responsibility to provide a healthier diet for children, but would create incentives for the food industry to improve the nutrition of leading products, or to re-direct advertising dollars towards healthier foods.

In Australia, evidence continues to demonstrate that energy-dense, non-core foods are heavily advertised during children's peak television viewing times [124–126]. In the US, in 2006, 44 food companies spent over US$1.6 billion promoting food and beverages to children and adolescents, predominantly carbonated beverages, quick-serve restaurant food and breakfast cereals [127].

Although there is a positive association between the amount of television watched and increased consumption of commonly advertised foods, and between exposure to television and obesity, both for adults [128, 129] and children [78, 130–132], the argument that this link is mediated by the impact of food advertising depends upon a distinct chain of reasoning. For children, this includes the assertion that food advertising alters preferences and purchase requests [133], which attach to higher-energy, advertised foods that crowd out and replace the more energy-dilute foods the child would have eaten if not exposed to advertising. While it is logical to assume that 'fast-food restaurants would not choose to advertise if advertising did not increase the demand for their products' [134], proving a causative link – as distinct from demonstrating correlations between a cluster of behaviours – has not been straightforward. In a recent paper, Boyland and colleagues reported that children preferred to select high-fat and high-carbohydrate foods after viewing food commercials, and that this effect was more pronounced among children who were habitual television viewers [135]. The authors point out that their findings support the argument that food advertising not only alters brand choice but alters generic food preferences in favour of energy-dense, nutrient-poor foods.

A consistent theme in food advertising is the presence of voluntary, industry-designed schemes that are promoted as accommodating community concerns about childhood obesity and obviating the need for direct government involvement. In the US, evidence suggests that as a result of pledges made under the Council of Better Business Bureau's Children's Food and Beverage Advertising Initiative [136], television food advertisements viewed by children aged two to 11 declined by 12% between 2004 and 2008. However, by 2010, exposure to food advertising increased by 9% over 2008, and in 2010 children viewed 39% more ads for fast food and other restaurants than in 2002 [137]. Adolescent exposure to food advertising increased by 23% during 2004 to 2010; adult exposure increased at an even higher rate [138]. Another study found that in 2009, over two-thirds of all food advertising by signatories to the Children's Food and Beverage Advertising Initiative was for non-core ('once-in-a-while') foods, and that healthy food advertising was invisible [139].

In 2009, the US Congress authorised an appropriation to establish the Interagency Working Group on Food Marketed to Children comprising representatives of the Federal Trade Commission (FTC), Food and Drug Administration, the Centers for Disease Control and Prevention, and the Department of Agriculture. The working group was tasked with developing a set of food marketing principles to guide industry self-regulation that would improve the nutritional profile of food marketed to children aged two to 17 years [140]. From 2016, the working group's proposed principles would require all food products falling within the ten most heavily marketed product categories to comply with two nutrition principles. These set maximum values for 'negative' nutrients including saturated fat, added sugars and sodium, and secondly, require all marketed foods to 'provide a meaningful contribution to a healthful diet' by containing minimum amounts of either fruit, vegetables, whole grains, low-fat milk or a number of other food categories [140]. Although the final principles are voluntary, they will represent a credible consensus of relevant federal agencies on permissible forms of food advertising to children, which these agencies will expect the food industry to implement by 2016. If the food marketing principles are widely ignored, this could encourage the FTC to explore the full reach of its powers to regulate food marketing to children (subject to First Amendment, tailoring and evidential challenges) and theoretically, could provide support for the restoration of the FTC's rule-making powers under the unfairness doctrine [141]. By setting normative standards, engaging with the food industry, and monitoring and reporting on its compliance, the FTC could encourage both improvements in food marketing practices, and the reformulation of heavily advertised foods.

In its submission to the Interagency Working Group in July 2011, the Children's Food and Beverage Advertising Initiative (CFBAI) announced new uniform nutrition criteria, to be implemented by 31 December 2013, which define the nutritional characteristics for foods advertised to children under 12 across ten product categories [142]. Arguing that the Interagency Working Group's proposed principles are 'not realistic and thus ... not aspirational' [143], the CFBAI argued that the application of the Interagency Working Group's principles to children and adolescents aged two to 17 is 'overly broad and inappropriate', whereas the CFBAI 'properly focuses on advertising primarily directed to children under 12' [143, p23].

Australia's co-regulatory approach to children's food advertising begins with the *Children's Television Standards* 2009 (CTS) prescribed by the Australian Communications and Media Authority (ACMA) [144, 145]. The CTS apply to the designated children's (C) and preschool (P) programming that broadcasters are required to broadcast under their licences (CTS 6–19). Compliance with the CTS is a license condition for commercial television broadcasters [146]. The CTS provide that where advertisements contain premium offers, such as toys offered for sale with advertised foods, the advertisement must not make reference to the premium 'in a way that is more than merely incidental' to the advertised product (CTS 33(2)). The CTS prevent the repetition of advertisements within any 30-minute period (CTS 29), and prohibit the promotion of commercial products by popular characters, including animated, cartoon and movie characters (CTS 35). Food advertisements may not contain misleading or incorrect information about the nutritional value of the product (CTS 32(7)).

Evidence suggests that food advertisers have regularly ignored the CTS in the past [147, 148]. In a review of the 2005 version of the CTS, completed in 2009, ACMA decided against imposing any additional restrictions on food advertising during children's designated programming, concluding that 'the relative contribution of advertising to childhood obesity is difficult to quantify and the causal relationship between these may not be possible to determine' [149, p9]. ACMA also carried out economic modelling which showed that banning the advertising of foods high in fat, salt or sugar (HSSF foods) could significantly affect the revenues and profitability of broadcasters [149, p6]. As Ingleby and colleagues point out, the revenue consequences of restricting unhealthy food advertising 'becomes less attractive as a proposition when it is translated into an argument that children should be exposed to harm as the price of having television programs made for them' [150].

The *Children's Television Standards* are supplemented by the co-regulatory *Commercial Television Industry Code of Practice* [151] which is registered as a code of practice under the *Broadcasting Services Act* 1992 [152]. This code provides that food advertisements directed to children shall not promote an unhealthy lifestyle, or the excessive or compulsive consumption of foods or beverages [151, para 6.23]; it also requires compliance with the *Code for Advertising & Marketing Communications to Children* adopted by the Australian Association of National Advertisers (AANA Code) [153]. Neither code is designed to restrict the frequency, timing or placement of advertisements for energy-dense, nutrient-poor foods directed to children [154]. Leaving aside the fact that both codes rely wholly on consumer complaints, and lack independent monitoring, both codes also consist of generally expressed principles which recent practice suggests are exceedingly difficult to break. Neither code restricts the cumulative impact of unhealthy food advertising on children's preferences and expectations [154, pp134–38].

As evidence and community concern about food marketing to children have continued to grow, the food industry has sought to manage the political risk of regulation by developing additional self-regulatory schemes. Recent initiatives include the Responsible Children's Marketing Initiative developed by the Australian Food and Grocery Council (AFGC) [155], which came into operation during the period when ACMA was reviewing the *Children's Television Standard* (2005). The AFGC Initiative applies to designated children's and preschool programming, and G-rated programs where >50% of the audience are children under 12 years, but not other programming where children are nevertheless a significant share of the audience. In 2009, when the National Preventative Health Taskforce recommended phasing out the marketing of energy-dense, nutrient-poor (ENDP) food on free-to-air and pay TV before 9pm, together with premium offers and the use of competitions, cartoons and promotional characters, the Australian Government responded that it would continue to monitor the effectiveness of voluntary codes including the AANA Code, the AFGC Initiative, and a similar initiative by the Quick Service Restaurant Industry [59, pp46–47].

King and colleagues evaluated non-core food advertising before and after the introduction of the AFGC's Responsible Children's Marketing Initiative. They found that while signatories to the AFGC initiative reduced their rate of non-core food advertising, there was no reduction in the rate of non-core advertisements overall (which continue to dominate peak viewing times), since non-signatories to the initiative increased their rate of non-core food advertising [124]. Nor should it be assumed that exposure would be dramatically reduced if more advertisers implemented the AFGC principles, given their focus on programs directed to children, rather than children's peak viewing periods. Hebden and colleagues found that the introduction, in August 2009, of the children's marketing initiative of the Quick Service Restaurant Industry made no difference to the frequency of non-core fast food advertisements broadcast during peak children's viewing periods [156].

Handsley and colleagues have argued that if the goal is to actually reduce children's *exposure* to non-core food advertising, restrictions based on time of day will be required, not merely restrictions on advertising within designated children's programming [157]. In the UK, broadcast advertising is regulated by the *UK Code of Broadcast Advertising* (BCAP Code), which was written and is reviewed by an industry body, the Broadcast Committee of Advertising Practice (BCAP) under delegation from OfCom, the telecommunications regulator [158, 159]. In 2006, the Food Standards Agency (FSA) advocated a complete ban on all advertising of foods high in salt, sugar and fat on television before 9pm [160]. After a lengthy inquiry, OfCom did implement a ban on HSSF food advertising [158, section 32.5], based on the nutrient profiling model developed by the FSA [161]. The ban applies specifically to advertising of foods high in salt, sugar and fat in 'programmes commissioned for, principally directed at or likely to appeal to' audiences below the age of 16. OfCom has contracted out the enforcement of the BCAP Code to the Advertising Standards Authority [162].

The significant difference between 'children's programs' or 'programs targeted at children', and 'peak children's viewing periods' illustrates the political and philosophical difficulty of implementing an effective ban, which would require the value of commercial speech to adults to be balanced with the benefits of encouraging healthier diets for children and adolescents. Other important variables include whether advertising restrictions apply to children and adolescents, or only to children; the nutritional parameters of foods that attract any ban; and whether or not the administering authority is a government agency, industry or independent body. While there is substantial evidence in Australia showing that the food advertising children are exposed to does not support a healthy diet, governments are reluctant to take on the food industry, and regulation will only improve things to the extent that it addresses the criteria above.

(3) Economic incentives to encourage investment in workplace-based risk prevention and health promotion programs

> Goal: To exploit the workplace, in both the private and public sectors, as a setting for disease prevention and health promotion programs encompassing smoking cessation, obesity prevention and healthy eating

Although calls for a 'fat tax' are regularly made and are the best-known example of an economic strategy for obesity prevention [163], there is a wide range of options for altering the policy environment in ways that could indirectly influence food consumption patterns at the population level. These include imposing a levy on television advertising of energy-dense, non-core foods that do not meet minimum nutritional criteria [164], eliminating the tax deductibility of food advertising costs for non-core foods [134], as well as financing initiatives to make fresh fruit and vegetables more accessible and affordable to low-income and remote populations [165]. In 2010, the Australian Government rejected the recommendation of the National Preventative Health Taskforce to commission a review of economic policies, including the use of taxation, grants, pricing, incentives and subsidies to promote access and consumption of healthier foods and greater levels of physical activity [59, p37]. The wide-ranging Henry review of Australia's future tax system also rejected the notion of a fat tax, because of the difficulty of accurately estimating the health and productivity costs attributable to particular (less healthy) food or product constituents, and because of the multiple influences – besides food choices – on obesity, including genetic, social and economic factors [166]. The population health effects of the dietary changes that could result from a tax on certain classes of food or food ingredients are also not well understood [167].

Like schools, and healthcare encounters, the workplace is an important setting for disease prevention. A growing body of research evaluates the business case for workplace-based disease prevention and health promotion programs, and seeks to identify the optimal design elements, spending and managerial requirements of successful programs [168, 169]. Since risk reduction and better employee health offers the promise of reductions in future healthcare costs and sick leave, and improved productivity and morale, workplace-based risk prevention programs provide the opportunity for alignment between the economic goals of business, the public health goals of government, and the interests of individual employees. At the global level, the World Economic Forum hosts the Workplace Wellness Alliance and promotes corporate wellness initiatives as an opportunity for multinational companies to contribute to the prevention of chronic disease [170, 171].

In the US, employers have a direct financial incentive to invest in evidence-based wellness programs, not only because absenteeism and low productivity affect the bottom line, but also because employees' health insurance premiums are typically paid for or are heavily subsidised by employers. In 2010, 69% of non-federal private and public employers offered health benefits to employees. Of these, nearly three-quarters of employers offered 'wellness programs'. Services typically included in these programs include: weight-loss and smoking cessation programs, personal health coaching, gym membership discounts, nutrition and healthy living classes, and online resources [172, p170]. Increases in healthcare premiums, including employee contributions [172, pp20–21], combined with the economic downturn and the imperatives of deficit reduction, are driving a longer-term trend towards government policies to encourage workplace-based health promotion programs, with sharper financial incentives for employees to participate in them. For employees, this typically means submitting to a health risk assessment, followed by the development of an individualised risk reduction program, with annual review.

President Obama's Patient Protection and Affordable Care Act (PPACA), signed in 2010, authorises grants to small businesses (<100 employees) to establish comprehensive wellness programs [173], and provides for the development of reporting requirements for group health plans to report on wellness and health promotion initiatives, including smoking cessation, weight management, diabetes management and nutrition [174]. It also requires the Centers for Disease Control and Prevention to conduct a periodic national survey of workplace-based health programs and to provide technical assistance to employers in evaluating such programs [175].

Federal law currently restricts employers from varying health insurance premium contributions according to the health status of the particular employee [176]. However, an important exception permits premium discounts or rewards of up to 20% of the cost of the employee's premium contribution where the employee has complied with the requirements of a wellness program that is 'reasonably designed to promote health or prevent disease' [177, 178]. From 2014, this incentive is increased to 30%, and up to 50% if the Secretaries of Health and Human Services, Labor and the Treasury so determine [179, 180]. The point at which financial incentives for participation in wellness programs (in both private and state-funded health insurance schemes) become intrusive and coercive, remains a matter of debate [181]. From 2014, the PPACA guarantees the availability and renewability of health insurance cover for employers and individuals, prescribes the grounds on which premiums may vary, and further restricts discrimination based on an individual's health status [182]. PPACA requires all plans to include an 'essential benefits package' (including specified preventive and wellness services and chronic disease management) [183], and sets up a number of risk adjustment processes to allocate payments to plans with high-risk enrolees. In this environment, the central role of health promotion and risk prevention programs in reducing healthcare costs, with financial incentives to encourage participation, seems set to continue.

One bill not passed by Congress in 2009 would have offered tax credits to businesses setting up comprehensive wellness programs, for a period of ten years [184]. One of the primary goals of the US-based Workplace Wellness Alliance is to 'develop and advocate for tax-credit and other legislation that promotes worksite health promotion programs and other health management initiatives' [185].

The twin factors that are helping to drive investment in wellness programs in the US – that is, the direct financial burden on employers who either self-insure or pay the larger share of employees' health insurance premiums, coupled with financial incentives for employees – are absent in Australia. Australians enjoy taxpayer-funded, rather than employer-funded, national healthcare coverage through Medicare, and private health insurance is community rated [186]. Any reversal of community rating would likely undermine the market for private health insurance and increase demand for Medicare-funded services, something the Australian Government would be keen to avoid.

In 2009, the National Preventative Health Taskforce argued that public sector organisations at all levels of government should lead by example by introducing, identifying and replicating successful workplace-based health promotion programs that could serve as 'models of good practice to the employment sector as a whole' [67, p53]. To encourage uptake within the private sector, they suggested that health promotion programs should be exempt from fringe benefits tax, free of goods and services tax (GST), and tax deductible. The Australian Government did not respond directly to these recommendations, although it has indicated it does not support exempting employer-funded smoking cessation programs from fringe benefits tax [59, p73].

From 1 July 2011, under the National Partnership Agreement on Preventive Health [187], the Commonwealth is providing up to A$289 million in funding to the states to develop healthy living initiatives in the workplace [188]. The NSW Healthy Workers Initiatives, for example, will comprise advice, support and resources for businesses (including a website, phone service and onsite assistance), as well as a coaching service for individuals [189]. For its part, the Commonwealth is developing a National Healthy Workplace Charter with peak business groups, national standards, and an awards scheme for best practice in workplace health programs.

Despite the differences in health insurance arrangements, the US experience has clear implications for Australia. The workplace offers a rare opportunity for a win–win partnership between government, business and public health stakeholders, yet what is absent are economic drivers. Australian employers are largely protected from the direct healthcare costs of employee ill-health, and unless there is compelling evidence to demonstrate that a healthy workers initiative dramatically improves productivity in the short to medium term, uptake is unlikely to be on the scale required to substantially contribute to disease prevention goals. What the current voluntary model overlooks is that workplace-based initiatives are not merely a vehicle for improving business productivity by enlightened businesses; rather, the workplace is an important setting for reaching a large proportion of the working population.

This suggests two priorities. Firstly, the Australian Government should act on the recommendation of the National Preventative Health Taskforce by reconsidering how the taxation system could best support the uptake of healthy worker programs, encompassing smoking cessation, obesity prevention and improved nutrition. Secondly, governments, as employers, should lead by example, implementing comprehensive programs for the benefit of government employees, and using their purchasing and contracting powers to impose accreditation standards to drive improvements in the nutritional quality of foods sold in government buildings, hospitals and other public sector settings.

(4) A co-regulatory approach to food reformulation

> Goal: To moderate overconsumption of saturated fat, sugar and salt at the population level by providing a statutory underpinning to food reformulation negotiations encompassing food manufacturers, retailers, government, and public health stakeholders

The availability of 'cheap, palatable, energy-dense foods' that are skilfully marketed and high in fat, sugar or salt, is an important change in the environment that has driven the upward trend in population weight gain over the past few decades [190]. Reformulation of food products is a population-level 'superpolicy' that could improve nutrition by reducing the amount of overconsumed nutrients. Some major food manufacturers and retailers, such as Pepsico [191] and Wal-Mart [192], are already taking steps to improve the nutritional profile of their portfolio of products.

Prevailing beliefs about the importance of free markets, limited government regulation, consumer choice and personal responsibility support the view that it would be inappropriate for a government agency to prescribe mandatory standards for nutrients (salt, sugar, saturated fat) for the food sector. A competing view might hold that regulation has a legitimate role to play in setting the ground rules for a multi-stakeholder process to drive nutritional improvements within the food supply. There are several factors that, in combination, suggest a growing role for government in public health nutrition.

Firstly, although the status of good nutrition, as a value within Australian food regulation, remains ambiguous, anyone familiar with the Food Standards Code cannot fail to acknowledge that nutrients in food are already regulated prescriptively and in almost forensic detail, in order to reduce health risks, to set parameters for health and nutrient claims, and to avoid confusion, misunderstanding and deceptive advertising [193].

Secondly, consumers cannot make healthy choices in circumstances where only a minority of products (for example, snacks and beverages) meet 'healthy' nutritional criteria [194] *and* where there is no evaluative food labelling scheme to assist consumers to rapidly distinguish between products based on their nutrition [104]. Thirdly, in the light of evidence of its role in cardiovascular disease, New York City, followed by a range of US states and cities, has banned trans fats in restaurant cooking [195, 196].

Over time, salt reduction also has the potential to significantly re-shape assumptions about the legitimate limits of food regulation. Around three quarters of salt intake in most high-income countries comes from added salt in processed foods and pre-cooked meals [197]. This eliminates choice and, since most individuals are unaware of their high-salt intake, hampers personal efforts to moderate consumption. The benefits of salt reduction in controlling hypertension and reducing cardiovascular disease at the population level is strongly supported by evidence, but requires gradual – and more than trivial – reductions in salt levels across those product categories that most contribute to excess levels [198, 199]. Many countries have adopted voluntary targets for reductions in population salt intake, managed by government [200] or, as in Australia, through a Food and Health Dialogue that includes government, the food industry and public health groups [201]. A measure of resistance (passive or active) to substantial reductions in salt targets, by at least some sections of the food industry, is predictable. For example, evidence suggests that salt reduction will reduce sales of sugar-sweetened soft drinks (which could assist in obesity prevention) [202]. Habituation to highly salty foods encourages demand for cheaply produced, profitable snacks, while water-binding chemicals in combination with salt can increase the water content, and thus the weight, of meat [199, pp377–78].

In 2009, the UK government set voluntary targets for salt reduction for the food industry to meet by 2012 [203], while New York City is coordinating a National Salt Reduction Initiative that includes 44 cities and states [204]. In Australia, the National Preventative Health Taskforce recommended that the Australian Government establish a Healthy Food Compact to drive changes in the food supply, with voluntary targets for reductions in salt, saturated and trans fats, and sugar [67, pp106–09, 144]. In a muted response, the Australian Government has committed A$900 000 over three years to 'develop the evidence base and rationale for future food reformulation activities' under the existing, voluntary, Food and Health Dialogue [59, pp38–40].

There is growing academic interest in regulatory strategies for reducing salt intake at the population level [205, 206]. In 2010, the Institute of Medicine recommended that the Food and Drug Administration revoke the 'generally recognised as safe' status of salt and set mandatory national standards for added salt to foods. These would be implemented in a step-wise manner, allowing consumer taste preferences to adapt and industry to resolve technical challenges [207].

One way of ensuring that food reformulation negotiations achieve an adequate level of momentum is through a co-regulatory approach that adds a statutory underpinning to what is currently a purely voluntary process. Consistent with the prevailing model of 'responsive regulation' – which favours 'soft', voluntary measures and only escalates to more direct forms of regulation and enforcement when voluntary strategies fail [67, pp57–58] – participation in the food reformulation dialogue could remain voluntary. In the absence of significant levels of participation from major food manufacturers and retailers, however, a voluntary process would stall. In that event, there should be a credible expectation that government will intervene more directly.

While the key components of a co-regulatory framework require further elaboration, they might begin by enshrining a Healthy Food Compact as a public process with a formal existence recognised in legislation or, at a minimum, in a code of practice developed by an appropriate host agency, such as the Australian National Preventive Health Agency [208] or Food Standards Australia New Zealand [209]. The code of practice could set out the goals of the dialogue for a defined five-year period, together with the roles, and respective obligations of government, manufacturers, retailers and industry associations, and community-based organisations, as participants in the dialogue. Major food manufacturers and retailers whose market share exceeds a prescribed minimum would be expected to become signatories to this process.

Signatories might also be offered choices; for example, between making prospective, binding commitments to reduce average levels of salt, saturated fat, and energy across priority food categories, and to increase levels of fibre and fruits, vegetables, nuts and legumes – versus participation in the dialogue for the relevant five-year term. Prospective commitments might be preferable for signatories that wish to maximise flexibility as well as reduced scrutiny of their product portfolio and manufacturing processes. Under the negotiated process, signatories would need to negotiate towards feasible targets for improvements in the nutrition of products within priority product lines against a credible expectation that if target levels were not achieved, default levels in some areas might be set through a government-appointed process. Progress would be monitored with public reporting.

While the focus of negotiations across the various priority categories within the food reformulation dialogue would be improved nutrition, the focus of negotiations involving retailers could involve commitments relating to the advertising and marketing of healthy foods, and increased visibility and shelf space for healthier products. Both streams would rely on the goodwill of those involved to work effectively: government, manufacturers, industry associations, consumer groups, and experts in public health and nutrition. The ground rules for the dialogue would need to balance public health goals with technical feasibility and consumer acceptability, pursuing significant change across the food supply, while minimising damage to existing brands.

Conclusion

I have argued in this chapter that governments have a critical role to play in the prevention of obesity and diabetes through the development of a 'plausible policy basket' that includes both regulatory and non-regulatory interventions. Significant improvements in health and wellbeing, not to mention productivity, are unlikely unless governments acknowledge this leadership role. Effective policies for obesity prevention require governments, in collaboration with other stakeholders, to recognise that improving the public's health is a legitimate goal for public policy, rather than delegating responsibility for health to individuals and private markets. At the same time, there is plenty of scope for reasonable people to disagree about the legitimate boundaries of law reform initiatives, since public health policies are difficult to keep separate from political philosophies.

Although a multi-level response is needed that addresses environments, lifestyles and healthcare services, the case studies presented in this chapter – governance reform, food advertising controls, incentives for disease prevention within the workplace, and a clearer structure for commercial food reformulation – are all directed at the environment, rather than at individuals and their behaviours per se. While this will not satisfy the critics, there is an important distinction here. Personal autonomy remains an important value in free, market-oriented societies. On any fair assessment, the case studies presented here do not involve dictating lifestyles or diets to individuals.

On the other hand, policies that create a more supportive environment for healthy living may very well conflict with the economic interests of those businesses that derive substantial revenues from current patterns of overeating, poor nutrition and physical inactivity. In tobacco control, public health advocates have learned that there are few, if any, opportunities for collaboration with tobacco companies [210, 211]. From a perspective of two or three decades, however, legislatures have literally driven over the top of the tobacco industry, dramatically reducing the scale of tobacco use (if not the profitability of tobacco companies themselves) in the process. Reducing the 'food economy' is not the goal of obesity prevention. On the other hand, it would be naive of the food industry, looking towards the next decade or so, to assume that governments will not seek to off-set rising healthcare costs and stagnating productivity by experimenting with regulatory measures to reduce the preventable component of chronic disease. While debate continues about whether the food and beverage industries can be genuine partners in strategies to improve diet and reduce energy intake [191, 212–215], the point is that the law of obesity prevention has already arrived and is likely to stay for some time. Its future remains to be written, debated, implemented and evaluated. That said, regulatory interventions, like those presented in the case studies above, may come sooner than many expect.

References

1. Martin R (2001). Domestic regulation of public health: England and Wales. In R Martin & L Johnson (Eds). *Law and the public dimension of health* (pp75–112). London: Cavendish (p79).

2. *South Australian Public Health Act* 2011 ss. 61–62.

3. Reynolds C (2004). Law and public health: addressing obesity. *Alternative Law Journal,* 29: 62–167.

4. Mello M, Studdert D & Brennan T (2006). Obesity: the new frontier in public health law. *New England Journal of Public Health,* 354: 2601–10.

5. Monroe J, Collins J, Hon. P.Maier, Merrill T, Benjamin G & Moulton A (2009). Legal preparedness for obesity prevention and control: a framework for action. *Journal of Law, Medicine & Ethics*, 37(Suppl. 1): 15–23.

6. Pomeranz J & Gostin L (2009). Improving laws and legal authorities for obesity prevention and control. *Journal of Law, Medicine & Ethics*, 37: 62–75.

7. Sacks G, Swinburn B & Lawrence M (2009). Obesity policy action framework and analysis grids for a comprehensive policy approach to reducing obesity. *Obesity Reviews*, 10: 76–86.

8. Magnusson R (2008). What's law got to do with it? Part 1: a framework for obesity prevention. *Australia and New Zealand Health Policy* 2008 [Online]. Available: www.anzhealthpolicy.com/content/5/1/10 [Accessed 20 October 2011].

9. Magnusson R (2008). What's law got to do with it? Part 2: legal strategies for healthier nutrition and obesity prevention. *Australia and New Zealand Health Policy* 2008 [Online]. Available: www.anzhealthpolicy.com/content/5/1/11 [Accessed 20 October 2011].

10. Wikler D (2002). Personal and social responsibility for health. *Ethics & International Affairs*, 16(2): 47–55.

11. Leichter H (2003). 'Evil habits' and 'personal choices': assigning responsibility for health in the 20th century. *The Milbank Quarterly*, 81: 603–26.

12. Le Grand J (2008). The giants of excess: a challenge to the nation's health. *Journal of the Royal Statistical Society Series* A, 171: 834–56.

13. Jesson J (2008). Weighing the wellness programs: the legal implications of imposing personal responsibility obligations. *Virginia Journal of Social Policy and the Law*, 15: 217–98.

14. Australian Institute of Health & Welfare (AIHW) (2010). *Australia's Health 2010*. Canberra: AIHW (p114).

15. Roberts L, Letcher T, Gason A & Lobstein T (2009). Childhood obesity in Australia remains a widespread health concern that warrants population-wide prevention programs. *Medical Journal of Australia*, 191: 46–47.

16. Victorian Department of Human Services (2008). *Future prevalence of overweight and obesity in Australian children and adolescents, 2005–2025,* Melbourne: Department of Human Services.

17. Begg S, Vos T, Barker B, Stevenson C, Stanley L & Lopez A (2007). *The burden of disease and injury in Australia, 2003*. Canberra: AIHW, (p39).

18. Kim S & Popkin B (2006). Commentary: understanding the epidemiology of overweight and obesity – a real global public health concern. *International Journal of Epidemiology*, 35: 60–67.

19. Access Economics Pty Ltd (2008). *The growing cost of obesity in 2008: three years on*. Report by Access Economics Pty Ltd to Diabetes Australia.

20. Flegal K, Carroll M, Ogden C & Johnson C (2002). Prevalence and trends in obesity among US adults, 1999–2000. *The Journal of the American Medical Association*, 288: 1723–27.

21. Flegal K, Carroll M, Ogden C & Curtin L (2010). Prevalence and trends in obesity among US adults, 1999–2008. *The Journal of the American Medical Association,* 303: 235–41.

22. Ogden C & Carroll M (2010. Prevalence of obesity among children and adolescents: United States, trends 1964–1965 through 2007–2008. Centers for Diseases Control and Prevention. National Center for Health Statistics [Online]. Available: www.cdc.gov/nchs/data/hestat/obesity_child_07_08/obesity_child_07_08.htm [Accessed 20 October 2011].

23. Wright J, Kennedy–Stephenson J, Wang C, McDowell M & Johnson C (2004). Trends in intake of energy and macronutrients – United States, 1971–2000. *The Journal of the American Medical Association,* 291: 1193–94.

24. Wright J & Wang C (2010). Trends in intake of energy and macronutrients in adults from 1999–2000 through 2007–2008. US Department of Health and Human Services. Centers for Disease Control and Pevention. NCHS Data Brief No. 49 [Online]. Available: www.cdc.gov/nchs/data/databriefs/db49.htm [Accessed 20 October 2011].

25. Stewart S, Cutler D & Rosen A (2009). Forecasting the effects of obesity and smoking on US life expectancy. *New England Journal of Medicine,* 361: 2252–60.

26. Peters A, Barendregt J, Willekens F, Mackenbach J, Al Mamun A & Bonneux L (2003). Obesity in adulthood and its consequences for life expectancy: a life-table analysis. *Annals of Internal Medicine,* 238: 24–32.

27. Olshansky S, Passaro D, Hershow R, Layden J, Carnes B, Brody J, et al. (2005). A potential decline in life expectancy in the United States in the 21st century. *New England Journal of Medicine,* 352: 1138–45.

28. D'Arcy J. Holman C & Smith F (2008). Implications of the obesity epidemic for the life expectancy of Australians. Report to the Public Health Advocacy Institute of Western Australia [Online]. Available: www.phaiwa.org.au/index.php/publications-mainmenu-125/reports-mainmenu-127/61-obesity-and-life-expectancy [Accessed 20 October 2011].

29. Colagiuri S, Lee C, Colagiuri R, Magliano D, Shaw J, Zimmet P & Caterson I. (2010). The cost of overweight and obesity in Australia. *Medical Journal of Australia,* 192: 260–264.

30. Goss J (2008). Projection of Australian healthcare expenditure by disease, 2003 to 2033. Cat. No. HWE 43. Canberra: AIHW, (p21).

31. Finkelstein E, Trogdon J, Cohen J & Dietz W (2009). Annual medical spending attributable to obesity: payer- and service-specific estimates. *Health Affairs – Web Exclusive,* 28(5): w822–w831.

32. RAND Corporation (2007). *Obesity and disability: the shape of things to come* (RAND Health, Research Highlights), 2007 [Online]. Available: www.rand.org/pubs/research_briefs/2007/RAND_RB9043-1.pdf [Accessed 20 October 2011].

33. World Health Organization (2000). *Obesity: preventing and managing the global epidemic.* WHO Technical Report Series 894, Geneva: World Health Organisation.

34. Yusuf S, Hawken S, Ôunpuu S, Dans T, Avenzum A, Lanas F, et al. (2004). Effect of potentially modifiable risk factors associated with myocardial infarction in 52 countries (the INTERHEART Study): case-control study. *The Lancet,* 364: 937–52.

35. Reeves M & Rafferty A (2005). Healthy lifestyle characteristics among adults in the United States, 2000. *Archives of Internal Medicine,* 165: 854–57.

36. Hopkins J (2005). Only 3% of US citizens follow good health advice. *British Medical Journal,* 330: 1044.

37. Atlantis E, Barnes E & Ball K (2007). Weight status and perception barriers to healthy physical activity and diet behavior. *International Journal of Obesity,* 32: 343–52.

38. Australian Broadcasting Corporation (2005). Transcript of Interview with the Hon. Tony Abbott MP. *Four Corners.* 17 October [Online]. Available: www.abc.net.au/4corners/content/2005/s1480656.htm [Accessed 20 October 2011].

39. Wakefield M, Loken B & Hornik R (2010). Use of mass media campaigns to change health behaviour. *The Lancet,* 376: 1261–71.

40. Johnson-Taylor W, Fisher R, Hubbard V, Starke-Reed P & Eggers P (2008). The change in weight perception of weight status among the overweight: comparison of NHANES III (1988–1994) and 1999–2004 NHANES. *International Journal of Behavioral Nutrition and Physical Activity,* 5: 9 [Online]. Available: www.ijbnpa.org/content/5/1/9 [Accessed 20 October 2011].

41. Johnson F, Cooke L, Croker H & Wardle J (2008). Changing perceptions of weight in Great Britain: comparison of two population surveys. *British Medical Journal,* 337: a494.

42. Giskes K & Siu J (2008). Do Australians perceive their weight status differentially and accurately? Implications for health promotion. *Australian and New Zealand Journal of Public Health,* 32: 183–84.

43. Bleich S (2008). Public perception of overweight. *British Medical Journal,* 337: 243–44 (p243).

44. Australian Institute of Health & Welfare (AIHW) (2004). *Australia's health 2004.* Canberra: AIHW. Cat. No. AUS 44 (p122).

45. Australian Government (2011). Personally controlled electronic health record system: legislation issues paper [Online]. Available: www.yourhealth.gov.au/internet/yourhealth/publishing.nsf/Content/pcehr-legals [Accessed 21 October 2011].

46. *Healthcare Identifiers Act* 2010 (Cth).

47. Commonwealth of Australia (2009). *Building the foundations for an e-health future: update on proposals for healthcare identifiers.* Issued by the Australian Health Ministers' Conference.

48. New York City, N.Y., Title24, Health Code §13.04.

49. New York City of Health and Mental Hygiene. The New YorkCity A1C Registry [Online]. Available: www.nyc.gov/html/doh/html/diabetes/diabetes-nycar.shtml [Accessed 21 October 2011].

50. Steinbrook R (2006). Facing the diabetes epidemic: mandatory reporting of glycosylated hemoglobin values in New York City. *New England Journal of Medicine,* 354: 545–48.

51. Mariner W (2007). Medicine and public health: crossing legal boundaries. *Journal of Health Care Law & Policy,* 10: 121–51.

52. Australian Institute of Health and Welfare (2006). *Chronic diseases and associated risk factors in Australia, 2006.* Canberra: AIHW. AIHW Cat. No. PHE 81.

53. Tong B & Stevenson C (2007). *Comorbidity of cardiovascular disease, diabetes and chronic kidney disease in Australia.* Cardiovascular Disease Series no. 28. Cat. no. CVD 37. Canberra: AIHW.

54. Weiss C, Boyd C, Yu Q, Wolff J & Leff B (2007). Patterns of prevalent major chronic disease among older adults in the United States. *Journal of the American Medical Association,* 298: 1160–62.

55. Turrell G, Stanley L, de Looper M & Oldenburg B (2006). *Health inequalities in Australia: morbidity, health behaviours, risk factors and health service use.* Health Inequalities Monitoring Series No. 2. AIHW Cat. No. PHE 72. Canberra: Queensland University of Technology & AIHW.

56. King T, Kavanagh A, Jolley D, Turrell G & Drawford D (2006). Weight and place: a multilevel cross-sectional survey of area-level social disadvantage and overweight/obesity in Australia. *International Journal of Obesity,* 30: 281–87.

57. Kiim M, Berger D & Matte T (2006). *Diabetes in New York City: public health burden and disparities.* New York: New York City Department of Health and Mental Hygiene.

58. Medicare Benefits Schedule items 701, 703, 705, 707 [Online]. Available: www9.health.gov.au/mbs/search.cfm [Accessed 21 October 2011].

59. Australian Government (2010). Taking preventative action: a response to *Australia: the healthiest country by 2020: the report of the National Preventative Health Taskforce* [Online]. Available: www.preventativehealth.org.au/ [Accessed 21 October 2011].

60. Ashworth M & Jones R (2008). Pay for performance systems in general practice: experience in the United Kingdom. *Medical Journal of Australia,* 189: 60–61.

61. Scott A, Sivey P, Ait Ouakrim D, Willenberg L, Naccarella L, Furler J & Young D (2011). The effect of financial incentives on the quality of healthcare provided by primary care physicians. *Cochrane Database of Systematic Reviews.* Issue 9, Art. No.: CD008451.

62. Australian Government. Department of Health and Ageing. Practice Incentives Program [Online]. Available: www.medicareaustralia.gov.au/provider/incentives/pip/index.jsp [Accessed 21 October 2011].

63. Young D, Scott A & Best J (2010). For love or money? Changing the way GPs are paid to provide diabetes care. *Medical Journal of Australia,* 193: 67–68.

64. Australian Government. Department of Health and Ageing. Australian Primary Care Collaboratives Program (APCCP). [Online]. Available: www.health.gov.au/internet/main/publishing.nsf/Content/health-pcd-programs-apccp-index.htm [Accessed 21 October 2011].

65. Australian Primary Care Collaboratives (APCC). [Online]. Available: www.apcc.org.au/[Accessed 21 October 2011].

66. Australian Government. Department of Health and Ageing (2010). Medicare Locals: discussion paper on governance and functions [Online]. Available: www.yourhealth.gov.au/internet/yourhealth/publishing.nsf/content/MedicareLocalsDiscussionPaper [Accessed 21 October 2011].

67. National Preventative Health Taskforce. *Australia: the healthiest country by 2020. The report of the National Preventative Health Strategy: the roadmap for action.* 30 June 2009 [Online]. Available: www.yourhealth.gov.au/internet/yourhealth/publishing.nsf/Content/nphs-report-roadmap [Accessed 21 October 2011].

68. Balen A, Dresner M, Scott E & Drife J (2006). Should obese women with polycistic ovary syndrome receive treatment for infertility? *British Medical Journal*, 332: 434–35.

69. Peters M & Glantz L (2007). Should smokers be refused surgery? *British Medical Journal*, 334: 20–21.

70. Buyx A (2008). Personal responsibility for health as a rationing criterion: why we don't like it and why maybe we should. *Journal of Medical Ethics*, 34: 871–74.

71. Onishi N (2008). Japan, seeking trim waists, measures millions. *New York Times*, 13 June 2008.

72. Thaler R & Sunstein C (2008). *Nudge: improving decisions about health, wealth, and happiness*. New Haven: Yale University Press.

73. Gostin L (2007). General justifications for public health regulation. *Public Health*, 121: 829–34.

74. Marteau T, Oliver A & Ashcroft R (2008). Changing behaviour through state intervention. *British Medical Journal*, 337: a2543.

75. Finkelstein E, Ruhm C & Kosa K (2005). Economic causes and consequences of obesity. *Annual Review of Public Health*, 26: 239–57.

76. James W (2007). The fundamental drivers of the obesity epidemic. *Obesity Reviews*, 9(Suppl. 1): 6–13.

77. Moodie R, Swinburn B, Richardson J & Somaini B (2006). Childhood obesity: a sign of commercial success, but a market failure. *International Journal of Pediatric Obesity*, 1(3): 133–38.

78. Jordan A & Robinson T (2008). Children, television viewing, and weight status: summary and recommendations from an expert panel meeting. *Annals of the American Academy of Political and Social Science*, 615: 119–32.

79. Rose G (1985). Sick individuals and sick populations. *International Journal of Epidemiology*, 14: 32–38 (p37).

80. Frank J, Lomax G, Baird P & Lock M (2006). Interactive role of genes and the environment. In J Heymann, C Hertzman, M Barer & R Evans (Eds). *Healthier societies: from analysis to action* (pp11–34). New York: Oxford University Press (p19).

81. World Health Organisation (2003). *Diet, nutrition and the prevention of chronic diseases*. World Health Organization Technical Report Series 916. Geneva, World Health Organization (pp54–71).

82. Kumanyika S (2007). Obesity prevention concepts and frameworks. In S Kumanyika & R Brownson (Eds). *Handbook of obesity prevention* (pp85–114). New York: Springer (p102).

83. Egger G & Swinburn B (1997). An 'ecological' approach to the obesity pandemic. *British Medical Journal*, 315: 477–80.

84. McKinlay J & Marceau L (2000). To boldly go … *American Journal of Public Health*, 90: 25–33 (pp28–29).

85. Sallis J, Cervero R, Ascher W, Henderson K, Kraft M & Kerr J (2006). An ecological approach to creating active living communities. *Annual Review of Public Health*, 27: 297–322.

86. Campbell I (2003). The obesity epidemic: can we turn the tide? *Heart*, 89(Suppl. II): ii22–ii24.

87. Rose G (1981). Strategy of prevention: lessons from cardiovascular disease. *British Medical Journal*, 282: 1847–51.

88. Lang T & Rayner G (2007). Overcoming policy cacophony on obesity: an ecological public health framework for policymakers. *Obesity Reviews*, 8(Suppl. 1): 165–81.

89. Jain A (2005). Treating obesity in individuals and populations. *British Medical Journal*, 331: 1387–90.

90. Epstein R (2005). What (not) to do about obesity: a moderate Aristotelian answer. *Georgetown Law Journal*, 93: 1361–86.

91. Epstein R (2003). Let the shoemaker stick to his last: a defense of the 'old' public health. *Perspectives in Biology and Medicine*, 46(3): S138–59.

92. Sullum J (2004). The war on fat: is the size of your butt the government's business? *Reason*, 8: 20–31.

93. Hall M (2003). The scope and limits of public health law. *Perspectives in Biology and Medicine*, 46(3): S199–S209.

94. Leeder S (2004). Ethics and public health. *Internal Medicine Journal*, 34: 435–39 (pp436–37).

95. Christakis N & Fowler J (2007). The spread of obesity in a large social network over 32 years. *New England Journal of Medicine*, 357: 370–79.

96. Jochelson K (2006). Nanny or steward? The role of government in public health. *Public Health*, 120: 1149–55.

97. Daube M, Stafford J & Bond L (2008). No need for nanny. *Tobacco Control*, 17: 426–26.

98. Hon. Tony Abbott MHR. Former Minister for Health and Ageing (Australia). Address to the Queensland Obesity Summit. 3 May 2006 [Online]. Available: www.health.gov.au/internet/ministers/publishing.nsf/Content/health-mediarel-yr2006-ta-abbsp030506.htm?OpenDocument&yr = 2006&mth = 5 [Accessed 21 October 2011].

99. Dorfman L & Wallack L (2007). Moving nutrition upstream: the case for reframing obesity. *Journal of Nutrition Education and Behaviour*, 39: S45–S50.

100. Warner K (2006). Tobacco policy research: insights and contributions to public health policy. In Warner K (Ed). *Tobacco control policy* (pp3–86). San Francisco: Jossey-Bass (p18).

101. Oliver T (2006). The politics of public health policy. *Annual Review of Public Health*, 27: 195–33.

102. Kersh R & Morone J (2002). The politics of obesity: seven steps to government action. *Health Affairs*, 21: 142–53.

103. Gostin L (2007). Law as a tool to facilitate healthier lifestyles and prevent obesity. *Journal of the American Medical Association*, 197: 87–90.

104. Magnusson R (2010). Obesity prevention and personal responsibility: the case of front-of-pack food labelling in Australia. *BMC Public Health*, 10: 662 [Online]. Available: www.biomedcentral.com/1471-2458/10/662 [Accessed 21 October 2011].

105. Roberto C, Schwartz M & Brownell K (2009). Rationale and evidence for menu-labeling legislation. *American Journal of Preventive Medicine*, 37: 546–51.

106. Patient Protection and Affordable Care Act (US). H.R. 3590, §4205 (Nutrition Labeling of Standard Menu Items at Chain Restaurants and of Articles of Food Sold From Vending Machines).

107. *Food Act* 2003 (NSW). ss. 106K–106R.

108. McCarthy M (2004). The economics of obesity. *The Lancet,* 364: 2169–70.

109. Brownell K & Frieden T (2009). Ounces of prevention: the public policy case for taxes on sugared beverages. *New England Journal of Medicine,* 360: 1805–08.

110. Institute of Medicine (2009). *Local government actions to prevent childhood obesity.* Washington DC: The National Academies Press (pp4–11).

111. New York City Department of Health and Mental Hygiene. NYC Green Cart.[Online]. Available: www.nyc.gov/html/doh/html/cdp/cdp_pan_green_carts.shtml [Accessed 21 October 2011].

112. Tester J, Stevens S, Yen I & Laraia B (2010). An analysis of public health policy and legal issues relevant to mobile food vending. *American Journal of Public Health,* 100: 2038–46.

113. Coombes R (2011). Trans fats: chasing a global ban. *British Medical Journal,* 343: d5567.

114. Australian Institute of Health and Welfare (AIHW) (2010). *Health expenditure Australia 2008–09.* Health and Welfare Expenditure Series No. 425; Canberra: AIHW (pp8, 77).

115. World Health Organization (2004). *Global strategy on diet, physical activity and health.* WHA57.17.

116. National Obesity Prevention Act of 2008, H.R. 7179, 110th Congress, 2nd session, introduced into the House of Representatives, 27 September 2008 [Online]. Available: www.govtrack.us/congress/bill. xpd?bill = h110-7179 [Accessed 21 October 2011].

117. Patient Protection and Affordable Care Act (US). (P.L. 111–148), Title IV (§4001).

118. National Prevention Council (2011). *National prevention strategy: America's plan for better health and wellness.* Rockville, Maryland: Office of the Surgeon General [Online]. Available: www.healthcare. gov/centre/councils/nphpphc [Accessed 21 October 2011].

119. Department of Health (UK) (2003). Tackling health inequalities: a program for action (p37). [Online]. Available: www.dh.gov.uk/en/publicationsandstatistics/publications/ publicationspolicyandguidance/dh_4008268 [Accessed 21 October 2011].

120. *Australian National Preventive Health Agency Act* 2010 (Cth). s 11.

121. MacKay S, Antonopoulos N, Martin J & Swinburn B (2011). A comprehensive approach to protecting children from unhealthy food advertising and promotion. Obesity Policy Coalition; Melbourne [Online]. Available: www.opc.org.au/ [Accessed 21 October 2011].

122. Morley B, Chapman K, Mehta K, King L, Swinburn B & Wakefield M (2008). Parental awareness and attitudes about food advertising to children on Australian television. *Australian and New Zealand Journal of Public Health,* 32: 341–47.

123. Singh A, Mulder C, Twisk J, van Mechelen W & Chinapaw M (2008). Tracking of childhood overweight into adulthood: a systematic review of the literature. *Obesity Reviews,* 9: 474–88.

124. King L, Hebden L, Grunseit A, Kelly B, Chapman K & Venugopal K (2011). Industry self regulation

of television food advertising: responsible or responsive? *International Journal of Pediatric Obesity,* 6: e390–98.

125. Kelly B, Chapman K, King L & Hebden L (2011). Trends in food advertising to children on free-to-air television in Australia. *Australian and New Zealand Journal of Public Health,* 35: 131–34.

126. Hebden L, King L, Chau J & Kelly B (2011). Food advertising on children's popular subscription television channels in Australia. *Australian and New Zealand Journal of Public Health,* 35: 127–30.

127. Federal Trade Commission (2008). Marketing food to children and adolescents: a review of industry expenditures, activities, and self-regulation: a report to Congress. Federal Trade Commission.

128. Banks E, Jorm L, Rogers K, Clements M & Bauman A (2010). Screen-time, obesity, ageing and disability: findings from 91 266 participants in the 45 and up study. *Public Health Nutrition,* 14: 34–43.

129. Scully M, Dixon H & Wakefield M (2008). Association between commercial television exposure and fast-food consumption among adults. *Public Health Nutrition,* 12: 105–10.

130. Utter J, Scragg R & Schaaf D (2006). Associations between television viewing and consumption of commonly advertised foods among New Zealand children and young adolescents. *Public Health Nutrition,* 9: 606–12.

131. Wiecha J, Peterson K, Ludwig D, Kim J, Sobol A & Gortmaker S (2006). When children eat what they watch. *Archives of Pediatric Adolescent Medicine,* 160: 436–42.

132. Hesketh K, Wake M, Graham M & Waters E (2007). Stability of television viewing and electronic game/computer use in a prospective cohort study of Australian children: relationship with body mass index. *International Journal of Behavioral Nutrition and Physical Activity,* 4: 60 [Online]. Available: www.ijbnpa.org/content/4/1/60 [Accessed 21 October 2011].

133. Institute of Medicine (2006). *Food marketing to children and youth: threat or opportunity.* Washington DC: The National Academies Press.

134. Chou S, Rashad I & Grossman M (2008). Fast-food restaurant advertising on television and its influence on childhood obesity. *Journal of Law and Economics,* 51: 599–618 (p602).

135. Boyland E, Harrold J, Kirkham T, Corke C, Cuddy J, Evans D, et al. (2011). Food commercials increase preference for energy-dense foods, particularly in children who watch more television. *Pediatrics,* 128: e93–e100.

136. The Council of Better Business Bureaus. The Children's Food and Beverage Initiative [Online]. Available: www.bbb.org/us/about-children-food-beverage-advertising-initiative/ [Accessed 21 October 2011].

137. Harris J, Weinberg M, Schwartz M, Ross C, Ostroff J & Brownell K (2010). *Trends in television food advertising: progress in reducing unhealthy marketing to young people?* Yale University: Rudd Center for Food Policy & Obesity.

138. Harris J & Sarda V (2011). Trends in television food advertising to young people. 2010 Update. Yale University: Rudd Center for Food Policy & Obesity [Online]. Available: www.yaleruddcenter.org/briefs.aspx [Accessed 21 October 2011].

139. Kunkel D, McKinley C & Wright P (2009). The impact of industry self-regulation on the nutritional quality of foods advertised on television to children. Commissioned by Children Now [Online]. Available: www.childrennow.org/index.php/learn/reports_and_research/article/576 [Accessed 21 October 2011].

140. Interagency Working Group on Food Marketed to Children (2011). Preliminary proposed nutrition principles to guide industry self-regulatory efforts: request for comments [Online]. Available: www.ftc.gov/opa/2011/04/foodmarket.shtm [Accessed 21 October 2011].

141. Mello M (2010). Federal Trade Commission regulation of food advertising to children: possibilities for a reinvigorated role. *Journal of Health Politics, Policy and Law*, 35: 227–76.

142. Kolish E (2011). The children's food and beverage advertising initiative white paper on CFBAI's Uniform Nutrition Criteria [Online]. Available: www.bbb.org/us/children-food-beverage-advertising-initiative/info/ [Accessed 21 October 2011].

143. The Council of Better Business Bureaus (2011). Comments to the Interagency Working Group on food marketing to children [Online]. Available: www.bbb.org/us/children-food-beverage-advertising-initiative/info/comments/ [Accessed 21 October 2011].

144. Australian Media and Communications Authority (2009). *Children's television standards 2009* [Online]. Available: www.acma.gov.au/WEB/STANDARD/pc = PC_310262 [Accessed 21 October 2011].

145. Jolly R (2011). *Marketing obesity? Junk food, advertising and kids.* Parliamentary Library Research Paper no. 9, 2010–11.

146. *Broadcasting Services Act* 1992 (Cth). s.122.

147. Kelly B & Chau J (2007). Children's television sub-standards: a call for significant amendments. *Medical Journal of Australia*, 186: 18 (letter).

148. Chapman K, Nicholas P & Supramaniam R (2006). How much food advertising is there on Australian television? *Health Promotion International*, 21: 172–80.

149. Australian Communications and Media Authority (2009). *Review of the children's television standards, 2005: final report of the review.* Canberra: ACMA [Online]. Available: www.acma.gov.au/WEB/STANDARD/pc = PC_90095 [Accessed 21 October 2011].

150. Richard Ingleby, Lauren Prosser & Elizabeth Waters (2008). UNCROC and the prevention of childhood obesity: the right not to have food advertisements on television. *Journal of Law and Medicine*, 16: 49–56 (pp55–56).

151. Free TV Australia (2010). *2010 commercial television industry code of practice* [Online]. Available: www.freetv.com.au/content_common/pg-code-of-practice.seo [Accessed 21 October 2011].

152. *Broadcasting Services Act* 1992 (Cth). s.123.

153. Australian Association of National Advertisers (2009). *Code for advertising & marketing communications to children*; August 2009 [Online]. Available: www.aana.com.au/codes.html [Accessed 21 October 2011].

154. MacKay S (2009). Food advertising and obesity in Australia: to what extent can self-regulation protect the interests of children? *Monash University Law Review*, 35: 118–46 (p134).

155. Australian Food and Grocery Council (2009). The responsible children's marketing initiative [Online]. Available: www.afgc.org.au/industry-codes/advertising-kids.html [Accessed 21 October 2011].

156. Hebden L, King L, Grunseit A, Kelly B & Chapman K (2011). Advertising of fast food to children on Australian television: the impact of industry self-regulation. *Medical Journal of Australia,* 195: 20–24.

157. Handsley E, Mehta K, Coveney J & Nehmy C (2009). Regulatory axes on food advertising to children on television. *Australia and New Zealand Health Policy,* 6: 1.

158. The UK Code of Broadcast Advertising (BCAP Code) (2010). [Online]. Available: www.cap.org.uk/The-Codes/BCAP-Code.aspx [Accessed 21 October 2011].

159. The Contracting Out (Functions Relating to Broadcast Advertising) and Specification of Relevant Functions Order 2004 (UK). [Online]. Available: www.legislation.gov.uk/uksi/2004/1975/pdfs/uksi_20041975_en.pdf [Accessed 13 December 2011].

160. Derbyshire D (2006). Ban all junk food ads before 9pm, says watchdog. *The Telegraph* (UK). 15 June [Online]. Available: www.telegraph.co.uk/news/uknews/1521313/Ban-all-junk-food-ads-before-9pm-says-watchdog.html [Accessed 21 October 2011].

161. Food Standards Agency (UK) (2009). Guide to using the nutrient profiling model [Online]. Available: food.gov.uk/healthiereating/advertisingtochildren/nutlab/nutprofmod [Accessed 21 October 2011].

162. Advertising Standards Authority (ASA). [Online]. Available: asa.org.uk/ [Accessed 21 October 2011].

163. Bond M, Williams M, Crammond B & Loff B (2010). Taxing junk food: applying the logic of the Henry Tax Review. *Medical Journal of Australia,* 193: 472–73.

164. Harper T & Mooney G (2010). Prevention before profits: a levy on food and alcohol advertising. *Medical Journal of Australia,* 192: 400–02.

165. Giang T, Karpyn A, Laurison H, Hillier A & Perry R (2008). Closing the grocery gap in underserved communities: the creation of the Pennsylvania Fresh Food Financing Initiative. *Journal of Public Health Management Practice,* 14: 272–79.

166. Commonwealth of Australia (2009). *Australia's future tax system – report to the Treasurer: part two, detailed analysis, volume 1 (The Henry Review)* (pp320–22).

167. Mytton O, Gray A, Rayner M & Rutter H (2007). Could targeted food taxes improve health? *Journal of Epidemiology and Community Health,* 61: 689–94.

168. Goetzel R & Ozminkowski R (2008). The health and cost benefits of work site health-promotion programs. *Annual Review of Public Health,* 29: 303–23.

169. Baicker K, Cutler D & Song Z (2009). Workplace wellness programs can generate savings. *Health Affairs,* 29: 304–11.

170. World Economic Forum. Workplace Wellness and Chronic Disease Prevention [Online]. Available: members.weforum.org/en/initiatives/Wellness/index.htm. [Accessed 21 October 2011].

171. World Economic Forum. Workplace Wellness Alliance [Online]. Available: www.weforum.org/issues/workplace-wellness-alliance. [Accessed 21 October 2011].

172. The Kaiser Family Foundation and Health Research & Educational Trust (2010). Employer health benefits 2010 annual survey [Online]. Available: ehbs.kff.org/ [Accessed 21 October 2011].

173. Patient Protection and Affordable Care Act (US). P.L. No. 111–148 (2009). s.10408.

174. Patient Protection and Affordable Care Act (US). P.L. No. 111–148 (2009). s.1001, inserting s. 2717 into the Public Health Service Act.

175. Patient Protection and Affordable Care Act (US). P.L. No. 111–148 (2009). s. 303.

176. 45 C.F.R. §146.121(b).

177. 45 C.F.R. §146.121(f).

178. Rothstein M & Harrell H (2009). Health risk reduction programs in employer-sponsored health plans: part II – law and ethics. *Journal of Occupational and Environmental Medicine,* 51: 951–57.

179. Patient Protection and Affordable Care Act (US). P.L. No. 111–148 (2009). s.1201, inserting s. 2705 into the Public Health Service Act.

180. Volpp K, Asch D, Galvin R & Loewenstein G (2011). Redesigning employee health incentives: lessons from behavioral economics. *New England Journal of Medicine,* 365: 388–90.

181. Jesson J (2008). Weighing the wellness programs: the legal implications of imposing personal responsibility obligations. *Virginia Journal of Social Policy and the Law,* 15: 217–98.

182. Patient Protection and Affordable Care Act (US). P.L. No. 111–148 (2009). s.1201, inserting ss.2702–03 into the Public Health Service Act.

183. Patient Protection and Affordable Care Act (US). P.L. No. 111–148 (2009). ss.1301–02.

184. The Healthy Workforce Act of 2009. S. 803/H.R. 1897 [Online]. Available: www.govtrack.us/congress/bill.xpd?bill = h111-1897 [Accessed 21 October 2011].

185. US Workplace Wellness Alliance [Online]. Available: www.uswwa.org/ [Accessed 21 October 2011].

186. *Private Health Insurance Act* 2007 (Cth). s. 55.5.

187. Council of Australian Governments (COAG) (2008). National partnership agreement on preventive health. Signed by Australian Governments. December [Online]. Available: www.anpha.gov.au/internet/anpha/publishing.nsf/Content/publications [Accessed 21 October 2011].

188. National Partnership Agreement on Preventive Health: National implementation plan 2009–15, (pp38–48). [Online]. Available: www.anpha.gov.au/internet/anpha/publishing.nsf/Content/publications [Accessed 21 October 2011].

189. NSW Health. Centre for Health Advancement (2010). NSW Healthy Workers Initiative: discussion paper. Centre for Health Advancement [Online]. Available: www.health.nsw.gov.au/Initiatives/healthyworkers/index.asp [Accessed 21 October 2011].

190. Swinburn B, Sacks G, Hall K, McPherson K, Finegood D, Moodie M, et al. (2011). The global obesity pandemic: shaped by global drivers and local environments. *The Lancet,* 378: 804–14 (p807).

191. Yach D, Khan M, Bradley D, Hargrove R, Kehoe S & Mensah G (2010). The role and challenges of the food industry in addressing chronic disease. *Globalization and Health,* 6: 10 [Online]. Available: www.globalizationandhealth.com/content/6/1/10 [Accessed 21 October 2011].

192. Stolberg S (2011). Wal-Mart shifts strategy to promote healthy foods. *New York Times,* 20 January 2011.

193. Food Standards Australia New Zealand (FSANZ). Food standards code [Online]. Available: www.foodstandards.gov.au/foodstandards/foodstandardscode.cfm [Accessed 21 October 2011].

194. Walker K, Woods J, Rickard C & Wong C (2007). Product variety in Australian snacks and drinks: how can the consumer make a healthy choice? *Public Health Nutrition,* 11: 1046–53.

195. New York City, Department of Health and Mental Hygiene. Board of health approves regulation to phase out artificial trans fat [Online]. Available: www.nyc.gov/html/doh/html/cardio/cardio-transfat-healthcode.shtml [Accessed 21 October 2011].

196. Mello M (2009). New York City's war on fat. *New England Journal of Medicine,* 360: 2015–20.

197. Brown I, Tzoulaki I, Candeias V & Elliott P (2009). Salt intakes around the world: implications for public health. *International Journal of Epidemiology,* 38: 791–813 (p807).

198. He F & MacGregor G (2009). A comprehensive review of salt and health and current experience of worldwide salt reduction programmes. *Journal of Human Hypertension,* 23: 363–84.

199. He F & MacGregor G (2010). Reducing population salt intake worldwide: from evidence to implementation. *Progress in Cardiovascular Diseases,* 52: 363–82.

200. Cappuccio F, Capewell S, Lincoln P & McPherson K (2011). Policy options to reduce population salt intake. *British Medical Journal,* 343: d4995.

201. Australian Government. Department of Health and Ageing. Food and health dialogue [Online]. Available: www.foodhealthdialogue.gov.au/internet/foodandhealth/publishing.nsf/Content/Home [Accessed 24 October 2011].

202. He F, Marrero N & MacGregor G (2008). Salt intake is related to soft drink consumption in children and adolescents: a link to obesity? *Hypertension,* 51: 629–34.

203. Food Standards Agency (UK) (2009). Salt reduction targets. 18 May [Online]. Available: www.food.gov.uk/scotland/scotnut/salt/saltreduction [Accessed 24 October 2011].

204. New York City. Department of Health and Mental Hygiene. Cutting salt, improving health [Online]. Available: www.nyc.gov/html/doh/html/cardio/cardio-salt-initiative.shtml [Accessed 24 October 2011].

205. Forshee R (2008). Innovative regulatory approaches to reduce sodium consumption: could a cap-and-trade system work? *Nutrition Reviews,* 66: 280–85.

206. Sugarman S (2009). Salt, high blood pressure, and performance-based regulation. *Regulation & Governance,* 3: 84–102.

207. Institute of Medicine (IOM) (2010). *Strategies to reduce sodium intake in the United States.* Washington, DC: The National Academies Press (pp8–15ff).

208. *Australian National Preventive Health Agency Act* 2010 (Cth). s. 11.

209. *Food Standards Australia New Zealand Act* 1991 (Cth). s. 17.

210. Malone R (2010). The tobacco industry. In W Wiist (Ed). *The bottom line or public health: tactics corporations use to influence health and health policy, and what we can do to counter them* (pp155–91). New York: Oxford University Press.

211. World Health Organization (2008). Guidelines for implementation of Article 5.3 of the *WHO Framework Convention on Tobacco Control* – on the protection of public health policies with respect to tobacco control from commercial and other vested interests of the tobacco industry. Decision FCTC/COP3(7). November.

212. Roberts I (2008). Corporate capture and Coca-Cola. *The Lancet,* 372: 1934–35.

213. Chopra M & Darnton-Hill I (2004). Tobacco and obesity epidemics: so different after all? *British Medical Journal,* 328: 1558–60

214. Ludwig D & Nestle M (2008). Can the food industry play a constructive role in the obesity epidemic? *Journal of the American Medical Association,* 300: 1808–11.

215. Yach D (2008). Food companies and nutrition for better health. *Public Health Nutrition,* 11: 109–11.

14

Whole of society approaches to preventing obesity and diabetes

Philayrath Phongsavan,[1] Chris Rissel,[1] Lesley King[1] and Adrian Bauman[1]

The current diabetes and obesity epidemic is largely a *societally and environmentally constructed* health problem. Physical inactivity and excessive intake of nutrient-poor and energy-dense foods are the two most important proximal behavioural contributors to the unprecedented diabetes and obesity levels currently facing many nations. Traditionally, individual behaviour change approaches and counselling, often combined with judicious use of evidence-based pharmacological agents, have been the mainstay of efforts to reduce these health risks. A newer socio-ecological approach refocuses solutions on tackling broader environmental causes of obesity and type 2 diabetes. This chapter examines promising societal and environmental responses that enable and support regular physical activity and healthy eating across populations. These approaches include redesigning the built environment, providing active transport options, promoting the availability and accessibility of healthy food choices, restricting promotion of unhealthy foods, and implementing ongoing social marketing strategies to influence sustained healthy eating and physical activity behaviours. Implications for policy development and how public health can work with various sectors of society to halt the rise in obesity and diabetes are discussed.

If it takes a village to raise a child, it takes the organised efforts of a society to ensure that all of its children grow up to be healthy. A public health approach, by definition, involves 'the science and art of preventing disease, prolonging life and promoting health through the organized efforts and informed choices of society, organizations, public and private, communities and individuals' [1].

Diabetes mellitus, in its commonest form known as type 2 diabetes, and obesity, share some of the same modifiable risk factors, such as low physical activity, prolonged sitting, and too much energy-dense, nutrient-poor foods. As a society, we have created a social and physical environment that facilitates being sedentary and encourages excessive food consumption. High-kilojoule convenience foods are readily available and more affordable than fresh food, and heavily marketed to all ages. We have designed transport systems to minimise physical effort, and prioritised private motor vehicles over public transport by building motorways instead of railways or rapid bus transit corridors. Unchecked development on urban fringes

---

1   Prevention Research Collaboration, Sydney School of Public Health, University of Sydney.

creates a vast suburban sprawl, making distances too great for walking and cycling. These structural problems facilitate and reinforce individual behaviours, with inactive options logistically easier, and unhealthy food choices cheaper and more accessible. This chapter examines the way this has occurred, and suggests ways to reorganise the efforts of society to create a healthier physical and social environment.

A socio-ecological perspective as a societal solution to preventing obesity and diabetes

Until recently, most obesity and diabetes prevention strategies have involved behaviour change programs that focus on the biology and psychology of the individual. This approach has some limitations. First, even optimal interventions that persuade individuals to eat better and be more physically active tend to have either weak or short-lived effects [2, 3]. This, together with the rapid rise in obesity and diabetes globally over the past three decades [4], suggests that the causes of obesity and diabetes are beyond individual biology and psychology. Second, individual and education-based programs tend to have low population reach, and usually enrol motivated individuals or those with already high levels of risk. While this strategy yields great effects for high-risk individuals, it has minimal effects on population levels of obesity and diabetes because it does not reach the largest numbers of people, those who are at average risk. As the causes of obesity and diabetes are likely to be linked to broader environmental and societal changes [5–7] that can impact populations, there is a need for a shift in thinking and solutions to these problems.

To achieve large and sustained public health gains through the prevention of diabetes and obesity, the whole population needs to be targeted regardless of their current health status. Even small shifts in the average level of a risk factor within a population would result in large population effects overall [8]. Optimal public health strategies then would encourage everyone in the community to make small shifts in lifestyle habits every day [9].

Socio-ecological perspectives describe the multilevel influences on individual health behaviour [10, 11]. Figure 1 shows these influences, conceptually drawn as concentric circles of influences from proximal to distal. Individual characteristics, beliefs and attitudes comprise the inner circle, surrounded by immediate influences of friends and family. Institutional environmental influences then come into play, such as the food environment and physical environment at workplaces, schools and places where people spend most of their time. Broader outer circles reflect the urban community environment, and the economic and cultural environments in which people live; these can influence social norms, food production and availability, public open space provision, and the existence of active transport options in communities and cities.

The socio-ecological perspective posits that prevention programs and policies that change people's knowledge, attitudes and skills without changing the societal and physical environments in which people work, live and play, are unlikely to be effective. Prevention strategies must operate on multiple levels, including individually targeted and tailored behaviour change components, as well as environment and social support strategies to make it easier for individuals to adopt healthy practices. Becoming more physically active is easier where there are safe walking/cycling paths in the neighbourhood, exercise stations or quality playgrounds in local parks. Healthy food choices are facilitated by neighbourhood shops that stock affordable and nutritious food. Interventions that cultivate social norms about the benefits of physical activity and healthy eating, policies that ensure physical activity programs are available in parks, or initiatives that emphasise the provision of comprehensible nutrition information at point of purchase all have potential important benefits. The following sections examine some promising societal and environmental responses that facilitate regular physical activity and healthy eating across populations.

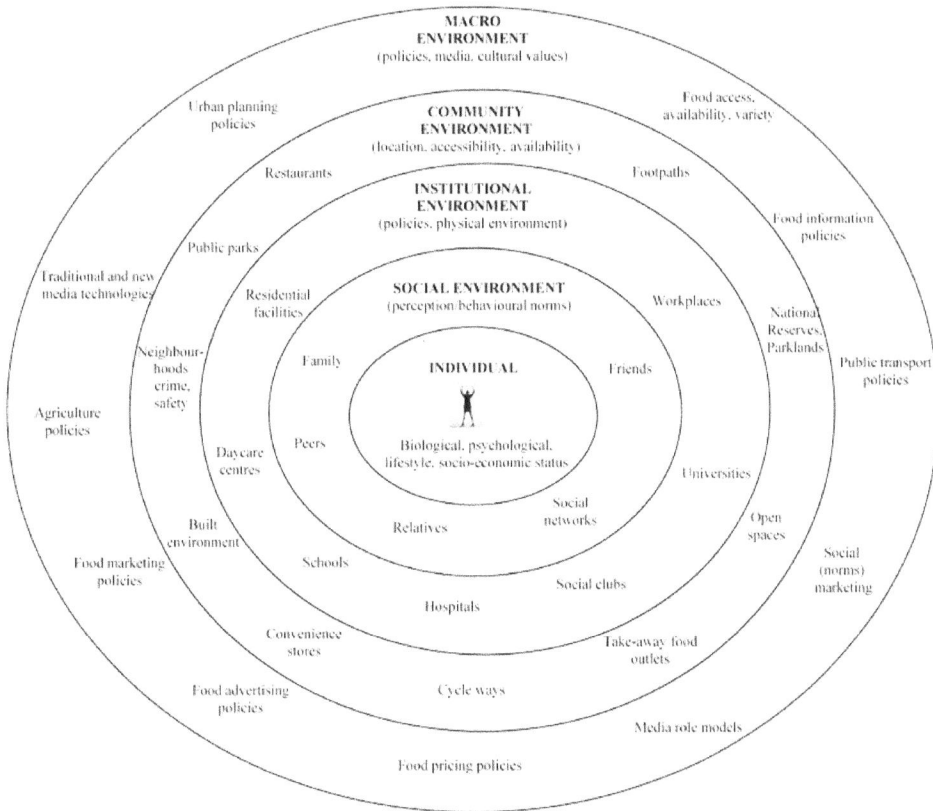

Figure 1. Socio-ecological perspective for obesity and diabetes prevention across societal levels [10, 11]

Physical activity environments

Redesigning the built environment for walking and cycling

Over half the Australian population is not reaching minimal recommendations of around 150 minutes per week (2.5 hours) of moderate–vigorous physical activity for health benefits [12]. This equates to approximately half an hour of activity accumulated over at least five separate sessions on most days each week. The target amount of 150 minutes per week can also be accrued in short bouts of ten minutes or more. Recommendations for weight maintenance or weight loss are substantially greater, typically around 60 to 90 minutes daily [13].

A key contributor to decreased daily physical is increased reliance on motor vehicles. Over 75% of Australians live in an urban setting [14], with a third of all car trips under three kilometres and a half under five kilometres, distances that could easily be walked or cycled. Short trips by bicycle can in fact be faster in an inner city context than driving [15]. If available, public transport as an alternative to driving can also provide some physical activity. Catching a bus or train generally involves a walk at either end of the trip. Walking, cycling or using public transport is often called 'active travel'.

Cycling is an important form of active travel. However, while about 10% of Australians will cycle in any given year, only 1%–2% cycle daily [16]. The opportunity to cycle depends on good cycling infrastructure, with a network of well-connected bicycle lanes and routes. This is particularly needed to overcome the perception of the dangers of cycling, ideally by separating cyclists from mainstream car traffic [17]. Recent cycling infrastructure development in central Sydney that applied these guidelines has resulted in an increase in the observed numbers of daily bicycle trips [18].

It is also important to encourage walking as a form of active travel. Walking accounts for two-thirds of women's and one-half of men's health enhancing physical activity [19], yet, the built environment in urban areas discourages walking. More sustained walking and cycling behaviours can be encouraged by urban design that creates a physical environment more conducive to cycling and walking. For example, occasional or non-regular riders do not ride long distances for utilitarian purposes. One way to reduce trip distances is to develop cities with higher density and greater mixed land use (having residential zoning near commercial areas). Urban planners and transport engineers could create more walkable physical environments through medium-density housing, connection of street networks and having mixed-use destinations (having local shops, businesses and residential dwellings in the same neighbourhood) [20]. This means more people can live near where they work, removing the need to commute long distances. Most people will choose the easiest, cheapest and most convenient way to get to work. If pedestrian and cycling footpaths were available, active transport is more likely.

While there is some truth in the idea of 'build it and they will come', the optimal approach is for good cycling and walking infrastructure to be built and promoted to the public and prospective users. A community-based project in Western Sydney to encourage cycling and the use of existing bicycle paths found a significant increase as a result of social marketing and behavioural programs [21, 22]. Similarly, there is a need to create and then promote walkable environments to the community, and change community perceptions around walking as a mode of transport.

Redesigning public spaces for active living and recreational activities

Active living refers to opportunities for people to incorporate active travel and recreational activities into their everyday lives. Town and city residents rely on public spaces such as natural reserves and public parks as venues for outdoor recreational activities [23]. Theoretically, public spaces are more likely to be used by the general population than indoor sport and exercise facilities such as the gym [24]. Epidemiological evidence shows that people living in activity-friendly environments with green spaces, playgrounds and walking/jogging paths tend to be more physically active [25–28], and both adults and children have reduced obesity risk [29, 30]. A recent systematic review found open space preservation to be associated with increased physical activity levels, primarily walking [31]. Yet, public spaces such as neighbourhood parks are an underutilised environmental setting for promoting physical activity. This reflects a research area in evolution, with much research describing associations between park characteristics and physical activity [27]. Limited evidence notwithstanding, the evidence to date supports the notion of neighbourhood parks as a promising environmental setting for promoting recreational activities. Since public spaces are amenable to change, improving their conduciveness to physical activity has good potential to improve the quality of community life [32].

Two 'naturalistic' studies in Sydney evaluated the impact of park improvements on physical activity levels. One study in Western Sydney did not reach conclusive findings about the impact of improving the environment in three parks on physical activity participation [33]. Another study in an inner Sydney suburb found improving children's playgrounds increased usage [34]. Despite their potential policy implications, intervention evidence from these naturalistic studies, so called because they aimed to evaluate the effectiveness of environmental changes opportunistically, remains limited [35, 36].

Even though improving facilities and amenities is an important step, the socio-ecological perspective would propose that an integrated approach would comprise promotion to increase awareness, and organised activity programs in renovated public spaces are also needed to motivate community use [35, 37]. Local councils and governments are in the position to define public space (re)design for supporting community-wide physical activity participation, and ensure that appropriate recreational programs are provided and promoted to the community.

Narrowing the health inequality gap through environmental strategies

Health inequalities between neighbourhoods have been well documented in Australia [38]. People living in socioeconomically disadvantaged areas have higher rates of chronic diseases and lower leisure-time physical activity than those in more affluent neighbourhoods [39]. One benefit of a socio-ecological perspective in a comprehensive multilevel prevention obesity/diabetes program is that the interventions can impact whole populations, not just motivated individuals who attend clinics or specific programs. Based on this perspective, the development of public infrastructure could contribute to reducing the differences in health behaviours between poor and wealthy areas [40–43].

Positive relationships between access to quality public spaces and increased physical activity and reduced obesity risk are most apparent among residents living in socioeconomically disadvantaged areas, the elderly and homemakers [27, 30]. This suggests that improving the quality of public spaces (eg access, aesthetics, functionality, proximity, perceived safety), may counter the effects of neighbourhood socioeconomic disadvantage, and contribute to narrowing the diabetes and obesity inequality gap between areas [44].

Summary of physical activity environments

Living in activity-friendly communities can facilitate active transport and recreation for every person regardless of their socioeconomic status. Although more evidence is needed to demonstrate direct links between specific environmental infrastructure and physical activity, public health experts consider the evidence sufficient to recommend policy interventions to reshape approaches to urban planning and built environment designs for supporting active living [45]. Increasing incidental and everyday physical activities through environmental approaches may contribute sufficiently to increase total energy expenditure, and to have a role in obesity and diabetes prevention.

Food environments

Despite living in a society that has a plentiful supply of nutritious foods, the majority of Australian adults and children do not eat in accordance with dietary guidelines, and in particular consume excessive amounts of energy-dense, nutrient-poor (EDNP) foods. Energy-dense, nutrient-poor foods refer to foods high in total energy, fat and/or sugar and with little positive nutritional value. Examples include many fast foods, fried foods, fatty meats, cakes, confectionery and sweetened drinks.

Population increases in the prevalence in overweight and obesity indicate that a significant proportion of adults and children consume more energy than they require on a regular basis. In 2007, EDNP foods contributed to 35% of the daily energy intake of children aged two to 16 years, which is twice the recommended limit of 5%–20% [46]. For adults, EDNP comprised 36% of energy intake in 1995 [47].

As with physical activity, the science of nutrition education started with programs and clinicians providing advice to individuals. The approach has broadened to encompass the food environment, social norms and broader environmental influences, as highlighted by the socio-ecological framework. Food consumption patterns reflect the interactions between individual factors, such as food preferences and disposable income, and environmental factors, such as food availability, price and marketing. Despite the positive aspects of our food supply, our food environment in fact promotes excessive food consumption, particularly of EDNP foods. Energy-dense, nutrient-poor foods are widely available and extensively marketed, through multiple media as well as at point of sale [48]. These environmental influences are particularly strong, as nutrition information about specific food products is not highly accessible at point of sale. As such, there are many barriers to 'making healthy choices easier choices'.

Redesigning environments to improve the availability of healthy foods

People's access to healthy foods is influenced by the availability of healthy foods in their neighbourhood, or their access to transport to travel to more distant food retail outlets. A landmark study of 221 census areas with over 10 000 residents in the US found that residents increased their fruit and vegetable consumption by 32% for each additional supermarket in their census area [49]. Further studies in both Australia and other developed countries have consistently found that supermarkets offer a predictably large range of healthier food items and at lowest costs [50, 51].

Much of the work exploring food environments has focused on access differentials between more and less socioeconomically advantaged areas as a possible explanation of social gradients in the prevalence of obesity. This corresponds to the concept of 'deprivation amplification', where disadvantages arising from poorer quality environments amplify individual disadvantages in ways that are detrimental to health [52].

Some international studies have described reduced food availability and quality, and increased price of healthier foods in more disadvantaged neighbourhoods and rural areas [53, 54]. However, this has not been a consistent finding, and healthy food availability probably also depends on other factors such as population density and urban planning.

Two studies from the UK prospectively examined the impact of introducing a supermarket into an area which did not previously have one. Whilst one study found a substantial increase in nearby residents' consumption of fruit and vegetables [55], the other only found a change in those residents who switched to do all their shopping at the new supermarket [56]. A US study which followed 5115 people in several cities for 15 years, found that easy access to fresh food stores did not improve food choices [57]. The study also found that living near fast-food outlets was associated with increased consumption of fast food. Thus, limiting the availability and access to fast foods may be as important as increasing the availability and access of healthy food.

Altogether, the body of research on community food availability reinforces the public health value of mixed land use, with convenient location of supermarkets, and public transport routes, active transport infrastructure and community transport options to ensure people have good access to supermarket destinations [58].

Redesigning the nutrition information environment: food and menu labelling

People's access to healthy foods is also influenced by their ability to identify healthier food products. Thus, nutrition information systems are considered by public health professionals as important communication tools to inform and potentially influence consumers. They are also of interest to the food industry as promotional and marketing tools which offer opportunities for communicating both factually and persuasively.

Recently, front-of-pack (FOP) signposting schemes have been proposed as a consumer-friendly tool to assist consumers in making at-a-glance decisions about a product's nutritional composition [59]. The value of a FOP system has been clearly identified, and research indicates that shoppers achieve higher accuracy in determining product healthiness with simpler nutritional formats, particularly traffic light systems [60]. However, the public health and food industry interests in nutritional labelling have led to a plethora of FOP labelling systems over recent years, and there is now evidence that the simultaneous operation of multiple systems creates confusion and lack of trust in such information [61]. The need to have a single, consistent system in operation provides a strong argument for a mandatory labelling system. Researchers have also shown that the use of uniform FOP labelling may have indirect impacts on food supply, and may influence reformulation or development of healthier products [62].

As Australians are increasingly purchasing and relying on foods prepared outside the home, there has also been increased research and policy emphasis on the provision of nutrition information at point of purchase in food service outlets, despite inconclusive evidence regarding the effects of such labelling on purchasing and consumption [63]. In the interests of consumer information, the New South Wales (NSW) government has introduced legislation requiring all chain restaurants with 20 or more locations in NSW or 50 or more locations nationally to include kilojoule labelling on their menu boards for all 'standard menu items' from 2012. This follows the introduction of state menu nutrition labelling policies across the US since 2003, and a national bill in March 2010.

Redesigning the nutrition information environment: limiting food marketing

Whilst public health seeks to provide consumers with nutrition information, food marketing is designed to persuade consumers to buy specific food products, and tends to undermine public health nutrition efforts. The specific concern arises as food marketing is highly pervasive and the majority of foods advertised are EDNP [46].

Australian and international studies indicate that reductions in advertising of unhealthy foods and beverages are likely to be a cost-effective (and probably cost-saving) strategy for obesity prevention and chronic disease prevention [64, 65].

Many governments and international agencies have concerns about the marketing of foods and non-alcoholic drinks to children. In May 2010 the World Health Organization stipulated that governments should develop appropriate policies and set clear definitions for key components of restrictions on marketing of foods and drinks to children [66]. On the basis of the evidence, the Australian Government's National Preventative Health Task Force (2009) recommended government restrictions to reduce children's exposure to advertising of unhealthy foods [67]. In response, the Australian Government decided it would monitor the impact of self-regulation on 'reducing children's exposure to advertising of energy-dense, nutrient-poor foods and beverages', before any further government action [68].

Since then, studies indicate that industry self-regulation remains inadequate in reducing Australian children's exposure to junk food advertising on television, and children still see the same amount of television advertising for unhealthy foods as they did before industry self-regulation was introduced in 2009 [69, 70]. The lack of impact partially reflects the voluntary participation and lenient specifications of the industry self-regulatory standards [71]. For example, food companies were found to consistently stipulate higher thresholds for negative nutrients (saturated fats, added sodium and sugars) compared with existing professional criteria [72].

The rationale for government action to limit food marketing to children is gaining momentum. Only government is in the position to set a framework of advertising standards defining the types of foods and drinks deemed appropriate for advertising to children based on a food or drink's nutrient profile, and assessed using a standardised, independent nutrient-profiling tool; and ensure that these standards apply to all food companies.

Summary of food environments

Redesigning food environments to make them more conducive to healthy eating is fundamental to promoting nutrition at a population level. Individuals need to be informed about healthy food options, but the broader environment that promotes, advertises and creates accessible food purchasing also need to be influenced, if population dietary patterns are to be changed. Policies can ensure that healthy foods are widely available and accessible, that people have easy access to accurate nutritional information in order to identify healthier foods, and that this information is not undermined by persuasive marketing. These actions can contribute to a comprehensive approach to public health nutrition and obesity prevention.

Creating societal norms for active living and healthy eating

Even environmental and policy changes may not be sufficient to motivate people to become physically active or eat healthily. Cultural values and social norms also play a key role in the types and quantities of food and drinks consumed; and how much and where physical activity is incorporated into daily living. When individuals engage in active modes of travel, some may do so because they see others doing it, and consider such behaviour the norm in their society. Accordingly, striving for healthy eating habits and regular physical activity can be more difficult if such practices are not valued or perceived to be desirable within a society.

In this context, social marketing is well placed to augment the benefits of environmental and policy changes in ways that are consistent with a socio-ecological framework [67, 73]. Geoffrey Rose reminded us that 'It makes little sense to expect individuals to behave differently from their peers; it is more appropriate to seek a general change in behavioural norms and in the circumstances which facilitate their adoption' [74]. Diverse and complementary chronic disease prevention initiatives therefore must be supported by consistent messages to reshape cultural values and social norms. This includes promoting practical, simple everyday changes in lifestyles [75], as well as cultivating political and social movements for active communities and a healthy food supply. In this situation, social marketing to change social norms has an advocacy component, including targeting key decision-makers about a policy development or resource allocation decision [76]. This strategy has been widely used in tobacco control, where there is already strong community support for tobacco control legislation. In obesity and diabetes prevention, the goal is to replace the 'obesogenic' features of environment with environments that make it easier for individuals to be active and make healthy nutrition choices.

Preventing obesity and type 2 diabetes is a shared responsibility

The socio-ecological approach provides a framework to implement a broad range of environmental and policy initiatives across multiple levels of society. This involves directing physical activity and nutrition initiatives at infrastructure (eg active living communities), institutions (eg retail settings, workplaces), policies and regulations (eg food marketing to children), media (eg coverage of health issues), and social norms (eg relationships, behaviours). Building footpaths and regulating availability of fast food outlets are more permanent strategies, and can impact larger numbers of people than individual-based health education programs that target smaller numbers of motivated individuals with high risks. Making these changes at the whole population level is a necessary antecedent to diabetes prevention and to weight maintenance and obesity prevention.

The reality of widespread societal and environmental initiatives will require committed and sustained advocacy and resources, with positive population-wide changes in obesity and diabetes taking several years to manifest. Acknowledging this complexity, solving the obesity and diabetes 'epidemics' will require building multidisciplinary collaborations between scientists and policy-makers. Strengthening the research translation pathways, from findings to practice and policy enactment will be an important component of such collaborations. It is important to recognise that all tiers of government and various sectors of society shape beliefs and practices about physical activity and eating. As such, all are responsible for society's health. Organised public health efforts involve collaborations across government sectors and with different groups in society, such as industry, consumer groups, civil society and the media. As the City of Sydney has shown, urban renewal for active living across the life span and for all sub-population groups is possible in Australia. Government leadership, social planning and urban renewal that engages communities, businesses and relevant stakeholders is fundamental to the process. Only then will a society be able to hardwire regular physical activity and healthy eating into its everyday fabric and ensure more sustainable healthy behaviours to prevent obesity, diabetes and other chronic diseases.

References

1. Winslow CE (1920). The untilled fields of public health. *Science,* 51(1306): 23–33.

2. Centers for Disease Control and Prevention (CDC) (2010). *Guide to community preventive services: promoting good nutrition* [Online]. Available: www.thecommunityguide.org/nutrition/index.html [Accessed 23 July 2011].

3. Foster C, Hillsdon M & Thorogood M (2005). *Interventions for promoting physical activity.* Chichester, UK: John Wiley & Sons, Ltd.

4. World Health Organization (2005). *Preventing chronic disease: a vital investment. WHO global report*. Geneva: World Health Organization.

5. Bauman A, Ma G, Cuevas F, Omar Z, Waqanivalu T, Phongsavan P, Keke K & Bhushan A (2011). Cross-national comparisons of socioeconomic differences in the prevalence of leisure-time and occupational physical activity, and active commuting in six Asia-Pacific countries. *Journal of Epidemiology and Community Health,* 65(1): 35–43.

6. Suhrcke M, Nugent RA, Stuckler D & Rocco L (2006). *Chronic disease: an economic perspective*. London: Oxford Health Alliance.

7. Trinh OTH, Nguyen ND, Phongsavan P, Dibley MJ & Bauman AE (2009). Prevalence and risk factors with overweight and obesity among Vietnamese adults: Caucasian and Asian cut-offs. *Asia Pacific Journal of Clinical Nutrition,* 18(2): 226–33.

8. Rose G (2001). Sick individuals and sick populations. *International Journal of Epidemiology,* 30(3): 427–32.

9. World Health Organization (2004). *Global strategy on diet, physical activity and health*. Geneva: World Health Organization.

10. McLeroy KR, Bibeau D, Steckler A & Glanz K (1988). An ecological perspective on health promotion programs. *Health Education Quarterly,* 15(4): 351–77.

11. Stokols D (1992). Establishing and maintaining healthy environments: toward a social ecology of health promotion. *American Psychologist,* 47(1): 6–22.

12. Australian Institute of Health and Welfare (2010). *Australia's health 2010*. Australia's health series no. 12. Sydney: AIHW.

13. Haskell WL, Lee IM, Pate RR, Powell KE, Blair SN, Franklin BA, Macera CA, Heath GW, Thompson PD & Bauman A (2007). Physical activity and public health: updated recommendations for adults from the American College of Sports Medicine and the American Heart Association. *Medicine & Science in Sports Exercise,* 39(8): 1423–34.

14. Australian Government (2010). *Our cities: building a productive, sustainable and liveable future*. Discussion paper. Sydney: Infrastructure Australia.

15. Australian Bicycle Council (2010). *The Australian national cycling strategy 2011–2016*. Sydney: Austroads.

16. Merom D, van der Ploeg HP, Corpuz G & Bauman AE (2010). Public health perspectives on household travel surveys active travel between 1997 and 2007. *American Journal of Preventive Medicine,* 39(2): 113–21.

17. Daley M, Rissel C & Lloyd B (2007). All dressed up and no-where to go? A qualitative research study of the barriers and enablers to cycling in inner Sydney. *Road and Transport Research,* 16: 42–52.

18. City of Sydney (2011). *Bike riding booms around Sydney's new cycleways*. Sydney: City of Sydney.

19. Merom D, Bauman A & Ford I (2004). The public health usefulness of the exercise recreation and sport survey (ERASS) surveillance system. *Journal of Science and Medicine in Sport,* 7(1): 32–37.

20. Bauman AE & Bull FC (2007). *Environmental correlates of physical activity and walking in adults and children: a review of reviews.* London: National Institute of Health and Clinical Excellence [Online]. Available: www.nice.org.uk [Accessed 14 June 2011].

21. Bauman A, Rissel C, Garrard J, Kerr I, Speidel R & Fishman E (2008). *Cycling: getting Australia moving. Barriers, facilitators and interventions to get more Australians physically active through cycling.* Melbourne: Cycling Promotion Fund.

22. Rissel C, New C, Wen LM, Merom D, Bauman AE & Garrard J (2010). The effectiveness of community-based cycling promotion: findings from the Cycling Connecting Communities project in Sydney, Australia. *International Journal of Behavioral Nutrition and Physical Activity,* 7(1): 8.

23. Sydney Urban Parks Education and Research Group (2002). *Research report: Sydneysiders' use of parks and gardens, 2001.* Sydney: Centre for Visitor Studies.

24. Bendimo-Rung AL, Mowen AJ & Cohen DA (2005). The significance of parks to physical activity and public health: a conceptual model. *American Journal of Preventive Medicine,* 28: 159–68.

25. Brownson RC, Baker EA, Housemann RA, Brennan LK & Bacak SJ (2001). Environmental and policy determinants of physical activity in the United States. *American Journal of Public Health,* 91(12): 1995–2003.

26. Davidson KK & Lawson C (2006). Do attributes of the physical environment influence children's level of physical activity? *International Journal of Behavioral Nutrition and Physical Activity,* 3(19): 1–17.

27. Kaczynski AT & Henderson KA (2007). Environmental correlates of physical activity: a review of evidence about parks and recreation. *Leisure Sciences,* 29: 315–54.

28. Owen N, Humpel N, Leslie E, Bauman A & Sallis JF (2004). Understanding environmental influences on walking: review and research agenda. *American Journal of Preventive Medicine,* 27(1): 67–76.

29. Bell JF, Wilson JS & Liu GC (2008). Neighborhood greenness and 2-year changes in body mass index of children and youth. *American Journal of Preventive Medicine,* 35(6): 547–53.

30. Nielson TS & Hansen KB (2007). Do green areas affect health? Results from a Danish survey on the use of green areas and health indicators. *Health & Place,* 13: 839–50.

31. Durand CP, Andalib M, Dunton GF, Wolch J & Pentz MA (2011). A systematic review of built environment factors related to physical activity and obesity risk: implications for smart growth urban planning. *Obesity Reviews,* 12(5): e173–82.

32. Maller C, Townsend M, Brown P & St Leger L (2002). *Healthy parks healthy people: the health benefits of contact with nature in a part context. A review of current literature.* Melbourne: Deakin University.

33. NSW Department of Health (2002). *Walk it: active local parks. The effect of park modification on physical activity participation. Summary report.* Sydney: NSW Health Department.

34. Bohn-Goldbaum EE, Phongsavan P, Merom D & Bauman AE (under review). Does playground improvement result in increased physical activity among children?

35. Cohen DA, Golinelli D, Williamson S, Sehgal A, Marsh T & McKenzie TL (2009). Effects of park improvements on park use and physical activity: policy and programming implications. *American Journal of Preventive Medicine*, 37(6): 475–80.

36. Tester J & Baker R (2009). Making the playfields even: evaluating the impact of an environmental intervention on park use and physical activity. *Preventive Medicine*, 48: 316–20.

37. Cohen DA, Marsh T, Williamson S, Pitkin Derose K, Martinez H, Setodji C & McKenzie TL (2010). Parks and physical activity: why are some parks used more than others? *Preventive Medicine*, 50: S9–S12.

38. Turrell G, Kavanagh AM, Draper G & Subramanian SV (2007). Do places affect the probability of death in Australia? A multilevel study of area-level disadvantage, individual-level socioeconomic position and all-cause mortality, 1998–2000. *Journal of Epidemiology and Community Health*, 61(1): 13–19.

39. Kavanagh AM, Goller JL, King T, Jolley D, Crawford D & Turrell G (2005). Urban area disadvantage and physical activity: a multilevel study in Melbourne, Australia. *Journal of Epidemiology and Community Health*, 59(11): 934–40.

40. Coen SE & Ross NA (2006). Exploring the material basis for health: characteristics of parks in Montreal neighborhoods with contrasting health outcomes. *Health & Place*, 12(4): 361–71.

41. Giles-Corti B & Donovan RJ (2002). Socioeconomic status differences in recreational physical activity levels and real and perceived access to a supportive physical environment. *Preventive Medicine*, 35(6): 601–11.

42. Moore LV, Diez Roux AV, Evenson KR, McGinn AP & Brines SJ (2008). Availability of recreational resources in minority and low socioeconomic status areas. *American Journal of Preventive Medicine*, 34(1): 16–22.

43. Timperio A, Ball K, Salmon J & Crawford RD (2007). Is availability of public open space equitable across areas? *Health & Place*, 13: 335–40.

44. McLaren L, McIntyre L & Kirkpatrick S (2010). Rose's population strategy of prevention need not increase social inequalities in health. *International Journal of Epidemiology*, 39(2): 372–77.

45. Centers for Disease Control and Prevention (CDC) (2010). *Guide to community preventive services: promoting physical activity: Environmental and policy approaches* [Online]. Available: www.thecommunityguide.org/pa/environmental-policy/index.html [Accessed 23 July 2011].

46. Rangan A, Kwan J, Flood V, Louie J & Gill T (2011). Changes in 'extra' food intake among Australian children between 1995 and 2007. *Obesity Research & Clinical Practice*, 5: e55–e63

47. Rangan AM, Randall D, Hector DJ, Gill TP & Webb KL (2009). Consumption of 'extra' foods by Australian children: types, quantities and contribution to energy and nutrient intakes. *European Journal of Clinical Nutrition*, 62(3): 356–64.

48. Story M, Kaphingst KM, Robinson-O'Brien R & Glanz K (2008). Creating healthy food and eating environments: policy and environmental approaches. *Annual Review of Public Health*, 29: 253–72.

49. Morland K, Wing S & Diez Roux A (2002). The contextual effect of the local food environment on residents' diets: the atherosclerosis risk in communities study. *American Journal of Public Health*, 92(11): 1761–67.

50. Burns CM, Gibbon P, Boak R., Baudinette S & Dunbar JA (2004). Food cost and availability in a rural setting in Australia. *Rural Remote Health,* 4(4): 311.

51. Cummins S & Macintyre S (2002). A systematic study of an urban foodscape: the price and availability of food in greater Glasgow. *Urban Studies,* 39(11): 2115–30.

52. Macintyre S (2007). Deprivation amplification revisited; or, is it always true that poorer places have poorer access to resources for healthy diets and physical activity? *International Journal of Behavioral Nutrition and Physical Activity,* 4(32).

53. Cummins S, Smith DM, Taylor M, Dawson J, Marshall D, Sparks L & Anderson AS (2009). Variations in fresh fruit and vegetable quality by store type, urban-rural setting and neighbourhood deprivation in Scotland. *Public Health Nutrition,* 12(11): 2044–50.

54. Giskes K, Turrell G, van Lenthe FJ, Brug J & Mackenbach J P (2006). A multilevel study of socioeconomic inequalities in food choice behaviour and dietary intake among the Dutch population: the GLOBE study. *Public Health Nutrition,* 9(1): 75–83.

55. Wrigely N, Warm D & Margetts B (2003). Deprivation, diet and food retail access: findings from the Leeds 'Food Deserts' study. *Environment and Planning,* 35: 151–88.

56. Cummins S, Petticrew M, Higgins C, Sparks L & Findlay A (2004). *Reducing inequalities in health and diet: the impact of a food retail development. A pilot study.* London: MRC Social and Public Health Sciences Unit.

57. Boone-Heinonen J, Gordon-Larsen P, Kiefe CI, Shikany JM, Lewis CE & Popkin BM (2011). Fast food restaurants and food stores longitudinal associations with diet in young to middle-aged adults: the CARDIA Study. *Archives of Internal Medicine,* 171(13): 1162–70.

58. Burns C & Inglis A (2007). Measuring food access in Melbourne: access to healthy and fast food by car, bus and foot in Melbourne. *Health & Place,* 13: 877–85.

59. Blewett N, Goddard N, Pettigrew S, Reynolds C & Yeatman H (2011). *Labelling logic: review of food labelling law and policy* [Online]. Available: www.foodlabellingreview.gov.au/internet/foodlabelling/publishing.nsf/content/labelling-logic. [Accessed 4 May 2011].

60. Gorton D (2007). Nutrition labelling: update of scientific evidence on consumer use and understanding of nutrition labels and claims [Online]. Available: www.foodsafety.govt.nz/elibrary/industry/signposting-nutrition-study-research-projects/signs-literature-review-report_final-2.pdf [Accessed 5 May 2011].

61. Malam S, Cleg S, Kirwan S & McGinigal S (2009). *Comprehension and use of UK nutrition signpost labelling schemes.* London UK: Food Standards Agency.

62. Vyth EL, Steenhuis IH, Roodenburg AJ, Brug J & Seidell JC (2010). Front-of-pack nutrition label stimulates healthier product development: a quantitative analysis. *International Journal of Behavioral Nutrition and Physical Activity,* 7: 65.

63. National Heart Foundation of Australia (2010). *Rapid review of the evidence: the need for nutritional labelling on menus.* National Heart Foundation of Australia.

64. Cecchini M, Sassi F, Lauer JA, Lee YY, Guajardo-Barron V & Chisholm D (2010). Tackling unhealthy diets, physical inactivity, and obesity: health effects and cost-effectiveness. *The Lancet,* 376(9754): 1775–84.

65. Vos T, Carter R, Barendregt J, Mihalopoulos C, Veerman JL, Magnus A, Cobiac L, Bertram MY, Wallace AL & ACE-Prevention Team (2010). *Assessing cost-effectiveness in prevention (ACE-Prevention): final report.* Melbourne: Deakin University and Brisbane: University of Queensland.

66. World Health Organization (2010). *Set of recommendations on the marketing of foods and non-alcoholic beverages to children.* Geneva: World Health Organization.

67. National Preventive Health Taskforce (2009). *Australia: the healthiest country by 2020. The report of the National Preventative Health Strategy: the roadmap for action.* Canberra: Commonwealth of Australia.

68. National Preventative Health Taskforce (2010). *Taking preventative action. A response to* Australia: the healthiest country by 2020. The report of the National Preventative Health Strategy: the roadmap for action. Canberra: Commonwealth of Australia.

69. Hebden LA, King L, Grunseit A, Kelly B & Chapman K (2011). Advertising of fast food to children on Australian television: the impact of industry self-regulation. *Medical Journal of Australia,* 195(1): 20–24.

70. King L, Hebden L, Grunseit A, Kelly B, Chapman K & Venugopal K (2011). Industry self-regulation of television food advertising: Responsible or responsive? *International Journal of Pediatric Obesity,* 6(2–2): e390–e98.

71. Hebden L, King L, Kelly B, Chapman K & Innes-Hughes C (2010). Industry self-regulation of food marketing to children: reading the fine print. *Health Promotion Journal of Australia,* 21(3): 229–35.

72. Hebden L, King L, Kelly B, Chapman K & Innes-Hughes C (2010). Regulating the types of foods and beverages marketed to children: how useful are food industry commitments. *Nutrition & Dietetics,* 67(4): 258–66.

73. Maibach EW, Abroms LC & Marosits M (2007). Communication and marketing as tools to cultivate the public's health: a proposed 'people and places' framework. *BMC Public Health,* 7: 88.

74. Rose G (1992). *The strategy of preventive medicine.* Oxford: Oxford University Press.

75. Australian Government. Swap it, don't stop it [Online]. Available: www.swapit.gov.au [Accessed 23 July 2011].

76. Wallack W, Dorfman L, Jernigan D & Themba M (1993). *Media advocacy and public health: power for prevention.* Newbury Park: Sage.

Treatment

15

How self-perception, emotion and beliefs influence eating and weight-related behaviour

Brooke Adam[1] and Elizabeth Rieger[2]

This chapter examines the psychological and environmental factors contributing to the self-perception of obese individuals and its impact on weight-related behaviour. Emotional functioning, environmental factors, physical health, eating and weight-related attitudes, beliefs and behaviour are explored. The impact of these factors on meaningful short- and long-term treatment outcomes is discussed.

A wealth of knowledge and research exists which attests to the pervasive and often serious physical consequences of obesity. Examining the health problem of obesity at a surface level, one might feel puzzled as to why some obese patients experience marked difficulty, often over an extended period of time, to make relatively modest behaviour change in exchange for significant improvements in physical and psychological health and associated quality of life. Clinically, obesity is associated with a range of psychosocial problems such as depression, low self-esteem, guilt, shame, body dissatisfaction, social withdrawal and isolation, stigmatisation and discrimination [1–3]. However, not all obese persons will experience psychological problems. The obese population is heterogeneous in terms of aetiology, maintaining factors, and psychological and physiological concomitants [4, 5]. As such, over recent years the question of whether those who are obese have psychological difficulties has shifted to who will experience psychological problems and in what ways [1]? This chapter will examine the main psychological difficulties experienced by obese individuals, some of the factors known to contribute to these difficulties, and how these difficulties in turn impact on weight-related behaviours and, as such, should be included as a key component of treatment.

The range of psychological problems associated with obesity

Psychological difficulties are already evident in obese children and adolescents, a finding which emphasises the importance of preventing and treating paediatric obesity [6]. Given that obesity is increasing in childhood and adolescence, its psychological and social

1 Boden Institute of Obesity, Nutrition, Exercise and Eating Disorders, University of Sydney.

2 Department of Psychology, Australian National University.

consequences (such as teasing, peer exclusion, body dissatisfaction and poor self-esteem) are also of rising importance [7].

Clear evidence is emerging of the concerning association between obesity and the self-perception of children and adolescents. In a 2006 study [8], 2813 children with a mean age of 11.3 years completed self-report measures of self-perception and body shape perception, and their body mass index (BMI) was calculated. Results clearly indicated that obesity has a negative association with self-esteem. Specifically, obese girls and boys possessed lower perceived athletic competence, physical appearance and global self-worth than their normal-weight counterparts. The association between obesity and negative self-perception was particularly evident in girls, with obese girls reporting significantly decreased social acceptance and satisfaction with physical appearance than healthy weight peers. Overall, it was found that obese children were two to four times more likely than normal weight children to have low self-worth.

Given the cross-sectional nature of these data, it is unclear whether negative self-esteem is a cause and/or consequence of obesity. However, a longitudinal study by Strauss (2000) [9] was able to provide stronger support for the causal role of obesity in negatively impacting self-esteem. This study similarly found that female childhood obesity at nine years of age was associated with impaired self-esteem. At the four-year follow-up, obese girls experienced significant, decreasing self-esteem, which was associated with sadness, loneliness, anxiety and risk-taking behaviour (eg smoking and alcohol consumption).

In addition to poor self-esteem, adult obese individuals are more likely to have a psychological disorder, with a higher prevalence of mood, anxiety, alcohol use, personality and eating disorders among the obese [10, 11]. Of the various psychological disorders, binge-eating disorder (BED) has the strongest connection with obesity. BED is characterised by frequent episodes of binge eating in which the person consumes a large amount of food in a discrete period of time, coupled with a sense of a loss of control. It is very different from an episode of overeating, in terms of the amount of food consumed and the driven, compulsive nature of the behaviour [1]. In BED, there is no immediate compensatory behaviour (such as purging or excessive exercise) as seen in bulimia nervosa. BED is common in individuals with obesity; estimates are that approximately one-third of the obese population undergoing treatment for weight-loss experience binge eating symptomatology [12]. Similarly, the prevalence of obesity among individuals with BED may be as high as 65% [13] which is much higher than the prevalence in the general adult population [14].

Yet the most consistent finding in terms of the psychological problems associated with obesity is that obese individuals experience higher levels of body image disturbance than their normal-weight counterparts [15]. This may take the form of experiencing high levels of dissatisfaction with their appearance, being excessively preoccupied with their appearance, believing that their appearance proves something negative about their worth as a person, avoiding many social situations because of their weight, and being overly concerned about hiding or disguising their body. One of the largest studies to date that has investigated body satisfaction at various BMI categories was conducted by Frederick, Peplau and Lever (2006)

[16]. This study involved 52 677 men and women who were asked to rate their level of body satisfaction on a scale ranging from 'I have a great body' to 'I find my body unattractive'. The results indicated that rating one's body as unattractive was higher among obese male and female participants compared with the other BMI categories: 69% of women and 54% of men with a BMI ≥35 felt unattractive compared to 5% of women and 6% of men with a BMI between 18.5 and 21.7. Across most BMI categories, women reported greater body dissatisfaction than men except in the underweight categories (due to men's desire to be larger). Particularly for women, a desire to lose weight is strongly associated with a desire to change appearance and physical shape, and in turn feel more attractive or experience greater body satisfaction. Women and men report that one factor they find motivating to lose weight is to be able to have more choice in the range of clothing available to wear that they regard as more flattering and fashionable [17].

While not all obese individuals experience elevated body dissatisfaction, two subgroups of obese individuals who are particularly vulnerable in this regard are people with BED and those seeking gastric banding [15–17]. In addition, it is important to note that factors other than seeking to improve body satisfaction may drive the desire to achieve a thinner physique (such as the belief that weight loss will improve the individual's relationships) and that treatment should assist individuals to improve these other factors in addition to interventions aimed at achieving weight loss [18].

Factors contributing to the negative impact of obesity on self-perceptions: thin ideal internalisation and stigma

The negative impact of obesity on self- and body-esteem has been attributed in part to internalisation of Western society's 'thin ideal' [19, 20]. The psychological and behavioural consequences of societal pressure to be thin are considerable. An increasing number of children and adolescents in Western societies report that they engage in dieting behaviour to lose or maintain weight [21]. However, dieting in pre-adulthood leaves individuals at greater risk of subsequent weight gain compared to non-dieters [22]. One explanation is that dieting often precedes the onset of binge eating, and an increased risk of other eating disorder pathology, weight gain and obesity in later adulthood [23, 24].

In addition to internalisation of the thin ideal, obese individuals are known to experience considerable stigma and discrimination which in turn is likely to have a negative influence on self-perceptions. There is a wealth of data demonstrating the existence of a pervasive stigma towards obese individuals, with discrimination documented in all domains of life including social life, parenting practices, education, employment and healthcare. Indeed, as Puhl and Brownell (2002) [25, p108] state, negative attitudes and behaviours towards obese people 'constitute one of the last socially acceptable forms of discrimination'.

In the social domain, strongly negative attitudes regarding obese individuals are already evident in pre-school and primary school-aged children. In one study, Latner and Stunkard (2003) [26] presented ten- and 11-year-old boys and girls with drawings of six children: a healthy child, a child using crutches, a child in a wheelchair, a child with no left hand, a child with a slight facial deformity, and an obese child. The children were asked to rank the drawings in terms of the child they liked best to worst. It was found that children ranked the healthy child as the most preferred and the obese child as the least preferred. Compared to when the same study was conducted in 1961, the obese child was ranked as even less desirable by the children in the 2003 study, indicating that negative attitudes towards obese children have become stronger over time. This study highlights that obese children and adults are implicitly perceived as a devalued social group.

Parenting practices are another domain in which negative attitudes towards obese individuals have been documented. For instance, in one study, parents were given three pictures of children (an average-weight child, an obese child and a handicapped child) and were asked to tell a story about each picture to their own child [27]. There were striking differences in the rate of successful outcomes at the end of each story: the outcome was happy for the average-weight child on 45% of occasions, 80% for the handicapped child and on zero occasions for the obese child.

In addition, research has found evidence of negative attitudes and behaviours towards obese students in their education. For example, obese students are less likely to be accepted into college than average-weight students despite having equivalent academic records and making the same number of college applications [25]. In a prospective study, women who were overweight in adolescence had completed fewer years of school, were less likely to be married, had lower household incomes and had higher rates of poverty than women who had not been overweight in adolescence [28]. Moreover, negative attitudes and practices have been documented for obese people at virtually every stage of the employment process [29]. Overweight applicants are evaluated more negatively than average-weight applicants and are less likely to be hired. Once employed, negative attitudes continue, with overweight employees being perceived as lazy, sloppy, less competent, lacking in self-discipline and disagreeable. They are also seen as poor role models. At the termination stage, there is evidence from legal case documentation that obese employees have been fired due to their weight even if they hold positions for which weight is irrelevant (eg computer analysts) and despite formal recognition for fine job performance.

In the domain of healthcare, negative attitudes towards obese patients have been found among doctors, nurses and medical students. In one particularly concerning study, 12% of nurses reported that they were reluctant to touch obese patients while 24% stated that they found obese patients to be 'repulsive' [30]. Being aware of negative attitudes towards them may result in obese individuals delaying seeking medical care (eg obese women delaying getting a breast examination), which obese patients have attributed to embarrassment about their weight and previous negative experiences with healthcare professionals.

The impact of psychological difficulties on weight-related behaviours and obesity

While obesity can result in negative self-perceptions, psychological problems can in turn influence weight-related behaviours and obesity. One psychological factor that may result in weight gain and ultimately obesity is if the individual has a low level of motivation for weight control. A highly influential model in current understandings of health-related behaviours is the stages of change model [31]. According to this model, there are two main factors that contribute to an individual's level of motivation to engage in a healthy behaviour: decisional balance and self-efficacy. Decisional balance is defined as the relative balance between the potential gains (pros) and losses (cons) of engaging in a health-related behaviour such as reducing fat consumption and doing more physical activity. According to the model, people are motivated to engage in these health behaviours when the pros of reducing dietary fat or increasing exercise outweigh the cons. This is precisely what the research shows: for individuals with lower levels of motivation to engage in these health behaviours, the cons of reducing dietary fat (eg 'Eating less fat would mean not eating my favourite foods') or increasing exercise ('Trying to do more exercise would add to my time-pressure') outweigh the pros ('Eating less fat and exercising more would help me to feel more energetic and attractive') [32]. However, by the time people are highly motivated and are actively working to reduce their fat consumption and increase their exercise levels, the pros of these behaviours outweigh the cons [32].

Self-efficacy is the other main factor contributing to an individual's motivation to engage in health-related behaviours. Self-efficacy refers to the individual's level of confidence that she/he can successfully engage in a health behaviour, even in challenging situations where there is a high level of temptation to engage in an unhealthy behaviour. If the individual lacks confidence that she/he can perform the healthy behaviour, then little or no attempt will be made to do so. Self-efficacy is a strong predictor of the degree to which people engage in weight-control behaviours, such as their amount of fruit and vegetable consumption [33] as well as their success at weight management [34].

In addition to low levels of motivation to engage in weight-control behaviours, another psychological problem that may contribute to obesity is negative affect. According to the affect-regulation model, individuals who are prone to experiencing negative emotions such as depression, anxiety, anger or stress may eat in an attempt to provide comfort or distraction from these distressing emotions. In support of the affect-regulation model, Stice and colleagues (2005) [35] conducted a study in which 496 adolescent girls (aged from 11 to 15 years) were followed up over four years. Girls who reported higher levels of depression and body image disturbance at baseline were significantly more likely to be obese four years later.

This finding has been replicated in adults. For example, in a study by Block et al. [4], 1355 American men and women between the ages of 25 and 64 years had their BMI and stress levels across various life domains (job-related demands, relationship strains and financial stress) assessed at baseline and then followed up over nine years. Stress in certain domains (eg job-related demands and difficulty paying bills for men and women; strains in family relationships for women) predicted more weight gain over the next nine years, mainly among individuals who were already obese at baseline. In contrast, individuals who had a normal BMI at baseline lost weight or gained less weight as stress increased. This study highlights that individuals differ in their appetitive and eating behaviour in response to life stress. This individual variation may contribute to the inconsistent findings in the research, with some studies finding that negative emotions predict obesity [35] while others do not [36].

Given this connection between life stress and weight gain, it is perhaps not surprising that the stress to which obese individuals are exposed to as a result of negative societal attitudes and behaviours can worsen their obesity. Adams and Bukowski [37] found that the victimisation (ie bullying) experienced by obese 12- to 13-year-old girls predicted a deterioration in their body image by the age of 14 to 15 years which in turn predicted an increase in depression and BMI by the age of 16 to 17 years. In another longitudinal study examining mood and weight changes over a 12-month period after controlling for baseline BMI, depression at baseline was found to be predictive of adolescent obesity one year later [38]. These results are in keeping with the association between negative affect and overeating mentioned previously.

Another psychological factor that may result in people becoming obese is the presence of BED. A five-year prospective study conducted by Fairburn and colleagues (2003) [39] compared individuals with BED and bulimia nervosa. In this study, 48 individuals with BED and 102 individuals with bulimia nervosa who were not in treatment for their disorder were assessed at 15-month intervals regarding their eating disorder symptoms and general psychiatric symptoms. At the five-year time-point, a higher proportion of the BED group (39%) was obese compared to the bulimic group (20%). Indeed the rates of obesity had nearly doubled in the BED group during the five years of the study.

Implications for treatment

The effectiveness of interventions for obesity must be assessed based on a comprehensive range of outcomes that look beyond weight loss, such as increased motivation, improved mood and self-esteem, and decreased social isolation. Not only will attention to these factors improve the individual's quality of life, but will directly impact on weight control if these psychological issues are involved in maintaining the individual's obesity.

Most patients present for treatment of obesity wanting to lose 20%–30% of their pre-treatment body weight, which is unrealistic in the context of the modest weight loss (ie 5%–10% of pre-treatment body weight) that a significant subset of obese patients have difficulty achieving using behavioural treatments [41]. As Cooper and Fairburn (2001) [40] point out, obese patients' weight goals seem entirely reasonable in our Western society which promotes the idea that weight is highly controllable. In the media we are bombarded with stories and images of significant weight losses achieved in very short periods of time, from the television program *The biggest loser* through to the increasing obsession with celebrity post-baby bodies. Further, as mentioned above, the thin-ideal internalisation and social pressure to be slim also contributes to an expectation of achieving an unrealistically low weight in treatment.

Behavioural weight-loss treatment (BWT) addresses eating habits and levels of physical activity, with an emphasis on making sustainable lifestyle changes with the aim of resulting in sustained weight loss. The results of group-based BWL treatment are well established; this form of treatment generally results in weight loss between 7%–10% of initial body weight over the typical 16- to 24-week treatment period [42]. However, the pattern of weight loss and maintenance in patients who engage in this form of treatment is remarkably consistent: the point of maximum weight loss is usually reached six months after commencement of treatment, then weight regain begins gradually and consistently until weight stabilises at around baseline levels by five years for most patients [43, 44].

To augment successful maintenance of weight losses, motivational enhancement therapy (MET) strategies may prove beneficial as there is a strong theoretical and empirical rationale for the role of motivation in successful long-term weight control. As previously stated, individuals are motivated to change their behaviour when they experience alterations in decisional balance (ie when the advantages of change are perceived to outweigh the disadvantages) and self-efficacy (ie when they are confident that they can successfully change). Compared to the weight-loss phase, the weight-maintenance phase may have particularly adverse effects on both decisional balance and self-efficacy and hence motivation for weight control. Firstly, the amount of weight loss achieved during treatment and its impact on other domains of life (such as improved health, body satisfaction, and relationships with others) may be less than hoped for, thereby diminishing the perceived advantages of continuing to engage in strenuous weight-control behaviours [41]. Secondly, given the consistent pattern of weight regain, most patients will have a history of weight-control failures, thus undermining a sense of confidence or self-efficacy regarding their ability to achieve long-term success [5]. Unfortunately, the negative alterations in decisional balance and self-efficacy associated with weight maintenance occur at a time when the patient's self-motivation for weight control is paramount, given the reduction or cessation in external support from treating clinicians that occurs at this time. Indeed, research indicates that problems in sustaining motivation are associated with poorer long-term weight control for obese patients [45]. In addition, overweight and obese patients' levels of motivation to increase their physical activity, increase their consumption of fruit and vegetables, and decrease their dietary fat intake are predictors of their level of engagement in these weight-control behaviours one year later [46]. Thus, both theoretical and empirical work suggests that enhancing the motivation of obese patients to control their weight may have benefits for their long-term weight management.

While clinical guidelines highlight the key importance for treatment success of enhancing patients' motivation to control their weight [47], the research base from clinical trials to support such recommendations is sparse. This stands in marked contrast to the considerable research undertaken on MET in the treatment of other health behaviours, particularly alcohol problems. In the largest of these studies, a four-session MET intervention resulted in substantial and sustained (over three years) reductions in drinking behaviour among patients with severe drinking problems and achieved comparable effects to interventions of longer duration [48]. One of the few studies to have employed MET in the treatment of obesity found that the addition of three MET sessions to a standard BWL program resulted in significantly better treatment adherence and glucose control at post-treatment relative to standard treatment in obese women with type 2 diabetes [49]. In another study, obese patients who received up to 15 MET sessions after failing to lose a significant amount of weight in a BWL program, subsequently lost significantly more weight and engaged in significantly more weekly exercise than those who did not receive the MET intervention [50]. Yet since neither of these studies included a follow-up assessment, the effectiveness of MET for the maintenance of weight loss remains unknown.

In a pilot study assessing the efficacy of MET for weight maintenance in obesity, 22 obese adults (68% of whom were classified in the extreme/severe obesity range) participated in a 20-session behavioural weight-loss program, which included three MET sessions [51]. The patients experienced a significant reduction in weight from pre- to post-treatment (a mean weight loss of 5% of initial body weight) with no significant increase in weight from post-treatment to the one-year follow-up. Patients also reported significant improvements in obesity-related quality of life, impulsive eating tendencies, body dissatisfaction, and maladaptive cognitions at post-treatment that were maintained at the one-year follow-up. Importantly, reported utilisation of MET strategies by patients was significantly correlated with the degree of weight-loss maintenance. These results suggest MET can assist obese patients in maintaining their weight losses and make sustained improvements in terms of quality of life, impulsive eating tendencies, body dissatisfaction and maladaptive cognitions.

The evidence we have at hand demonstrating the significant association between obesity and negative self/body-esteem already at a very young age, points to the need to address this in treatment explicitly. Cooper and Fairburn (2001) [41] outline promising cognitive behavioural strategies to treat obese patients who avoid body exposure, engage in frequent body checking, or have ongoing, frequent critical thoughts about their appearance, with the overarching goal to foster greater self-acceptance.

Conclusions

It is clear that there are a range of psychological problems associated with obesity, such as low self-esteem, body dissatisfaction, depression and eating disorder pathology. Although we are currently unable to identify clear and causal relationships between obesity and the known comorbid psychological problems outlined in this chapter, we can be certain that the impact of these problems is broad-reaching. Longitudinal data, in addition to research examining the trajectory of obesity and psychological comorbidities in older adults given the relatively recent onset of the obesity epidemic, will be important in uncovering more precisely the causal relationships and longer-term impacts that exist between these problems. A growing body of research points to the need to integrate motivational enhancement therapy and self-acceptance modules into obesity treatment, in order to achieve maintained improvements in the physical and psychological health of obese patients in the months and years following treatment.

Acknowledgements

The authors wish to thank Sarah Horsfield for her comments on this chapter.

References

1. Friedman MA & Brownell KD (2002). Psychological consequences of obesity. In CG Fairburn & KD Brownell (Eds). *Eating disorders and obesity: a comprehensive handbook* (pp393–98). 2nd edn. New York: The Guildford Press.

2. Friedman KE, Reichmann SK, Costanzo PR, Zelli A, Ashmore JA & Musante G J (2005). Weight stigmatization and ideological beliefs: Relation to psychological functioning in obese adults. *Obesity Research,* 13(5): 907–16.

3. Puhl RM & Brownell KD (2003). Psychosocial origins of obesity stigma: toward changing a powerful and pervasive bias. *Obesity Reviews*, 4(4): 213–27.

4. Block JP, He Y, Zaslavsky AM Ding L & Ayanian JZ (2009). Psychosocial stress and weight change among US adults. *American Journal of Epidemiology*, 170(2): 181–92.

5. DiLillo V, Siegfried NJ & Smith West D (2003). Incorporating motivational interviewing into behavioral obesity treatment. *Cognitive and Behavioral Practice*, 10: 120–30.

6. Goldfield GS & Epstein LH (2002). Management of obesity in children. In CG Fairburn & KD Brownell (Eds.). *Eating disorders and obesity: a comprehensive handbook* (pp573–77). 2nd edn. New York: The Guildford Press.

7. Magarey AM, Daniels LA & Boulton JC (2001). Prevalence of overweight and obesity in Australian children and adolescents: reassessment of the 1985 and 1995 data against new standard international definitions. *The Medical Journal of Australia*, 174: 561–64.

8. Franklin J, Denyer G, Steinbeck KS, Caterson ID & Hill AJ (2006). Obesity and risk of low self-esteem: a statewide survey of Australian children. *Pediatrics,* 118(6): 2481–87.

9. Strauss RS (2000). Childhood obesity and self-esteem. *Pediatrics,*105(1): 1–5.

10. Marcus MD & Wildes JE (2009). Obesity: is it a mental disorder? *International Journal of Eating Disorders*, 42(8): 739–53.

11. Petry NM, Barry D, Pietrzak RH & Wagner JA (2008). Overweight and obesity are associated with psychiatric disorders: results from the national epidemiologic study on alcohol and related conditions. *Psychosomatic Medicine*, 70(3): 288–97.

12. Yanovski SZ (2002). Binge eating in obese persons. In CG Fairburn & KD Brownell (Eds). *Eating disorders and obesity: a comprehensive handbook* (pp403–10). 2nd edn. New York: The Guildford Press.

13. Striegel-Moore RH, Cachelin FM, Dohm F, Pike KM, Wilfley DE & Fairburn CG (2001). Comparison of binge eating disorder and bulimia nervosa in a community sample. *International Journal of Eating Disorders*, 29(2): 157–65.

14. Cameron AJ, Welborn TA, Zimmet PZ, Dunstan DW, Owen N, Salmon J, Dalton M, Jolley D & Shaw JE (2003). Overweight and obesity in Australia: the 1999–2000 Australian diabetes, obesity and lifestyle study (AusDiab). *Medical Journal of Australia*, 178(9): 427–32.

15. Rosen JC (2002). Obesity and body image. In CG Fairburn & KD Brownell (Eds). *Eating disorders and obesity: a comprehensive handbook* (pp309–402). 2nd edn. New York: The Guildford Press.

16. Frederick DA, Peplau LA & Lever J (2006). The swimsuit issue: correlates of body image in a sample of 52 677 heterosexual adults. *Body Image*, 3(4): 413–19.

17. Hrabosy JI, Masheb RM, White MA, Rothschild BS, Burke-Martindale CH & Grilo CM (2006). Prospective study of body dissatisfaction and concerns in extremely obese gastric bypass patients: 6- and 12- month postoperative outcomes. *Obesity Surgery*, 16(12): 1615–621.

18. Cooper Z & Fairburn CG (2001). A new cognitive behavioral approach to the treatment of obesity. *Behaviour Research and Therapy*, 39(5): 499–511.

19. Stice E & Shaw HE (1994). Adverse effects of the media portrayed thin-ideal on women and linkages to bulimic symptomatology. *Journal of Social and Clinical Psychology*, 13(3): 288–308.

20. Klaczynski PA, Goold KW & Mudry JJ (2004). Culture, obesity stereotypes, self-esteem and the 'thin ideal': a social identity perspective. *Journal of Youth and Adolescence*, 33(4): 307–17.

21. Neumark-Sztainer D, Story M, Hannan PJ, Perry CL & Irving LM (2002). Weight-related concerns and behaviours among overweight and non-overweight adolescents: implications for preventing weight-related disorders. *Archives of Pediatric and Adolescent Medicine*, 156(2): 171–78.

22. Field AE, Austin SB, Taylor CB, Malspeis S, Rosner B, Rockett HR, Gillman MW & Colditz GA (2003). Relation between dieting and weight change among preadolescents and adolescents. *Pediatrics*, 112(4): 900–6.

23. Grilo, CM (2002). Binge eating disorder. In CG Fairburn & KD Brownell (Eds). *Eating disorders and obesity: a comprehensive handbook* (Second Edition) (pp178–82). New York: The Guildford Press.

24. Neumark-Sztainer D, Wall M, Haines J, Story M & Eisenberg MA (2007). Why does dieting predict weight gain in adolescents? Findings from Project EAT-II: a 5-year longitudinal study. *Journal of the American Dietetic Association*, 107(3): 448–55.

25. Puhl R & Brownell KD (2002). Stigma, discrimination and obesity. In CG Fairburn & KD Brownell (Eds). *Eating disorders and obesity: a comprehensive handbook* (pp108–12). 2nd edn. New York: The Guildford Press.

26. Latner JD & Stunkard AJ (2003). Getting worse: the stigmatization of obese children. *Obesity Research*, 11(3): 452–56.

27. Adams GR, Hicken M & Salehi M (1988). Socialization of the physical attractiveness stereotype: parental expectations and verbal behaviours. *International Journal of Psychology*, 23(1, 6): 137–49.

28. Gortmaker SL, Must A, Perrin JM, Sobol AM & Dietz WH (1993). Social and economic consequences of overweight in adolescence and young adulthood. *New England Journal of Medicine*, 329(14): 1008–12.

29. Roehling MV (1999). Weight-based discrimination in employment: psychological and legal aspects. *Personnel Psychology*, 52(4): 969–1016.

30. Brown I (2006). Nurses' attitudes towards adult patients who are obese: literature review. *Journal of Advanced Nursing*, 53(2): 221-32.

31. DiClimente, CC & Prochaska, JO (1998). Towards a comprehensive, transtheoretical model of change: stages of change and addictive behaviours. In WR Miller & N Heather (Eds). *Treating addictive behaviours* (pp3–24). New York: Plenum Press.

32. Prochaska JO, Velicer WF, Rossi JS, Goldstein MG, Marcus BH, Rakowski W, Fiore C, Harlow LL, Redding CA, Rosenbloom D & Rossi SR (1994). Stages of change and decisional balance for 12 problem behaviours. *Health Psychology*, 13(1): 39–46.

33. Shaikh AR, Yaroch AL, Nebeling L, Yeh MC & Resnicow K (2008). Psychosocial predictors of fruit and vegetable consumption in adults: a review of the literature. *American Journal of Preventative Medicine*, 34(6): 535–43.

34. Elfhag K & Rossner S (2005). Who succeeds in maintaining weight loss? A conceptual review of factors associated with weight loss maintenance and weight regain. *Obesity Reviews*, 6(1): 67–85.

35. Stice E, Presnell K, Shaw H & Rohde P (2005). Psychological and behavioural risk factors for obesity onset in adolescent girls: a prospective study. *Journal of Consulting and Clinical Psychology*, 73(2): 195–202.

36. Roberts RE, Seleger S, Strawbridge WJ & Kaplan GA (2003). Prospective association between obesity and depression: evidence from the Alameda County Study. *International Journal of Obesity*, 27(4): 514–21.

37. Adams RE & Bukowski WM (2008). Peer victimization as a predictor of depression and body mass index in obese and non-obese adolescents. *The Journal of Child Psychology and Psychiatry*, 49(8): 858–66.

38. Goodman E & Whitaker RC (2002). A prospective study of the role of depression in the development and persistence of adolescent obesity. *Pediatrics*, 110(3): 497–504.

39. Fairburn CG, Stice E, Cooper Z, Doll HA, Norman PA & O'Connor ME (2003). Understanding persistence in bulimia nervosa: a 5-year naturalistic study. *Journal of Consulting and Clinical Psychology*, 71(1): 103–9.

40. Jeffrey RW, Wing RR & Mayer RR (1998). Are smaller weight losses or more achievable weight loss goals better in the long-term for obese patients? *Journal of Consulting and Clinical Psychology*, 66(4): 641–45.

41. Cooper Z & Fairburn CG (2001). A new cognitive behavioural approach to the treatment of obesity. *Behavior Research and Therapy*, 39(5): 499–511.

42. Wilson GT & Brownell KD (2002). Behavioral treatment for obesity. In CG Fairburn & KD Brownell (Eds). *Eating disorders and obesity: a comprehensive handbook* (pp524–28). 2nd edn. New York: The Guildford Press.

43. Fabricatore AN & Wadden TA. (2006). Obesity. *Annual Review of Clinical Psychology*, 2(1): 357–77.

44. Jeffrey RW, Drewnowski A, Epstein LH, Stunkard AJ, Wilson GT, Wing RR & Hill DR (2000). Long-term maintenance of weight loss: current status. *Health Psychology*, 19(1): 5–16.

45. Williams GC, Grow VM, Freedman ZR, Ryan RM & Deci EL (1996). Motivational predictors of weight loss and weight maintenance. *Journal of Personality and Social Psychology*, 70(1): 115–26.

46. Robinson AH, Norman GJ, Sallis JF, Calfas KJ, Rock CL & Patrick K (2008). Validating stage of change measures for physical activity and dietary behaviours for overweight women. *International Journal of Obesity*, 32(7):1137–44.

47. National Health and Medical Research Council (2003). *Clinical practice guidelines for the management of overweight and obesity in adults.* Canberra: National Health and Medical Research Centre, Australia.

48. Carroll KM, Connors GJ, Cooney NL, DiClemente CC, Donovan DM, Kadden RR, Longabaugh RL, Rounsaville BJ, Wirtz PW & Zweben A (1998). Internal validity of project MATCH treatments: discriminability and integrity. *Journal of Clinical and Consulting Psychology*, 66(2): 290–303.

49. Smith DE, Heckemeyer CM, Kratt PP & Mason DA (1997). Motivational interviewing to improve adherence to a behavioural weight-control program for older obese women with NIDDM: a pilot study. *Diabetes Care*, 20(1): 52–4.

50. Carels R, Darby L, Cacciapaglia HM, Konrad K, Coit C, Harper J, Kaplar ME, Young K, Baylen CA & Versland A (2007). Using motivational interviewing as a supplement to obesity treatment: a stepped-care approach. *Health Psychology*, 26(3): 369–74.

51. Rieger E, Dean HY, Steinbeck KS, Caterson ID & Manson E (2009). The use of motivational enhancement studies for the maintenance of weight loss among obese individuals: a preliminary investigation. *Diabetes, Obesity and Metabolism*, 11(6): 637–40.

16

The role of physical activity in the prevention and treatment of diabetes

Klaus Gebel,[1] Hidde P van der Ploeg,[1] Maria Fiatarone Singh[2] and Adrian Bauman[1]

This chapter is concerned with the role of physical activity and exercise prescription as components in the prevention and treatment of diabetes. First, the evidence for the diabetes-specific health benefits of physical activity is summarised and the physiological mechanisms are pointed out. Studies of medical comorbidities of diabetes are discussed. Recommendations for physical activity and exercise in the prevention and control of type 2 diabetes are provided, and challenges in the implementation of such strategies are discussed.

The health benefits of regular moderate-intensity physical activity are well known. In particular, epidemiological evidence has shown that an active lifestyle is beneficial in the prevention and treatment of more than 20 health conditions including coronary heart disease, stroke, type 2 diabetes and some cancers [1–3].

Physical activity is defined as body movement produced by skeletal muscle that results in energy expenditure above resting level [2], and can be accumulated at any time, for example during work, housework, transportation or during leisure time. Exercise is a subset of 'leisure time physical activity' that is usually structured, planned, repetitive, and has the purpose of providing recreation, improving or maintaining physical fitness, or enhancing other components of health or wellbeing (see Figure 1). Physical fitness includes cardio-respiratory fitness, muscle strength, body composition and flexibility [4, 5]. Metabolic fitness is also increasingly recognised as an important component of fitness which is closely related to physical activity levels, as well as cardiovascular and musculoskeletal fitness [6].

For the general adult population the American College of Sports Medicine recommends to accumulate at least 30 minutes of at least moderate-intensity physical activity on five, preferably all, days of the week, or vigorous-intensity aerobic physical activity for at least 20 minutes on three days per week [1, 3, 7]. However, even though physical activity confers numerous health benefits, large parts of the adult population are not sufficiently active [8–13].

---

1 Sydney School of Public Health, University of Sydney.

2 Discipline of Exercise and Sports Science, Faculty of Health Science, University of Sydney.

Type 2 diabetes is related to genetic, environmental and behavioural factors. Particularly, lack of physical activity and visceral obesity are considered to be major contributors to the global diabetes epidemic.

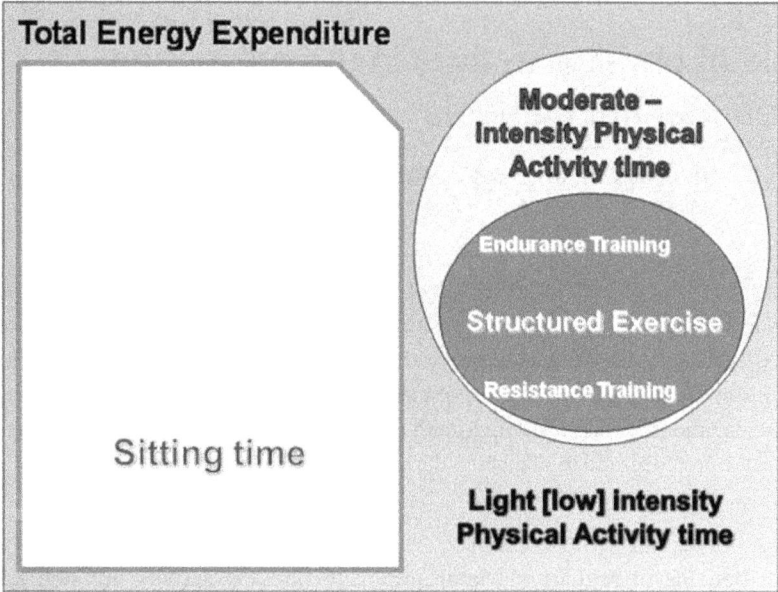

Figure 1. Energy expenditure in humans subdivided into sedentary behaviour, physical activity and the various forms of exercise.

This chapter is concerned with the role of physical activity and exercise prescription as components in the prevention and treatment of diabetes [14, 15]. First, the evidence for the diabetes-specific health benefits of physical activity will be summarised. Recommendations for physical activity and exercise in the prevention and control of type 2 diabetes will be provided, and challenges in the implementation of such strategies will be discussed.

Prevention of type 2 diabetes

Physical inactivity and overweight/obesity are both risk factors for the development of type 2 diabetes. Regular physical activity improves insulin sensitivity, and reduces glucose levels [16]. The role of obesity in the development of diabetes type 2 is likely to work through adipocytes releasing adipocytokines into the circulation, including leptin, adipsin, resistin and interleukin-6 (IL-6) [17], some of which are associated with insulin resistance [18, 19]. There are indications that obesity plays a larger role than physical activity in the development of diabetes [20–22]. However, physical activity has been shown to be beneficial in the prevention of type 2 diabetes independent of weight loss [16]. Besides the beneficial effects of physical activity on the development of type 2 diabetes, it can also be effective in prevention of the metabolic syndrome [16, 23], and during pregnancy in the prevention of gestational diabetes [24, 25], and has independent benefits in reducing cardiovascular risk [1]. The following sections summarise the evidence from observational and intervention studies on the role of physical activity in the primary and secondary prevention of type 2 diabetes.

Diabetes prevention evidence: observational studies

The evidence for primary prevention comes from observational epidemiology; these are usually from large population-based cohort studies that examined whether exposure to occupational, commuting and leisure-time physical activity was related to the subsequent risk of developing type 2 diabetes.

A meta-analysis synthesised the findings from ten prospective cohort studies from the US, the UK, Finland and Japan regarding the exposure to moderate-intensity physical activity and the risk of developing type 2 diabetes [26]. These studies included 301 221 participants and 9367 incident cases of diabetes. The pooled relative risk for diabetes in those who regularly engaged in moderate physical activity was 0.69 (95% CI 0.58–0.83) compared with inactive participants. Similarly, the relative risk of those who walked regularly was 0.70 (0.58–0.84) compared with almost no walking. The associations remained significant when adjusted for BMI [26].

Likewise, a recent report summarised the results from 25 prospective cohort studies and found a similar inverse relationship between physical activity and diabetes incidence. This relationship applied to men and women, different age groups and ethnicities. The reduction in relative risk for type 2 diabetes ranged from 15%–60% for those that were physically active compared with their more inactive peers [16]. It also appears that several domains of physical activity (occupational, commuting and leisure-time physical activity) are all inversely related to the risk of developing type 2 diabetes. Based on these studies, at least 30 minutes per day (210 minutes per week) of at least moderate-intensity physical activity is sufficient to achieve a significant reduction in diabetes incidence [16].

A new area of research has developed around total 'sitting' time. These studies have indicated that prolonged sitting time, including measures of television watching, might be associated with the risk of developing type 2 diabetes, independent of leisure-time physical activity [27–29]. Furthermore, breaks in sitting time have been associated with improvements in waist circumference, triglycerides, and two-hour plasma glucose levels [30]. Two large cohort studies have observed that each two-hour increment per day in watching TV, as a proxy measure of sitting time, was associated with a 14%–20% increase in diabetes incidence, even after adjustment for physical activity participation [31, 32].

Diabetes prevention: the evidence from intervention studies

The strongest evidence for the benefits of physical activity and exercise in the prevention of type 2 diabetes comes from community-based lifestyle intervention trials. To date, at least six randomised trials have examined whether lifestyle interventions, including physical activity, reduce the risk of developing type 2 diabetes among adults with impaired glucose tolerance. These trials are:

- Diabetes Prevention Program (DPP), US
- Diabetes Prevention Study (DPS), Finland
- Da Qing IGT and Diabetes Study (DQS), China
- Diabetes Prevention Program (IDPP), India
- Diabetes Prevention Program (JDPP), Japan
- Västerbotten Intervention Program (VIP), Sweden.

All these trials demonstrated that structured lifestyle modification programs reduced the incidence of type 2 diabetes compared to controls or usual care. For these programs, exercise was usually an independent predictor of improved metabolic control or reduced diabetes incidence, and varied modes of exercise were usually included (see Table 1).

In the Da Qing study in China, 577 middle-aged men and women with impaired glucose tolerance were randomised to a diet only, exercise only, diet and exercise, or control group. The unsupervised exercise prescription ranged from 140 minutes per week for those over 50 years to 280 minutes per week for younger participants. After six years, the diet, exercise, and combined diet and exercise interventions achieved 31%, 46%, and 42% reductions in the risk of developing diabetes compared with the control group [33]. At 20-year follow-up, a sustained preventive benefit was still observed, with the likelihood of diabetes 43% lower among those allocated to the lifestyle interventions [34].

In the US Diabetes Prevention Program (DPP) 3324 overweight and obese participants with impaired glucose tolerance were randomised into three groups (placebo, metformin therapy, and lifestyle). The lifestyle modification intervention aimed to increase physical activity to at least 150 minutes per week (primarily unsupervised brisk walking, but with availability of two sessions of supervised exercise per week) and reduce weight by at least 7%. After a follow-up of three years the lifestyle intervention showed a 58% reduction in the risk of developing diabetes compared to the placebo group, while the metformin group had a risk reduction of only 31% [35]. At ten-year follow-up, compared to controls, the lifestyle intervention maintained a 34% lowered risk of diabetes, and the metformin group maintained an 18% reduction [36].

The Finnish Diabetes Prevention Study ($n = 522$) showed similar results to the US DPP. This lifestyle intervention comprised 210 minutes per week of exercise (including three sessions per week of supervised aerobic and resistance/power training) and diet-induced weight loss of 5%–7%, resulting in a four-year diabetes risk reduction of 58% ($p < .001$). In this study, those who failed to meet the weight-loss goal, but accumulated four hours of weekly moderate exercise, had a significantly lower risk of diabetes than the control group [37]. Three years after the program, intervention group participants maintained many lifestyle changes and their risk for diabetes was still 36% lower than among controls [38].

Table 1. Lifestyle change goals in the intervention groups in diabetes prevention programs. Adapted from Baker M et al. 2011.

Study (country)	Exercise / physical activity							Diet / nutrition			
	Duration (min/wk)	Intensity	Structured exercise	Supervised exercise	Aerobic activity	PRT activity※	Occupational activity	Portion control	Fat	Alcohol	Fibre
DPP (US)	≥150*	Moderate	✓	✓	✓	✓	✓	✓	✓	✓	✗
DPS (Finland)	≥210	Moderate to strenuous	✓	✓	✓	✓	✓	✗	✓	✗	✓
DQS (China)	≥35–420†	Light to very strenuous	✓	✗	✓	✗	✗	✓	✓	✓	✗
IDPP (India)	≥210	Moderate	✓	✗	✓	✗	✓	✓	✓	✗	✓
JDPP (Japan)	210–280	Moderate	✓	✗	✓	✗	✗	✓	✓	✓	✗
VIP (Sweden)	≥150‡	Low-Moderate	✓	✓	✓	✓	✗	✓	✓	✓	✓

* Energy expenditure ≥700 kcal/week was the primary objective, and the target volume (min/week) was allowed to be increased/decreased based on the intensity of activities performed.

† 35–210 min/week for persons ≥50 years; 70–420 min/week for persons <50 years.

‡ 2.5 hours per day prescribed as supervised exercise in the first month.

PRT = Progressive resistance training; DPP = Diabetes Prevention Program (US); DPS = Diabetes Prevention Study (Finland); DQS = Da Qing IGT and Diabetes Study (China); IDPP = Diabetes Prevention Program (India); JDPP = Diabetes Prevention Program (Japan); VIP = Västerbotten Intervention Program (Sweden).

※ PRT: progressive resistance training.

The Indian Diabetes Prevention Study (n = 531) comprised a physical activity target of unsupervised brisk walking for at least 30 minutes each day (210 min/week). After three years the relative risk reduction for diabetes was 28.5% for the lifestyle intervention, 26.4% for metformin, and 28.2% for the combination of both interventions compared to the control group [39].

A non-randomised lifestyle intervention among middle-aged males in Sweden included a substantial physical activity component. Over six years of follow-up, the lifestyle intervention achieved a 63% risk reduction for the development of diabetes compared with the control group [40]. A more recent Swedish study randomised 194 middle-aged adults with impaired glucose tolerance to lifestyle intervention or usual care, and observed metabolic indicators and insulin resistance improvements at 12 months, with some improvements maintained at five years (VIP program) [41].

The Japanese Diabetes Prevention Program (JDPP) followed 458 men for four years. Twenty percent of participants were randomised to an intensive intervention group of diet and physical activity advice, and the others were assigned to the standard intervention (control) group. The JDPP prescribed 30 to 40 minutes per day (ie 210 to 280 minutes per week) of unsupervised moderate intensity physical activity [42]. This prescription included sport and active commuting, and reduced diabetes incidence by 68% at four-year follow-up.

Summary of diabetes prevention evidence

The net results of these diverse trials in people at risk of diabetes show a clear secondary prevention benefit of lifestyle interventions [43]. There appear to be independent protective benefits of both weight loss and physical activity. A recent Cochrane review summarised these results, and in a meta-analysis of randomised controlled diabetes prevention trials, showed that exercise and diet interventions reduced the risk of type 2 diabetes by 37% [44]. Although most lifestyle trials did not distinguish benefits attributed to weight loss or to physical activity [45], several studies did observe effects of activity independent of weight loss, suggesting these risk factors partly operate independently of each other [33, 39].

Limitations of these trials include self-report of physical activity participation. However, in epidemiological studies where measurement error in exposure occurs, the observed relative risk is likely to underestimate the true relative risk, so these 'physical activity self report' estimates are likely to underestimate the preventive relationship between activity and diabetes incidence. Objective measurement would be better [46], and in epidemiological studies, fitness measures show a strong protective relationship to diabetes incidence [47–49].

Recommendations for diabetes prevention

For at-risk individuals, a minimum dose of at least 150 minutes per week, and possibly substantially more, of 'at least moderate-intensity physical activity' is recommended to prevent diabetes. This is in addition to recommendations for a healthy diet and weight loss.

Physical activity advice should form part of every clinical counselling session with individuals at risk of diabetes, and a clear plan should be developed. People can accumulate physical activity in different settings: through active commuting, and in their leisure time through structured or unstructured exercise programs. Higher levels of physical activity, up to an hour a day of moderate-intensity activity, yield even greater reductions in the incidence of type 2 diabetes [1, 43, 50]. Resistance training regimens, which are important in diabetes management, should also be considered, especially for older adults [3], and three of the RCTs of diabetes prevention (DPP, DPS, VIP) have specifically included this exercise modality. It also appears that long uninterrupted periods of sitting should be avoided.

As previously mentioned, obesity is an independent risk factor for diabetes. However, while a minimum of 30 minutes of physical activity per day (150 to 210 minutes per week) appears to be sufficient for a significant risk reduction in type 2 diabetes, this may not be sufficient for weight maintenance or weight loss [3, 51]. At least 60 to 90 minutes of moderate-intensity physical activity daily is needed for weight maintenance in previously overweight or obese people [51–53]. Therefore, engaging in more than 30 minutes of moderate-intensity physical activity per day would not only reduce the risk of developing diabetes directly, but for those who are overweight or obese also by influencing body weight and improving fat distribution.

1.5 Challenges in implementation

The epidemiological evidence relates to both the primary and secondary prevention of diabetes. The primary prevention of diabetes involves a whole-population approach, which requires actions in both clinical and community settings. This means that all clinical encounters need to recommend physical activity/exercise, in the same way that tobacco cessation is almost universally recommended. Unfortunately, many primary care physicians remain reluctant to adopt this area of preventive counselling [54]. Advice regarding moderate intensity physical activity may have better compliance rates than vigorous-intensity prescriptions [55], so that the initial goal is to ensure all sedentary and low active individuals reach at least the minimal threshold of 150 minutes of activity each week, preferably across five or more days. In addition, clinicians need to become advocates for physical activity programs and facilities across the community [56], in the same way that they rapidly adopted and disseminated an anti-smoking stance in the 1980s.

The secondary prevention goal requires identification of those at risk for diabetes, which is itself a challenge. For these individuals, more structured and evidence-based lifestyle advice is important. Patient advice should highlight the importance of physical activity in diabetes prevention, and include referral to appropriate structured exercise programs; in addition, some increases in incidental lifestyle activities are recommended to increase total energy expenditure, including active transport, increasing active chores and being active in one's local environment.

Management of type 2 diabetes

Apart from its role in the prevention of type 2 diabetes, physical activity and exercise have important roles in the treatment and management of diabetes [57–60]. This role remains largely unincorporated into mainstream clinical management of type 2 diabetes [61]. Given that exercise has an effect as potent as most oral hypoglycaemic agents [62], this is a critical gap in clinical care.

In this section, the health benefits of physical activity and exercise for individuals with type 2 diabetes will be discussed. Firstly, the evidence for the health benefits from various physical activity and exercise interventions for individuals with type 2 diabetes will be described. Then, physical activity and exercise recommendations for the care of diabetes will be outlined. Lastly, challenges in the implementation of strategies to increase levels of physical activity participation among those with diabetes will be discussed.

Diabetes management evidence: aerobic training

The majority of studies on the role of physical activity in the management of type 2 diabetes have focused on the effects of aerobic training [63]. Aerobic exercise involves the usage of large muscles and relies on aerobic levels of energy expenditure (eg brisk walking, cycling, jogging, swimming). Aerobic exercise alone is associated with clinically significant reductions in the glycosylated haemoglobin level [64, 65]. The physiological adaptations responsible for improvements in glucose control through aerobic training include increased capillary density, glucose transport (GLUT4) proteins in muscle, protein kinase B content, and glycogen synthase activity, as well as a shift from low-oxidative type 2b muscle fibres to moderate-oxidative, more insulin-sensitive type 2a muscle fibres [63, 66], and decreased inflammatory cytokines which impair insulin signalling in skeletal muscle [67, 68].

Aerobic training improves fitness levels and insulin sensitivity, and also results in redistribution of visceral adiposity [69]. Even in the absence of weight loss, vigorous activity can improve insulin sensitivity [70], decrease insulin resistance and reduce arterial stiffness [71]. Diabetes markers improved by exercise include insulin resistance, but also HDL and lipid profiles, as well as glycosylated haemoglobin levels and systemic inflammation in some studies [72, 73].

A meta-analysis pooled the results of seven randomised controlled trials on the effects of structured aerobic exercise interventions on cardio-respiratory fitness in adults with type 2 diabetes ($n = 266$). Participants in the exercise groups increased their fitness (VO_2max) by 11.8%, compared to 1% in control groups ($p < 0.003$). Interventions with higher intensities tended to yield larger improvements in fitness. Moreover, exercise intensity predicted weighted mean difference in glycosylated haemoglobin better than exercise volume [62]. A recent large-scale randomised trial from the US ($n = 4376$ overweight and obese individuals with type 2 diabetes) also found increases in cardio-respiratory fitness to be significantly higher in a combined physical activity and diet intervention than in a diabetes support and education group [74].

Diabetes management evidence: resistance training

Traditionally, aerobic training has been used as the main exercise modality to manage type 2 diabetes [75]. However, in recent years resistance training has been gaining wide acceptance as an important strategy in the treatment of diabetes [63]. In resistance training muscles work against a resistive load or weight leading to hypertrophy and improved muscular strength. With increasing age adults have decreases in muscle mass, functional capacity, resting metabolic rate, and increases in adiposity, and insulin resistance. Resistance training is associated with improvements in bone mineral density, muscle strength and muscle hypertrophy and can thereby help in the prevention of osteoporosis and sarcopenia and in the maintenance of functional status [7, 76]. However, only a small number of well-controlled intervention studies have examined the benefits of resistance training for people with type 2 diabetes [63]. The most recent meta-analysis of resistance training by Strasser et al. [77] included 13 RCTs in which resistance training reduced glycosylated haemoglobin (HbA(1c)) by 0.48% (95% CI −0.76, −0.21; $p = 0.0005$), fat mass by 2.33 kg (95% CI −4.71, 0.04; $p = 0.05$) and systolic blood pressure by 6.19 mmHg (95% CI −11.38, −1.00; $p = 0.02$). It has been hypothesised that the improved glucose uptake is not only due to an increase in muscle mass that is associated with resistance training, but probably also due to qualitative changes in muscles that enhance insulin signalling and thereby sensitivity [78]. Furthermore, progressive resistance training (PRT) has been found to positively influence insulin resistance [79, 80]. Based on this evidence, resistance training should be recommended in the management of type 2 diabetes and metabolic disorders.

The strongest evidence for the health benefits of resistance training in type 2 diabetes comes from two trials that used multiple exercises at relatively high intensities and showed a decrease in glycosylated haemoglobin of 1.1%–1.2% in the intervention group compared to no significant change in the control group [81, 82]. However, even studies that used relatively low volumes and intensities of resistance training achieved positive effects on glucose control [79, 83–87]. This is particularly important for individuals who are totally sedentary and are not likely to participate in programs involving strenuous aerobic or resistance training [63]. This could apply to older adults, who may find it difficult to get to, or participate in, structured aerobic programs.

Other health benefits of resistance training in diabetes are an improved body composition, increases in total fat-free mass, reduced blood pressure [82], improved muscular strength [85], lipid profiles [84], bone mineral density and metabolic rate at rest, and a preferential mobilisation of visceral and subcutaneous adipose tissue in the abdominal region [63]. Resistance training can also help in reducing the required insulin-sensitising medication dose and thereby limit side effects [82, 88], and benefits depression [89] and cognitive impairment [90], both of which are more prevalent in those with diabetes.

While there is substantial evidence for the health benefits of resistance training for people with type 2 diabetes, a Canadian study showed that 88% of individuals with diabetes do not carry out resistance training activities [91]. This shows the unrealised potential of wide-scale interventions to promote resistance training among people with diabetes.

Diabetes management evidence: aerobic and resistance training

Resistance and aerobic training have similar beneficial effects on insulin sensitivity and metabolic control in type 2 diabetes [58, 64, 92]. However, some studies compared combinations of both resistance and aerobic exercise versus only one of the two exercise modalities. A Canadian study (n = 28) compared the effects of a combined aerobic and resistance training program to aerobic training only in postmenopausal women with type 2 diabetes. There were no differences in weight loss, fitness, or blood lipids, but the combined group showed better glucose uptake and larger increases in muscle mass compared to the aerobic only group [87]. Similarly, an American study also reported on benefits of combining resistance and aerobic training on glycaemic control, fitness and lean tissue mass [65]. Another Canadian study showed that while both aerobic and resistance training alone were effective in reducing glycosylated haemoglobin, the combination of both exercise modalities was more effective [64]. However, in this study, the combined group had twice the volume of exercise, which may have been responsible for the added efficacy of this treatment, as noted by the authors. Furthermore, an Italian study (n = 120) that combined aerobic and resistance training showed more general improvements in cardiovascular risk factors than studies that used resistance training only as the intervention [93]. Finally, a meta-analysis found that the differences in the benefits of aerobic, resistance and combined training for people with diabetes were small. However, combined training generally showed advantages over aerobic or resistance training alone [94]. This leads to the optimal clinical recommendation of both modalities, but either may be more convenient or accessible for different patient groups.

Clinically, there are many patients with multiple comorbidities who cannot tolerate the dose of aerobic exercise that has proven effective in RCTs. Resistance training improves aerobic capacity, osteoarthritis pain and disability, depression, functional status, gait and balance impairments, bone density, and insomnia, thus addressing the spectrum of associated clinical disorders in older type 2 adults with diabetes [95], and providing a strong rationale for its utility in this condition. Notably, high intensity PRT is feasible even when robust aerobic exercise is impossible due to frailty, balance disorders, osteoarthritis or advanced peripheral vascular disease for example, making it particularly suitable for the typical older adult with type 2 diabetes. In addition, only PRT attenuates the loss of lean tissue (muscle and bone) accompanying weight loss diets typically prescribed for overweight adults with diabetes [96], thus minimising weight cycling related to lowered basal metabolic rate. By contrast, aerobic exercise is *not* anabolic, and does not increase muscle mass, precluding the associated metabolic and clinical benefits such a shift in body composition produces [13].

Diabetes management evidence: patho-physiological mechanisms

A Cochrane review and a meta-analysis, both synthesising the results of 14 randomised controlled trials of aerobic and resistance exercise programs, found that levels of glycosylated haemoglobin were reduced by around 0.6% in the exercise groups, while there were no differences between the groups in body mass index [97, 98]. Khaw et al. found that each 1% increase in glycosylated haemoglobin with levels between 5%–6.9% was associated with a 28% increase in mortality risk, independent of other risk factors, including age, blood pressure, serum cholesterol and body mass index [99]. It was suggested that much of the excess mortality risk of diabetes in men could be profiled by the biomarker of increased glycosylated haemoglobin.

The limited impact on the body mass index in exercising groups may be due to increases in muscle mass, that keep body mass relatively constant [97], particularly in trials of resistance training. It seems likely that muscle and adipose tissue distribution plays a crucial role in glucose metabolism, rather than body mass itself. It has been shown that an increase in lean body mass is inversely correlated with changes in glycosylated haemoglobin [83, 100], which might be due to increased storage of glucose in the skeletal muscle [76]. Muscle hypertrophy is not only associated with an increase in insulin sensitivity, but also with an increase in resting metabolic rate, exercise tolerance and functional mobility [65]. Furthermore, exercise-induced reductions in abdominal subcutaneous and visceral adipose tissue distributions are related to increased insulin sensitivity, without changes in overall body weight [69, 87]. Adipose tissue is associated with secretion of adipocytokines, which can negatively influence insulin resistance [101]. In conclusion, exercise-induced increases in fat-free mass and reductions in adipose tissue, as well as shifts in anabolic-catabolic hormonal profile are beneficial for glucose control and other aspects of metabolic health, regardless of changes in body weight. These relationships are demonstrated in Figure 2.

Summary of diabetes management evidence

Numerous trials have demonstrated the health benefits of physical activity and exercise in the treatment of type 2 diabetes. Physical activity is associated with improved insulin sensitivity and glucose control independent of weight loss [97]. Moreover, regular physical activity leads to a decrease in blood lipids and blood pressure, and has independent protective benefits on coronary heart disease risk, which is elevated among those with diabetes. The benefits achieved by aerobic and resistance training seem apparent shortly after starting a structured exercise program. Activity needs to be regular; the frequency of exercise sessions is optimally at least three or more times per week to maintain metabolic benefits. This is due to the known acute bout effect of exercise on insulin resistance, which wanes between 24 and 96 hours after exercise, and is responsible for a portion of the long-term training benefits [102]. In general, both higher volumes and higher intensities of exercise result in greater metabolic improvements [43].

There are a few limitations in studies on physical activity in diabetes management, including trials in small selected samples. Similar to studies about the prevention of diabetes, some trials used interventions of combined physical activity, nutrition and medication [74, 103]. In order to isolate the independent effect of physical activity in diabetes management interventions, one needs to compare exercise alone versus other therapeutic modalities [97]. Current trials are underway examining the long-term efficacy of exercise and dietary

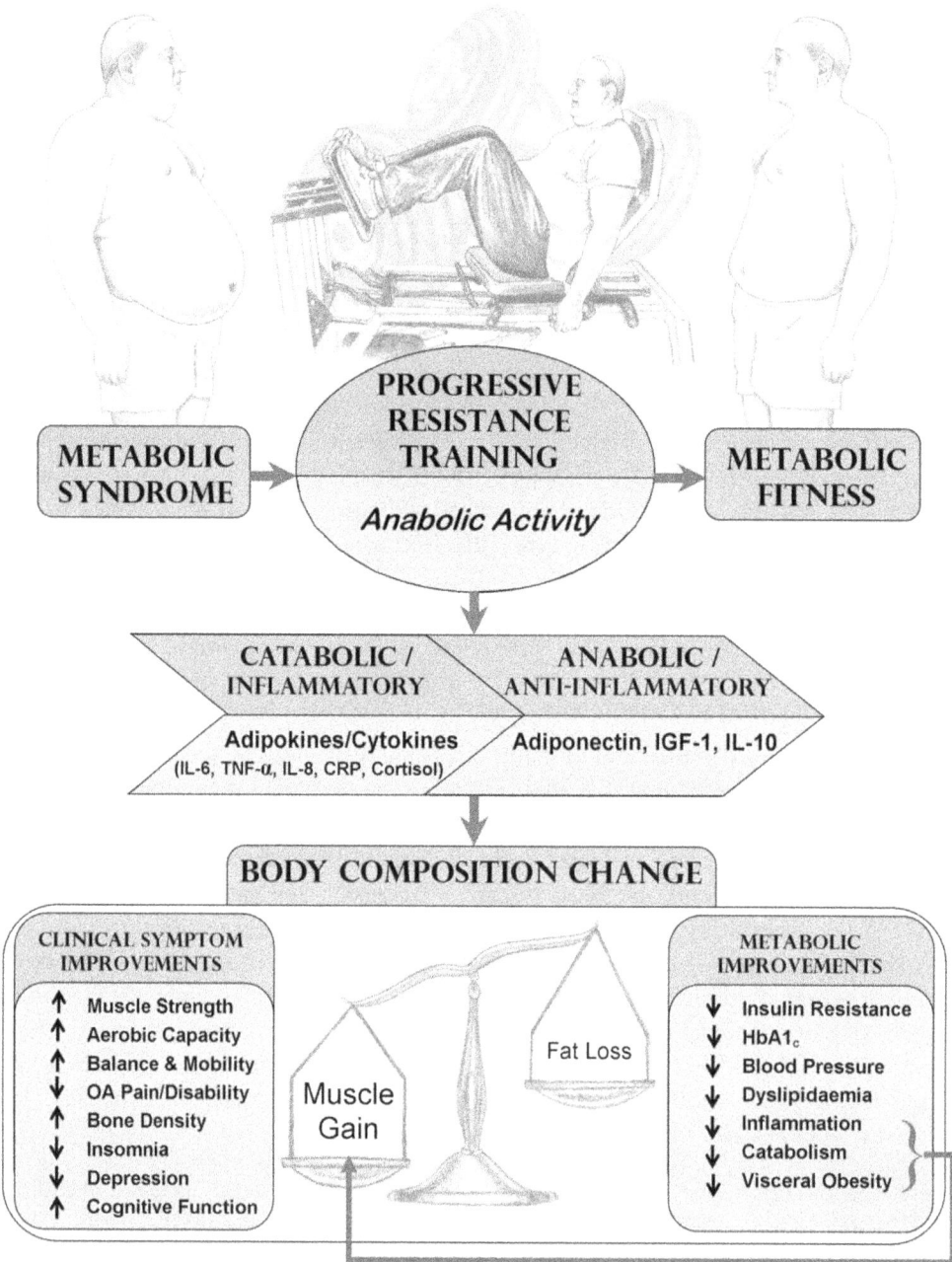

Figure 2. Schematic representation of PRT and its role in metabolic fitness.
Legend: OA osteoarthritis; HbA1c glycosylated haemoglobin.

In summary, because of its manifold benefits, physical activity has been described as an important 'medicine' for the treatment of type 2 diabetes [108]. Moreover, the non-pharmacological nature of physical activity and the low cost of exercise programs also makes this intervention appealing [97]. Nevertheless, physical activity is still underutilised in clinical settings to manage diabetes [60, 109–111].

Recommendations for diabetes management

Individually tailored and structured physical activity programs are important in the management of diabetes [110]. For instance, the patient's age, aerobic fitness, muscle strength, body composition, previous level of physical activity, timing and doses of insulin and oral hypoglycaemic agents, and comorbidities and diabetic complications should be considered in exercise prescriptions for individuals with type 2 diabetes [43, 58]. In particular, co-existent osteoarthritis, cardiovascular disease, orthostatic hypotension, peripheral vascular disease, and peripheral neuropathy, all common in type 2 diabetes, will influence the modality and intensity of exercise, the need for supervision, and other specific recommendations.

To improve glycaemic control, support weight maintenance, and reduce the risk of cardiovascular disease, the American Diabetes Association (ADA) and the Amercian College of Sports Medicine (ACSM) recommends individuals with type 2 diabetes to engage in at least 150 minutes per week of moderate-intensity physical activity (40%–60% of VO_2max, which equates to 50%–70% of the maximum heart rate) or at least 60 minutes per week of vigorous aerobic exercise (>60% of VO_2max or >70% of maximum heart rate) [43, 112]. Engaging in moderate to vigorous aerobic and/or resistance training yields greater benefits in the reduction of cardiovascular risk than lower volumes of physical activity [43], and an increased volume of activity is required for weight loss [43, 51]. Depending on the duration and intensity of physical activity the increased insulin sensitivity lasts for 24 to 72 hours after an activity session [113]. This underlines the importance of regular physical activity and therefore it is recommended that individuals with type 2 diabetes should not have more than two consecutive days without physical activity [43, 112].

Physical activity recommendations for adults with type 2 diabetes traditionally focused on aerobic activities, such as walking [114]. However, recent evidence has highlighted the effects of resistance training in addition to aerobic activities. Based on the substantial evidence that highlights the benefits of resistance and aerobic training, a combination of both exercise modalities appears optimal [76]. This is also stated in the recommendations for the general population of the American College of Sports Medicine, the American Diabetes Association, the American Heart Association, and the US Department of Health and Human Services that highlight the importance of incorporating resistance training into physical activity, especially for older adults [1, 3, 7, 112].

Pre-exercise screening should be considered for patients with type 2 diabetes. Screening should consider retinal disease, osteoarthritis, orthostatic hypotension, occult cardiovascular disease, peripheral vascular disease, peripheral neuropathy and diabetic foot disease, depression, cognitive impairment and gait and balance disorders to reduce potential risks and guide the specific exercise recommendations relevant to each individual.

There have been some concerns among medical practitioners about health risks associated with high-intensity resistance training for older adults. Particularly, these concerns are about acute elevation of blood pressure and an increase in risk of stroke, myocardial infarction, and retinal haemorrhage. However, there is no evidence that resistance training actually increases the risk of such events [43]. In fact, chronic resistance training is associated with lower blood pressure [77, 115] and lower risk of cardiovascular events and mortality [116].

Physical activity and diabetes complications

People with diabetes have at least twice the risk of incident and fatal cardiovascular events compared to the general population [117–119]. Furthermore, people with diabetes with low cardio-respiratory fitness have a higher risk of overall mortality than those with higher fitness levels [120]. Physical activity improves fitness and reduces the risk of cardiovascular disease substantially, which makes an active lifestyle particularly important for people with diabetes [74].

Additionally, diabetes is associated with other medical comorbidity, including retinopathy, peripheral neuropathy, orthostatic hypotension, mobility impairment, osteoarthritis, peripheral vascular disease and renal disease. These can limit exercise capacity among patients with diabetes. Therefore, it is of particular importance for people with diabetes in the early stages to commence regular exercise [121]. Specific exercise regimens may be required in the presence of diabetic complications. For instance, patients with peripheral neuropathy may benefit from non-weight-bearing activities, such as resistance training, swimming or cycling [43]. Among patients with autonomic neuropathy or receiving beta-blockers, perceived exertion rather than the heart rate should be used to adjust the intensity of physical activity [109], and pre-exercise cardiac testing should be carried out before embarking on vigorous activity regimens in anyone with elevated cardiovascular risk, which includes most people with type 2 diabetes [88].

There are no known adverse effects of either resistance or aerobic training on vision or the progression of diabetic retinopathy. However, for patients with proliferative or severe non-proliferative retinopathy, moderate physical activity is recommended as vigorous exercise could potentially trigger vitreous haemorrhage or retinal detachment [43].

Blood glucose monitoring may be important before, during and after prolonged exercise. Acute bouts of exercise may require adjustment of medications on exercise days to prevent hypoglycaemia, the latter which may otherwise occur during exercise or many hours afterwards including nocturnally. Exercise may be timed for the post prandial peak in blood glucose; this will reduce the risk of exercise-related hypoglycaemia as well as reduce post-prandial hyperglycaemia and hyperinsulinemia [43, 122].

Challenges in implementation

There is substantial evidence for the health benefits of physical activity and exercise in the management of type 2 diabetes. However, as reported in studies from the US [123], Canada [59, 124] and Australia [110] the proportion of people with type 2 diabetes meeting the minimal physical activity recommendations is significantly lower than in the age-matched general population. An Australian population study reported significant gaps in physical activity recommendations and uptake as part of widespread diabetes management [110].

The principles of behaviour change are needed to encourage physical activity in the treatment of diabetes [59, 91, 111, 125]. Factors that facilitate or impede aerobic or resistance training need to be identified and addressed in clinical counselling. For example, older adults with diabetic complications may have difficulties engaging in more vigorous aerobic activities, and resistance training might be a better option. A frequent barrier is program costs, or the cost of resistance training equipment, and the daunting prospects of activity among sedentary individuals [76]. Since it is difficult to provide ongoing one-on-one supervision in resistance or aerobic training, understanding the maintenance of skills is required in the transition from supervised to independent training. Some resistance training interventions show long-term effects on muscle strength and body composition, but not on glycaemic control [114, 126].

Conclusion

Physical activity and exercise are effective in both prevention and treatment of diabetes, metabolic syndrome and cardiovascular disease. Both aerobic and resistance training have important roles in diabetes prevention and treatment, and the choice depends upon patient preferences, the need for supervision and the availability of exercise facilities. Higher doses and intensities of exercise are generally more effective, although there is benefit in starting at low to moderate levels of exercise intensity and volume, in order to reduce high drop-out rates and prevent overuse injuries [75]. For some patients, exercise regimens should commence with moderate-intensity physical activities such as brisk walking [127, 128]. High volumes of exercise and incidental physical activity are required for weight loss, but activity can produce losses of the metabolically critical visceral fat compartment without overall change in body weight, and this can be of substantial benefit. On account of the acute bout effects, exercise frequency should be at least three days per week or more.

In summary, exercise is as potent as oral hypoglycaemic agents for glucose homeostasis, does not cause weight gain like insulin and oral agents, and provides additional benefits for fitness, functional independence, body composition, and vascular comorbidities which cannot be gained with pharmacologic or nutritional treatment alone. Thus, it should be seen as core to the prevention and treatment of type 2 diabetes, rather than an optional additional management strategy.

References

1. US Department of Health and Human Services (2008). *2008 physical activity guidelines for Americans.* Washington, DC: US Department of Health and Human Services.

2. US Department of Health and Human Services (1996). *Physical activity and health: a report of the surgeon general.* Atlanta: Centers for Disease Control and Prevention.

3. Haskell WL, Lee IM, Pate RR, Powell KE, Blair SN, Franklin BA, Macera CA, Heath GW, Thompson PD & Bauman A (2007). Physical activity and public health: updated recommendation for adults from the American College of Sports Medicine and the American Heart Association. *Medicine and Science in Sports and Exercise*, 39(8): 1423–34.

4. Caspersen CJ, Powell KE & Christenson GM (1985). Physical activity, exercise, and physical fitness: definitions and distinctions for health-related research. *Public Health Reports*, 100(2): 126–31.

5. Thompson PD, Buchner D, Pina IL, Balady GJ, Williams MA, Marcus BH, Berra K, Blair S, Costa F, Franklin B, Fletcher G, Gordon N, Pate R, Rodriguez B, Yancy A & Wenger N (2003). Exercise and physical activity in the prevention and treatment of atherosclerotic cardiovascular disease: a statement from the Council on Clinical Cardiology (Subcommittee on Exercise, Rehabilitation, and Prevention) and the Council on Nutrition, Physical Activity, and Metabolism (Subcommittee on Physical Activity). *Circulation*, 107(24): 3109–16.

6. Hassinen M, Lakka TA, Hakola L, Savonen K, Komulainen P, Litmanen H, Kiviniemi V, Kouki R, Heikkilä H & Rauramaa R (2010). Cardiorespiratory fitness and metabolic syndrome in older men and women: the dose responses to exercise training (DR's EXTRA) study. *Diabetes Care*, 33(7): 1655–57.

7. Nelson ME, Rejeski WJ, Blair SN, Duncan PW, Judge JO, King AC, Macera CA & Casteneda-Sceppa C (2007). Physical activity and public health in older adults: recommendation from the American College of Sports Medicine and the American Heart Association. *Medicine and Science in Sports and Exercise*, 39(8): 1435–45.

8. Bauman A, Bull F, Chey T, Craig CL, Ainsworth BE, Sallis JF, Bowles HR, Hagströmer M, Sjöström M, Pratt M & The IPS Group (2009). The international prevalence study on physical activity: results from 20 countries. *International Journal of Behavioral Nutrition and Physical Activity*, 6(1): 21.

9. Sjöström M, Oja P, Hagströmer M, Smith B & Bauman AE (2006). Health-enhancing physical activity across European Union countries: the Eurobarometer study. *Journal of Public Health*, 14(5): 291–300.

10. Stamatakis E, Ekelund U & Wareham NJ (2007). Temporal trends in physical activity in England: the health survey for England 1991 to 2004. *Preventive Medicine*, 45(6): 416–23.

11. Troiano RP, Berrigan D, Dodd KW, Masse LC, Tilert T & McDowell M (2008). Physical activity in the United States measured by accelerometer. *Medicine and Science in Sports and Exercise*, 40(1): 181–88.

12. Asia-Pacific Physical Activity Network (2008). *Regional physical activity prevalence in the Asia-Pacific region*. Sydney: Asia-Pacific Physical Activity Network.

13. Chau J, Smith BJ, Bauman A, Merom D, Eyeson-Annan M, Chey T & Farrell L (2008). Recent trends in physical activity in New South Wales: is the tide of inactivity turning? *Australian and New Zealand Journal of Public Health*, 32(1): 82–5.

14. Zimmet P (2000). Globalization, coca-colonization and the chronic disease epidemic: can the doomsday scenario be averted? *Journal of Internal Medicine*, 247(3): 301–10.

15. LaMonte MJ, Blair SN & Church TS (2005). Physical activity and diabetes prevention. *Journal of Applied Physiology*, 99(3): 1205–13.

16. Hu G, Lakka TA & Tuomilehto J (2009). Physical activity, fitness, and the prevention of type 2

diabetes. In IM Lee, S Blair, J Manson & RS Paffenbarger Jr (Eds). *Epidemiologic methods in physical activity studies* (pp 201–24). New York: Oxford University Press.

17. Chandran M, Phillips SA, Ciaraldi T & Henry RR (2003). Adiponectin: more than just another fat cell hormone? *Diabetes Care*, 26(8): 2442–50.

18. Pittas AG, Joseph NA & Greenberg AS (2004). Adipocytokines and insulin resistance. *Journal of Clinical Endocrinology and Metabolism*, 89(2): 447–52.

19. Simpson KA & Singh MA (2008). Effects of exercise on adiponectin: a systematic review. *Obesity*, 16(2): 241–56.

20. Weinstein AR, Sesso HD, Min Lee I, Cook NR, Manson JE, Buring JE & Gaziano JM (2004). Relationship of physical activity vs body mass index with type 2 diabetes in women. *Journal of the American Medical Association*, 292(10): 1188–94.

21. James SA, Jamjoum L, Raghunathan TE, Strogatz DS, Furth ED & Khazanie PG (1998). Physical activity and NIDDM in African-Americans: the Pitt County study. *Diabetes Care*, 21(4): 555–62.

22. Hu FB, Sigal RJ, Rich-Edwards JW, Colditz GA, Solomon CG, Willett WC, Speizer FE & Manson JE (1999). Walking compared with vigorous physical activity and risk of type 2 diabetes in women: a prospective study. *Journal of the American Medical Association*, 282(15): 1433–39.

23. Orchard TJ, Temprosa M, Goldberg R, Haffner S, Ratner R, Marcovina S, Fowler S & The Diabetes Prevention Program Research Group (2005). The effect of metformin and intensive lifestyle intervention on the metabolic syndrome: the Diabetes Prevention Program randomized trial. *Annals of Internal Medicine*, 142(8): 611–19.

24. Dempsey JC, Butler CL & Williams MA (2005). No need for a pregnant pause: physical activity may reduce the occurrence of gestational diabetes mellitus and preeclampsia. *Exercises and Sport Science Reviews*, 33(3): 141–49.

25. Hegaard HK, Pedersen BK, Nielsen BB & Damm P (2007). Leisure time physical activity during pregnancy and impact on gestational diabetes mellitus, pre-eclampsia, preterm delivery and birth weight: a review. *Acta Obstetricia et Gynecologica*, 86(11): 1290–96.

26. Jeon CY, Lokken RP, Hu FB & van Dam RM (2007). Physical activity of moderate intensity and risk of type 2 diabetes. *Diabetes Care*, 30(3): 744–52.

27. Healy GN, Dunstan DW, Salmon J, Cerin E, Shaw JE, Zimmet PZ & Owen N (2007). Objectively measured light-intensity physical activity is independently associated with 2-h plasma glucose. *Diabetes Care*, 30(6): 1384–89.

28. Hamilton MT, Healy GN, Dunstan DW, Zderic TW & Owen N (2008). Too little exercise and too much sitting: inactivity physiology and the need for new recommendations on sedentary behavior. *Current Cardiovascular Risk Reports*, 2(4): 292–98.

29. Owen N, Bauman A & Brown W (2009). Too much sitting: a novel and important predictor of chronic disease risk? *British Journal of Sports Medicine*, 43(2): 81–83.

30. Healy GN, Dunstan DW, Salmon J, Cerin E, Shaw JE, Zimmet PZ & Owen N (2008). Breaks in sedentary time: beneficial associations with metabolic risk. *Diabetes Care*, 31(4): 661–66.

31. Hu FB, Leitzmann MF, Stampfer MJ, Colditz GA, Willett WC & Rimm EB (2001). Physical activity and television watching in relation to risk for type 2 diabetes mellitus in men. *Archives of Internal Medicine*, 161(12): 1542–48.

32. Hu FB, Li TY, Colditz GA, Willett WC & Manson JE (2003). Television watching and other sedentary behaviors in relation to risk of obesity and type 2 diabetes mellitus in women. *Journal of the American Medical Association*, 289(14): 1785–91.

33. Pan XR, Li GW, Hu YH, Wang JX, Yang WY, An ZX, Hu ZX, Lin J, Xiao JZ, Cao HB, Liu PA, Jiang XG, Jiang YY, Wang JP, Zheng H, Zhang H, Bennett PH & Howard BV (1997). Effects of diet and exercise in preventing NIDDM in people with impaired glucose tolerance: the Da Qing IGT and Diabetes Study. *Diabetes Care*, 20(4): 537–44.

34. Li G, Zhang P, Wang J, Gregg EW, Yang W, Gong Q, Li H, Jiang Y, An Y, Shuai Y, Zhang B, Zhang J, Thompson TJ, Gerzoff RB, Roqlic G, Hu Y & Bennett PH (2008). The long-term effect of lifestyle interventions to prevent diabetes in the China Da Qing Diabetes Prevention Study: a 20-year follow-up study. *The Lancet*, 371(9626): 1783–89.

35. Diabetes Prevention Program Research Group (2002). Reduction in the incidence of type 2 diabetes with lifestyle intervention or metformin. *New England Journal of Medicine*, 346(6): 393–403.

36. Diabetes Prevention Program Research Group (2009). 10-year follow-up of diabetes incidence and weight loss in the Diabetes Prevention Program Outcomes Study. *Lancet*, 374(9702): 1677–86.

37. Tuomilehto J, Lindström J, Eriksson JG, Valle TT, Hämäläinen H, Ilanne-Parikka P, Keinänen-Kiukaanniemi S, Laakso M, Louheranta A, Rastas M, Salminen V, Aunola S, Cepaitis Z, Moltchanov V, Hakumäki M, Mannelin M, Martikkala V, Sundvall J & Uusitupa M (2001). Prevention of type 2 diabetes mellitus by changes in lifestyle among subjects with impaired glucose tolerance. *New England Journal of Medicine*, 344(18): 1343–50.

38. Lindström J, Ilanne-Parikka P, Peltonen M, Aunola S, Eriksson JG, Hemiö K, Hämäläinen H, Härkönen P, Keinänen-Kiukaanniemi S, Laakso M, Louheranta A, Mannelin M, Paturi M, Sundvall J, Valle TT, Uusitupa M & Tuomilehto J (2006). Sustained reduction in the incidence of type 2 diabetes by lifestyle intervention: follow-up of the Finnish Diabetes Prevention Study. *Lancet*, 368(9548): 1673–79.

39. Ramachandran A, Snehalatha C, Mary S, Mukesh B, Bhaskar AD & Vijay V (2006). The Indian Diabetes Prevention Programme shows that lifestyle modification and metformin prevent type 2 diabetes in Asian Indian subjects with impaired glucose tolerance (IDPP-1). *Diabetologia*, 49(2): 289–97.

40. Eriksson KF & Lindgarde F (1991). Prevention of type 2 (non-insulin-dependent) diabetes mellitus by diet and physical exercise: the 6-year Malmo feasibility study. *Diabetologia*, 34(12): 891–98.

41. Lindahl B, Nilssön TK, Borch-Johnsen K, Røder ME, Söderberg S, Widman L, Johnson O, Hallmans G & Jansson JH (2009). A randomized lifestyle intervention with 5-year follow-up in subjects with impaired glucose tolerance: pronounced short-term impact but long-term adherence problems. *Scandinavian Journal of Public Health*, 37(4): 434–42.

42. Kosaka K, Noda M & Kuzuya T (2005). Prevention of type 2 diabetes by lifestyle intervention: a Japanese trial in IGT males. *Diabetes Research and Clinical Practice*, 67(2): 152–62.

43. Sigal RJ, Kenny GP, Wasserman DH, Castaneda-Sceppa C & White RD (2006). Physical activity/exercise and type 2 diabetes: a consensus statement from the American Diabetes Association. *Diabetes Care*, 29(6): 1433–38.

44. Orozco LJ, Buchleitner AM, Gimenez-Perez G, Figuls MRI, Richter B & Mauricio D (2008). Exercise or exercise and diet for preventing type 2 diabetes mellitus. *Cochrane Database of Systematic Reviews*, 3: CD003054.

45. Yates T, Khunti K, Bull F, Gorely T & Davies MJ (2007). The role of physical activity in the management of impaired glucose tolerance: a systematic review. *Diabetologia*, 50(6): 1116–26.

46. Montoye HJ, Kemper HCG, Saris WHM & Washburn RA (1996). *Measuring physical activity and energy expenditure*. Champaign: Human Kinetics.

47. Carnethon MR, Gidding SS, Nehgme R, Sidney S, Jacobs DR, Jr & Liu K (2003). Cardiorespiratory fitness in young adulthood and the development of cardiovascular disease risk factors. *Journal of the American Medical Association*, 290(23): 3092–100.

48. Sawada SS, Min Lee I, Naito H, Noguchi J, Tsukamoto K, Muto T, Higaki Y, Tanaka H & Blair SN (2010). Long-term trends in cardiorespiratory fitness and the incidence of type 2 diabetes. *Diabetes Care*, 33(6): 1353–57.

49. Sieverdes JC, Sui X, Lee DC, Church TS, McClain A, Hand GA & Blair SN (2010). Physical activity, cardiorespiratory fitness and the incidence of type 2 diabetes in a prospective study of men. *British Journal of Sports Medicine*, 44(4): 238–44.

50. Kesaniemi YK, Danforth E, Jr, Jensen MD, Kopelman PG, Lefebvre P & Reeder BA (2001). Dose-response issues concerning physical activity and health: an evidence-based symposium. *Medicine and Science in Sports and Exercise*, 33(Suppl. 6): S351–58.

51. Jakicic JM, Otto AD, Polzien K & Davis K (2009). Physical activity and weight control. In I Min Lee, S Blair, J Manson & RS Paffenbarger Jr, (Eds). *Epidemiologic methods in physical activity research* (pp225–45). New York: Oxford University Press.

52. Hill JO & Wyatt HR (2005). Role of physical activity in preventing and treating obesity. *Journal of Applied Physiology*, 99(2): 765–70.

53. Jakicic JM, Clark K, Coleman E, Donnelly JE, Foreyt J, Melanson E, Volek J & Volpe SL (2001). American College of Sports Medicine position stand: appropriate intervention strategies for weight loss and prevention of weight regain for adults. *Medicine and Science in Sports and Exercise*, 33(12): 2145–56.

54. van der Ploeg HP, Smith BJ, Stubbs T, Vita P, Holford R & Bauman AE (2007). Physical activity promotion: are GPs getting the message? *Australian Family Physician*, 36(10): 871–74.

55. Duncan GE, Anton SD, Sydeman SJ, Newton RL Jr, Corsica JA, Durning PE, Ketterson TU, Martin AD, Limacher MC & Perri MG (2005). Prescribing exercise at varied levels of intensity and frequency: a randomized trial. *Archives of Internal Medicine*, 165(20): 2362–69.

56. Bauman A, Murphy N & Lane A (2009). The role of community programmes and mass events in promoting physical activity to patients. *British Journal of Sports Medicine*, 43(1): 44–46.

57. Rosenberg DE, Jabbour SA & Goldstein BJ (2005). Insulin resistance, diabetes and cardiovascular risk: approaches to treatment. *Diabetes Obesity & Metabolism*, 7(6): 642–53.

58. Praet SFE & van Loon LJC (2007). Optimizing the therapeutic benefits of exercise in type 2 diabetes. *Journal of Applied Physiology*, 103(4): 1113–20.

59. Boudreau F & Godin G (2009). Understanding physical activity intentions among French Canadians with type 2 diabetes: an extension of Ajzen's theory of planned behaviour. *International Journal of Behavioral Nutrition and Physical Activity*, 6(110): 35.

60. Kirk A, Barnett J, Leese G & Mutrie N (2009). A randomized trial investigating the 12-month changes in physical activity and health outcomes following a physical activity consultation delivered by a person or in written form in type 2 diabetes: Time2Act. *Diabetic Medicine*, 26(3): 293–301.

61. Plotnikoff RC, Karunamuni ND, Johnson JA, Kotovych M & Svenson LW (2008). Health-related behaviours in adults with diabetes: associations with healthcare utilization and costs. *Canadian Journal of Public Health*, 99(3): 227–31.

62. Boule NG, Kenny GP, Haddad E, Wells GA & Sigal RJ (2003). Meta-analysis of the effect of structured exercise training on cardiorespiratory fitness in type 2 diabetes mellitus. *Diabetologia*, 46(8): 1071–81.

63. Tresierras MA & Balady GJ (2009). Resistance training in the treatment of diabetes and obesity: mechanisms and outcomes. *Journal of Cardiopulmonary Rehabilitation & Prevention*, 29(2): 67–75.

64. Sigal RJ, Kenny GP, Boule NG, Wells GA, Prud'homme D, Fortier M, Reid RD, Tulloch H, Coyle D, Phillips P, Jennings A & Jaffey J (2007). Effects of aerobic training, resistance training, or both on glycemic control in type 2 diabetes: a randomized trial. *Annals of Internal Medicine*, 147(6): 357–69.

65. Marcus RL, Smith S, Morrell G, Addison O, Dibble LE, Wahoff-Stice D & LaStayo PC (2008). Comparison of combined aerobic and high-force eccentric resistance exercise with aerobic exercise only for people with type 2 diabetes mellitus. *Physical Therapy*, 88(11): 1345–54.

66. Wang Y, Simar D & Fiatarone Singh MA (2009). Adaptations to exercise training within skeletal muscle in adults with type 2 diabetes or impaired glucose tolerance: a systematic review. *Diabetes Metabolism Research and Reviews*, 25(1): 13–40.

67. Yang H, Youm YH, Vandanmagsar B, Ravussin A, Gimble JM, Greenway F, Stephens JM, Mynatt RL & Dixit VD (2010). Obesity increases the production of proinflammatory mediators from adipose tissue T cells and compromises TCR repertoire diversity: implications for systemic inflammation and insulin resistance. *Journal of Immunology*, 185(3): 1836–45.

68. Olefsky JM & Glass CK (2010). Macrophages, inflammation, and insulin resistance. *Annual Review of Physiology*, 72: 219–46.

69. Mourier A, Gautier JF, De Kerviler E, Bigard AX, Villette JM, Garnier JP, Duvallet A, Guezennec CY & Cathelineau G (1997). Mobilization of visceral adipose tissue related to the improvement in insulin sensitivity in response to physical training in NIDDM. Effects of branched-chain amino acid supplements. *Diabetes Care*, 20(3): 385–91.

70. Kirwan JP, Solomon TP, Wojta DM, Staten MA & Holloszy JO (2009). Effects of 7 days of exercise training on insulin sensitivity and responsiveness in type 2 diabetes mellitus. *American Journal of Physiology, Endocrinology and Metabolism*, 297(1): E151–56.

71. Yokoyama H, Emoto M, Fujiwara S, Motoyama K, Morioka T, Koyama H, Shoji T, Inaba M & Nishizawa Y (2004). Short-term aerobic exercise improves arterial stiffness in type 2 diabetes. *Diabetes Research & Clinical Practice*, 65(2): 85–93.

72. Sykes K, Yeung TLV & Ko GTC (2004). A 12-week prospective randomized controlled trial to investigate the effects of aerobic training on type 2 diabetes patients. *American Journal of Recreation Therapy*, 3(3): 36–42.

73. Ribeiro IC, Iborra RT, Neves MQ, Lottenberg SA, Charf AM, Nunes VS, Negrão CE, Nakandakare ER, Quintão EC & Passarelli M (2008). HDL atheroprotection by aerobic exercise training in type 2 diabetes mellitus. *Medicine and Science in Sports and Exercise*, 40(5): 779–86.

74. Jakicic JM, Jaramillo SA, Balasubramanyam A, Bancroft B, Curtis JM, Mathews A, Pereira M, Regensteiner JG & Ribisl PM (2009). Effect of a lifestyle intervention on change in cardiorespiratory fitness in adults with type 2 diabetes: results from the Look AHEAD Study. *International Journal of Obesity*, 33(3): 305–16.

75. Praet SF, van Rooij ES, Wijtvliet A, Boonman-de Winter LJ, Enneking T, Kuipers H, Stehouwer CD & van Loon LJ (2008). Brisk walking compared with an individualised medical fitness programme for patients with type 2 diabetes: a randomised controlled trial. *Diabetologia*, 51(5): 736–46.

76. Eves ND & Plotnikoff RC (2006). Resistance training and type 2 diabetes: considerations for implementation at the population level. *Diabetes Care*, 29(8): 1933–41.

77. Strasser B, Siebert U & Schobersberger W (2010). Resistance training in the treatment of the metabolic syndrome: a systematic review and meta-analysis of the effect of resistance training on metabolic clustering in patients with abnormal glucose metabolism. *Sports Medicine*, 40(5): 397–415.

78. Holten MK, Zacho M, Gaster M, Juel C, Wojtaszewski JF & Dela F (2004). Strength training increases insulin-mediated glucose uptake, GLUT4 content, and insulin signaling in skeletal muscle in patients with type 2 diabetes. *Diabetes*, 53(2): 294–305.

79. Ishii T, Yamakita T, Sato T, Tanaka S & Fujii S (1998). Resistance training improves insulin sensitivity in NIDDM subjects without altering maximal oxygen uptake. *Diabetes Care*, 21(8): 1353–55.

80. Misra A, Alappan NK, Vikram NK, Goel K, Gupta N, Mittal K & Bhatt SL (2008). Effect of supervised progressive resistance-exercise training protocol on insulin sensitivity, glycemia, lipids, and body composition in Asian Indians with type 2 diabetes. *Diabetes Care*, 31(7): 1282–87.

81. Dunstan DW, Daly RM, Owen N, Jolley D, De Courten M, Shaw J & Zimmett P (2002). High-intensity resistance training improves glycemic control in older patients with type 2 diabetes. *Diabetes Care*, 25(10): 1729–36.

82. Castaneda C, Layne JE, Munoz-Orians L, Gordon PL, Walsmith J, Foldvari M, Roubenoff R, Tucker KL & Nelson ME (2002). A randomized controlled trial of resistance exercise training to improve glycemic control in older adults with type 2 diabetes. *Diabetes Care*, 25(12): 2335–41.

83. Eriksson J, Taimela S, Eriksson K, Parviainen S, Peltonen J & Kujala U (1997). Resistance training in the treatment of non-insulin-dependent diabetes mellitus. *International Journal of Sports Medicine*, 18(4): 242–46.

84. Honkola A, Forsen T & Eriksson J (1997). Resistance training improves the metabolic profile in individuals with type 2 diabetes. *Acta Diabetologica*, 34(4): 245–48.

85. Dunstan DW, Puddey IB, Beilin LJ, Burke V, Morton AR & Stanton KG (1998). Effects of a short-term circuit weight training program on glycaemic control in NIDDM. *Diabetes Research and Clinical Practice*, 40(1): 53–61.

86. Maiorana A, O'Driscoll G, Goodman C, Taylor R & Green D (2002). Combined aerobic and resistance exercise improves glycemic control and fitness in type 2 diabetes. *Diabetes Research and Clinical Practice*, 56(2): 115–23.

87. Cuff DJ, Meneilly GS, Martin A, Ignaszewski A, Tildesley HD & Frohlich JJ (2003). Effective exercise modality to reduce insulin resistance in women with type 2 diabetes. *Diabetes Care*, 26(11): 2977–82.

88. Kavookjian J, Elswick BM & Whetsel T (2007). Interventions for being active among individuals with diabetes: a systematic review of the literature. *The Diabetes Educator*, 33(6): 962–88.

89. Singh NA, Stavrinos TM, Scarbek Y, Galambos G, Liber C & Fiatarone Singh MA (2005). A randomized controlled trial of high versus low intensity weight training versus general practitioner care for clinical depression in older adults. *The Journals of Gerontology. Series A, Biological Sciences and Medical Sciences*, 60(6): 768–76.

90. Perrig-Chiello P, Perrig WJ, Ehrsam R, Staehelin HB & Krings F (1998). The effects of resistance training on wellbeing and memory in elderly volunteers. *Age and Ageing*, 27(4): 469–75.

91. Plotnikoff RC (2006). Physical activity in the management of diabetes: population-based perspectives and strategies. *Canadian Journal of Diabetes*, 30(1): 52–62.

92. Ivy JL (1997). Role of exercise training in the prevention and treatment of insulin resistance and non-insulin-dependent diabetes mellitus. *Sports Medicine*, 24(5): 321–36.

93. Balducci S, Leonetti F, Di Mario U & Fallucca F (2004). Is a long-term aerobic plus resistance training program feasible for and effective on metabolic profiles in type 2 diabetic patients? *Diabetes Care*, 27(3): 841–42.

94. Snowling NJ & Hopkins WG (2006). Effects of different modes of exercise training on glucose control and risk factors for complications in type 2 diabetic patients: a meta-analysis. *Diabetes Care*, 29(11): 2518–27.

95. Fiatarone Singh M (2002). Exercise comes of age: rationale and recommendations for a geriatric exercise prescription. *The Journals of Gerontology. Series A, Biological Sciences and Medical Sciences*, 57(5): M262–M82.

96. Daly RM, Dunstan DW, Owen N, Jolley D, Shaw JE & Zimmet PZ (2005). Does high-intensity resistance training maintain bone mass during moderate weight loss in older overweight adults with type 2 diabetes? *Osteoporosis International*, 16(12): 1703–12.

97. Thomas DR, Elliott EJ & Naughton GA (2006). Exercise for type 2 diabetes mellitus. *Cochrane Database of Systematic Reviews*, 3: CD002968.

98. Boule NG, Haddad E, Kenny GP, Wells GA & Sigal RJ (2001). Effects of exercise on glycemic control and body mass in type 2 diabetes mellitus: a meta-analysis of controlled clinical trials. *Journal of the American Medical Association*, 286(10): 1218–27.

99. Khaw KT, Wareham N, Luben R, Bingham S, Oakes S, Welch A & Day N (2001). Glycated haemoglobin, diabetes, and mortality in men in Norfolk cohort of European Prospective Investigation of Cancer and Nutrition (EPIC-Norfolk). *British Medical Journal*, 322(7277): 15–18.

100. Baldi JC, Snowling N (2003). Resistance training improves glycaemic control in obese type 2 diabetic men. *International Journal of Sports Medicine*, 24(6): 419–23.

101. Lee SH, Park SA, Ko SH, Yim HW, Ahn YB, Yoon KH, Cha BY & Kwon HS (2010). Insulin resistance and inflammation may have an additional role in the link between cystatin C and cardiovascular disease in type 2 diabetes mellitus patients. *Metabolism*, 59(2): 241–46.

102. Wojtaszewski JF & Richter EA (2006). Effects of acute exercise and training on insulin action and sensitivity: focus on molecular mechanisms in muscle. *Essays in Biochemistry*, 42: 31–46.

103. Krook A, Holm I, Pettersson S & Wallberg-Henriksson H (2003). Reduction of risk factors following lifestyle modification programme in subjects with type 2 (non-insulin dependent) diabetes mellitus. *Clinical Physiology and Functional Imaging*, 23(1): 21–30.

104. Rubin RR, Gaussoin SA, Peyrot M, DiLillo V, Miller K, Wadden TA, West DS, Wing RR & Knowler WC (2010). Cardiovascular disease risk factors, depression symptoms and antidepressant medicine use in the Look AHEAD (Action for Health in Diabetes) clinical trial of weight loss in diabetes. *Diabetologia*, 53(8): 1581–89.

105. Wing RR, Rosen RC, Fava JL, Bahnson J, Brancati F, Gendrano IN, Kitabchi A, Schneider SH & Wadden TA (2010). Effects of weight loss intervention on erectile function in older men with type 2 diabetes in the Look AHEAD trial. *Journal of Sexual Medicine*, 7(1 Pt 1): 156–65.

106. Curtis JM, Horton ES, Bahnson J, Gregg EW, Jakicic JM, Regensteiner JG, Ribisl PM, Soberman JE, Stewart KJ & Espeland MA (2010). Prevalence and predictors of abnormal cardiovascular responses to exercise testing among individuals with type 2 diabetes: the Look AHEAD (Action for Health in Diabetes) study. *Diabetes Care*, 33(4): 901–07.

107. Albu JB, Heilbronn LK, Kelley DE, Smith SR, Azuma K, Berk ES, Pi-Sunyer FX, Ravussin E & Look AHEAD Adipose Research Group (2010). Metabolic changes following a 1-year diet and exercise intervention in patients with type 2 diabetes. *Diabetes*, 59(3): 627–33.

108. Tucker PS, Fisher-Wellman K & Bloomer RJ (2008). Can exercise minimize postprandial oxidative stress in patients with type 2 diabetes? *Current Diabetes Review*, 4(4): 309–19.

109. Albright A, Franz M, Hornsby G, Kriska A, Marrero D, Ullrich I & Verity LS (2000). American College of Sports Medicine position stand: exercise and type 2 diabetes. *Medicine and Science in Sports and Exercise*, 32(7): 1345–60.

110. Neville L & Bauman A (2004). Self-reported risk factors and management strategies used by people with diabetes mellitus identified from the 1997 and 1998 NSW Health Surveys. *NSW Public Health Bulletin*, 15(4): 57–62.

111. Kirk AF, Barnett J & Mutrie N (2007). Physical activity consultation for people with type 2 diabetes. Evidence and guidelines. *Diabetic Medicine*, 24(8): 809–16.

112. American College of Sports Medicine and American Diabetes Association (2010). Exercise and

type 2 diabetes. American College of Sports Medicine and the American Diabetes Association: joint position statement. *Medicine and Science in Sports and Exercise*, 42(12): 2282–303.

113. Wallberg-Henriksson H, Rincon J & Zierath JR (1998). Exercise in the management of non-insulin-dependent diabetes mellitus. *Sports Medicine*, 25(1): 25–35.

114. Dunstan DW, Daly RM, Owen N, Jolley D, Vulikh E, Shaw J & Zimmet P (2005). Home-based resistance training is not sufficient to maintain improved glycemic control following supervised training in older individuals with type 2 diabetes. *Diabetes Care*, 28(1): 3–9.

115. Fagard RH & Cornelissen VA (2007). Effect of exercise on blood pressure control in hypertensive patients. *European Journal of Cardiovascular Prevention & Rehabilitation*, 14(1): 12–17.

116. Tanasescu M, Leitzmann MF, Rimm EB, Willett WC, Stampfer MJ & Hu FB (2002). Exercise type and intensity in relation to coronary heart disease in men. *Journal of the American Medical Association*, 288(16): 1994–2000.

117. Meltzer S, Leiter L, Daneman D, Gerstein HC, Lau D, Ludwig S, Yale JF, Zinman B, Lillie D & Steering and Expert Committees (1998). 1998 clinical practice guidelines for the management of diabetes in Canada. Canadian Diabetes Association. *Canadian Medical Association Journal*, 159(Suppl. 8): S1–29.

118. Skerrett PJ & Manson JE (2002). Reduction in risk of coronary heart disease and diabetes. In N Ruderman, JT Devlin, SH Schneider & A Kriska (Eds). *Handbook of exercise in diabetes* (pp 155–81). Alexandria, VA: American Diabetes Association.

119. Buse JB, Ginsberg HN, Bakris GL, Clark NG, Costa F, Eckel R, Fonseca V, Gerstein HC, Grundy S, Nesto RW, Pignone MP, Plutzky J, Porte D, Redberg R, Stitzel KF, Stone NJ, American Heart Association & American Diabetes Association (2007). Primary prevention of cardiovascular diseases in people with diabetes mellitus: a scientific statement from the American Heart Association and the American Diabetes Association. *Diabetes Care*, 30(1): 162–72.

120. Church TS, Cheng YJ, Earnest CP, Barlow CE, Gibbons LW, Priest EL & Blair SN (2004). Exercise capacity and body composition as predictors of mortality among men with diabetes. *Diabetes Care*, 27(1): 83–88.

121. Constantini N, Harman-Boehm I & Dubnov G (2005). Exercise prescription for diabetics: more than a general recommendation. *Harefuah*, 144(10): 717–23, 50.

122. Hayes C & Kriska A (2008). Role of physical activity in diabetes management and prevention. *Journal of the American Dietetic Association*, 108(4): S19–S23.

123. Nelson KM, Reiber G & Boyko EJ (2002). Diet and exercise among adults with type 2 diabetes: findings from the third national health and nutrition examination survey (NHANES III). *Diabetes Care*, 25(10): 1722–28.

124. Plotnikoff RC, Taylor LM, Wilson PM, Courneya KS, Sigal RJ, Birkett N, Raine K & Svenson LW (2006). Factors associated with physical activity in Canadian adults with diabetes. *Medicine and Science in Sports and Exercise*, 38(8): 1526–34.

125. Plotnikoff R, Lippke S, Courneya K, Birkett N & Sigal R (2008). Physical activity and social

cognitive theory: a test in a population sample of adults with type 1 or type 2 diabetes. *Applied Psychology: An International Review*, 57(4): 628–43.

126. Plotnikoff RC, Eves N, Jung M, Sigal RJ, Padwal R & Karunamuni N (2010). Multicomponent, home-based resistance training for obese adults with type 2 diabetes: a randomized controlled trial. *International Journal of Obesity*, 34(12): 1733–41.

127. Eyler AA, Brownson RC, Bacak SJ & Housemann RA (2003). The epidemiology of walking for physical activity in the United States. *Medicine and Science in Sports and Exercise*, 35(9): 1529–36.

128. Li F, Fisher KJ, Brownson RC & Bosworth M (2005). Multilevel modelling of built environment characteristics related to neighbourhood walking activity in older adults. *Journal of Epidemiology and Community Health*, 59(7): 558–64.

17

Nutrition therapy in the treatment of diabetes

Jennie Brand-Miller[1,2] and Geoffrey Ambler[3,4]

The optimal nutrition therapy for diabetes, like that of obesity, remains controversial because of the lack of high quality studies. There is increasing evidence that the conventional low-fat, high-carbohydrate diet is not ideal. Recent randomised controlled trials suggest that alternative dietary strategies with moderately lower carbohydrate content, including those with a lower glycaemic index, or higher fat (Mediterranean-style) or higher protein content are equally or more effective for managing diabetes. Observational studies suggest that such dietary approaches will also reduce the risk of complications. In Australia, consideration of both quantity and type of carbohydrate (carbohydrate counting, glycaemic index and glycaemic load) is an established part of diabetes management.

There is universal support for dietary therapy as an integral part of the treatment of both type 1 and type 2 diabetes. Although there are aspects of management unique to type 1 diabetes, much is similar because both types share the need to manage hyperglycaemia and hypoglycaemia on a day-to-day basis and to manage weight effectively. They both give rise to similar microvascular and macrovascular complications through common mechanisms arising from suboptimal glycaemic and metabolic control.

There is controversy surrounding the optimal diet or dietary pattern for diabetes because of lack of high quality studies. Current dietary recommendations are largely based on historical consensus and include limiting total fat, saturated fat and trans fatty acids, choosing high fibre and wholegrain foods, and monitoring and regulating carbohydrate intake to assist with glycaemic control. Moderate weight loss achieved through energy restriction and regular physical activity markedly improves glycaemia and cardiovascular risk factors in those who are overweight [1]. Unfortunately, on their own, these recommendations have been largely unsuccessful in practice in achieving good blood glucose control or maintenance of weight loss over the long term. For this reason, studies employing alternate strategies (eg high protein, low carbohydrate, vegetarian, Mediterranean-style, low glycaemic index/glycaemic load) have been explored.

---

1   School of Molecular Bioscience, University of Sydney.

2   Boden Institute of Obesity, Nutrition, Exercise and Eating Disorders, University of Sydney.

3   Institute of Endocrinology and Diabetes, Children's Hospital at Westmead.

4   Discipline of Paediatrics, University of Sydney.

The rationale

While there is now unequivocal evidence that dietary advice in conjunction with exercise can prevent or delay the development of type 2 diabetes in at-risk individuals (ie those with prediabetes) [2, 3], the role and type of dietary advice following the diagnosis is much less clear. In this chapter, we argue that the optimal diet composition for managing diabetes is not one judged simply by improvements in glycaemic control. Rather we contend that diets for diabetes should have proven efficacy in *all* of the following parameters:

- Optimising glucose metabolism (improving HbA1c, reducing postprandial glycaemia, reducing frequency and risk of hypoglycaemia, reducing glucose variability)
- Achieving appropriate weight loss in overweight or obese individuals or healthy weight maintenance in those not overweight
- Maintaining weight targets over the long term (years)
- In children and adolescents who are growing, providing appropriate energy intake and nutrients for optimal growth and development, while preventing or treating excessive weight gain
- Improving insulin sensitivity, even in the absence of weight loss
- Improving markers of the metabolic syndrome
- Improving markers of inflammation
- Reducing the future risk of cardiovascular disease and other complications linked to diabetes
- Being enjoyable and sustainable over the long term
- Maintaining healthy attitudes to food and avoiding eating disorders
- Being compatible with sustainable agricultural practices.

On this basis, there is evidence that some diets fare better than others. In the remainder of this review, we describe the best evidence available for different dietary approaches. We use randomised controlled trials in individuals with diabetes as our gold standard, and where not available, long-term prospective observational studies in large cohorts. Not all studies have been undertaken in individuals with diabetes, but the findings in overweight and obese individuals can be assumed to be indicative. It is also important to recognise that large-scale, long-term quality dietary composition studies are difficult to achieve in diabetes and obesity because of cost, patient-adherence factors, confounding concomitant therapies and other practical issues.

Improving HbA1c and glucose metabolism

A 2007 Cochrane systematic review [4] concluded that there were no high quality dietary studies that demonstrated the efficacy of any form of dietary treatment in type 2 diabetes. Indeed, in their view, there was no good evidence that diet alone (usually low-fat, high-carbohydrate advice) improved glycated haemoglobin, a long-term measure of blood glucose control, at one year. They found that very low-calorie diets were associated with a rise in glycated haemoglobin at 12 months. In contrast, adoption of exercise (± diet) was highly effective, reducing glycated haemoglobin by a significant 1%. That review considered there was insufficient data to compare one form of dietary advice with another, although their criteria excluded studies shorter than six months. In a more recent Cochrane review [5], Thomas and Elliott identified 11 high quality studies of low glycaemic index (GI) or low glycaemic load (GL) diets lasting one to 12 months. They concluded that on average, glycated haemoglobin decreased by 0.5% and hypoglycaemic episodes declined more on the low GI/GL diets compared to the conventional low-fat advice. Since then, Jenkins et al. have published the largest study to date, showing that a low GI diet was more effective at improving glycated haemoglobin than a high cereal fibre diet in 210 individuals with type 2 diabetes. While some small-scale studies [6, 7] suggest that high-protein, low-carbohydrate diets are more effective than other diets in improving glucose metabolism, there is a lack of high quality data. In a two-year trial, Shai found that changes in fasting glucose and insulin levels were more favourable among the diabetic participants assigned to the Mediterranean diet than those assigned to the low fat.

In addition to long-term goals, the optimisation of day-to-day blood glucose levels is also an important consideration, particularly the control of postprandial hyperglycaemia and avoidance of hypoglycaemia. Type 2 diabetes subjects (and type 1 subjects, discussed later) treated with insulin or other hypoglycaemic agents are at risk of hypoglycaemia which poses significant health and social risks, and these risks need to be minimised. There is also some evidence from observational data for adverse effects of blood glucose fluctuations (independent of overall glycaemic control) on diabetes complications [8]. For these reasons, monitoring and regulating the amount and type of carbohydrate on a daily basis (or carbohydrate counting) is recommended in diabetes management [9]. Such approaches have been more intensively applied to type 1 diabetes and are discussed below, but are also widely used in type 2 diabetes.

Reduce weight

In adults with type 2 diabetes, weight loss and weight-loss maintenance are essential components of management yet only in the last decade have diets of different composition been given the degree of scientific study and scrutiny they deserve. Ideally, the management goal would be normalisation and maintenance of weight, BMI and abdominal circumference to within the normal healthy range; however it is recognised that this is currently a rarely achievable goal and therefore modest weight loss of 5% to 10% is an initial target [10]. In overweight children and adolescents who are still growing, weight maintenance is usually the initial goal, which translates into improved BMI as they grow, although modest weight loss that still allows normal linear growth is desirable in the obese [11]. Prevention of progression to overweight or obesity is also a primary goal at all ages in type 2 and type 1 diabetes.

Several meta-analyses and reviews have concluded that low-carbohydrate, high-protein diets [12–15] and low GI or low glycaemic load diets [5, 16, 17] may be more successful for weight loss than traditional low-fat, high-carbohydrate diets. Similar benefits have recently been suggested for Mediterranean-style diets [18, 19]. Indeed, in our view, a conventional low-fat, high-carbohydrate diet appears to be one of the slowest ways to lose weight. However, one high-quality, long-term study found no difference in weight-loss outcomes between high vs low protein, high vs low fat, or high carbohydrate vs low carbohydrate diets at two years [16]. Only ~15% of subjects maintained a weight loss of 10% at the two-year mark. Notably, carbohydrate quality (high vs low GI) was not a variable.

Maintain weight loss over the longer term

The ability of different diets to maintain weight loss is arguably the most important attribute of a diet but there is little research to date to guide recommendations. Some evidence suggests that alternative dietary approaches may also be more successful for maintenance of the achieved weight loss than low-fat, high-carbohydrate diets [10–14]. In the Diogenes Study [17], ~800 overweight and obese individuals were randomised to one of five *ad libitum* diets after 8% of body weight loss had been achieved by means of a very low-energy diet. Two levels of protein and two levels of GI were studied. After six months, the high-protein and low GI diets were shown to be equally successful, but the combination of both high protein *and* low GI, produced the greatest absolute weight-loss maintenance and the lowest study drop-out rate. Importantly, this large well-designed study found that the conventional low-fat diet with average protein and GI was associated with the fastest rate of weight re-gain.

Improving insulin sensitivity

Improving insulin sensitivity is arguably the defining attribute of a good diet because insulin resistance is a fundamental contributor to the pathogenesis of type 2 diabetes. Indeed, insulin resistance combined with a defect in pancreatic insulin secretion, cause a relative insulin deficiency that occurs in most people with type 2 diabetes. The modifiable factors that worsen insulin resistance are excessive body weight, physical inactivity and smoking. Increasing muscle mass and lowering abdominal fat both markedly improve insulin sensitivity. Hence a combination of weight loss and physical activity, particularly resistance exercise, is the ideal lifestyle intervention to reduce the risk of type 2 diabetes.

However, diet composition has been shown to have a separate additional effect on insulin sensitivity. Observational studies and intervention trials have shown the macronutrient distribution (ie the ratio of fat:carbohydrate:protein energy) and the quality of individual macronutrients directly influence insulin sensitivity.

The effect of dietary fat and carbohydrate on insulin sensitivity have been debated for decades. Some of the controversy stems from divergent findings in animals versus humans, and in differing study designs. Insulin resistance can be induced in animal models by diets high in fat, sucrose or fructose. However, a single bout of exercise or high starch meal can completely reverse the defect. In humans, some studies suggest that a high intake of fat is associated with impaired insulin sensitivity but this may be modified by the type of fat and by the type of subject. Several studies indicate that a high-saturated-fat diet may be especially deleterious in physically inactive, sedentary individuals, while short (three to four weeks), studies in lean, healthy subjects have shown no effects on insulin sensitivity [18]. The KANWU study included 162 healthy subjects who received isoenergetic diets for three months containing either a high proportion of saturated fatty acids (SAFA) or mono-unsaturated (MUFA) acids [19]. Within each group there was a second assignment to fish oil supplements or placebo. Insulin sensitivity was significantly impaired by the SAFA diet (–10%) but did not change on the MUFA diet. However, the beneficial effects of MUFA were *not* seen when total fat intake exceeded 37%E (the median level of participants). Addition of n-3 fatty acids did not influence insulin sensitivity, and neither diet altered insulin secretion. Taken together, these and other findings suggest that at fat intake close to average in industrialised nations (ie ~35% E), it is preferable to maintain the *higher* fat intake but to reduce relative saturated fat intake and thus increase the proportion of MUFA or PUFA fatty acids, rather than increase the percentage energy derived from carbohydrate.

The quantity and quality of carbohydrate can also influence insulin sensitivity. In a cross-sectional analysis of ~3000 individuals in the Framingham Offspring Study, wholegrains, total fibre from all sources, as well as fibre from cereals and fruit, were inversely related to insulin resistance [20], but there was no relationship with total carbohydrate intake. Dietary glycaemic index (GI) and glycaemic load (GL) were also directly related to insulin resistance with approximately 10% more insulin resistance in the highest quintile of GI than in the lowest.

Some high-carbohydrate diets appear to have beneficial effects on insulin sensitivity. In healthy, young persons, isoenergetic substitution of *high fibre* carbohydrate foods for saturated fatty acids improves insulin sensitivity within four weeks [21]. Indeed, carbohydrates consumed without fibre may produce detrimental effects [22]. In individuals with diabetes, higher-carbohydrate intake has the potential to raise postprandial glucose and increase insulin demand, an effect that might worsen insulin resistance. Low GI diets, however, in which the carbohydrates are more slowly digested and absorbed, resulting in lower postprandial glycaemia, have improved insulin sensitivity in some studies. Insulin sensitivity was 45% higher as judged by euglycaemic clamp procedure in type 2 diabetes patients who ate a low GI diet for four weeks compared with a macronutrient-matched high GI diet [23]. The alpha-glucosidase inhibitor, ecarbose, which slows carbohydrate digestion but is not absorbed into the systemic circulation, also produces improvements in insulin sensitivity [24]. Low GI diets also improve insulin sensitivity in overweight women with polycystic ovarian syndrome [25].

The evidence for wholegrains vs refined grains to improve insulin sensitivity is inconsistent. A well-designed but small intervention study, compared six to ten servings of breakfast cereal, bread, rice, pasta, muffins, cookies and snacks from either whole or refined grains (in both cases mostly ground to flour) in a conventional high-carbohydrate, low-fat diet. Using the glucose clamp, insulin sensitivity was higher after six weeks on the wholegrain diet compared with a similar period on the refined grain diet [26]. Unfortunately, this finding was not confirmed in the larger WHOLEheart Study in which 60 g to 120 g per day wholegrain foods were ingested for up to 16 weeks by overweight individuals [27].

The effect of fructose and sucrose on insulin sensitivity also remains controversial. Studies in animals, often fed extremely high intakes (eg 70% of total calories), have shown a detrimental effect of fructose and sucrose compared with starch or glucose [28]. When fructose and glucose were compared directly, fructose was found to be the culpable moiety.

The evidence in humans, however, suggests that fructose and sucrose in *realistic* amounts have beneficial effects on insulin sensitivity. In lean, young healthy males, a diet containing 25% sucrose produced higher insulin sensitivity as assessed in a two-step clamp procedure than a diet containing 1% sucrose [29]. Similarly, a study in patients with type 2 diabetes showed that a diet with 10% fructose produced a 34% improvement in insulin sensitivity measured by the glucose clamp [30]. In this study, patients lived in a hospital environment and all food was provided. Finally, using the glucose clamp, no effects on insulin sensitivity were noted after three months of a 13% fructose vs sucrose diet in type 2 diabetes [31]. It is conceivable, however, that at very high intakes (>30% E), sucrose and fructose have adverse effects.

Improving markers of the metabolic syndrome

The best evidence that dietary changes can improve the metabolic syndrome comes from landmark studies in which intensive lifestyle interventions prevented or delayed progression from impaired glucose tolerance to type 2 diabetes mellitus [2, 3, 36]. Both studies employed low-fat, high-carbohydrate diets (30% of energy from fat, 10% from saturated fat) in combination with physical activity to achieve the goal of weight loss. Mistakenly, these findings have since been perceived as a rational basis for recommending low-fat, high-carbohydrate diets. Unfortunately, weight loss *per se* likely played the most important role, such that the superiority of low-fat diets for people with diabetes and the metabolic syndrome is questionable.

In intervention trials, increased carbohydrate intake is well known to increase serum triglycerides and lower HDL, two markers of the metabolic syndrome [32]. Indeed, the similarity implies that high carbohydrate diets of a certain nature play an etiological role in the metabolic syndrome. Several meta-analyses and reviews have concluded that low-carbohydrate, high-protein diets [12], low-GI or low-GL diets [5, 33, 34] and Mediterranean-style diets [35] may be more effective (or just as effective) for improving markers of the metabolic syndrome as traditional low-fat, high-carbohydrate diets. This higher effectiveness holds true over both the shorter and the longer term.

Improving inflammatory markers

Chronic low-grade inflammation plays a recognised role in the development and the progression of both type 2 diabetes and vascular disease [36]. Inflammation is also the likely intermediary between aspects of carbohydrate nutrition and chronic disease. A single glucose challenge has been shown to increase the production of reactive oxygen molecules with mitochondria and activation of pro-inflammatory transcription factors, such as nuclear factor-kappaB (NF-kB). In individuals with impaired glucose tolerance, obese or persons with type 2 diabetes, the result is pronounced and lasts longer (>2–3 h) than in non-diabetic persons [37]. Indeed, in individuals with type 2 diabetes, glucose fluctuations during postprandial periods have a more specific triggering effect on oxidative stress than chronic sustained hyperglycaemia [38]. High GI/GL diets that are associated with greater postprandial glucose excursions may therefore promote low-grade inflammation.

In short-term metabolic ward studies in healthy individuals, the consumption of high GI foods has been directly linked to the creation of oxidative stress, as judged by higher activation of NF-kB and increased generation of nitrotyrosine. The presence of oxidative stress can also be detected by an acute decline in antioxidant concentrations in plasma following a meal. Botero et al. [39] observed differences in fasting and postprandial total antioxidant capacity over the course of a five-hour observation period following one week on a low or high GI diet in overweight men. Plasma total antioxidant capacity in response to diet may therefore be the first metabolic adaptation linking carbohydrate nutrition to type 2 diabetes.

Reducing future risk of microvascular and macrovascular complications

There are no intervention studies examining the risk of diabetes complications for diets of differing composition. In their absence, large, long-term prospective observational studies in healthy individuals can be regarded as indicative. In meta-analyses, replacing saturated fat with polyunsaturated fat is associated with a 26% reduction in risk of cardiovascular disease [40]. In contrast, replacing saturated fat with carbohydrate is linked to a non-significant increase in risk. Carbohydrate intake (whether high or low) is not usually an independent predictor of the development of type 2 diabetes mellitus. In meta-analyses, however, quality of carbohydrate intake as assessed as the GI, GL and dietary fibre shows a consistent positive relationship to the risk of type 2 diabetes mellitus and cardiovascular disease (CVD), despite non-significant findings in some individual prospective studies [41]. The highest relative risks (>2) are observed among those with both a higher dietary GI or GL and lower (cereal) fibre intake. Recently, some prospective cohort studies have demonstrated that higher intake of high GI carbohydrates, but not low GI carbohydrates, is associated with greater risk of developing CVD [42]. Similarly, there is increased risk of type 2 diabetes mellitus and overweight associated with dietary patterns that are characterised by higher intakes of refined grains or white bread, ready-to-eat breakfast cereals, sugar-sweetened beverages, potatoes or French fries, sweets or sweet bakery products [43]. In contrast, a protective pattern commonly included carbohydrate choices such as fruits, vegetables, legumes, wholemeal or wholegrain bread and high-fibre breakfast cereals.

The dietary approaches that reduce the risk of developing type 2 diabetes, obesity or CVD are likely to be the same as those that reduce the risk of complications in individuals with diabetes. Interestingly, the apparently protective diets share a unifying mechanism of reducing postprandial glycaemia and insulinaemia, despite variable macronutrient distribution. Thus it is possible but remains unproven at present whether any diet that facilitates a reduction in postprandial glycaemia without worsening dyslipidemia, is likely to improve insulin sensitivity and relieve the burden on the beta cell, thereby reducing the risk of complications. The least effective diet will be one that increases postprandial glycaemia and places extra demands on beta-cell function. These adverse effects will be most detrimental for individuals with severe insulin resistance, that is, many individuals with diabetes.

Enjoyable and sustainable diets

In the short term, a wide variety of diets will reduce weight and improve cardiovascular risk factors under realistic clinical conditions. But only a minority of individuals have been found to sustain dietary adherence over the longer term. There is no single diet that is associated with satisfactory dietary adherence, although a high protein–low GI diet was associated with significantly higher completion rates in the Diogenes Study of weight-loss maintenance [17]. More extreme diets, such as very low carbohydrate diets (Atkins) or very low-fat diets (eg Ornish) are more likely to be discontinued [44]. To manage the epidemic of obesity and diabetes, practical techniques to increase dietary adherence are urgently needed.

One way to do this is to offer a broad range of healthy diet options, to better match individual patient preferences, lifestyles and cultural backgrounds. Dansinger et al. [44] found that only one in four individuals were adherent one year after counselling, yet those individuals who sustained the greatest weight loss and risk reduction were those who were able to comply, no matter what the diet composition. Thus a diet's ease of adoption, rather than diet composition per se, is an important attribute of an effective diet. These findings challenge the assumption that one type of diet is appropriate for everyone and that popular diets can be ignored.

Another way to increase adherence is to offer intensive, systematic and individualised dietary counselling. In the Diabetes Prevention Program, freely available intensive dietary counselling was effective in sustaining weight loss, and cardiovascular and diabetes risk reduction over a three-year period, irrespective of ethnicity, socioeconomic group or cultural background [2]. Only 7.5% of individuals dropped out of the study despite the large number of face-to-face visits over a long period. While dietary counselling requires more resources from the health system, cost-effectiveness analyses show that the intensive lifestyle interventions cost no more than drug interventions [45]. Moreover, over the long term, we can expect fewer side effects and more benefits (eg reduced risk of other lifestyle diseases) associated with adherence to a healthy diet.

Vegetarian diets for diabetes

A vegetarian or semi-vegetarian diet, with emphasis on plant foods such as wholegrains, legumes, nuts, fruits, vegetables, is widely believed to have a number of *nutritional* benefits over a meat-based diet for the management of diabetes. Vegetarian diets can be (but not necessarily) lower in saturated fat, higher in dietary fibre and richer in micronutrients such as magnesium, ie factors that are associated with higher insulin sensitivity. Observational studies show that a vegetarian or vegan diet is associated with reduced risk of development of type 2 diabetes and lower risk of complications in those with existing diabetes. The European Prospective Investigation into Cancer and Nutrition study found that among participants with diabetes, there was a significant inverse association between cardiovascular mortality and intake of total vegetables, legumes and fruit [46]. In women with type 2 diabetes, frequent consumption of nuts was associated with a 50% reduction in the risk of CVD and a more favourable lipid profile [47]. One long-term intervention study, in which animal protein was partly replaced with soy protein, reported significant improvements in total cholesterol, LDL cholesterol, triglycerides and CRP levels in individuals with diabetes [48]. Nonetheless, it is difficult to separate vegetarianism from other healthy lifestyle behaviours, which also improve risk factors. Some evidence suggests it is the absence of processed meat products from vegetarian diets rather than meat per se that offers benefits.

Compatibility with sustainable agricultural practices

Some health authorities have recommended vegetarian diets over meat-based diets on the grounds of environmental sustainability. However, the issue is debated even among the experts. Much of Australia is classed as arid or semi-arid, with vast areas that are unsuitable for crop agriculture, but suitable for grazing. In the Australian context, most agriculturalists and those who are knowledgeable consider extensive, free-range grazing systems with relatively low stocking rates and a rotation of cropping and pastures as sustainable. Such relatively low input–low output systems have been sustained for decades, eg the sheep-wheat-legume-based pasture systems in south-eastern Australia. The animal/ pasture component in the rotation actively promotes sustainability. In Australia, Good Agricultural Practice and Best Management Practice production systems are widely recognised and used.

The notion that we should not eat meat or dairy for environmental reasons may in itself be a flawed argument because avoidance of meat requires the production of more grain to obtain the same nutrition. Animal source foods are nutrient dense and generally are able to nourish the human population more effectively than plants. Overconsumption and waste are profoundly more important for both sustainability and health than simply considering plant vs animal consumption. At present, over a quarter of all foods consumed are 'non-core foods', ie foods that are not essential to good health, yet demand a disproportionately large amount of scarce resources such as water, and generate large amounts of greenhouse gases.

Particular aspects of nutrition therapy for type 1 diabetes

Although the underlying pathogenesis is initially different in type 1 vs type 2 diabetes (absolute insulin deficiency vs relatively greater insulin resistance, respectively) and mean age of onset differ, the subsequent metabolic derangements that stem from chronic hyperglycaemia and that are involved in the pathogenesis of diabetes complications are common to both. The principles discussed above for the nutritional management of type 2 diabetes therefore also apply to the management of type 1 diabetes, particularly as they relate to weight control, avoidance of hyperglycaemia and hypoglycaemia and optimisation of metabolic control and insulin sensitivity. There are some particular considerations for type 1 diabetes, mainly relating to carbohydrate counting and type of carbohydrate.

Type 1 diabetes has an acute and earlier age of onset than type 2 diabetes, with the majority of cases diagnosed in children and adolescents after a short duration of symptoms. Most people diagnosed with type 1 diabetes are not obese, even prior to the weight loss that often occurs before the diagnosis. Because all type 1 subjects require insulin therapy, nutritional management commences with a different focus. A major priority is to have a nutritional and insulin plan that meets short- and long-term glycaemic goals, including control of hyperglycaemia, and minimises hypoglycaemia and glucose fluctuations. Additional goals are long-term maintenance of a healthy weight and prevention or reduction in risk of long-term complications that are not usually present at diagnosis (but can often be in type 2 diabetes). Not surprisingly, in line with trends to increasing prevalence of overweight and obesity in society, children diagnosed with type 1 diabetes are heavier and taller than their peers [49] and this has been postulated to be associated with the earlier onset of type 1 diabetes seen in various registries and termed the 'accelerator hypothesis'. This hypothesis suggests that the relative insulin resistance associated with being overweight or obese accelerates the progression to clinical onset of type 1 diabetes in those that are genetically predisposed [50]. There is also evidence that in the longer term, those with type 1 diabetes are heavier than their non-diabetic peers [51]. There is also a subgroup with type 1 diabetes who have significant inherent insulin resistance in addition to that associated with obesity; the term 'double diabetes' has been used for this group and they are often considered for co-treatment with insulin sensitising agents. Therefore the management of overweight and obesity in young people with type 1 diabetes is a frequent necessity.

Carbohydrate counting has become an established part of the nutritional management in type 1 diabetes and is a necessary component of flexible multiple daily injection plans and insulin pump therapy. There has been a movement away from recommending relatively fixed carbohydrate intake (or carbohydrate prescription) to more flexible and physiological approaches in which subjects are taught to match their insulin doses with their desired and counted carbohydrate intake. There is reasonable evidence to conclude that the use of carbohydrate counting with flexible insulin to carbohydrate ratio is associated with improved HbA1c and quality of life, but no conclusions regarding effects on body weight or severe hypoglycaemia [52, 53]. The DAFNE study demonstrated that adult type 1 diabetes subjects using such an approach achieved a significant improvement in HbA1c and quality of life over six months, without worsening severe hypoglycaemia or cardiovascular risk. However, there are not yet comparable data in children and adolescents. Despite such studies, there are limited data on the best methods and teaching to employ or the degree of accuracy required in carbohydrate counting. While trends have been to aim for more accurate matching of insulin to carbohydrate, one study demonstrated that postprandial BGL control was not affected by variations of up to 17% in the carbohydrate amount covered by the same insulin dose [54]. With insulin pump therapy, the only available randomised prospective study recently demonstrated that in adults, accurate carbohydrate counting had advantages over empirical estimation of doses in a number of parameters over 24 weeks, including HBA1c, BMI, waist circumference and quality of life [55].

There is also evidence that the type of carbohydrate as well as the quantity is important in minimisimg glucose fluctuations and hypoglycaemia; these are the concepts of glycaemic index and glycaemic load [4]. While there are no data in children and adolescents, the conclusions from the adult studies cited above should also be applicable to young people and their diabetes nutritional plans should incorporate these concepts.

Conclusions

The findings of recent, high quality studies have been surprising and yet remarkably consistent. The conventional low-fat diet is probably *not* the optimal diet for managing diabetes, weight or risk factors for cardiovascular disease. Rather, there appear to be superior dietary patterns that offer good diabetes control, more flexibility and greater ability for individuals to choose a diet that they enjoy and can sustain over the longer term. These alternative nutritional strategies include those with a moderately lower carbohydrate content, those with a lower glycaemic index, or higher fat (Mediterranean-style), or higher protein content. Very low-carbohydrate diets (with higher protein and fat) cannot be recommended to people with type 1 diabetes because of adverse effects on renal function. In individuals with type 2 diabetes, there is a lack of long-term dietary studies that go beyond the measurement of risk factors (eg glycated haemoglobin) to assess hard outcomes such as death and diabetes-related complications. Unfortunately, such studies are difficult and expensive to conduct, not amenable to patent generation and unlikely to eventuate. Long-term prospective observational studies in healthy individuals remain our best guide. At the present time, diets low in saturated fat and trans fats, with a lower GI and GL, and higher fibre content, represent our best advice for increasing life expectancy and quality of life in individuals with diabetes. With current insulin delivery methods in type 1 diabetes, carbohydrate counting and consideration of glycaemic index and glycaemic load remain an important component of the nutritional plan.

References

1. American Diabetes Association (2008). Nutrition recommendations and interventions for diabetes. *Diabetes Care*, 31(Suppl. 1): S61–S78.

2. Diabetes Prevention Program Research Group (2002). Reduction in the incidence of type 2 diabetes with lifestyle intervention or metformin. *The New England Journal of Medicine*, 346(6): 393–403.

3. Tuomilehto J, Lindstrom J, Eriksson JG, Valle TT, Hamalaninen H, Ilanne-Parikka P, et al. (2001). Prevention of type 2 diabetes mellitus by changes in lifestyle among subjects with impaired glucose tolerance. *The New England Journal of Medicine*, 344: 1343–50.

4. Thomas D & Elliott E (2009). Low glycaemic index, or low glycaemic load, diets for diabetes mellitus. *Cochrane Database of Systematic Reviews*.[Online]. Available: onlinelibrary.wiley.com/doi/10.1002/14651858.CD006296.pub2/pdf [Accessed 12 December 2011].

5. Nield L, Moore H, Hooper L, Cruickshank K, Vyas A, Whittaker V, et al. (2009). Dietary advice for treatment of type 2 diabetes mellitus in adults. *Cochrane Database of Systematic Reviews* [Online].

Avaliable: onlinelibrary.wiley.com/doi/10.1002/14651858.CD004097.pub4/pdf [Accessed 12 December 2011].

6. Boden G, Sargrad K, Homko C, Mozzoli M & Stein TP (2005). Effect of a low-carbohydrate diet on appetite, blood glucose levels, and insulin resistance in obese patients with type 2 diabetes. *Annals of Internal Medicine*, 142(6): 403–11.

7. Gannon MC & Nuttall FQ (2004). Effect of a high-protein, low-carbohydrate diet on blood glucose control in people with type 2 diabetes. *Diabetes*, 53(9): 2375–82.

8. Nalysnyk L, Hernandez-Medina M & Krishnarajah G (2010). Glycaemic variability and complications in patients with diabetes mellitus: evidence from a systematic review of the literature. *Diabetes*, 12(4): 288–98.

9. American Diabetes Association (2011). Standards of medical care in diabetes. *Diabetes Care*, 34(Suppl. 1): S11–61.

10. Bantle JP, Wylie-Rosett J, Albright AL, Apovian CM, Clark NG, Franz MJ Hoogwerf BJ, Lichtenstein AH, Mayer-Davis E, Mooradian AD & Wheeler ML (2008). Nutrition recommendations and interventions for diabetes: a position statement of the American Diabetes Association. *Diabetes Care*, (Suppl. 1): S61–78.

11. Smart C, Aslander-van Vliet E & Waldron S (2009). Nutritional management in children and adolescents with diabetes. *Pediatric Diabetes*, (Suppl .12): 100–17.

12. Halton TL & Hu FB (2004). The effects of high protein diets on thermogenesis, satiety and weight loss: a critical review. *Journal of the American College of Nutrition*, 23(5): 373–85.

13. Krieger JW, Sitren HS, Daniels MJ & Langkamp-Henken B (2006). Effects of variation in protein and carbohydrate intake on body mass and composition during energy restriction: a meta-regression 1. *The American Journal of Clinical Nutrition*, 83(2): 260–74.

14. Nordmann AJ, Nordmann A, Briel M, Keller U, Yancy WS Jr., Brehm BJ & Bucher HC (2006). Effects of low-carbohydrate vs low-fat diets on weight loss and cardiovascular risk factors: a meta-analysis of randomized controlled trials. *Archives of Internal Medicine*, 166(3): 285–93.

15. Samaha F, Foster G & Makris A (2007). Low-carbohydrate diets, obesity, and metabolic risk factors for cardiovascular disease. *Current Atherosclerosis Reports*, 9(6): 441–47.

16. Sacks FM, Bray GA, Carey VJ, Smith SR, Ryan DH, Anton SD, et al. (2009). Comparison of weight-loss diets with different compositions of fat, protein, and carbohydrates. *New England Journal of Medicine*, 360(9): 859–73.

17. Larsen TM, Dalskov SM, van Baak M, Jebb SA, Papadaki A, Pfeiffer AFH, et al. (2010). Diets with high or low protein content and glycemic index for weight-loss maintenance. *New England Journal of Medicine*, 363(22): 2102–13.

18. Vessby B (2000). Dietary fat and insulin action in humans. *British Journal of Nutrition*, 83: S91–S6.

19. Vessby B, Uusitupa M, Hermansen K, Riccardi G, Rivellese A, Tapsell L, et al. (2001). Insulin sensitivity in healthy men and women: the KANWU study. *Diabetologia*, 44(3): 312–19.

20. McKeown N, Meigs J, Liu S, Saltzman E, Wilson P & Jacques P (2004). Carbohydrate nutrition,

insulin resistance, and the prevalence of the metabolic syndrome in the Framingham offspring cohort. *Diabetes Care*, 27(2): 538–46.

21. Perez-Jimenez F, Lopez-Miranda J, Pinillos M, Gomez P, Paz-Rojas E, Montilla P, et al. (2001). A Mediterranean and a high carbohydrate diet improve glucose metabolism in healthy young persons. *Diabetologia*, 44(11): 2038–43.

22. Due A, Larsen TM, Mu H, Hermansen K, Stender S, Astrup A (2008). Comparison of 3 ad libitum diets for weight-loss maintenance, risk of cardiovascular disease, and diabetes: a 6-month randomized, controlled trial. *The American Journal of Clinical Nutrition*, 88(5): 1232–41.

23. Rizkalla S, Taghrid L, Laromiguiere M, Huet D, Boillot J, Rigoir A, et al. (2004). Improved plasma glucose control, whole-body glucose utilization, and lipid profile on a low-glycemic index diet in type 2 diabetic men: a randomized controlled trial. *Diabetes Care*, 27(8): 1866–72.

24. Holman RR, Cull CA & Turner RC (1999). A randomized double-blind trial of acarbose in type 2 diabetes shows improved glycemic control over 3 years (UKPDS 44). *Diabetes Care*, 22(6): 960–64.

25. Marsh KA, Steinbeck KS, Atkinson FS, Petocz P & Brand-Miller JC (2010). Effect of a low glycemic index compared with a conventional healthy diet on polycystic ovary syndrome. *The American Journal of Clinical Nutrition*, 92(1): 83–92.

26. Pereira M, Jacobs D, Pins J, Raatz S, Gross M, Slavin J & Seaquist, ER (2002). Effect of wholegrains on insulin sensitivity in overweight hyperinsulinemic adults. *The American Journal of Clinical Nutrition*, 75(5): 848–55.

27. Brownlee IA, Moore C, Chatfield M, DP R, Ashby P, Kuznesof SA, Jebb SA & Seal CA (2010). Markers of cardiovascular risk are not changed by increased wholegrain intake: the WHOLEheart study, a randomised, controlled dietary intervention. *British Journal of Nutrition*, 104(1): 125–34.

28. Daly ME, Vale C &Walker M (1997). Dietary carbohydrates and insulin sensitivity: a review of the evidence and clinical implications. *The Amercian Journal of Clinical Nutrition*, 66(5): 1072–85.

29. Kiens B & Richter E (1996). Types of carbohydrate in an ordinary diet affect insulin action and muscle substrates in humans. *The American Journal of Clinical Nutrition*, 63(1): 47–53.

30. Koivisto VA & Yki-Jarvinen H (1993). Fructose and insulin sensitivity in patients with type 2 diabetes. *Journal of Internal Medicine*, 233(2): 145–53.

31. Thorburn A, Crapo P, Beltz W, Wallace P, Witztum J & Henry R (1989). Lipid metabolism in non-insulin-dependent diabetes: effects of long-term treatment with fructose-supplemented mixed meals. *The American Journal of Clinical Nutrition*, 50: 1015–22.

32. Garg A (1998). High-mono-unsaturated-fat diets for patients with diabetes mellitus: a meta-analysis. *The American Journal of Clinical Nutrition*, 67(Suppl. 3): 577S–82S.

33. Livesey G, Taylor R, Hulshof T & Howlett J (2008). Glycemic response and health a systematic review and meta-analysis: relations between dietary glycemic properties and health outcomes. *The American Journal of Clinical Nutrition*, 87(1): 258S–68.

34. Thomas D, Elliott E & Baur L (2007). Low glycaemic index or low glycaemic load diets for overweight and obesity. *Cochrane Database of Systematic Reviews*, Issue 3: Art. No.: CD005105. DOI: 10.1002/14651858.CD005105.pub2.

35. Shai I, Schwarzfuchs D, Henkin Y, Shahar DR, Witkow S, Greenberg I, et al. (2008). Weight loss with a low-carbohydrate, mediterranean, or low-fat diet. *New England Journal of Medicine*, 359(3): 229–41.

36. Couzin-Frankel J (2010). Inflammation bares a dark side. *Science*, 330(6011): 1621.

37. Kempf K, Rose B, Herder C, Kleophas U, Martin S, Kolb H (2006). Inflammation in metabolic syndrome and type 2 diabetes. *Annals of the New York Academy of Sciences*, 1084: 30-48.

38. Monnier L, Mas E, Ginet C, Michel F, Villon L, Cristol J-P, Colette C (2006). Activation of oxidative stress by acute glucose fluctuations compared with sustained chronic hyperglycemia in patients with type 2 diabetes. *The Journal of the American Medical Association*, 295(14): 1681-87.

39. Botero D, Ebbeling CB, Blumberg JB, Ribaya-Mercado JD, Creager MA, Swain JF, et al. (2009). Acute effects of dietary glycemic index on antioxidant capacity in a nutrient-controlled feeding study. *Obesity*, 17(9): 1664–70.

40. Jakobsen MU, O'Reilly EJ, Heitmann BL, Pereira MA, BälterK, Fraser GE, et al. (2009). Major types of dietary fat and risk of coronary heart disease: a pooled analysis of 11 cohort studies. *The American Journal of Clinical Nutrition*, 89(5): 1425–32.

41. Barclay A, Petocz P, McMillan-Price J, Flood V, Prvan T, Mitchell P, et al. (2008). Glycemic index, glycemic load and chronic disease risk: a meta-analysis of observational studies. *The American Journal of Clinical Nutrition*, 87(3): 627–37.

42. Sieri S, Krogh V, Berrino F, Evangelista A, Agnoli C, Brighenti F, et al. (2010). Dietary glycemic load and index and risk of coronary heart disease in a large Italian cohort: the EPICOR Study. *Archives of Internal Medicine*, 170(7): 640–47.

43. Buyken A, Mitchell P, Ceriello A & Brand-Miller J (2010). Optimal dietary approaches for prevention of type 2 diabetes: a lifecourse perspective. *Diabetologia*, 53(3): 406–18

44. Dansinger ML, Gleason JA, Griffith JL, Selker HP & Schaefer EJ (2005). Comparison of the Atkins, Ornish, Weight Watchers and Zone Diets for weight loss and heart disease risk reduction. *The Journal of the American Medical Association*, 293(1): 43–53.

45. The Diabetes Prevention Progrom Research Group (2003). Within-trial cost-effectiveness of lifestyle intervention or metformin for the primary prevention of type 2 diabetes. *Diabetes Care*, 26(9): 2518–23.

46. Nothlings U, Schulze MB, Weikert C, Boeing H, van der Schouw YT, Bamia C, et al. (2008). Intake of vegetables, legumes, and fruit, and risk for all-cause, cardiovascular, and cancer mortality in a European diabetic population. *Journal of Nutrition*, 138(4): 775–81.

47. Li TY, Brennan AM, Wedick NM, Mantzoros C, Rifai N & Hu FB (2009). Regular consumption of nuts is associated with a lower risk of cardiovascular disease in women with type 2 diabetes. *Journal of Nutrition*, 139(7): 1333–38.

48. Azadbakht L, Atabak S & Esmaillzadeh A (2008). Soy protein intake, cardiorenal indices, and C-reactive protein in type 2 diabetes with nephropathy: a longitudinal randomized clinical trial. *Diabetes Care*, 31(4): 648–54.

49. Knerr I, Wolf J, Reinehr T, Stachow R, Grabert M, Schober E, et al. (2005). The 'accelerator hypothesis': relationship between weight, height, body mass index and age at diagnosis in a large cohort of 9248 German and Austrian children with type 1 diabetes mellitus. *Diabetologia*, 48(12): 2501–04.

50. Wilkin TJ (2009). The accelerator hypothesis: a review of the evidence for insulin resistance as the basis for type 1 as well as type 2 diabetes. *International Journal of Obesity*, (7): 716–26.

51. Mortensen HB, Robertson KJ, Aanstoot HJ, Danne T, Holl RW, Hougaard P, et al. (1998). Insulin management and metabolic control of type 1 diabetes mellitus in childhood and adolescence in 18 countries. Hvidøre Study Group on Childhood Diabetes. *Diabetic Medicine*, 15(9): 752–59.

52. Gilbertson HR, Brand-Miller JC, Thorburn AW, Evans S, Chondros P & Werther GA (2001). The effect of flexible low glycemic index dietary advice versus measured carbohydrate exchange diets on glycemic control in children with type 1 diabetes. *Diabetes Care*, 24(7): 1137–43.

53. DAFNE Study Group (2002). Training in flexible, intensive insulin management to enable dietary freedom in people with type 1 diabetes: dose adjustment for normal eating (DAFNE) randomised controlled trial. *British Medical Journal*, 325(7367): 746.

54. Smart CE, Ross K, Edge JA, Collins CE, Colyvas K & King BR (2009). Children and adolescents on intensive insulin therapy maintain postprandial glycaemic control without precise carbohydrate counting. *Diabetic Medicine*, 26(3): 279–85.

55. Laurenzi A, Bolla AM, Panigoni G, Doria V, Uccellatore A, Peretti E, et al. (2011). Effects of carbohydrate counting on glucose control and quality of life over 24 weeks in adult patients with type 1 diabetes on continuous subcutaneous insulin infusion: a randomized, prospective clinical trial (GIOCAR). *Diabetes Care*, 34(4): 823–27.

18

Current therapies and pharmacy programs for obesity and diabetes

Carol Armour,[1] Betty Chaar,[2] Michael Murray,[2] Geoffrey Ambler[3,4] and Ines Krass[2]

A growing body of Australian and international literature has reported the benefits and improved health outcomes resulting from various trials of pharmaceutical care, self-management support and other cognitive services in chronic conditions such as diabetes and obesity. This review will focus on existing medications, the reasons why they might not work for some individuals and the potential for new ways to treat both diseases. It will also review novel ways to manage the diseases, including using community pharmacy as a site for intervention, once effective therapies are available.

The burden of diabetes and obesity for individuals and for the community is high. The complications of both diseases are related and of the order that adequate treatment and control are vital to limit an epidemic of severe morbidity and mortality. Medications and how they are used play a key role in the management of these chronic conditions. Current antidiabetic therapies enhance insulin secretion by pancreatic beta-cells, reducing insulin resistance, modulating glucose metabolism or in type 1 diabetes or refractory type 2 diabetes, replacing insulin. Although several subclasses of non-insulin agents have been in use for some time, detailed information on their modes of action, use in various combinations and factors that prevent their optimal use are only recently emerging and require further understanding. Pharmacotherapy is also being increasingly used as a component of preventive programs targeting insulin resistance and obesity before onset of diabetes ('prediabetes'), especially in children and adolescents. Pharmacists contribute significantly to quality use of medicines when they provide information, advice and recommendations to patients and providers to optimise therapeutic outcomes. In recent years, pharmacists have also sought to develop an expanded role in contributing to the management of chronic diseases to meet the needs of this growing patient population.

1 Woolcock Institute of Medical Research, Sydney Medical School, University of Sydney.

2 Faculty of Pharmacy, University of Sydney.

3 Discipline of Paediatrics, University of Sydney.

4 Institute of Endocrinology and Diabetes, Children's Hospital, Westmead.

Diabetes

Type 2 diabetes mellitus (T2DM), the most common form of diabetes, is now an escalating worldwide epidemic. It contributes significantly to premature mortality, morbidity and disability through the development of micro- and macrovascular complications of uncontrolled disease. In Australia, the 2007–2008 National Health Survey estimated that 818 200 Australians (4%) have diabetes, based on self-reports [1]. The earlier national Australian Diabetes, Obesity and Lifestyle study found that approximately 1.2 million (7.4%) of Australians aged 25 years and over had diabetes with half of the respondents unaware [1]. A further 16% of Australians have been estimated to have impaired glucose metabolism or prediabetes [2]. The total economic burden is estimated at A\$6 billion annually (2003) arising mainly from the costs associated with the treatment of complications [3].

The incidence and prevalence of T2DM in adolescents is increasing globally, but especially in those of non-white European descent [4]. The International Diabetes Federation estimates that 285 million people around the world have diabetes. This total is expected to rise to 438 million within 20 years. Highest risk groups are those of black African descent, native North American, Hispanic, Asian, South Asian and Native Pacific Islanders. These groups have higher genetic risk factors with the clinical expression of T2DM being accelerated by increasing rates of childhood and adolescent overweight and obesity [5]. While T2DM is being seen in increasing prevalence in younger age groups, it is rarely seen until the second decade of life since it requires the trigger of the physiological increase in insulin resistance that occurs with puberty [4].

Obesity

Obesity is a major global public health and economic problem as it is associated with significant morbidity and mortality. In 2005, the World Health Organisation reported approximately 1.6 billion adults as overweight; 400 million of those were obese [6]. Australia is one of the most overweight developed nations [7], with a growing incidence over the last 12 years, approximately 68% of adult men and 55% of adult women were overweight or obese in 2007–2008 [8]. The total cost of obesity in 2008 was A\$58.2 billion which included the costs attributable to associated diseases [9].

Overweight and obesity are both disease states and risk factors for many other chronic conditions. Overweight is defined as a body mass index (BMI) ≥25 in adults or 85th percentile in children and adolescents and obesity as a body mass index ≥30 in adults or the 95th percentile in children and adolescents. Higher body mass was responsible for 7.5% of the total burden of disease and injury in 2003, ranked behind tobacco (7.8%) and high blood pressure (7.6%) [10].

Excess body mass predicts higher mortality and/or morbidity in cardiovascular disease, T2DM, some cancers and increasingly, osteoarthritis [11]. Obesity is also strongly associated with back, reproductive and mental health problems, and obstructive sleep apnoea. Modest weight losses of 5% to 10% have been shown to improve hypertension and dyslipidaemia [10, 12].

In response to this problem the Australian Government recommended in June 2009, strategies for the treatment, management and prevention of obesity in 'Weighing it up – obesity in Australia', as well as better regulation of weight-loss products and programs to ensure safety and efficacy[9].

Addressing the problems

Evidence-based strategies addressing the problem of T2DM support the benefits of early interventions in prediabetes and strict control of glycaemia, blood pressure and lipids in established diabetes to reduce the risk and delay the onset of the complications such a cardiovascular and kidney disease [13–15]. In recent years, a plethora of clinical and management guidelines which recommend therapeutic targets to optimise disease control have become widely available to healthcare practitioners. This, coupled with advances in understanding of the pathophysiology of T2DM and the introduction of a range of new management therapies in the past decade, have ushered in the possibility of reducing the disease burden associated with T2DM and its complications.

There is broad agreement that the most appropriate first-line therapy for overweight and obesity in all age groups is behavioural and lifestyle interventions, including nutritional and exercise interventions [16]. This is particularly so in children and adolescents in whom the problem is generally less entrenched and has fewer complications. Also, there is lower availability of licensed drugs for the use of obesity in children and adolescents and greater reluctance to use pharmacotherapy in the young because of concern about long-term side effects. The lessons of history have shown these concerns to be justified.

Management of T2DM

The clinical management of T2DM aims to achieve control of glycaemia, as well as other risk factors such as blood pressure, dyslipidaemia and obesity to prevent or reduce the progression of the micro- and macrovascular complications associated with the condition. Initial and then ongoing management involves recommended modifications to diet and physical activity to address blood glucose as well as cholesterol and blood pressure. For blood glucose, if satisfactory glycaemic control is not achieved through weight loss and increased physical activity alone, pharmacotherapy is indicated. The current guidelines recommend that pharmacological therapy is commenced with metformin [17]. However, over time beta-cell function progressively declines, usually necessitating the addition of additional agents which include sulfonylureas, meglitinides, thiazolidinediones, and potentially incretin mimetics such as the oral DPPIV inhibitors, injectable agents such as exenatide, or insulin. The therapeutic use of each of these classes is discussed in the next section.

T2DM is a complex condition to manage, requiring all elements of the biopsychosocial model to be considered. Addressing lifestyle issues such as diet and exercise, as well as care in commencing and up-titrating medications, and vigilance in monitoring of the disease including achieving and sustaining blood glucose and other targets in therapy, is demanding on the person with diabetes, their families and on healthcare resources. The membership of the health professional team that supports the person with T2DM is broad, and depending upon individual patient's needs may include the general practitioner, practice nurse and dietitian, as well as the diabetes nurse educator, specialist endocrinologist, podiatrist, optometrist, ophthalmologist and psychologist. As described in later parts of this chapter the pharmacist can, and should, be an integral member of the healthcare team supporting the care of the person with diabetes.

The rest of this chapter will focus on pharmacotherapy for blood glucose in T2DM and pharmacotherapy in obesity, and management of these diseases in adults and adolescents. Commercial programs available for obesity management will be discussed, as well as optimising management of T2DM and obesity in our current health system and the evidence and potential role of pharmacy in improving outcomes for these diseases.

Optimisation of current therapies for diabetes

Current antidiabetic agents enhance the secretion of insulin by pancreatic beta-cells, improve insulin resistance in tissues or modulate glucose metabolism. Although several classes of drugs have been used in the treatment of diabetes for some time it is only recently that detailed information on their modes of action and the factors that prevent their optimal use in patients have emerged.

Major classes of antidiabetic agents

(a) Insulin secretagogues

ATP is generated during mitochondrial glucose metabolism and modulates the opening of ATP-sensitive potassium channels on the plasma membrane. These channels are composed of eight polypeptides: four sulfonylurea receptor (SUR1) subunits that are members of the ATP-binding cassette transporter family and four Kir6 subunits that are members of the inwardly rectifying potassium channel family [18]. Hypoglycaemic sulfonylureas, such as glibenclamide, glipizide and tolbutamide, stimulate insulin secretion by interaction with SUR1. SUR1-induced closure of the ATP-sensitive potassium channel mediated by sulfonylureas depolarises the plasma membrane and promotes the release of insulin [19].

The meglitinides, such as repaglinide and nateglinide, are non-sulfonylurea insulin secretagogues whose mechanism of action resembles that of the sulfonylureas but is mediated through a different binding site on SUR1 [20]. Unlike the sulfonylureas, the meglitinides stimulate first-phase insulin release in a glucose-sensitive manner [21]. These properties enhance the control of serum glucose and insulin concentrations.

(b) Insulin sensitisers

The storage of lipid in adipocytes and other cells is dysregulated in T2DM and desensitises insulin signalling. As a result, adipocytes do not store triglycerides adequately or release adipokines that regulate food intake. Thiazolidinediones are agonists for the nuclear peroxisome proliferator-activated receptor-gamma (PPAR-gamma), which regulates lipid storage in adipocytes [22]. These agents enhance insulin sensitivity by modulating the production of adipokines, including leptin, adiponectin, resistin and tumour necrosis factor-alpha, by adipocytes. By activating PPAR-gamma thiazolidinediones alter the transcription of genes that regulate glucose and lipid metabolism, such as lipoprotein lipase, fatty acyl-CoA synthase, glucokinase and the glucose transporter GLUT4.

Although PPAR-gamma appears to be an important target for thiazolidinediones the receptor is expressed primarily in adipocytes. That these drugs improve insulin resistance in other cells that do not express PPAR-gamma suggests that there may be additional targets. Thus, thiazolidinediones may also target the adenosine monophosphate-activated protein kinase (AMPK), which is an important fuel sensor that regulates glucose and lipid metabolism.

(c) Biguanides

The most important biguanide in current use is metformin but its mechanism of action is not entirely clear. In diabetic patients metformin decreases hepatic glucose output by decreasing gluconeogenesis and by increasing glucose uptake by skeletal muscle. However, it has also been shown that metformin activates AMPK in liver and muscle [23]. AMPK inhibits acetyl-coenzyme A carboxylase, which is the rate-limiting step of lipogenesis and down-regulates hepatic sterol-regulatory-element-binding-protein-1, which is a major regulator of lipogenic genes. This decreases triglyceride synthesis and facilitates the normalisation of lipid and glucose metabolism.

(d) Incretin mimetics

Exenatide is the only drug in this group currently available in Australia. Exenatide binds to the human GLP-1 receptor, which provides glycaemic control via various mechanisms [24]. It is an insulin secretagogue that stimulates glucose dependent insulin secretion and therefore only works during hyperglycaemia but not during hypoglycaemia. The functioning of pancreatic beta-cells in patients with T2DM may also be improved by exenatide [24]. The secretion of glucagon is suppressed by exenatide, which lowers the blood glucose levels in both fasting and postprandial periods.

Furthermore, exenatide delays gastric emptying in patients with T2DM [24]. This is very important in the regulation of postprandial blood glucose control, since the latter is strongly determined by the delivery of nutrients from the stomach to the small intestine. Exenatide also suppresses appetite, leading to a reduction in food intake and a decrease in body weight in the longer term usually of some kilograms.

It is indicated in Australia as adjunctive therapy to improve glycaemic control in patients with T2DM who are taking metformin, a sulfonylurea, or a combination of metformin and a sulfonylurea but are not achieving adequate glycaemic control.

(e) DPP-IV inhibitors

Another new class of oral antidiabetic agents are the dipeptidyl peptidase IV inhibitors (DPP-IV) or 'incretin enhancers'. They work by delaying the degradation of GLP-1 and thus extend the action of insulin in a glucose dependent manner, while also suppressing the release of glucagon [24]. There are currently three agents in this class approved in Australia: saxagliptin, sitagliptin and vildagliptin.

(f) Alpha-glucosidase inhibitors

These agents, acarbose and miglitol, are taken orally and slow absorption of glucose by inhibiting alpha-glucosidases in the upper GI tract. These enzymes are responsible for converting complex polysaccharide carbohydrates into monosaccharides in a dose dependent fashion. They are less potent than other oral agents with an HbA1c lowering effect of 0.4% to 0.9% generally reported and are usually used in combination with other agents rather than as monotherapy [25].

(g) Insulin

Historically, insulin has been used late in the therapeutic cascade in T2DM after trial and failure to achieve targets through lifestyle modification and oral medications. Since decline in beta-cell function and reduced effectiveness of other agents over time is common in the pathophysiology of T2DM, many if not most patients will require insulin therapy, usually within ten years of the diagnosis of T2DM. In general, physicians have been reluctant to add insulin to therapy because of concerns about increased complexity, risk of hypoglycaemia and patient acceptance, and the possible need to commence insulin injections has been used as a motivator or 'threat' to improve lifestyle factors [26]. Yet insulin is the most efficacious agent to lower blood glucose levels in diabetes mellitus. A variety of insulin regimens are employed including simple basal supplements (with isophane, insulin-glargine or insulin-detemir) to suppress hepatic glucose production, with the addition of prandial doses (regular human insulin or rapid-acting analogue) if needed to control meal-related hyperglycaemia. Premixed insulin combinations are also frequently used. To date, insulin pump therapy has not been generally recommended as a means of insulin delivery in T2DM because simpler injection regimens are effective and cheaper; however increasing use is likely in subgroups with T2DM who have blood glucose levels that are difficult to stabilise.

(h) Combination therapy

The agents outlined above are frequently used in combination, especially if glycaemic targets are not being met with single agents. As yet, there is no clear evidence as to which combinations are most effective or the order in which they are used and often the decision relates to individual patient factors and physician preference. The American Diabetes Association and the European Association for the Study of Diabetes have published a consensus algorithm for the metabolic management of T2DM [27]. The NHMRC of Australia has also published an algorithm as part of the *Evidence-based clinical care guidelines in blood glucose control in type 2 diabetes* [28]. In each of these guidelines, metformin is a cornerstone of therapy, often with the addition of a secretagogue agent as a second line and then the addition or substitution of insulin. A number of combination medications are available that combine metformin with a sulphonylurea, or with a DPP-IV inhibitor. We can expect changes in these drug therapy paradigms as experience is gained with newer agents such as incretin mimetics and the safety concerns with other agents (eg thiazolidinediones) are clarified.

Adverse effects of current therapies and pharmacokinetic considerations

(a) Insulin secretagogues

The major side effect of sulfonylureas and meglitinides is hypoglycaemia, but this is usually mild and by definition is self-treated. Additional adverse effects of meglitinides include upper respiratory tract infections, rhinitis, bronchitis, dizziness and headache.

Pharmacokinetic studies have shown that serum concentrations of sulfonylureas and meglitinides are subject to marked inter-individual variation. Hepatic cytochromes P450 (CYPs) 2C8, 2C9 and 2C19 mediate the phase I oxidation of most of these drugs. These CYPs exhibit polymorphisms that give rise to altered drug pharmacokinetics. The two major variant alleles of CYP2C9 – CYP2C9*2 and CYP2C9*3 – occur at frequencies of ~11% and ~7%, respectively, in Caucasians, but exhibit lower incidence in African-Americans and Asians [29]. These CYP2C9 polymorphisms influence the apparent clearance of tolbutamide, glimepiride and glibenclamide and may complicate therapy in Caucasians in particular [29]. In contrast, *in vivo* pharmacokinetics of gliclazide were dependent on CYP2C19. The poor metaboliser phenotype for CYP2C19 is important in Asians due to the higher incidence of defective CYP2C19*2 and *3 alleles (~20% in Asians, but only 2% in Caucasians).

Repaglinide is eliminated by CYP2C8 and, to a lesser extent, CYP3A4-mediated oxidation to inactive phase I metabolites and by UDP-glucuronosyltransferases to the acyl glucuronide [30]. The CYP2C8*1/*3 genotype has been associated with decreased plasma concentrations of repaglinide. In comparison, nateglinide is metabolised by CYP2C9 and CYP3A4. However, the concordance between CYP2C alleles and the pharmacodynamics of these drugs is imperfect [29], and CYP2C genotyping to direct drug and dose selection is not currently indicated.

(b) Insulin sensitisers

Adverse effects of thiazolidinediones such as rosiglitazone and pioglitazone include weight gain and increase in peripheral fat mass, oedema, anaemia, pulmonary oedema, congestive heart failure and myocardial ischaemia [31]. Oedema is a drug class effect that precludes the use of the thiazolidinediones in patients with evidence of cardiac failure. The incidence of peripheral oedema was about 27% in one Australian study, which was reportedly somewhat higher than in other studies [31]. This was attributed to broader inclusion criteria or to the concurrent use of drugs such as non-steroidal anti-inflammatory drugs and calcium-channel blockers.

CYP2C8 is primarily responsible for the hydroxylation and N-demethylation of rosiglitazone in the human liver, with minor contributions from CYP2C9 [32]. By comparison, pioglitazone is oxidised by CYP2C8 and to a lesser extent by CYP3A4 [33]. The involvement of CYP3A4 in these pathways increases the potential for drug–drug interactions because this enzyme is involved in the metabolism of most drugs. CYP3A4 is also inducible by coadministered drugs including anti-epileptic agents and St John's wort. Thus, avoidance of potent CYP3A4 inducers in patients receiving thiazolidinediones is advisable.

The future role of thiazolidinediones is increasingly uncertain because of safety issues, which also include an increased risk of fracture and osteoporosis as well as exacerbation of diabetic macular oedema in some patients [28]. Predominantly because of concerns about myocardial ischaemia risk, the use of rosiglitazone has been suspended in the European Union and restricted in the US [34] and additional warnings have been added in other countries, including Australia [35]. Recently pioglitazone has been reported to be associated with an increased risk of bladder cancer in those with the longest cumulative exposure; a safety warning has been issued by the FDA [36] and its use has been suspended in some countries. An earlier agent, troglitazone, was discontinued in 2000 because of concerns of liver toxicity [37].

(c) Biguanides

The most serious potential adverse effect of the biguanide class of oral hypoglycaemic agents is lactic acidosis. Phenformin was withdrawn some years ago because of high risk of lactic acidosis. However, metformin is safer than phenformin, and the risk of developing lactic acidosis is low, at less then one in 10 000 patients prescribed the agent [28], providing the drug is not used in patients from high-risk groups. Metformin itself causes few adverse effects with gastrointestinal upset the most common.

Metformin does not undergo oxidative biotransformation and is excreted unchanged by the kidneys [38]. In normal renal function, metformin is unlikely to accumulate but is contraindicated in patients with risk factors for lactic acidosis or drug accumulation because of kidney, liver or cardiac dysfunction. Recently, it has been recognised in guidelines that metformin can be prescribed with vigilance, in people with stable chronic kidney disease down to an eGFR of 30 ml/min [28].

As per the product information, metformin may also lower serum vitamin B12 levels by reducing B12 absorption, and, while this vitamin is stored long term in the liver, it is prudent to assess the blood vitamin B12 level each couple of years to ensure it remains in the health range.

(d) Incretin mimetics

Subcutaneously administered exenatide is generally well tolerated. The most frequently reported adverse effect is nausea which leads to a discontinuation of treatment in about 2%–4% of patients although it usually improves with time [39]. The incidence of nausea is higher during the initial weeks of treatment and declines thereafter. The observed weight loss in patients using exenatide is not associated with the occurrence of nausea. Other, usually minor and transient gastrointestinal complications such as vomiting and diarrhoea are also reported. Further adverse effects include feeling jittery, dizziness and headache [24, 39].

Severe hypoglycaemia causing unconsciousness, is rare in patients using exenatide. However, mild to moderate hypoglycaemia might occur more often with this agent, especially when used in combination with a sulphonylurea [24]. Similar to nausea, the incidence of hypoglycaemia peaks during the initiation of treatment and decreases over time.

Because exenatide delays gastric emptying, it can influence the efficacy of agents that require rapid gastrointestinal absorption. Therefore, medications that depend on threshold concentrations such as oral contraceptives and antibiotics should be administered at least one hour before exenatide.

Exenatide is administered by subcutaneous injection. The initial dosage should be 5 µg twice daily and if tolerated, should be increased to 10 µg twice daily after one month of treatment. Elimination of exenatide occurs mainly via glomerular filtration, hence the use of this agent is not recommended in patients with a severely impaired renal function.

(e) DPP-IV inhibitors

These agents are generally well tolerated. The most common side effects are upper respiratory tract infection and headache. Use is also associated with abdominal pain, nausea and diarrhoea. A key advantage is that this class do not cause hypoglycaemia at nearly the rate of the sulphonylureas, nor do they cause weight gain [24].

(f) Alpha-glucosidase inhibitors

Flatulence and diarrhoea are the main, very common side effects of this class of drugs which often limit their use [25].

(g) Insulin

The predominant adverse effects with insulin therapy are risk of hypoglycaemia and weight gain. One target of therapy in people requiring insulin treatment is that hypoglycaemia should be minimised. Mild hypoglycaemia occurs in ~30% of people at least once a year. Severe hypoglycaemia, which may be life-threatening, through causing trauma or triggering heart events such as myocardial infarct, occurs in 1%–2% yearly [28]. Occurrence of severe hypoglycaemia should be a 'red flag' to the diabetes healthcare team that the entire treatment approach needs revision, to identify the precipitating and predisposing factors and prevent recurrence.

Variations in genes that influence the pharmacodynamics of antidiabetic drugs

(a) Insulin secretagogues

There is considerable inter-individual variation in the response to these drugs. Several SUR1 variants have been identified including common polymorphisms in exon 16 and 18. It has been suggested that the Ser1369Ala variant of the ABCC8 gene that encodes SUR1 and also the Glu23Lys variant of Kir6.2 may be associated with the development of T2DM, especially if additional risk factors such as obesity are present [40].

(b) Insulin sensitisers

PPAR-gamma forms transcriptionally active heterodimers with RXR-beta so that defects in one or both genes may constitute an increased risk of insulin resistance. Thus, the common Pro12Ala variant of PPAR-gamma may contribute to the insulin resistant phenotype [41]. Obese individuals carrying the Ala-12 variant were at higher risk, especially if their dietary mono-unsaturated fatty acid intake was low. The observation that carriers of the RXR-beta C51T genotype who had a high body mass index also had an increased risk of gallstones may be relevant since both obesity and diabetes are important risk factors for gallstones [42]. Apart from possible contributions to disease development, as yet there is little information regarding the action of thiazolidinediones at variant PPAR-gamma.

(c) Biguanides

It now appears that AMPK is also a target for the biguanides. AMPK is a heterotrimeric complex containing a catalytic (alpha) subunit and two regulatory subunits (beta and gamma). In AMPK alpha2-null mice body weight and fat mass were increased and insulin sensitivity was impaired when they were administered a high-fat diet [43]. Single nucleotide polymorphisms in the AMPK alpha2 subunit gene were associated with altered serum lipoprotein concentrations in a patient cohort [44]. Similarly, relationships between diabetes and the −26C/T and IVS1+43C/T polymorphisms of the AMPK gamma2 subunit gene were evaluated. Patients who were homozygous for the −26T allele were associated with a higher risk of developing T2DM and patients who carried the IVS1+43TT variant had higher serum concentrations of triglycerides and cholesterol [45]. To date, information on the role of AMPK beta-subunit gene variation and disease development have not been delineated. Moreover, how AMPK subunit polymorphisms influence metformin efficacy in T2DM is yet to be established.

(d) and (e) Incretin mimetics and DPP-IV inhibitors

A single nucleotide polymorphism in the GLP-1 gene that encodes the major GLP-1 receptor variant, in which threonine 149 is replaced by methionine, is activated differentially by GLP-1 *in vitro* [46]. This receptor variant could account, in part, for different responses to GLP-1 agonists such as exenatide, but this possibility has not yet been actively explored.

With the exception of saxagliptin the available DPP-IV agents are not CYP substrates and so are seldom associated with pharmacokinetic drug-drug interactions. Vildagliptin has a half-life of 2.8 hours and generates several metabolites by CYP-independent pathways [47], whereas the mean apparent half-life for plasma sitagliptin is 9–14 hours [48]. In contrast, saxagliptin is oxidised by CYPs 3A4 and 3A5 to a major metabolite that is pharmacologically active. Instead, renal excretion is the most important elimination pathway for the drugs. It has been established that dose adjustments are recommended for patients with renal impairment.

Management of type 2 diabetes in adolescents

The principles of T2DM therapy in adolescents are similar to those in adults, although a much more limited range of pharmacological agents are approved and used. Again, lifestyle modification including nutritional components, physical activity and weight loss are first-line management tools [4]. However, in many instances, these are insufficient to meet treatment goals and the addition of pharmacotherapy is needed. In most countries, insulin and metformin are the only drugs approved for use in children and adolescents. Sulphonylurea agents are approved in fewer countries, but other agents have generally not yet had adequate appraisal of safety and efficacy in children and adolescents, and are not approved. The treatment options for T2DM in Adolescents and Youth (TODAY) study [49] is a randomised trial evaluating three arms of pharmacological intervention for T2DM in newly diagnosed T2DM adolescents. It compares the efficacy of metformin alone or in combination with rosiglitazone or lifestyle intervention. However, as described earlier, there is increasing concern about emerging serious adverse effects of the thiazolidinediones in any age group and it is unlikely they will have a significant future role. In any case, their known class effect to cause weight gain [50] has always been a disincentive to their use in adolescents.

The choice of initial therapy in T2DM in adolescents depends on the clinical presentation including symptoms, severity of hyperglycaemia and presence or absence of diabetic ketoacidosis. The differentiation of type 1 from type 2 diabetes is not always clear at presentation in adolescents and T2DM can present with ketosis (up to 33%) or ketoacidosis (5%–25%) [51]. In those with severe hyperglycaemia and/or ketosis/ketoacidosis, initial treatment should always be with insulin for initial stabilisation and rapid metabolic control, in conjunction with lifestyle measures. Laboratory investigations (particularly type 1 diabetes related antibodies and C-peptide) and clinical course will help clarify the diagnosis and it is common practice to add metformin and wean insulin to the point of cessation if possible. Asymptomatic patients will usually have a trial of lifestyle modification without drug therapy, while those with mild-to-moderate symptoms without ketosis will usually be treated with metformin in addition to lifestyle modification [52, 53]. The adequacy of ongoing therapy is judged by a number of clinical criteria, but mainly HbA1c <7% and fasting plasma glucose <7 mmol/l.

The proportion of adolescents with T2DM treated with lifestyle modification alone is reported to be 11%–50% [53]. However, as in adults, failure of therapy increases with duration. When lifestyle modification alone is inadequate, metformin is commonly added. Surveys indicate that a substantial proportion of adolescents with T2DM take metformin

(28%–71%) [53]. Metformin is approved by the FDA and also recommended by the American Diabetes Association and the International Society for Paediatric and Adolescent Diabetes as the first-line pharmacological agent in adolescents with T2DM. Doses up to a maximum of 2000 mg per day are usually recommended [53], divided twice daily, although the whole dose can be taken once a day using an extended release preparation which may improve gastrointestinal tolerability and compliance [54]. Metformin is also used as an adjunct to therapy in type 1 diabetes in adolescents with significant insulin resistance. A recent systematic review [55] (including adults and adolescents) demonstrated reduced insulin requirement with metformin, but no improved metabolic outcome and no data on cardiovascular outcomes are available.

When lifestyles measures and metformin are inadequate, or metformin is not tolerated or is contraindicated, insulin is added or substituted. Randomised controlled trials (RCT) comparing various insulin regimens in T2DM in adolescents do not exist, however data from adult experience are generally applicable. A bedtime long-acting insulin analogue is commonly used as initial insulin therapy, but a wide range of other regimens are used according to local preference, including multiple daily injections. Some guidelines in adults [56] suggest that isophane insulin should be used first and insulin analogues reserved for special indications. However there are some data to suggest lower rates of hypoglycaemia with analogues [57] and they are favoured as first-line insulin therapy by paediatric endocrinologists [53]. At present, insulin pump therapy is generally not recommended in T2DM [58, 59]. This is largely due to the increased intensity and cost of therapy, and because targets can often be met with simpler insulin therapy. However lower rates of hypoglycaemia and increased sensitivity to insulin when delivered by pump are attractive potential benefits.

Drugs other than metformin or insulin for adolescents with T2DM are not approved by regulatory authorities, although surveys indicate significant usage by some providers [53]. Newer agents such as GLP1 agonists and DPP4 inhibitors [50] may play a future role, especially in more difficult clinical situations.

Management of obesity in adolescents

Lifestyle intervention through exercise and dietary modification should be the primary treatment for obesity in children and adolescents; drug therapy should be considered a secondary option in refractory situations and usually only in adolescents. Family-targeted behavioural and lifestyle intervention programs have been shown to have clinically significant benefits [16], although these benefits are not always sustained. Drug therapy used as an adjunct to lifestyle intervention in adolescents with obesity was analysed in a recent Cochrane review, including sibutramine, orlistat and metformin [16]. The use of sibutramine (a serotonin and noradrenaline reuptake inhibitor) in adolescents was examined in five studies, with data showing improved BMI over lifestyle alone; adverse events were greater in sibutramine than placebo-treated adolescents, but with low rates of any serious adverse events. Subsequently, however, sibutramine has been withdrawn from most parts of the world, including the US, Europe and Australia because of post-marketing surveillance data which indicated increased risk of myocardial infarction and stroke in patients with existing cardiovascular disease [60]. In two available RCTs of orlistat (a gastrointestinal lipase inhibitor) in combination with lifestyle measures in adolescents there was also a greater improvement in BMI over placebo; however orlistat-treated patients had a much higher prevalence of gastrointestinal adverse effects, particularly oily stool evacuation, cramps, abdominal pain and increased defaecation, but also increased asymptomatic gallstones in one study [61]. While orlistat is still available, in May 2010 the FDA warned about a possible link with severe liver injury in rare cases [62], and labelling was revised to include this.

The most relevant drug used as an adjunct to lifestyle measures in adolescents with obesity is metformin, a biguanide oral hypoglycaemic agent. There are now several studies indicating its safety and efficacy in adolescents with insulin resistance and obesity (or prediabetes). In a recent systematic review and meta-analysis that included five suitable RCTs [63], metformin was concluded to have moderate efficacy in reducing BMI and insulin in hyperinsulinaemic obese children and adolescents, although no long-term studies were available. In pooled analysis, metformin reduced BMI by a mean 1.42 mg/m^2 which was considered moderate compared to available data on subitramine (-1.66 kg/m^2) or orlistat (-0.76 kg/m^2) [16]. Gastrointestinal adverse events were more frequently reported in those receiving metformin (risk difference 10%–14%), but there were no serious adverse events. There is a need to further evaluate metformin in longer-term studies as an adjunct to more intensive lifestyle interventions [64]. Even without this further evidence, metformin is commonly used in clinical practice in adolescents with obesity, insulin resistance and other features of metabolic syndrome because of its favourable safety profile and its established use as pharmacotherapy in T2DM in adolescents.

Management of obesity in adults and commercial programs in Australia

There is a wide range of weight-loss programs available including commercial weight-loss programs provided in the pharmacy as well as Jenny Craig and Weight Watchers, internet-based programs, weight-loss products such as meal replacements available from supermarkets, and community-based weight-management or exercise programs. The Weight Management Council of Australia provides a voluntary code of practice for commercial weight-loss companies [65]. Although commercial weight-loss programs are very popular, they usually only induce large short-term changes in weight and these changes are mostly transient. There is a need to establish evidence-based practices that demonstrate efficacy, safety and long-term weight maintenance. At this point in time there is very little data on the efficacy or outcomes of the commercial weight-loss programs in Australia [75].

Various factors affect an individual's efforts in terms of short-term weight loss and maintenance [66]. The majority of overweight adults have a history of previous weight-loss treatments. A study by Burke et al. (2008) examined individuals' past experiences with weight-loss treatments [67]. Program features identified as least satisfying included dissatisfaction with diet product (20.4%) and concerns about safety of program or product

(17.2%). The most common reasons for difficulty in successfully losing weight that were identified were difficulty to make and maintain lifestyle change (38%), no time (32.4%) and lack of support (18.5%). Similarly, a study by Jeffery et al. (2004) examined how individuals' attitudes about weight-loss efforts change during weight loss [68]. Individuals who lost less weight during the six months reported feeling more negative reactions. Reported satisfaction in relation to weight-loss effort declined over time, and in the last two months, perceived benefits were approximately equal to perceived costs of weight change.

Various studies have shown that superior weight loss occurs when cognitive behavioural therapy is added to diet and exercise interventions. Health education is required to facilitate patients making informed choices about their health. A study by Swift et al. (2009) showed that intended weight loss and outcomes were positively associated with health beliefs [69]. The results of this study also suggest that healthcare professionals may find it productive to discuss the social and aesthetic benefits associated with weight management. Cognitive strategies that have been identified in weight management include increasing awareness of negative thoughts, problemsolving alternatives to negative self-talk and pre-intervention strategies such as motivational interviewing and establishing objective weight-loss outcomes [70]. Establishing readiness for change via motivational interviewing has been shown to predict sustained change efforts in physical exercise, dietary change and adherence [70].

In all of these programs there is a need to clarify patients' expectations for weight-loss outcomes, provide objective and realistic goals, and re-evaluate these goals over the course of management.

Management of type 2 diabetes and obesity in the health system

There are a variety of effective therapies available and new approaches to be trialled in future. Notwithstanding the availability of effective therapies and treatment guidelines, translation of evidence into practice and delivering optimal care represents a significant challenge to healthcare systems. Because of the nature of T2DM and the need for patients to understand and take control of their lifestyle in order to reduce their health risk, people with T2DM are especially vulnerable and need intensive chronic disease management and ongoing support. From a systems perspective, however, limited patient access to diabetes healthcare professionals, as a result of personnel shortages [71], especially in rural and remote areas, and lack of systems to support chronic disease management with continuity of care [72, 73], are well recognised barriers to achieving optimal health outcomes for diabetes. Hence, there is a need to develop cost-effective innovative models of diabetes and weight management care based on more intensive continuity of care [74] including self-management support, regular monitoring and follow-up in order to enable patients to achieve the recommended targets.

Pharmacists in type 2 diabetes care

In recent years, pharmacists, as highly trained healthcare professionals with expertise in medicines, have sought to develop an expanded role in diabetes care to meet the burgeoning needs of this growing patient population. There are compelling arguments which support this expanded involvement. Community pharmacies provide an established and visible network, extending to remote areas, of easily accessible healthcare professionals. Through regular and less formal contact than that with doctors, pharmacists are able to build strong relationships with patients and become a reliable source of information. Pharmacists can also have ongoing relationships with other healthcare providers and can serve as the 'bridge' between healthcare providers and the patients, thus ensuring continuity of care. Therefore visits to the community pharmacy offer an excellent opportunity to screen at-risk patients and to provide education and support to diagnosed T2DM patients, particularly if they do not regularly visit a general practitioner (GP) or diabetes educator. In addition, as medications play a key role in preventing the complications of T2DM, ensuring their effectiveness through monitoring and adherence support as well as screening for drug -related problems, is critical to achieving improved health outcomes.

Specific services that pharmacists have offered patients in T2DM include opportunistic screening for undiagnosed disease [76], diabetes self-management education, medication-adherence support and medication management such as the at-home medicines review, ensuring the quality and evidence-based use of medications, monitoring clinical outcome measures eg blood glucose levels, blood pressure, lipid levels, and reminding patients of the importance of regular examinations for diabetic complications [77].

Two recent systematic reviews of the effects of these pharmacist–outpatient interventions on adults with diabetes mellitus showed significant improvements in HbA1C for patients in a diverse group of clinical settings and countries. Overall, the results suggest that pharmacist interventions can reduce long-term costs by improving glycaemic control and thus diminishing future diabetes complications [78, 79].

Diabetes care in Australian pharmacy

In 1999, a specialised T2DM service, the Diabetes Medication Assistance Service (DMAS), was developed for delivery in Australian community pharmacy. Its focus was on the provision of self-management support through a series of regular visits with a credentialed pharmacist to assist people with T2DM more effectively self-manage their condition and improve their use of medicines. At each visit, the pharmacist tailored the consultation to the individual needs of the patient. By using motivational interviewing and goal setting, in combination with education, the pharmacist aimed to empower the patient to take better control of their diabetes [80].

A systematic program of research involving two pilot studies, an RCT and an implementation trial has provided a strong evidence base for the clinical efficacy and cost-effectiveness of the DMAS. The RCT used a multi-site, control versus intervention, repeated measures design within five states in Australia. Fifty-six community pharmacies, 28 interventions and 28 controls, were randomly selected from a representative sample of urban and rural areas. Intervention pharmacies delivered the DMAS to patients with T2DM during the course of five visits to the pharmacy over a period of six months. Control pharmacists assessed patients at birth and six months and delivered no intervention. A total of 289 patients (149 interventions and 140 controls) completed the study. Significantly greater improvements in glycaemic control were seen in the intervention group compared to the control, ie a mean reduction in HbA1c of –0.97% (95% CI: –0.8, –1.14) in the intervention group compared with –0.27% (95% CI: –0.15, –0.39) in the control group. Improvements were also seen in blood pressure control and quality of life in the intervention group. Pharmacists identified a range of interventions (4309 for 149 patients) to improve the care and wellbeing of their patients. Monitoring of the progress of the disease and as well as the outcomes of the interventions appeared to be the essential element of the disease state management process. Both pharmacists and patients identified the outstanding benefits of the service and expressed great satisfaction with service provision. The DMAS was shown to be cost-effective when compared to other government funded programs [75].

The RCT was followed by a national implementation trial, the Diabetes Pilot Program (DPP) which aimed to answer three further questions regarding the DMAS service: 1) what are the key barriers and facilitators to national implementation of the DMAS service 2) what is the optimal number of pharmacy visits and 3) what is the sustainability of clinical improvements beyond DMAS service delivery. A national quota sample of 90 community pharmacies in Australia were randomly assigned into Group 1 (six-month DMAS) or Group 2 (12-month DMAS) and subsequently recruited a total of 524 patients. The implementation process was carefully tracked with data collected through individual or group interviews with 100 patients, 28 pharmacists and 41 GPs at the beginning and at the end of DMAS to explore their experiences and perceptions of DMAS and to identify barriers and facilitators. A wide range of clinical (HbA1c, blood pressure, lipids) and quality of life outcome measures were assessed.

The results indicated that the DMAS may be successfully implemented in diverse community pharmacy settings providing: 1) the pharmacy has adequate staff and infrastructure; 2) there are good pharmacist-GP relationships; 3) the pharmacy has a pool of eligible patients; 4) there is effective promotion and integration of the DMAS within the healthcare sector; and 5) there is adequate remuneration for service delivery. The clinical outcomes of the implementation trial mirrored those of the RCT. Both the six-month and 12-month DMAS resulted in significant and similar reductions in HbA1c (–0.9; 95% CI:–0.65, –1.12), total cholesterol (–0.3; 95% CI:–0.07, –0.38), triglycerides (–0.3; 95% CI:–0.10, –0.53) and overall ten year CVD risk; moreover the benefits were sustained up to 12 months after the end of the DMAS [81]. The extent and sustainability of clinical improvements achieved by the DMAS together with the resulting reduction in cardiovascular risk should translate into future cost savings to healthcare systems by delaying and reducing diabetes related complications. Collectively these studies support the feasibility and efficacy of community pharmacy T2DM diabetes care in the Australian healthcare setting.

In addition to the effectiveness of pharmacy support for people with T2DM, several studies have also supported the feasibility and efficacy of opportunistic screening for T2DM in community pharmacy [82–84]. Community pharmacy provides a logical site with its established, expansive and visible network of easily accessible health professionals, able to access a broad population who are apparently healthy and who rarely come into contact with GPs or nurses.

Weight-management programs in community pharmacy

In the context of weight management in the UK, the government recognised the contribution that pharmacy can make in managing the obesity epidemic in the white paper *Pharmacy in England* [85]. In doing so, pharmacy contract negotiators recommended a government-funded national weight-management service initiative in community pharmacies [86].

Several other studies have illustrated that community pharmacists' involvement in weight-loss programs has been associated with successful weight loss. A study in Denmark reported the results of 'slimming courses' held at 19 community pharmacies for 269 obese patients [87]. Average weight loss was 5.3 kg for females and 6.2 kg for males. At one year follow-up 20% of the patients who had completed the course had maintained a weight loss of greater than five kilograms [87]. Community pharmacists could play a key role in providing holistic weight-loss programs and collaborating with healthcare professionals, rather than being seen as product suppliers [88].

A recent Pharmacy Pulse survey showed that more than 17% of pharmacies in Australia want to be known as a destination for a weight-loss solution [89]. In 2003, the National Pharmacy Database Project reported that 8.7% of 1131 Australian community pharmacies surveyed conducted weight-management programs by trained staff [90]. At present, the majority of commercial weight-loss programs are based on very low-calorie diets that are mostly achieved by meal replacement shakes and soups. Other factors necessary for weight change such as increased physical activity are supplementary to the weight-loss product and used to augment the product specifically. Most programs provide ongoing support either by in-store consultants, a website or telephone support services.

Lifeweight™ was the first nationally released weight-management program specifically designed for community pharmacy. The program combines the product Xenical® (orlistat) with pharmacist-delivered cognitive services to provide a holistic package [75].

It was launched in 2004, following the decision to down schedule Xenical® (orlistat) from a prescription to pharmacist-only medication. The program was developed in collaboration with the Pharmacy Guild of Australia, the Pharmaceutical Society of Australia, the Australian Institute of Pharmacy Management and Roche, the manufacturers of Xenical®. Training programs and resources were made available for pharmacists and pharmacy assistants to increase their skills in delivering the program. Content of the program is comprehensive and well structured, based on evidence-based material and is aligned with National Health and Medical Research Council guidelines [75]. Baseline and longitudinal patient data is collected including age, weight, body mass index, target weight, measured progress to target, final weight on completion of or withdrawal from the program. Adoption and uptake of Lifeweight™ in community pharmacies has declined in recent times, as both consumers and pharmacists have articulated a need for a well-planned, accredited, community pharmacy-based, remunerated service that would deliver a more comprehensive collaborative service [91]. Such a service would ideally not be based on a product but a wholistic, evidence-based program. This would allow for increased numbers of overweight and obese Australians to have access to a consistent, evidence-based, integrated healthcare weight-management program. Improvement in health for the overweight and obese, and better management of diabetes, hypertension, hypercholesterolemia and other obesity-related health issues would be the outcome. This would result in decreased costs to the healthcare system due to reduced mortality and morbidity attributed to the overweight and obese Australian population.

Conclusion

Innovation of service delivery is critical to address the burgeoning problems of T2DM, obesity and related diseases. The complications of these diseases place a considerable burden on the healthcare system.

The review of available pharmacotherapy for T2DM and obesity shows that there is considerable inter-individual variation in response to the various drug classes and the reasons for this are currently under investigation. In adolescents and children the approach to therapy is not merely a reflection of recommendations for adults. In terms of support for pharmacotherapy and lifestyle interventions, community pharmacy programs have provided evidence of effectiveness in T2DM, however at this point in time support for weight-loss programs has been inhibited by the focus on individual commercial products. Nevertheless, community pharmacists are a valuable resource of trained healthcare professionals that should be utilised to provide diabetes and obesity prevention and care services as part of an integrated primary care sector approach.

Acknowledgements

The authors would like to thank Kate LeMay for her careful editing of this chapter.

References

1. Australian Institute of Health and Welfare (2011). Diabetes [Online]. Available: www.aihw.gov.au/diabetes/ [Accessed 2 June 2011].

2. Diabetes Australia Victoria (2008). Diabetes facts [Online]. Available: www.diabetesvic.org.au/health-professionals/diabetes-facts [Accessed 2 June 2011].

3. Colagiuri S, Colagiuri R, Conway B, Grainger D & Davey P (2003). DiabCo$t Australia: assessing the burden of type 2 diabetes in Australia. Diabetes Australia, Canberra [Online]. Available: www.australiandiabetescouncil.com/AustralianDiabetesCouncil/media/PDFs/diabcost_finalreport.pdf [Accessed 2 June 2011].

4. Rosenbloom AL, Silverstein JH, Amemiya S, Zeitler P & Klingensmith GJ (2009). Type 2 diabetes in children and adolescents. *Pediatric Diabetes*, 10(12): 17–32.

5. Han JC, Lawlor DA & Kimm SY (2010). Childhood obesity. *The Lancet*, 375(9727): 1737–48.

6. World Health Organization (2006). Obesity and overweight fact sheet No 311 [Online]. Available: www.who.int/mediacentre/factsheets/fs311/en/index.html [Accessed 23 May 2010].

7. Australian Bureau of Statistics (2009). National health survey: summary of results, 2007–08. Canberra: Australian Bureau of Statistics.

8. National Preventative Health Task Force (2009). *Australia: the healthiest country by 2020. The report of the National Preventative Health Strategy: the roadmap for action.* Including addendum for October 2008 to June 2009 [Online]. Available: www.health.gov.au/internet/preventativehealth/publishing.nsf/Content/tech-obesity [Accessed 5 September 2011].

9. House of Representatives Standing Committee on Health and Ageing (2009). *Weighing it up: obesity in Australia.* Canberra: Commonwealth of Australia.

10. World Health Organization (2000). *WHO Technical Report Series 894. Obesity: preventing and managing the global epidemic.* Report of a World Health Organization consultation. Geneva: World Health Organization.

11. Australian Institute of Health and Welfare (2008). *Australia's health 2008* Cat. no. AUS 99. Canberra: Australian Institute of Health and Welfare.

12. National Health and Medical Research Council (2003). *Clinical practice guidelines for the management of overweight and obesity in adults.* Canberra: Commonwealth of Australia.

13. UK Prospective Diabetes Study (UKPDS) Group (1998). Intensive blood-glucose control with sulphonylureas or insulin compared with conventional treatment and risk of complications in patients with type 2 diabetes (UKPDS 33). *The Lancet*, 352(9131): 837–53.

14. Patel A, Group AC, MacMahon S, Chalmers J, Neal B, Woodward M, et al. (2007). Effects of a fixed combination of perindopril and indapamide on macrovascular and microvascular outcomes in patients with type 2 diabetes mellitus (the ADVANCE trial): a randomised controlled trial. *The Lancet*, 370(9590): 829–40.

15. Del Prato S (2009). Megatrials in type 2 diabetes: from excitement to frustration? *Diabetologia*, 52(7): 1219–26.

16. Oude Luttikhuis H, Baur L, Jansen H, Shrewsbury VA, O'Malley C, Stolk RP & Summerbell CD (2009). Interventions for treating obesity in children. *Cochrane Database of Systematic Reviews*, 2009(1):CD001872.

17. Diabetes Australia (2011). *Diabetes management in general practice.* 17th edn 2011–12 [Online]. Available: www.racgp.org.au/guidelines/diabetes [Accessed 27 July 2011].

18. Seino S (1999). ATP-sensitive potassium channels: a model of heteromultimeric potassium channel/receptor assemblies. *Annual Review of Physiology*, 61(88): 337–62.

19. Yokoshiki H, Sunagawa M, Seki T & Sperelakis N (1998). ATP-sensitive K+ channels in pancreatic, cardiac, and vascular smooth muscle cells. *American Journal of Physiology*, 274(1 Pt 1): C25–37.

20. Meyer M, Chudziak F, Schwanstecher C, Schwanstecher M & Panten U (1999). Structural requirements of sulphonylureas and analogues for interaction with sulphonylurea receptor subtypes. *British Journal of Pharmacology*, 128(1): 27–34.

21. Modi P (2007). Diabetes beyond insulin: review of new drugs for treatment of diabetes mellitus. *Current Drug Discovery Technologies*, 4(1): 39–47.

22. Lehmann JM, Moore LB, Smith-Oliver TA, Wilkison WO, Willson TM & Kliewer SA (1995). An antidiabetic thiazolidinedione is a high affinity ligand for peroxisome proliferator-activated receptor gamma (PPAR gamma). *Journal of Biological Chemistry*, 270(22): 12953–956.

23. Zhou G, Myers R, Li Y, Chen Y, Shen X, Fenyk-Melody J, et al. (2001). Role of AMP-activated protein kinase in mechanism of metformin action. *Journal of Clinical Investigation*, 108(8): 1167–74.

24. Campbell RK (2011). Clarifying the role of incretin-based therapies in the treatment of type 2 diabetes mellitus. *Clinical Therapeutics*, 33(5): 511–27.

25. Campbell LK, White JR & Campbell RK (1996). Acarbose: its role in the treatment of diabetes mellitus. *Annals of Pharmacotherapy*, 30(11): 1255–62.

26. Pevrot M, Rubin RR, Lauritzen T, Skovlund SE, Snoek FJ, Matthews DR, et al. (2005). Resistance to insulin therapy among patients and providers. *Diabetes Care*, 28(11): 2673–79.

27. Nathan DM, Buse JB, Davidson MB, Ferrannini ELE, Holman RR, Sherwin R, et al. (2009). Medical management of hyperglycaemia in type 2 diabetes: a consensus algorithm for the initiation and adjustment of therapy. A consensus statement of the American Diabetes Association and the European Association for the Study of Diabetes. *Diabetes Care*, 32(1): 193–203

28. Colagiuri S, Dickinson S, Girgis S & Colagiuri R (2009). *National evidence-based guidelines for blood glucose control in type 2 diabetes*. Canberra: Diabetes Australia and the NHMRC.

29. Kirchheiner J, Roots I, Goldammer M, Rosenkranz B & Brockmöller J (2005). Effect of genetic polymorphisms in cytochrome P450 (CYP) 2C9 and CYP2C8 on the pharmacokinetics of oral antidiabetic drugs: clinical relevance. *Clinical Pharmacokinetics*, 44(12): 1209–25.

30. Bidstrup TB, Bjørnsdottir I, Sidelmann UG, Thomsen MS & Hansen KT (2003). CYP2C8 and CYP3A4 are the principal enzymes involved in the human in vitro biotransformation of the insulin secretagogue repaglinide. *British Journal of Clinical Pharmacology*, 56(3): 305–14.

31. Hussein Z, Wentworth JM, Nankervis AJ, Proietto J & Colman PG (2004). Effectiveness and side effects of thiazolidinediones for type 2 diabetes: real-life experience from a tertiary hospital. *Medical Journal of Australia*, 181(10): 536–39.

32. Niemi M, Backman JT & Neuvonen PJ (2004). Effects of trimethoprim and rifampin on the pharmacokinetics of the cytochrome P450 2C8 substrate rosiglitazone. *Clinical Pharmacology and Therapeutics*, 76(3): 239–49.

33. Jaakkola T, Laitila J, Neuvonen PJ & Backman JT (2006). Pioglitazone is metabolised by CYP2C8 and CYP3A4 in vitro: potential for interactions with CYP2C8 inhibitors. *Basic and Clinical Pharmacology and Toxicology*, 99(1): 44–51.

34. US Food and Drug Administration (2010). FDA significantly restricts access to the diabetes drug Avandia [Online]. Available: www.fda.gov/Drugs/DrugSafety/PostmarketDrugSafetyInformationforPatientsandProviders/ucm226956.htm [Accessed 27 July 2011].

35. Therapeutics Goods Administration (2010). Rosiglitazone (Avandia/Avandamet). Advisory statement [Online]. Available: www.tga.gov.au/safety/alerts-medicine-rosiglitazone-100924.htm [Accessed 27 July 2011].

36. US Food and Drug Administration (2010). Actos (pioglitazone): ongoing safety review. Potential increased risk of bladder cancer [Online]. Available: www.fda.gov/Safety/MedWatch/SafetyInformation/SafetyAlertsforHumanMedicalProducts/ucm226257.htm [Accessed 27 July 2011].

37. US Food and Drug Administration (2010). Rezulin (troglitazone). [Online]. Available: www.fda.gov/Safety/MedWatch/SafetyInformation/SafetyAlertsforHumanMedicalProducts/ucm173081.htm [Accessed 27 July 2011].

38. Graham GG, Punt J, Arora M, Day RO, Doogue MP, Duong JK, et al. (2011). Clinical pharmacokinetics of metformin. *Clinical Pharmacokinetics*, 50(2): 81–98.

39. Amori RE, Lau J & Pittas AG (2007). Efficacy and safety of incretin therapy in type 2 diabetes. *Journal of the American Medical Association*, 298(2): 194–206.

40. Laukkanen O, Pihlajamäki J, Lindström J, Eriksson J, Valle TT, Hämäläinen H, et al. (2004). Polymorphisms of the SUR1 (ABCC8) and Kir6.2 (KCNJ11) genes predict the conversion from impaired glucose tolerance to type 2 diabetes: the Finnish diabetes prevention study. *Journal of Clinical Endocrinology and Metabolism*, 89(12): 6286–90.

41. Hasstedt SJ, Ren QF, Teng K & Elbein SC (2001). Effect of the peroxisome proliferator-activated receptor-g2 pro12Ala variant on obesity, glucose homeostasis, and blood pressure in members of familial type 2 diabetic kindreds. *Journal of Clinical Endocrinology and Metabolism*, 86(2): 536–41.

42. Chang SC, Rashid A, Gao YT, Andreotti G, Shen MC, Wang BS, et al. (2008). Polymorphism of genes related to insulin sensitivity and the risk of biliary tract cancer and biliary stone: a population-based case-control study in Shanghai, China. *Carcinogenesis*, 29(5): 944–48.

43. Fujii N, Ho RC, Manabe Y, Jessen N, Toyoda T, Holland WL, et al. (2008). Ablation of AMP-activated protein kinase a2 activity exacerbates insulin resistance induced by high-fat feeding of mice. *Diabetes*, 57(11): 2958–66.

44. Spencer-Jones NJ, Ge D, Snieder H, Perks U, Swaminathan R, Spector TD, et al. (2006). AMP-kinase a2 subunit gene PRKAA2 variants are associated with total cholesterol, low-density lipoprotein-cholesterol and high-density lipoprotein-cholesterol in normal women. *Journal of Medical Genetics*, 43(12): 936–42.

45. Xu M, Li X, Wang JG, Du P, Hong J, Gu W, et al. (2005). Glucose and lipid metabolism in relation to novel polymorphisms in the 5'-AMP-activated protein kinase g2 gene in Chinese. *Molecular Genetics and Metabolism*, 86(3): 372–78.

46. Beiborn M, Worrall CI, McBride EW & Kopin AS (2005). A human glucagon-like peptide-1 receptor polymorphism results in reduced agonist responsiveness. *Regulation Peptides*, 130(1–2): 1–6.

47. Tran HH, Smith PYH, Batard H, Wang Y, Einolf L, Gu H, et al. (2009). Absorption, metabolism, and excretion of [14C]vildagliption, a novel dipeptiful peptidase 4 inhibitor, in humans. *Drug Metabolism & Disposition*, 37(3): 536–44.

48. Herman GA, Mistry GC, Bergman YB, Wang AQ, Zeng W, Chen L, et al. (2011). Evaluation of pharmacokinetic parameters and dipeptidyl peptidase-4 inhibition following single doses of sitagliptin in healthy, young Japanese males. *British Journal of Clinical Pharmacology*, 71(3): 429–36.

49. Zeitler P, Epstein L, Grey M, Hirst K, Kaufman F, Tamborlane W, et al. (2007). Treatment options for type 2 diabetes in adolescents and youth: a study of the comparative efficacy of metformin alone or in combination with rosiglitazone or lifestyle intervention in adolescents with type 2 diabetes. *Pediatric Diabetes*, 8(2): 74–87.

50. Waugh N, Cummins E, Royle P, Clar C, Marien M, Richter B, et al. (2010). Newer agents for blood glucose control in type 2 diabetes: systematic review and economic evaluation. *NIHR Health Technology Assessment Journal*, 14(36): 1–248.

51. American Diabetes Association (2000). Type 2 diabetes in children and adolescents. *Diabetes Care*, 23(3): 381–89.

52. Laffel L & Svoren BM (2011). Management of type 2 diabetes in children and adolescents. UpToDate Inc [Online]. Available: www.uptodate.com/contents/management-of-type-2-diabetes-mellitus-in-children-and-adolescents?source=search_result&selectedTitle=1~150 [Accessed 17 June 2011 2011].

53. Flint A & Arslanian S (2011). Treatment of type 2 diabetes in youth. *Diabetes Care*, 34(Suppl. 2): S177–83.

54. Jabbour S & Ziring B (2011). Advantages of extended-release metformin in patients with type 2 diabetes mellitus. *Postgraduate Medicine*, 123(1): 15–23.

55. Vella S, Buetow L, Royle P, Livingstone S, Colhoun HM & Petrie JR (2010). The use of metformin in type 1 diabetes: a systematic review of efficacy. *Diabetologia*, 53(5): 809–20.

56. Adler AI, Shaw EJ, Stokes T & Ruiz F (2009). Newer agents for blood glucose control in type 2 diabetes: summary of NICE guidance. *British Medical Journal*, 338: b1668.

57. Nathan DM, Buse JB, Davidson MB, Heine RJ, Holman RR, Sherwin R, et al. (2006). Management of hyperglycemia in type 2 diabetes: a consensus algorithm for the initiation and adjustment of therapy. A consensus statement from the American Diabetes Association and the European Association for the Study of Diabetes. *Diabetes Care*, 29(8): 1963–72.

58. Cummins E, Royle P, Snaith A, Greene A, Robertson L, McIntyre L, et al. (2010). Clinical effectiveness and cost-effectiveness of continuous subcutaneous insulin infusion for diabetes: systematic review and economic evaluation. *NIHR Health Technology Assessment Journal*, 14(11): iii–iv, xi–xvi, 1–181.

59. Kirk SE (2003). Insulin pump therapy for type 2 diabetes. *Current Diabetes Reports*, 3(5): 373–77.

60. US Food and Drug Administration (2010). Meridia (sibutramine): market withdrawal due to risk of serious cardiovascular events [Online]. Available: www.fda.gov/safety/medwatch/safetyinformation/safetyalertsforhumanmedicalproducts/ucm228830.htm [Accessed 17 June 2011].

61. Chanoine JP, Hampl S, Jensen C, Boldrin M & Hauptman J (2005). Effect of orlistat on weight and body composition in obese adolescents: a randomized controlled trial. *Journal of the American Medical Association*, 293(23): 2873–83.

62. US Food and Drug Administration (2010). Orlistat (marketed as Alli and Xenical): labeling change [Online]. Available: www.fda.gov/Safety/MedWatch/SafetyInformation/SafetyAlertsforHumanMedicalProducts/ucm213448.htm [Accessed 17 May 2011].

63. Park MH, Kinra S, Ward KJ, White B & Viner RM (2009). Metformin for obesity in children and adolescents: a systematic review. *Diabetes Care*, 32(9): 1743–45.

64. Garnett SP, Baur LA, Noakes M, Steinbeck K, Woodhead HJ, Burrell S, et al. (2010). Researching effective strategies to improve insulin sensitivity in children and teenagers: RESIST. A randomised control trial investigating the effects of two different diets on insulin sensitivity in young people with insulin resistance and/or pre-diabetes. *BMC Public Health*, 10: 575.

65. Weight Management Council Australia (2005). *Weight management code of practice*. 3rd edn. East Melbourne: Weight Management Council Australia Limited.

66. Elfhag K & Rossner S (2005). Who succeeds in maintaining weight loss? A conceptual review of factors associated with weight loss maintenance and weight regain. *Obesity Reviews*, 6(1): 67–85.

67. Burke LE, Steenkiste A, Music E & Styn MA (2008). A descriptive study of past experiences with weight-loss treatment. *Journal of American Dietetic Association*, 108(4): 640–47.

68. Jeffery RW, Kelly KM, Rothman AJ Sherqood NE & Boutelle KN (2004). The weight loss experience: a descriptive analysis. *Annals of Behavioral Medicine*, 27(2): 100–06.

69. Swift JA, Glazebrook C, Anness A & Goddard R (2009). Obesity-related knowledge and beliefs in obese adults attending a specialist weight-management service: implications for weight loss over 1 year. *Patient Education and Counseling*, 71(1): 70–76.

70. Van Dorsten B & Lindley EM (2008). Cognitive and behavioral approaches in the treatment of obesity. *Endocrinology & Metabolism Clinics of North America*, 37(4): 905–22.

71. Burge MR, Lucero S, Rassam AG & Schade DS (2000). What are the barriers to medical care for patients with newly diagnosed diabetes mellitus? *Diabetes, Obesity and Metabolism*, 2: 351–54.

72. Georgiou A, Burns J, McKenzie S, Penn D, Flack J & Harris MF (2006). Monitoring change in diabetes care using diabetes registers: experience from divisions of general practice. *Australian Family Physician*, 35(1–2): 77–80.

73. Proudfoot J, Infante F, Holton C, Powell-Davies G, Bubner T, Beilby J, et al. (2007). Organisational capacity and chronic disease care: an Australian general practice perspective. *Australian Family Physician*, 36(4): 193–288.

74. Dennis SM, Zwar N, Griffiths R, Roland M, Hasan I, Powell Davies G, et al. (2008). Chronic disease management in primary care: from evidence to policy. *Medical Journal of Australia*, 188(Suppl. 8): S53–S56.

75. Rieck A, Clifford R & Everett A (2006). *Community pharmacy weight management project (Stages 1 and 2)*. Crawley: University of Western Australia.

76. Krass I & Armour CL (2011). Preventing disease: screening in the pharmacy. In Krska J (Ed). *Pharmaceutical public health* (pp221–44). London: Pharmacy Press.

77. Krass I, Armour CL, Mitchell B, Brillant M, Dienaar R, Hughes J, et al. (2007). The Pharmacy Diabetes Care Program: assessment of a community pharmacy diabetes service model in Australia. *Diabetic Medicine,* 24(6): 677–83

78. Wubben DP & Vivian EM (2008). Effects of pharmacist outpatient interventions on adults with diabetes mellitus: a systematic review. *Pharmacotherapy*, 28(4): 421–36.

79. George PP, Molina JA, Cheah J, Chan SC & Lim BP (2010). The evolving role of the community pharmacist in chronic disease management: a literature review. *Annals of the Academy of Medicine Singapore*, 39(11): 861–67.

80. Mitchell B, Armour C, Lee M, Song YJ, Stewart K, Peterson G, et al. (2011). Diabetes medication assistance service: the pharmacist's role in supporting patient self-management of type 2 diabetes (T2DM) in Australia. *Patient Education and Counseling*, 83(3): 288–94.

81. Krass I, Mitchell B, Song YJ, Stewart K, Peterson G, Hughes J, et al. (2011). Diabetes medication assistance service stage 1: impact and sustainability of glycaemic and lipids control in patients with Type 2 diabetes. *Diabetic Medicine*, 28(8): 987–93.

82. Hourihan F, Krass I & Chen TC (2003). Rural community pharmacy: a feasible site for a health promotion and screening service for cardiovascular risk factors. *Australian Journal of Rural Health*, 11(1): 28–35.

83. Hersberger KE, Botomino A, Mancini M & Bruppacher R (2006). Sequential screening for diabetes: evaluation of a campaign in Swiss community pharmacies. *Pharmacy World & Science*, 28(3): 171–79.

84. Krass I, Mitchell B, Clarke P, Brillant M, Dienaar R, Hughes J, et al. (2007). Pharmacy Diabetes Care Program: analysis of two screening methods for undiagnosed type 2 diabetes in Australian community pharmacy. *Diabetes Research and Clinical Practice*, 75(3): 339–47.

85. Department of Health (2008). *Pharmacy in England: building on strengths – delivering the future.* London: HM Government.

86. Blenkinsopp A, Anderson C & Armstrong M (2010). Community pharmacy's contribution to improving the public's health: the case of weight management. *International Journal of Pharmacy Practice*, 16(3): 123–25.

87. Toubro S DI, Hermansen I, Herborg H & Astrup A (1999). Dietary guidelines on obesity at Danish pharmacies: results of a 12-week course with a 1-year follow-up. *Ugeskrift for Laeger*, 161(38): 5308–13.

88. Maryon-Davis A (2005). Weight management in primary care: how can it be made more effective? *Proceedings of the Nutrition Society*, 64(1): 97–103.

89. Offord L (2009). Turning losses into healthy gains. *Australian Journal of Pharmacy*, 90(1065): 42–44, 46.

90. Berbatis CG, Sunderland VB, Mills CR & Bulsara M (2003). *National Pharmacy Database Project.* Perth: Curtin University of Technology of Western Australia.

91. Offord L (2006). Lifeweight's just like losing weight: stick to the program (The Lifeweight weight loss program). *The Australian Journal of Pharmacy*, 87: 30–33.

19

Diabetes healthcare strategies to cope with the growing epidemic

Marg McGill[1,2,3] and Jane Overland[1,2]

Globally, the spectrum of diabetes services varies from a single healthcare provider working in an isolated community setting, to small groups of primary care doctors and nurses working in health centres or district hospitals, through to highly sophisticated tertiary units in major urban areas with access to a range of specialists, nurses and other diabetes team members. In this chapter we explore how diabetes care may be best delivered at these various levels, taking into consideration political, cultural and economic environments. Not every case of diabetes can be looked after at the community level. Likewise, not every case of diabetes can be looked after at the specialist level. How to support and balance these two services to optimise healthcare delivery for the total community of people with diabetes, is one of the most important questions in organising diabetes care.

Diabetes care is becoming a priority for health systems as costs and health outcomes are being closely scrutinised. Traditional health systems are designed to provide symptom-driven responses to acute illnesses. Consequently, they are poorly configured to meet the needs of the chronically ill. Simply seeing more and more patients within the traditional model will lead to shorter consultations that can only focus on a quick review of blood glucose and providing a prescription. Models of care that are focused on outcomes and prevention of acute and chronic complications have been developed and proposed as viable alternatives to current care systems to address these problems.

Globally, the spectrum of diabetes services varies from a single healthcare provider working in an isolated community setting, to small groups of primary care doctors and nurses working in clinics, health centres or district hospitals, through to highly sophisticated tertiary units in major urban areas with access to a range of specialist physicians, nurses and other diabetes team members. In this chapter we explore how diabetes care may be best delivered at these various levels. Not every case of diabetes can be looked after at the community level. Likewise, not every case of diabetes can be looked after at the specialist

1   Diabetes Centre, Royal Prince Alfred Hospital.

2   Sydney Nursing School, University of Sydney.

3   Central Clinical School, University of Sydney.

level. How to support and balance these two extremes is one of the most important questions in organising diabetes care in Australia today. Irrespective of where diabetes care is being provided along the healthcare delivery continuum, services based on the chronic care model (CCM) [1] help healthcare systems provide more clinically effective and cost-efficient care.

The chronic care model

The CCM provides a paradigm shift from our current model of healthcare delivery, to a system that is prevention based and focused on avoiding long-term problems, including diabetes complications [2]. Due to its multi-faceted nature, quality diabetes care requires an integration of the person with diabetes into a health system that promotes long-term management. [3]. Unlike acute illnesses, diabetes encompasses behavioural, psychosocial, psychological, environmental and clinical factors, all of which require team-based support from a variety of healthcare disciplines [4–6]. The premise of the model is that quality diabetes care is not delivered in isolation, but with community resources, delivery system design, decision support and clinical information systems working in tandem leading to productive interactions between a proactive practice team and prepared activated patient [2]. Indeed, in a recent meta-analysis by Shojania et al. [7], the strategy most effective in improving diabetes care, as measured by HbA1c (glycated haemoglobin), is multi-disciplinary team-based care, a fundamental feature of the chronic care model. Other key elements of this model include:

1. Healthcare organisation – this provides the structural foundation (philosophically and literally) upon which the remaining four components of the CCM rely. Diabetes service providers who are able to gain the support of their health system and organisation are more likely to facilitate and sustain their programs.

2. Community resources and policies – provide individuals with diabetes, their caregivers, service providers with a variety of ancillary services that provide support for self-management.

3. Decision support – uses expertise to establish evidence-based clinical practice guidelines, standards and protocols which provide a framework to assure quality and consistency.

4. Self-management – engages the patient in the active self-management of their condition.

5. Clinical information systems – are necessary for collecting and housing timely, useful data about individual patients and populations of patients, using tools such as patient registries and databases. Diabetes service providers not only need to rely on information systems for patient monitoring, but to a larger extent for tracking and reporting data for practice and system's reports and feedback.

6. Delivery system design – affords opportunities to restructure practices to facilitate team care and define team roles, and delegates tasks such as exploration of reconfiguring the delivery of care in primary care, community clinic and hospital settings.

Diabetes in primary care

Primary care in the community forms an integral part of healthcare and is the first level of contact for the majority of people with diabetes. The sheer number of people with diabetes would dictate this to be a necessity. How we improve diabetes care at this level is therefore a matter of great importance.

Worldwide, primary care is usually provided by a doctor, acting alone and almost invariably also treating many other diseases. In many ways, diabetes is just a condition that the patient 'happens to have' and its management can be surreptitiously relegated to a lesser role than the clinical problem of the day. Various attempts have been made to overcome these issues and it is beyond the scope of this chapter to outline them all, but some examples will be mentioned here. In the UK, a 'mini-diabetes clinic' has been promoted within the auspices of general practice. Doctors are rewarded if the percentage of their diabetic patients reaching a target HbA1c level exceeds a predefined requirement.

In Australia, general practice is the mainstream of the primary care system, and is supported by a single government-controlled universal health insurance fund, Medicare. Together with the public hospital system and community health centres, the Medicare program provides non-user-pays access to medical services for all residents. Under this program the majority of medical practitioner services are funded on a Medicare fee-for-service basis and access to most specialist services is dependent on referral from a general practitioner. As such, general practitioners have always played an important role in managing people with chronic disease such as diabetes. A novel study in the late 1990s, which used Medicare data to look at health service utilisation for the population of New South Wales (NSW), showed that people with diabetes saw their general practitioners nearly twice as often as their non-diabetes counterparts [8].

Regardless of where care is provided, effective management of diabetes requires scheduled and regular patient visits for monitoring diabetes, detecting complications, adjusting medications, negotiating lifestyle changes and providing ongoing support; such visits are a critical element to successful outcomes. Until recently this level of care was not supported by general practitioner funding arrangements. There were also issues in relation to accessing non-medical healthcare professionals, who are well recognised as integral to diabetes healthcare teams. Access to a multidisciplinary team was only offered by hospitals, funded by state governments, and services provided by nursing and allied health professionals outside this setting were not covered by Medicare. As such, funding supported one-to-one medical service provision rather than multidisciplinary care.

However, in the last decade, Australian healthcare reform has seen a plethora of new Medicare benefits to support chronic disease management at the primary care level. In terms of diabetes, this reform provided funding to support general practitioners complete a diabetes annual cycle of care (DACC). As outlined in Table 1, the DACC encompasses routine measurement of glycaemic control and macrovascular risk factor parameters, assessment for diabetes-related eye, kidney and foot disease, and lifestyle education. It also includes medication review. In general, completion of the DACC requires the person with diabetes to attend multiple appointments with their general practitioner as well as, where indicated, appointments with specialists, diabetes educators, allied health professionals and laboratories. This can be inconvenient to the patient, so there is a risk that not all activities within the DACC are completed. To lessen this risk Medicare offers additional funding, as a service incentive payment, for each diabetic patient within a general practice who has completed the full cycle of care within a 13-month time frame [8]. This is further supplemented by an outcomes payment based on the proportion of patients with diabetes within a practice reaching general target levels of care each year [9]. These incentives, while welcomed, put increased pressure on general practitioners to ensure the delivery of effective primary care. To relieve this pressure, many practices have turned to nurses working in the general practice environment to help coordinate and complete the DACC. Today it appears these nurses have been accepted unequivocally by the Australian medical profession as a viable option to augment the services of general practitioners, with well over half of general practices in Australia now employing at least one practice nurse, thereby expanding the primary care team. Further to this, the federal government realised that better planned and coordinated care that looked beyond individual episodes of care to a more broad view was required, so Medicare funding of care plans was introduced in 1999.

In 2005 Medicare went a step further and provided a funding basis for team care arrangements, designed to enable general practitioners to shift from episodic fragmented care to whole person care that is integrated with other healthcare providers [10]. Under this initiative reduced fee allied health services (eg podiatry, dietetics, psychological counselling, etc) are available to patients for whom a care plan and team care arrangements have been written.

Funding of the DACC, care plans and team care arrangements are all intended to improve patient outcomes. To date, however, there is a paucity of published evidence that these initiatives have improved patient care, although some improvements in patients with diabetes have been noted [11, 12]. An audit of 230 patients by Zwar et al. in 2007 [12] found that patients were more likely to be involved in multidisciplinary care for diabetes after a care plan was written (47.8% before versus 63.5% after). Zwar also reported a statistically significant improvement in HbA1c, systolic and diastolic blood pressure, and total cholesterol in these patients. However, as admitted by the authors, some of the improvements were relatively small and may have been of limited clinical significance. Despite this, we have certainly noted the impact of these health reforms over recent years as an increasing number of patients referred to our Diabetes Centre at Royal Prince Alfred Hospital in Sydney already have a diabetes organ complication assessment performed in the primary care setting. As a result, diabetes specialist centres need to reassess their roles to avoid costly duplication of services.

Table 1. The diabetes annual cycle of care.

Activity	Frequency/description
Assess diabetes control by measuring HbA1c	At least once every cycle
Ensure that a comprehensive eye examination is carried out††	At least once every two years
Measure weight and height and calculate body mass index (BMI)†††	At least twice every cycle
Measure blood pressure	At least twice every cycle
Examine feet††††	At least twice every cycle
Measure total cholesterol, triglycerides and HDL cholesterol	At least once every cycle
Test for microalbuminuria	At least once every cycle
Provide self-care education	Patient education regarding diabetes management
Review diet	Reinforce information about appropriate dietary choices
Review levels of physical activity	Reinforce information about appropriate levels of physical activity
Check smoking status	Encourage cessation of smoking (if relevant)
Review of medication	Medication review

†† Not required if the patient is blind or does not have both eyes.

††† Initial visit: measure height and weight and calculate BMI as part of the initial assessment. Subsequent visits: measure weight.

†††† Not required if the patient does not have both feet.

Source: Department of Human Services (2011). Practice Incentives Program: Diabetes Incentive Guidelines. Australian Government [Online]. Available: www.medicareaustralia.gov.au/provider/incentives/pip/files/2709-4-diabetes-incentive-guidelines.rtf. [Accessed 12 January 2012].

In rural and remote Australia, primary care is often delivered through a system of health centres or clinics. Appropriately supported, these centres can provide routine diabetes management to the majority of people with diabetes within a local area, but require the ability to refer more complicated cases such as patients with newly diagnosed type 1 diabetes, or those with an active foot problem. The success of this approach was evidenced by a randomised cluster trial conducted in the Torres Strait, located between Australia and Papua New Guinea and inhabited by Indigenous Australians scattered over a wide area in small communities [14]. The study aimed to implement a sustainable system of care by providing basic training in clinical diabetes care to local Indigenous health workers employed in randomly selected health centres. The study team also assisted local staff within these centres to establish diabetes registers and recall systems, and to develop diabetes care plans. Diabetes specialist outreach services were established concurrently for all health centres within the Torres Strait, and were designed to facilitate referral and provide care to more complicated patients. It also provided a secondary benefit for local staff to learn up-to-date diabetes management principles through working alongside the diabetes specialist during visits to the health centres. It was found that diabetes care processes improved in all health centres and the intervention sites showed greatest progress, with significant improvements in weight, blood pressure and glycaemic control parameters. Moreover, people with diabetes managed by the intervention clinics were 40% less likely to be admitted to hospital for a diabetes-related condition. Over time, local service providers have assumed increasing responsibility for routine diabetes care, thus ensuring sustainability of the service. Similarly, the Royal Prince Alfred Hospital Diabetes Centre has recently established a collaborative partnership with the Maari Ma Health Aboriginal Cooperation in Far Western NSW to assist them in providing specialised team-based care within their local community to people with diabetes.

Traditional specialist care

The hospital clinic

In many urban areas around the world the majority of diabetes care is provided by a hospital, often characterised by a large inpatient unit supported by outpatient clinics. While some hospitals have diabetes-specific outpatient services, many people with diabetes are seen within the context of a large general medical clinic. Although specialists are often notionally in charge in this setting and the clinic is considered a 'specialised diabetes clinic', much of the time the duty of actually seeing people with diabetes is delegated to junior and rotating medical staff. Typically, nursing staff undertake process tasks such as preparing medical records, measuring the patient's height and weight and testing blood glucose levels. Many of these clinics are not prepared to cope with caring for people with a chronic disease, and are entrenched with unsuitable systems, often as a result of hospital regulations. For example, providing patients only with a few week's supply of medications means that clinics are overwhelmed by people attending to have a prescription written. This ultimately leads to shorter consultation times to cope with increased throughput of clinic attendees. As a consequence, care tends not to be patient-focused nor up-to-date, resulting in poor clinical outcomes.

Whilst these clinics in all likelihood will remain the backbone of specialist diabetes treatment for many countries, simple policy changes can improve diabetes care without imposing too much of a cost penalty. An example that can improve continuity of care is to link the rotating junior doctors' clinic with that of a more permanent senior doctor. In that way, patients will see someone familiar and if, for example, they have a specific difficult diabetic problem, the junior rotating doctor can be supervised in its management by the senior consultant. A further step that can improve diabetes care within the traditional system is to allocate nurses to the specialised position of diabetes educator or diabetes specialist nurse so they can complement and enhance what the doctors provide. For this to be successful, it is important their roles are separate from that of the clinic nurse, and not just be seen as 'an additional pair of hands' to help with routine clinic or ward duties. Rather, they should be employed to provide education regarding self-management principles to either in- or outpatients, or a combination of both. In some cases their role may be fully dedicated to educating patients; however, with further training, the specialist nurse can well provide many areas of diabetes management. These staff can be trained to make clinical decisions about the management of diabetes, including management of glycaemic control, hypertension and dyslipidaemia; provide self-management education; and coordinate team services to meet the patient's health needs. Utilising nursing staff to provide many of the routine clinical services is less expensive than using medical staff, and takes the load from the medical staff so they can concentrate on more complex cases. Indeed, a meta-analysis comparing clinical outcomes from protocol-driven, nurse-led clinics with traditional physician-led clinics has shown care is no worse in a nurse or allied health driven system [15]. However, the success of this approach may lie in the careful selection and training of staff. Recognising the advanced skills of the diabetes specialist nurse, both through a career structure and improved financial incentives, is important to ensure continuity of staff.

Traditional diabetes clinics have often been considered to be antiquated. However, they can be made to work and realistically will likely remain the backbone of specialist diabetes care worldwide. However, for them to be effective, there are organisational and system issues to which the senior doctor in the clinic must pay attention, rather than limiting his/her role to a medical one.

Medical specialist diabetes care provided in private practice

In Australia a system of private specialist diabetes care exists to offer choice and to reduce some of the burden on publicly funded services. Subsidy or insurance of private health services is available. However, patients may be faced with a co-payment if their diabetes practitioner charges above the subsidised fee. These costs are a major barrier to many patients receiving the level and type of care they require, particularly when multiple specialists are involved. In the majority of cases private services are run by solo practitioners and access to support services provided by allied health professionals can be difficult and also costly. In many ways similar to their primary care counterparts, the private specialists face the same difficulty of providing multidisciplinary care required by some diabetic patients.

Specialist team-based integrated care

Specialist diabetes care can also be provided in a more integrated and multidisciplinary manner, addressing not only glucose control but also complications and comorbidities of diabetes, involving doctors as well as allied health professionals. Such integrated care is often conveniently provided at a 'diabetes centre', an entity which is distinct from the diabetes clinic. To appreciate the full potential of such a diabetes centre, it is worthwhile noting its heterogeneous nature. Although many facilities may function under the same generic name, they can differ quite considerably if one scratches below the surface. Initially, the role of such diabetes centres in Australia was to provide diabetes education. For many this remains their primary function and hence 'diabetes education centre' is perhaps a more appropriate name. These education centres have generally been developed to support large diabetes clinics and are usually located separately from where medical consultations are made. In this model, clinical care is provided by physicians and patient self-management education and support is conducted by other diabetes team members. It is a system of care repeated in many countries around the world, and can be highly successful in meeting the clinical, educational and psychological needs of the person with diabetes and their family.

Toward the other end of the spectrum, a diabetes centre can incorporate clinical activities. In this manner the duties of doctors and other health professionals become more integrated, co-located and co-dependent. This is the model we have relied on extensively at Royal Prince Alfred Hospital in Sydney for the last three decades. Initially, a prime motive of such initiatives was initiation of insulin therapy and stabilisation of diabetes without the need for hospitalisation; in this system duties are largely provided by diabetes nurses but with the backing of doctors. Over the years more specialised clinical services, such as screening and management of diabetes complications, diabetic foot disease, diabetes in pregnancy, neuropathic pain and use of insulin pump treatment have been progressively added to the service provided by our Diabetes Centre. In many of these activities, the nursing and allied health professionals play such a specialised role that the doctor's function can become a supporting, as well as a supervisory, one. We have found nursing and allied health professionals to be better in these roles than rotating doctors, if for nothing else because patients appreciate more continuity. Conceptually, there is no reason why one single good doctor cannot provide all these services to his/her patients and we have indeed witnessed some who were able to do so, but in our experience it is logistically difficult. In many ways, in our system there are many specialists that make up the team but not all of them are doctors. This concept of, for example, a nurse being more 'specialised' in a clinical area of diabetes management than a doctor is sometime difficult for a traditionalist to understand or with which to feel comfortable.

Obviously to provide such specialised services, diabetes centre staff members require ongoing training which is at one time more specialised and yet also broader in scope, identical philosophically to that required by their medical counterparts undergoing specialist training.

By its very 'Rolls Royce' nature, this type of integrated specialist diabetes care is more resource hungry than diabetes in primary care. By creating such 'super centres' there will be constant ambivalence between balancing 'state of the art' services with providing day-to-day diabetes care to a large number of people. Due to resource constraints, this will always be a problem and it is even worse for a unit which is dependent on throughput for its funding. This dilemma will necessitate a rational debate of who needs specialist care.

Linking diabetes care between community care and specialist care

Many cases of diabetes management can be capably provided at the community level. It therefore makes sense for the majority of patients without complications or comorbidities of diabetes to be managed within the community. On the other hand, patients with more complicated disease warrant referral to the specialists, depending on their individual need. Whilst conceptually sound and obvious, a seamless delivery for such a division of labour is not easy to achieve.

Medicare Locals are a key part of the Labor government's national health reform measures in Australia. They will be primary healthcare organisations working to make it easier for patients to access the services they need by better linking local general practitioners, nursing and other health professionals, hospitals and aged care, and maintaining up-to-date local service directories.

Medicare Locals are designed to:

• Improve the patient journey through developing integrated and coordinated services
• Provide support to clinicians and service providers to improve patient care
• Identify the health needs of local areas and develop locally focused and responsive services
• Successfully implement primary healthcare initiatives and programs
• Be efficient and accountable with strong governance and effective management systems.

Over time, Medicare Locals will be provided with more flexible funding to target services to meet their local community's specific needs. This could mean, for example, supporting local diabetes care or anti-smoking activities. Exactly how this will be done and what an integrated system of care between Medicare Locals and other health service providers will look like is yet to be determined. Nevertheless it is clear that hospital-based diabetes services will need to be more community focused in their outlook. In response to healthcare reform they will need to develop and implement communication systems that enhance discussion between primary care and the hospital and offer complementary services to ensure that the individualised needs of the person with diabetes, their family and their healthcare providers are met, services are not duplicated and the gaps are filled.

How could we improve synergism between primary and specialist care?

A possible solution is the system we have used at the Diabetes Centre of Royal Prince Alfred Hospital in Sydney. We rely on a Shared Care System to partition responsibilities between primary care doctors and ourselves and in 1986 we established a Complication Assessment Service [16] to underpin such a sharing arrangement. A recent study comparing outcomes of patients cared for under our model with those of patients attending traditional specialist services found that the adherence to management guidelines in our shared care model was superior to traditional specialist care. Moreover, a significantly higher proportion of patients managed under the shared care model achieved an HbA1c within 1% of normal range, and/or a blood pressure at target [17]. This would suggest that the majority of patients with the most common form of diabetes known as type 2 diabetes, do not need to see a specialist service in the traditional three to four monthly cycle to receive a similar quality of care.

Apart from achieving good endpoints of glycaemic control and complication detection, this system is more cost-effective because specialists services to ophthalmologist, nephrologist, etc are generally only sought when recommended by a diabetes specialist.

It is worth noting a certain approaches can make such a system maximally effective. The specialist multidisciplinary team which examined the patients and reported to the primary care doctor at the Diabetes Centre must have good clinical skills and judgement in the various diabetes complications. This will allow the diabetes specialist to provide more precise recommendations about the timing of referrals to other specialists or indeed to provide appropriate treatment of some complications. For example, ability of the diabetes specialist to recognise not only retinopathy in a particular patient but also be confident that it is not vision threatening for the foreseeable future, may appropriately delay the referral until later. Another example is the ability to identify the occasional patient with non diabetes-related neuropathic pain may save many other patients with typical diabetes neuropathic pain from unnecessary referral to neurologists.

There are many other approaches to facilitate complementary primary and specialist diabetes care. For example, we have used telemedicine to make advice of our foot clinic staff more readily available to communities in rural and remote Australia [18].

What aspects of diabetes need specialist care?

One concern of diabetes healthcare professionals is that the current focus on funding diabetes care at the general practice level may be to the detriment of specialist care, particularly specialist and tertiary services. As discussed earlier, there are patients who, due to the nature or severity of their disease, need specialist care. People with type 1 diabetes are a case in point. Both national and international guidelines emphasise the critical importance of regular access to a specialist multidisciplinary team for people affected by this type of diabetes, particularly so for children and adolescents. Australia has the sixth highest rate of type 1 diabetes in children and adolescents in the world. Approximately 1000 children aged 14 years and younger are diagnosed in Australia each year and this continues to increase. There is evidence to suggest that this rise is already straining hospital resources and that increased caseloads on diabetes teams is placing young people in jeopardy of not receiving the recommended level of diabetes care. For example, a recent three-year longitudinal study by Hatherly et al. [19] found that the care provided to a sample of young people with type 1 diabetes living in the Australian Capital Territory and NSW fell significantly below recommended levels. Previous Australian research had identified that less than 25% of young people with type 1 diabetes living in the same area had achieved an HbA1c less than the recommended 7.5% [20, 21]. Results from the Hatherly study suggest that the number of young people achieving the target HbA1c had fallen even lower.

The study also showed that the attendance to healthcare professionals fell below what is recommended and declined over the three-year study period. Interestingly, where declines were seen, services were mainly provided in the public hospital setting. The authors suggested a number of possible contributing factors for this, including under-resourcing of these services. Their hypothesis was supported by the qualitative phase of Hatherly's study, where participants reported difficulties in making appointments especially for nursing and allied health services due to insufficient staff.

Issues were also raised in relation to accessing specialist care for those people living in rural areas. In Australia, as with most countries, specialist diabetes services are predominantly located within major urban centres. To address the issue of access, outreach services have been developed to help complement care provided by rural and regional healthcare providers. Under this 'shared care' model, endocrinologists from urban centres travel to regional sites around Australia. People are only seen by these specialists once or twice a year, if lucky, and all other diabetes care is provided by local medical professionals such as general practitioners, paediatricians or general physicians. Despite the widespread use of this shared-care approach to service delivery, there is a dearth of systematic evidence on its impact on diabetes outcomes. A recent study in young people found no differences with respect to the short-term impact of specialist versus shared care on glycaemic control [22]. However data are lacking on the development of diabetes complications and non-glycaemic risk factors. Despite this, the results of this study suggest that even minimal involvement of a specialist may play a role in improving health outcomes, an important finding given Australia's widely dispersed population.

To rationalise diabetes care, there are many areas which will need decisions about who is to do what and at which level. There is no single correct answer to this as the local situation will influence the decision, but some pertinent examples and relevant points can be raised.

For example, emotion would often dictate that the management of gestational diabetes should be at the specialist level. However, the large numbers of woman with this diagnosis now overwhelm diabetes pregnancy clinics. This places increased pressure on staff and means that women with pre-existing type 1 and type 2 diabetes may not get the level of care they need. The morbidity of gestational diabetes is relatively low in comparison with the type 1 and type 2 diabetes. A better use of resources would be to provide the care for woman with gestational diabetes in the community combined with appropriate protocols and guidelines to ensure referral to specialist services as required.

Treatment of diabetic foot disease is another example of how care between the community and the specialist services needs to be carefully partitioned, depending on the person's degree of risk. Guidelines often suggest that all people with diabetes should have their feet assessed and managed by podiatrists. This will place great stress on availability of podiatrists when their service is better directed to high-risk individuals, notably those with active foot lesions. It is better to assign the level of care depending on whether a patient has risk factors of foot ulceration such as impaired sensation or peripheral circulation and whether there are active foot lesions. This would allow patients with foot ulceration, severe foot infection and Charcot arthropathy to receive specialised attention that they need.

The care of people with type 1 diabetes is challenging for anyone. They need more multidisciplinary care and support such as dietary counselling of carbohydrate counting or intensive teaching for use of insulin infusion pumps. These skills are not readily available in the community. The lower prevalence of type 1 diabetes also means that most primary care doctors do not have enough exposure to this group of patients to gain experience. Therefore this group of individuals as adults are probably better managed at the specialist level and when in child or adolescent years, regularly by a specialist paediatrician skilled in diabetes care – usually a paediatric endocrinologist.

There is also the broader (and economically most important) question of who should look after the glycaemic control for the majority of people with type 2 diabetes. To date, there is a great deal of uncertainty about the optimal line of division between primary care and specialist care, both from medical and economical points of view.

The future: the way forward

The challenge ahead is to organise high-quality diabetes care that is accessible and affordable to an increasing number of people with diabetes. We need to document what we do and report outcomes so that effective models, specific to diabetes care in Australia, can be implemented widely. The evidence that team-based care provides the best outcomes needs to be embraced broadly, underpinned by expanding the roles of all health disciplines. If diabetes care is to achieve the healthcare benefits that the diabetes research described in this book has made possible, it must be tackled at both the community and specialist levels. In this regard, the complementarity between primary and specialist care plays a pivotal role, and a balanced approach is required by healthcare planners.

References

1. Wagner EH, Austin BT & Von Korfs M (1996). Improving outcomes in chronic illness. *Managed Care Quarterly,* 4(2): 12–25.

2. Wagner EH, Grothaus LX, Andhu N, et al. (2001). Chronic care clinics for diabetes in primary care: a system-wide randomized trial. *Diabetes Care,* 24: 695–700.

3. Wagner EH, Glasgow RE, Davis C, et al. (2001). Quality improvement in chronic illness care: a collaborative approach. *Joint Commission Journal on Quality and Patient Safety,* 27: 63–80.

4. Siminerio L, Funnell M, Peyrot M & Rubin R (2007). US nurses' perception of their role in diabetes care: results of the cross-national Diabetes, Attitudes, Wishes and Needs (DAWN) study. *The Diabetes Educator,* 33(1): 152–62.

5. Skovlund SE & Peyrot M (2005). DAWN International Advisory Panel: lifestyle and behavior: The Diabetes Attitudes, Wishes and Needs (DAWN) program: a new approach to improving outcomes of diabets care. *Diabetes Spectrum,* 18: 136–42.

6. Funnell MM, Peyrot MF, Rubin RR & Siminerio LM (2005). Steering toward a new DAWN in diabetes management: using diabetes nurse educators in primary care for patient empowerment, psychological support, and improved outcomes. *The Diabetes Educator,* 31(suppl.): 1–18.

7. Shojania K, Ranji SM, McDonald K, et al. (2006). Quality improvement strategies for type 2 diabetes. *Journal of the American Medical Association,* 296(22): 2681.

8. Department of Human Services (2010). GPII outcomes payment. Australian Government. 19 March [Online]. Available: www.medicareaustralia.gov.au/provider/incentives/gpii/outcome-payments.jsp [Accessed on 31 August 2011].

9. Department of Human Services (2010). GPII outcomes payment. Australian Government. 19 March [Online]. Available: www.medicareaustralia.gov.au/provider/incentives/gpii/outcome-payments.jsp [Accessed 31 August 2011].

10. Overland J, Yue DK & Mira M (2000). The pattern of diabetes care in New South Wales: a five-year analysis using Medicare occasions of service data. *The Australian and New Zealand Journal of Public Health,* 24(4): 389–93.

11. Wilkinson D, Mott K, Morey S, et al. (2003). *Evaluation of the Enhanced Primary Care (EPC) Medicare Benefits Schedule (MBS) items and General Practitioner Education, Support and Community Linkage Program (GPESCL). Final report.* Canberra: Australian Government Department of Health and Aging.

12. Zwar NA, Hermiz O, Comino EJ, et al. (2007). Do multidisciplinary care plans result in better care for type 2 diabetes? *Australian Family Physician,* 36(1–2): 85–89.

13. Georgiou A, Burns J, McKenzie S, et al. (2006). Monitoring change in diabetes care using diabetes registers: experience from divisions of general practice. *Australian Family Physician,* 35: 77–80

14. McDermott R, Tulip F, Schmidt B & Sinha A (2003). Sustaining better diabetes care in remote Indigenous Australian communities. *British Medical Journal,* 327(7412): 428–30.

15. Courtenay M & Carey N (2011). Nurse led interventions to improve control of blood pressure in people with hypertension: systematic review and meta-analysis. *British Medical Journal,* 341: c3995.

16. McGill M, Molyneaux DK & Yue JR (1993). A single visit diabetes complication assessment service: a complement to diabetes management at the primary care level. *Diabetic Medicine,* 10(4): 366–70.

17. Cheung N, Yue D, Kotowicz M, Jones P & Flack J (2008). A comparison of diabetes clinics with different emphasis on routine care, complications assessment and shared care. *Diabetic Medicine,* 25: 974–78.

18. McGill M, Constantino M & Yue DK (2000). Integrating telemedicine into a national diabetes footcare network. *Practical Diabetes,* 17(7): 235–38.

19. Hatherly K, Smith L, Overland J, Johnston C & Brown-Singh L (2011). Application of Australia clinical management guidelines: the current state of play in a sample of young people with type 1 diabetes in the state of New South Wales and the Australian Capital Territory. *Diabetes Research and Clinical Practice,* 93(3): 379–84.

20. Craig ME, Handelsman P, Donaghue KC, Chan A, Blades B, et al. (2002). Predictors of glycaemic control and hypoglycaemia in children and adolescents with type 1 diabetes from NSW and the ACT. *The Medical Journal of Australia,* 177(5): 235–38.

21. Handelsman P, Craig ME, Donaghue KC, Chan A, Blades B, et al. (2001). Homogeneity of metabolic control in New South Wales and the Australian Capital Territory, Australia. *Diabetes Care,* 24(9): 1690–91.

22. Hatherly K, Smith L, Overland J, Johnston C, Brown-Singh L, Waller D & Taylor S (2011). Glycemic control and type 1 diabetes: the differential impact of model of care and income. *Pediatric Diabetes,*12: 115–19.

20

Managing diabetes complications in the clinical arena

Stephen M Twigg[1,2] and Susan V McLennan[1,2]

In the absence of a complete prevention or cure for diabetes mellitus in all its forms, complications will occur in most people with diabetes. These are common and varied. The spectrum includes psychosocial as well as biological complications and they may be acute, as in those causing very low or high blood glucose. Chronic biological end-organ complications of diabetes include so-called microvascular complications of diabetic eye, kidney and nerve disease and the macrovascular complications of cardiovascular, cerebrovascular and peripheral vascular disease. Evidence from clinical trials indicates that using current healthcare and therapy standards, much can be done to prevent onset and progression of diabetes complications; indeed, over recent years, serial reductions in death rates in people with diabetes reflect such beneficial outcomes. This chapter will focus on trends and options in care as well as therapies that hold promise to improve complications outcomes in people with diabetes.

The spectrum of diabetes complications

Diabetes mellitus is essentially a syndrome where the hormone insulin is deficient in the body. As a result there is not enough insulin to prevent increases in blood glucose, or to normally regulate protein and body fat [1]. While blood glucose levels may be quite mildly elevated at certain times in some people with diabetes, if insulin is severely lacking it can rapidly lead to emergency, life-threatening conditions of diabetic ketoacidosis, where acid in the blood occurs, or hyperosmolar coma where blood glucose levels rise to very high levels and may cause coma [2].

A major breakthrough occurred in diabetes care when insulin was discovered as the hormone produced by the pancreas which is deficient in diabetes. A short time after that discovery in the early 1920s, people with diabetes, especially young children, had their lives saved by insulin injection treatment and emergency conditions such as diabetic ketoacidosis (DKA) were largely avoided, and quality of life was significantly improved [3]. The source of the insulin was initially isolated from animal pancreas, and was subsequently derived from human insulin made in the laboratory. However, after the discovery of insulin

---

1   Sydney Medical School, University of Sydney.

2   Department of Endocrinology, Royal Prince Alfred Hospital.

and its lifesaving role in therapy, it became increasingly clear over the subsequent years and decades that people with diabetes were at increased risk of developing a series of different complications from diabetes [4], namely damage to certain organs and tissues, especially the eyes, kidneys, nerves, heart and blood vessels. These complications are listed in Table 1. Research into the cause of diabetes complications and the mechanisms to prevent, detect and treat them, is the main focus of this chapter.

Table 1. The spectrum of diabetes complications, including acute and chronic, organic and psychosocial.

Time course	Complication grouping	Specific complications
Acute (usually hours to days)	Insulin lack	diabetic ketoacidosis, hyperosmolar non-ketotic coma
	Insulin excess	Hypoglycaemia
Chronic (usually years)	Microvascular	Diabetic retinopathy, diabetic nephropathy, diabetic neuropathy
	Macrovascular	Cardiovascular disease, cerebrovascular disease, peripheral arterial disease
	Other (see text for detailed list)	Including congenital malformations
Psychsocial	General	Depression, eating disorder
	Diabetes specific	Diabetes distress

Acute complications of diabetes

(i) Acute complications due to a lack of insulin

Amongst the three main types of diabetes mellitus – type 1, type 2, and gestational diabetes – the former two in the absence of a pancreas transplant, are incurable and persist, whereas the latter condition is transient. In type 1 diabetes there is absolute insulin deficiency. This means that in the absence of insulin therapy, cells in the body will become starved of glucose. Insulin is an important anabolic, or building-up, hormone that helps blood glucose move into tissues, and cells to create cellular energy, and it prevents breakdown of body fats and muscle. Insulin acts like a key to help glucose move into cells. In the complete absence of insulin, the cells in the body, especially the liver and skeletal muscle, cannot 'see' glucose outside the cell. As a result, the alternative form of stored glucose, known as glycogen, is rapidly broken down by fat and muscle. However glycogen is completely used up within 24 hours. The fat and muscle in the body are then broken down and the liver takes up fatty acids from the circulation to make an alternative form of energy for the body known as keto acids. While these acids, also known as ketone bodies, provide a source of energy to cells, over subsequent hours and days in the absence of any insulin the production of keto acids increases to severe levels [2]. The tissues and the circulation become progressively acidic, placing the defenses against pH imbalance at these sites under great physiologic stress. If the blood glucose is high, the blood is acidic and the blood or urine ketones are elevated, then a person is said to have 'diabetic ketoacidosis' (DKA). A person who develops DKA, will become 'hot and dry'; he or she will increasingly become dehydrated as large volumes of urine are passed due to elevated blood glucose, and will often be febrile due to having acid in the blood, causing an elevated body temperature. The person with DKA also attempts to breathe off carbon dioxide (CO_2) which is formed to excess in the body when CO_2 is produced from the alkali bicarbonate as a buffer combining with the excessive blood acid from ketones.

DKA is a medical emergency. If it is detected early enough, it can be readily treated with intravenous fluid and insulin and restoration of the body's ions, especially potassium, all with close monitoring [5]. Each year in Australia, some people with type 1 diabetes die due to diabetic ketoacidosis [6]. The risk of DKA in established type 1 diabetes is 1%–10% per patient per year [7]. The risk of DKA is increased in people with poor glycaemic control or previous episodes of DKA; peripubertal and adolescent girls; children with psychiatric disorders, including those with eating disorders; children with difficult or unstable family circumstances; children with limited access to medical services; and people who omit insulin [7]. Any death due to DKA is a disaster. If treatment is provided early enough, mortality should not occur, especially in people who have known type 1 diabetes. Increasingly, guidelines to help prevent DKA and to detect this acute complication early are being developed [8].

If a person with type 2 diabetes becomes severely deficient in insulin, the blood glucose levels may become markedly elevated over subsequent days and weeks [9]. For example, some people may develop levels of blood glucose above 50 mmol/L, compared with the normal non-diabetic range of about four to eight mmol/L. As blood glucose levels become elevated the glucose is lost into the urine, taking water with it and causing dehydration. The very high blood glucose levels affect consciousness and can cause confusion, and loss of consciousness or coma. This condition known as 'hyperosmolar non-ketotic coma', (or HONC), is life-threatening. It requires emergency room treatment and intensive care support. With careful rehydration and infusion of insulin, as well as treatment of the factor that may have destabilised diabetes, such as an infection, most people with HONC will survive.

Why people with type 2 diabetes may develop HONC, and yet people with type 1 diabetes can develop DKA, is an important clinical observation that has not been fully explained. In brief, it appears that in HONC, the body makes enough insulin to prevent keto acid formation but not enough to prevent blood glucose rising excessively, whereas the absolute insulin lack in type 1 diabetes leads to DKA. It has been observed repeatedly however that if some people with type 2 diabetes become severely acutely unwell, for example from a severe infection in the body or due to a heart attack (myocardial infarct), then DKA may transiently develop or they may develop a mix of HONC and DKA [9]. Distinguishing between type 1 and type 2 diabetes can be difficult and it is increasingly being recognised that some people with apparent type 2 diabetes, on careful assessment or in the course of time, develop a picture of type 1 diabetes [8].

(ii) Acute complications due to an excess of insulin

If blood glucose levels fall below the normal range, causing hypoglycaemia, it can make a person with diabetes feel unwell, with sweating and tremor and other symptoms, and in the most severe situation, loss of consciousness, known as 'hypoglycaemia coma'. Severe hypoglycaemia may be life-threatening, for example, by causing seizure, injury or precipitating heart attack or abnormal heart rhythm events [8, 10]. Essentially, hypoglycaemia occurs because treatments used for diabetes, either insulin or medications that cause increased insulin release from the pancreas, lower blood glucose excessively for the needs of the body at a certain point in time [11].

Hypoglycaemia of all forms is, understandably, feared by people with diabetes and their immediate carers and family [12]. Fear of hypoglycaemia and its consequences, including night-time episodes, is a major barrier to optimal blood glucose control in type 1 diabetes and in type 2 diabetes when insulin treatment is required [13]. For most people with type 1 diabetes, mild (ie self-treated) hypoglycaemia remains a regular occurrence. It may occur about twice weekly [14] and adversely affect quality of life. In contrast, severe hypoglycaemia occurs on average once every three or more years in type 1 diabetes [11, 14]. There is marked individual variation in the rate of severe hypoglycaemia. Some people never experience it, whereas in others it occurs multiple times a year, despite intensive diabetes support in management [11]. Nocturnal hypoglycaemia accounts for close to half of the episodes of severe hypoglycaemia in type 1 diabetes [14]. In type 2 diabetes, for people on insulin therapy, mild hypoglycaemia occurs in about 30% of people each year, and severe hypoglycaemia in 1%–2% [15]. Risk factors for severe hypoglycaemia in type 1 and type 2 diabetes include a long duration of diabetes and aiming for tighter blood glucose control [8, 11, 15].

Prevention of hypoglycaemia is an important aspect of diabetes care. In people with type 1 diabetes or type 2 diabetes on therapy that may lower blood glucose such as insulin, balancing blood glucose across the day by considering carbohydrate intake, physical activity and insulin dosage is a constant consideration [8, 11]. Some forms of insulin therapy and diabetes management regimens can help to prevent mild and severe hypoglycaemia. So too can insulin pump therapy, especially those that combine state of the art technology with real-time continuous blood glucose monitors [8].

Treatment of mild hypoglycaemia by oral glucose is usually highly effective, taking 15 to 20 minutes to begin to have effect [11]. In severe hypoglycaemia causing unconscious, intravenous treatment with glucose by a paramedic or a medical doctor, is usually effective. Alternatively, a hormone therapy known as glucagon, which mobilises glucose into the blood stream from glycogen stores in the liver, can be administered by intramuscular injection by a carer who has been educated in the administration, or by a health professional [13].

Table 2. Differing perspectives on diabetes complications.

More negative perspectives	More positive perspectives
Diabetes end-organ complications occur in most people with diabetes	Most diabetes complications that occur are mild to moderate in severity and complications can often be detected early and their progression prevented
Due to its high prevalence in Australia diabetes is the single commonest cause of kidney failure, and also working age blindness	Less than 2% of people with diabetes will develop end-stage kidney disease or blindness annually
More than 15% of people with diabetes will develop at least one foot ulcer in their life-time	The vast majority of foot ulcers that occur in people with diabetes will heal with proper care without requiring extensive amputation
The commonest cause of death in people with diabetes is cardiovascular disease	Yearly rates of death due to cardiovascular disease in people with diabetes have been falling by more than 50% in developed countries over recent decades, due likely to multiple improvements in patient care including blood cholesterol, blood pressure and blood glucose control
Routine screening for some diabetes complications on a regular basis is not yet established for some conditions such as diabetic cardiomyopathy or liver disease related to diabetes	Screening for some diabetes complications such as diabetic retinopathy, nephropathy and neuropathy and foot disease are well established and can help to prevent severe complications
Hypoglycaemia is common in people with diabetes and is due to doses of certain medications such as insulin causing an excessive lowering of blood glucose	While severe hypoglycaemia is ten to 20 times more common in those with type 1 compared with type 2 diabetes, most hypoglycaemia that occurs in all types of diabetes is mild, and severe hypoglycaemia can be prevented

Chronic diabetes complications

Diabetes complications can be divided into those affecting the small vessels of the body, so-called microvascular, and those affecting the larger vessels termed macrovascular. Microvascular complications are mainly those affecting eyes (diabetic retinopathy), kidneys (diabetic nephropathy) and nerves (diabetic neuropathy). Macrovascular complications are those of the heart (cardiovascular disease), brain vessels (cerebrovascular disease) and the limbs (peripheral arterial disease). There are other diabetes complications which may be mixed in type and are discussed subsequently.

In 2009, diabetes was among the top ten leading causes of death, being the direct cause of 3% of deaths in Australia, and contributing to another 7.1% of deaths [16]. In addition, the presence of diabetes complications increases the financial cost of diabetes at least twofold [10]. Diabetes is over-represented as a cause of death in the Indigenous population, where it was responsible for 8% of all Indigenous deaths, compared with 2.9% of deaths in non-

Indigenous people [16]. Probably due mainly to the increased prevalence of diabetes in the Australian community, the total number of deaths to which diabetes has contributed has progressively increased over the last 20 years [10, 16].

(i) Pathogenesis of diabetes complications

Why some organs, and tissues in them, are more susceptible to injury than others is not clear and is the subject of ongoing intensive research [17]. However, there are some common elements amongst the differing body parts that develop diabetes complications. In body sites affected by elevated blood glucose, tissues may become inflamed, or they may develop fibrosis/scar tissue or both [18]. Figure 1 indicates a schematic implicating biochemical pathways and adverse tissue changes that occur in diabetes complications. In inflammation, white cells are attracted into the tissue and inflammatory fluid may accumulate. The inflammation is persistent and of low intensity. In other cases the native cells in the tissue die and are replaced by scar tissue, also known as fibrosis, which involves new blood vessel growth and lay down of proteins termed extracellular matrix (ECM). Amongst the organs and tissues affected by diabetes complications, some may predominantly develop inflammation, some fibrosis, and others a mixture of the two. For example in diabetic nephropathy, there is evidence that inflammation in the kidney then leads to fibrosis with loss of kidney function [19].

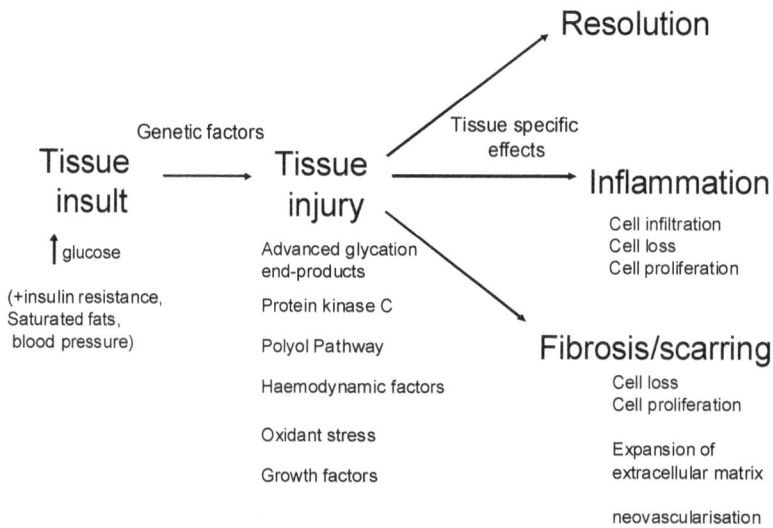

Figure 1. Schematic showing pathogenesis of diabetes complications based on biochemical and other cellular pathways activated (tissue injury), and tissue pathological change, which may lead to functional loss. High glucose interacts with genetic factors to cause tissue injury, tissue cell loss and in some cases, loss of function in a tissue. For further explanation refer to the text.

How elevated blood glucose in diabetes leads to diabetes complications is under intensive research [20, 21]. In brief, from a biochemical perspective, high glucose in the blood will ultimately diffuse into cells and cause elevated cell glucose. The main biochemical pathway that normally handles glucose, known as the glycolytic pathway, and the subsequent biochemical pathways known as the TCA cycle and oxidative phosphorylation, become overwhelmed by the excess glucose being metabolised and forced into it. As a result, a number of changes occur in the biochemistry of cells. The high activity in the oxidative phosphorylation pathway leads to dysfunction in the main energy forming part of the cell known as the mitochondria and to formation of excessive oxidative stress in cells. In addition, a number of overflow metabolic pathways that are not usually very active, become much more active as metabolites in the glycolytic pathway accumulate downstream of glucose. These overflow pathways include those termed the polyol pathway, the advanced glycation end-product pathway, the hexosamine pathway, and the diacylglycerol-protein kinase C related pathway [20]. Other factors that may mediate adverse effects of elevated glucose in cells and tissues are proteins known as growth factors and cytokines. For example, the growth factor known as connective tissue growth factor is induced by all of the glucose overflow pathways, and it can cause both inflammation and fibrosis in tissues affected by diabetes [18, 19]. Alterations in matrix degradation, in particular by matrix metalloproteinases and their regulators, also contribute to tissue damage in diabetes [22–24].

Despite the above knowledge, the development of diabetes complications remains somewhat of an enigma. Diabetes complications to some degree occur in practically every person who develops diabetes, although severe complications occur in only a minority [8]. For example, elevated blood and tissue glucose is only one important risk factor for diabetes complications. Amongst the microvascular complications, identical twin studies have shown that genetic factors account for one-third to one-half the variation in diabetes complications, and there are likely both protective genetic factors as well as susceptibility factors [25]. To date only some of these genetic factors have been identified. It is thought that the interaction between genetic susceptibility with the metabolic effects of elevated blood glucose causes the tissue complications of diabetes [21, 25]. It is notable that, while increasingly elevated blood glucose levels increase the risk of diabetes complications, some people with diabetes can have quite poor blood glucose levels long term and yet they develop minimal or no damage to tissues, whereas, in others, mildly elevated blood glucose can be associated with severe organ complications.

In addition to elevated glucose, there are other factors that can affect diabetes complications risk. Elevated fats, especially saturated fats, and abnormal cholesterol levels with low levels of 'good cholesterol' (termed high-density lipoprotein cholesterol or HDL-C) and elevated and reduced quality 'bad cholesterol' (termed low-density lipoprotein cholesterol or LDL-C), contribute especially to macrovascular complications risk [26]. Haemodynamic factors, especially elevated general body (systemic) blood pressure contribute to both micro- and macrovascular complications risk [26, 27]. Increased waist circumference and central body fat are associated with high blood pressure, abnormal fats and also resistance to the action of insulin. In people who have these characteristic features of insulin resistance, abnormal blood fats and cholesterol, and high blood pressure, the 'insulin resistance' or 'metabolic syndrome' is said to be present. Presence of the metabolic syndrome increases the risk and severity of complications in people with type 1 diabetes [27, 28].

In pregnancy, women who have pre-existing diabetes (type 1 or type 2) are at increased risk of having a pregnancy complicated by miscarriage, or certain birth defects, or having large babies due to effects of excess blood glucose on the developing fetus [29, 30]. In contrast, gestational diabetes, or GDM, develops in later pregnancy (usually 24+ weeks of gestation) and likely occurs due to metabolic effects of the placenta and pregnancy placing metabolic pressure on the mother's pancreas. GDM is usually a temporary form of diabetes and the elevated blood glucose tendency resolves after delivery. In pregnant women where the pancreas cannot make more insulin to overcome insulin resistance of the pregnancy, GDM develops. GDM increases the risk, in particular, of large babies at birth, leading potentially to obstetric complications at birth, stillbirth, and also increased risk of metabolic syndrome, overweight and obesity, and diabetes in later life [31, 32]. GDM also increases the risk of development of type 2 diabetes in the mother over subsequent years [32].

Research into diabetes complications occurs at the clinical and pre-clinical levels. As end-organ diabetes complications take many years to develop in humans, animal studies and cell-based research in the laboratory can help to examine diabetes complications in a more timely manner and to test differing interventions to prevent and treat diabetes complications [33]. The preclinical studies thus have advantages, although each is only a model of human diabetes and its complications, and are what is termed 'hypothesis generating'. Ultimately human clinical studies are required to determine best evidence methods to manage diabetes complications.

(ii) Specific organ diabetes complications described

A. Microvascular complications

Diabetic retinopathy

In the course of time, most people with diabetes will develop some form of change to the back of the eye (retina) [34]. The most common and non-vision-threatening type of diabetic retinopathy is termed 'non-proliferative', where neither growth of new vessels or severe leakiness of the retina is a concern. There are two vision-threatening types of diabetic retinopathy. One is proliferative, where new and fragile vessels grow in the retina, possibly as a result of poor oxygen supply from damaged initial blood vessels in the retina. The other, and most common, type of vision-threatening diabetic retinopathy is diabetic macular oedema where excessive leakiness of vessels occurs in the part of the retina that is critical to high-quality vision acuity termed the macula (and more centrally the fovea) [34]. In Australia, while diabetes remains the commonest cause of blindness in people of working age, less than 1% of people per year will develop blindness due to diabetes [35].

Diabetic nephropathy

While in each year only about 2% of people with diabetes develop very end-stage kidney disease (stage 5 chronic kidney disease), because diabetes mellitus is so common, diabetic nephropathy is the single commonest cause of end-stage kidney disease in Australia [35]. The damage to the kidney in diabetes may cause a progressive protein leak termed albuminuria, and also in the course of time, loss of kidney-filtering function (loss of the glomerular filtration rate). It is the combination of progressive albuminuria/proteinuria and loss of glomerular filtration rate that most clearly characterises diabetic nephropathy. It is thought that up to 30% of people with diabetes, in the course of time, will develop some nephropathy [36, 37]. In the early stages, small amounts of albumin loss in the urine, known as microalbuminuria, occur. Subsequently, the albumin and protein loss in the urine becomes more marked, and renal filtration function is lost. People with diabetic nephropathy not only have an increased risk of end-stage kidney failure developing but also increased cardiovascular disease risk – heart attack and heart failure [37].

Diabetic neuropathy

The commonest form of nerve damage in diabetes is to those supplying the feet. The sensory nerves are damaged more severely than the motor nerves. Loss of sensation in the feet increases the risk of foot ulceration in people with diabetes, and in their lifetime about 20% of people with diabetes will develop a foot ulcer, with less than 10% of these cases leading to the need for amputation [38]. In some people with diabetes, the feet and leg nerves become irritated and a painful form of neuropathy develops. This can be disabling, especially if prolonged, and requires specific medication to control, if not fully relieve, it.

There is debate as to whether the microvessels supplying the nerves (termed the 'vasa nervorum'), or the nerves themselves, are directly affected by elevated glucose, with evidence from animal and human studies that both may be involved [38].

In addition to peripheral neuropathy, there are other forms of nerve damage that can occur in diabetes. These forms of neuropathy include those involving the automatic nerves of the body known as autonomic neuropathy. Autonomic neuropathy can cause heart rhythm problems and a proneness to low blood pressure on standing, as well as stomach and bowel upset. Rarer forms of neuropathy, which often improve over some months, involve the cranial nerves or and the nerve plexus in the pelvis, known as 'diabetic amyotrophy' [38].

B. Macrovascular complications

Cardiovascular disease

The commonest cause of death in people with diabetes is heart disease, accounting for about half of the deaths [10]. The heart can be affected by disease of the coronary arteries, which is increased two- to six-fold in people with diabetes [39]. The presentation of heart disease may be through a classic history of chest pain known as angina, although in some people with diabetes the symptoms may be more subtle, such as new shortness of breath on less exertion.

Cerebrovascular disease

Lack of blood supply causing stroke is twice as common in people with diabetes as in the general population [40]. Large strokes can lead to death or major disability. In contrast, recurrent mini-strokes (causing damage to small parts of the brain known as 'lacunes'), can lead over the years to a form of vascular dementia, especially if blood pressure is elevated.

Peripheral artery disease

Peripheral artery disease is more common in people with diabetes. It can cause a number of health problems such as calf pain on walking, and delayed healing in people who develop foot ulcers, thus increasing the risk of amputation [41]. Smoking markedly increases the risk of peripheral artery disease in people with diabetes, and for this and many other reasons smoking avoidance and cessation is vital in diabetes care.

C. Other organ complications in diabetes

There are many other complications that are caused by diabetes or may be related to it. Diabetic foot disease occurs due to combinations of neuropathy, peripheral artery disease, ulceration and infection and foot deformity [42]. Cataract and glaucoma are increased in people with diabetes [34]. Erectile dysfunction (some degree of impotence) is common in men with diabetes due to nerve damage and blood vessel injury [43]. Limited joint mobility and skin thickening can occur in people with diabetes [44]. Diabetes is known to directly adversely affect heart muscle to cause 'diabetic cardiomyopathy' in at least one-third of people [45]. In type 2 diabetes, fatty liver known as non-alcoholic liver disease occurs in most, and diabetes accelerates its rate of deterioration to an inflammatory and scarring form known as non-alcoholic steatohepatitis and in some cases across decades, liver cirrhosis [46, 47]. People with type 1 diabetes have an increased risk of developing immune related conditions that may affect the thyroid gland to cause over- or under-activity, and also the small bowel condition known as coeliac disease, which is a where effects of gluten in the diet can cause a toxic effect on the bowel [8].

(iii) Psychosocial complications in diabetes

Diabetes places major psychological stress and self-care demands on the person with diabetes and the caring family members. People with diabetes have an increased rate of clinical depression and eating disorders, which can exacerbate adverse organ effects of diabetes and also adversely affect quality of life [8]. Suicide rates may be higher in young people with diabetes compared with the general population [6]. There is also a diabetes condition known as 'diabetes distress' that describes an underlying anxiety and psychological unwellness in people with diabetes [8]. Diabetes can adversely affect psychosocial development in children and adolescence [8]. The increased frequency of these conditions reflects that psychsocial support is commonly indicated in those with diabetes.

(iv) Clinical trials data in diabetes complications: metabolic control matters

While elevated blood glucose is a marker for increased diabetes complications risk, it took long-term clinical trials to prove that diabetes complications can be prevented by tight blood glucose control. Landmark studies in people with type 1 [8, 14] and type 2 diabetes [10, 48–52] have shown that better long-term average blood glucose, measured by a blood marker termed HbA1c or glycated haemoglobin, leads to reduced diabetes complications onset and in those who already have diabetes complications, their worsening. In studies varying from three to 10 years in duration, the onset and progression of microvascular complications were clearly prevented. For the macrovascular complications, cardiovascular events were shown to be prevented in longer-term studies of about 17 years' duration [53, 54]. In those longer-term studies, tight blood glucose control in the first six to 10 years led to sustained reduction in the subsequent ten years or so, indicating that the body has a 'memory' effect of elevated blood glucose. This 'metabolic memory' is intriguing. Some recent preclinical data suggest that glucose regulation of factors that control genes, so-called epigenetics, is involved in the memory effect [55].

A recent study in type 2 diabetes indicates that very tight blood glucose control long term in people with cardiovascular disease may lead to increased mortality [51]. The exact cause of death in the study was unclear, although severe hypoglycaemia episodes causing heart attacks or abnormal heart rhythms may at least partly explain the increased death rate. This study has led to the concept that tight blood glucose control and targets are indicated early in diabetes, but in people with a history of cardiovascular disease, especially if they require insulin therapy, the blood glucose targets should be more relaxed [10, 56].

(v) Blood pressure and cholesterol control also prevent diabetes complications

A number of important studies in type 1 and type 2 diabetes have shown that blood pressure control can prevent onset and worsening of microvascular complications, especially diabetic nephropathy and diabetic retinopathy, and all macrovascular complications, especially stroke. The class of medications known as angiotensin converting enzyme inhibitors and angiotensin receptor antagonists/blockers, appear to have special protective roles and are the preferred first-line agents in people with diabetes [57]. Other studies have shown that reduction in blood levels of bad (LDL) cholesterol, especially with medications known as 'statins', even in those without known cardiovascular disease, will reduce the risk of cardiovascular complications such as heart attack and stroke [58].

A study of people with type 2 diabetes in Denmark examined whether the combined simultaneous targeting of blood pressure, cholesterol and blood glucose would lead to improved outcomes [59]. It clearly demonstrated that targeting all three end-points over eight years or more, led to a more than 50% reduction in macro- and microvascular complications. These studies form the evidence for targeting blood glucose, blood pressure and cholesterol in people with diabetes.

(vi) Screening for diabetes complications

In people with diabetes, there is a clear evidence showing that screening to detect certain diabetes complications is important [8, 10]. This is because, in those developing complications, some therapies can be intensified to help prevent worsening of the complication to its end stages. For example, in diabetic retinopathy, vision-threatening forms (proliferative retinopathy or macular oedema) can be treated with laser therapy, or intraocular corticosteroids or anti-growth factor therapy, to help prevent vision loss. In diabetic nephropathy, even tighter blood pressure control (to less than 125/75 mmHg, rather than less than 130/80 mmHg) can help prevent its progression, and in people with diabetic foot disease, intensive patient education combined with protective foot wear and early treatment of foot ulcers, can help to prevent amputation.

The screening for diabetic retinopathy requires a thorough examination of the retinae and measurement of visual acuity. In diabetic nephropathy, urine tests for albumin and in some cases protein, as well as blood tests for renal function (glomerular filtration rate) are required. For neuropathy and foot problems, feet need to be carefully examined for sensation, pulses and mechanical foot problems as well as ulcers.

In people with type 2 diabetes, microvascular screening for complications should begin from diagnosis [10], as a delay in recognition of diabetes and diabetes diagnosis of some years is common in type 2 diabetes, and effects of high blood glucose often occur for many years before diabetes diagnosis. In type 1 diabetes, screening should occur after about three years of diabetes. In each case, screening should usually occur annually thereafter [8].

In terms of macrovascular disease, complications screening is usually by history taking and physical examination. The role for extensive heart investigations, including exercise tests, is unclear and studies have shown that unless a person has symptoms of heart disease, tight blood pressure, blood glucose and cholesterol control, as well as avoidance of smoking and possibly blood thinning (anti-platelet) therapy are the cornerstone of care.

In people with type 1 diabetes, screening approximately annually for autoimmune thyroid disease and also coeliac disease, each by blood test, is indicated in children and adults [8].

(vii) Major challenges in diabetes complications care

Managing diabetes and its complications has a number of inherent challenges. One dynamic tension is that long-term blood glucose control is important to prevent long-term organ complications of diabetes, yet tight blood glucose control can increase the risk of severe hypoglycaemia, especially in cases where insulin therapy is required, such as in all people with type 1 diabetes and in those with type 2 diabetes requiring insulin therapy. A second tension is that diabetes place major demands on a person's lifestyle in terms of healthy diet and exercise and, simultaneously, people with diabetes usually need to take multiple preventive medications to manage blood glucose, blood pressure and cholesterol. The person with diabetes needs to self-monitor blood glucose multiple times daily using a finger prick device and people with type 1 diabetes need to inject insulin four to five times daily. In people with type 1 diabetes this equates to more than 1000 blood glucose self-tests and more than 1000 insulin injections yearly. Diabetes is unrelenting and does not provide any 'holidays'.

Considering the demands that diabetes places on the person with diabetes and their families, the health professional support and healthcare delivery services required are extensive and high level. Services for people with diabetes need to be comprehensive yet individualised in their targets and emphasis [8, 10, 56, 60]. Multidisciplinary healthcare teams are required, involving a skilled doctor, diabetes nurse educator or practice nurse, and dietitian. In type 1 diabetes and complex type 2 diabetes, to support the general practitioner, an endocrinologist is indicated to help lead chronic care. Other members of the diabetes healthcare team will often include the podiatrist, exercise physiologist, psychologist or psychiatrist, orthotist, foot and vascular surgeon, renal physician, ophthalmologist, cardiologist and microbiologist. Care of the person with diabetes thus requires highly coordinated care in order to optimise targets in therapy and to ensure that regular diabetes complications screening is undertaken [8, 10, 56, 60].

(viii) Transplantation and diabetes complications

Kidney transplant is often an option in a person with diabetes who has end-stage renal failure requiring dialysis. Outcomes are good if cardiovascular disease and heart failure is not severe in a patient. Kidney transplant can be combined with pancreas transplant in some cases, resulting in reduced need for insulin therapy and a reduction in severe hypoglycaemia. There is also evidence that some forms of neuropathy and kidney disease can improve after pancreas transplant [61].

(ix) Reversibility of diabetes complications

While most diabetes complications are progressive, some are transient. The microvascular complications of diabetes may in some cases regress, especially with intensive therapy. For example, diabetic nephropathy in its early micro-albuminuria stages may regress to normo-albuminuria with treatment of blood pressure [62], and painful diabetic neuropathy symptoms may resolve with time and improved blood glucose control, as may early diabetic retinopathy. Even some changes of fibrosis in tissues such as the kidney may become less marked with tight control of blood pressure and blood glucose in diabetic nephropathy [61]. Most studies in diabetes complications to date have examined prevention of progression rather than regression of complications.

(x) Diabetes and obstetric care

It is beyond the scope of this chapter to address obstetric aspects of diabetes in detail. It should be noted however that in women with type 1 or type 2 diabetes, tight control of blood glucose before conception and across a pregnancy can lead to marked reduction in birth defects, stillbirth and large-at-birth babies [29, 30]. Outcomes are also improved for the baby in a mother with gestational diabetes, in terms of reduced complications at birth and possibly, less stillbirth [31]. The data from series of high quality studies, including Australian clinical trials [31], provides reassuring data that much can be achieved to prevent diabetes complications in pregnancies complicated by diabetes, whether it be type 1, type 2 or gestational diabetes in the mother.

(xi) Outcomes are improving in diabetes complications

Data from multiple databases in Australia and other developed countries have indicated that the rate of death in people with diabetes has reduced over the decades in both type 1 and type 2 diabetes [63, 64]. Factors that have likely contributed to this beneficial outcome include the increasing evidence to support more intensive control of cholesterol (with statins), blood pressure (with angiotensin converting enzyme inhibitors or angiotensin receptor blocker therapy) and blood glucose in people with diabetes, and possibly more complete screening for diabetes complications. Reductions in smoking rates have also likely helped. However, people with diabetes continue to have a reduced life expectancy on average compared with an age-matched general population and the earlier diabetes onset occurs, the greater the reduction in average life expectancy due to diabetes-related complications [63, 10]. This, combined with the end-stage complications that occur in diabetes and the morbidity complications caused and related healthcare costs [8, 10], demand no complacency in diabetes complications detection and its management.

(xii) Prospects in diabetes complications and related care

It is envisaged that healthcare services delivery will progressively be enhanced to ensure that most if not all people with diabetes have complications screening as clinically indicated and that they have their major risk factors of blood pressure, cholesterol and blood glucose tightly and safely controlled.

It may also be the case that an increasing focus on regression of diabetes complications will indicate whether actual regression of changes should be a target in treatment rather than just the prevention of worsening of complications. For example, regression of albuminuria may be shown in the course of time to predict fewer kidney and cardiovascular events than stabilisation of albuminuria levels alone. It may well be that our treatment of blood pressure improves with increasing and new combination of agents, as will our control of both good and bad cholesterol through combined therapies. In type 1 and type 2 diabetes improved knowledge in healthcare delivery and advances in technology, such as more sophisticated insulin pumps and blood glucose monitoring, will likely further help to improve long-term blood glucose diabetes and thus prevent organ complications and minimise severe hypoglycaemia.

Considering the adverse effects of high blood glucose on cells and cellular pathways to cause tissue injury (Figure 1), it is envisaged that therapies targeted at, for example, growth factors may increasingly help to prevent, stabilise and possibly reverse diabetes complications. Such is already being realised in diabetic retinopathy where anti-vascular endothelial growth factor therapy is becoming a reality for vision-threatening retinopathy to complement the traditional treatment of laser photocoagulation therapy [34]. As described in other chapters, the agent fenofibrate is showing remarkable effects in preventing microvascular complications of diabetes [65].

Lastly, as interventions for diabetic cardiomyopathy in prevention of heart failure and diabetes and liver disease develop, it is envisaged that screening for these two conditions will improve. Worldwide, despite the epidemic of obesity and diabetes, increased access to insulin and blood glucose monitoring through programs such as Insulin for Life [66], and to skilled teams of healthcare professionals, through the support of the International Diabetes Federation and United Nations spearheaded campaigns, are expected to improve global outcomes in diabetes.

References

1. World Health Organization (2006). Definition and diagnosis of diabetes mellitus and intermediate hyoerglycemia report of a World Health Organization/IDF consultation. Geneva: World Health Organization Press.

2. Balasubramanyam A, Nalini R, Hampe CS & Maldonado M (2008). Syndromes of ketosis-prone diabetes mellitus. *Endocrine Reviews*, 29(3): 292–302.

3. Banting FG & Best CH (1987 [1922]). The internal secretion of the pancreas. *The Journal of Laboratory and Clinical Medicine: Nutrition Classics*, 45(2): 55–57.

4. Deckert T, Poulsen JE & Larsen M. (1978). Prognosis of diabetics with diabetes onset before the age of thirty-one. *Diabetologia*, 14: 363–77.

5. Foster DW & McGarry JD (1983). The metabolic derangements and treatment of diabetic ketoacidosis. *New England Journal of Medicine*, 309(3): 159–69.

6. Tu E, Twigg SM, Duflou C & Semsarian C (2008). Causes of death in young Australians with type 1 diabetes: a review of coronial post-mortem cases. *Medical Journal of Australia,*188(12): 699–702.

7. Wolfsdorf J, Craig ME, Daneman D, Dunger D, Edge J, Lee W, Rosenbloom A, Sperling M & Hanas R (2009). Diabetic ketoacidosis in children and adolescents with diabetes. *Pediatric Diabetes*, 10(Suppl. 12): 118–33.

8. Craig ME, Twigg SM, Donaghue KC, Cheung NW, Cameron FJ, Conn J, Jenkins AJ, Silink M, for the Australian Type 1 Diabetes Guidelines Expert Advisory Group (in press accepted 16 August, 2011). National evidence-based clinical care guidelines for type 1 diabetes in children, adolescents and adults. Canberra: Australian Government Department of Health and Ageing.

9. Kitabchi AE & Nyenwe EA (2006). Hyperglycemic crises in diabetes mellitus: diabetic ketoacidosis and hyperglycemic hyperosmolar state. *Endocrinology and Metabolism Clinics of North America,* 35(4): 725–51.

10. Colagiuri S, Dickinson S, Girgis S & Colagiuri R (2009). *National evidence based guideline for blood glucose control in type 2 diabetes*. Canberra: Diabetes Australia and the NHMRC.

11. Cryer PE, Axelrod L, Grossman AB, Heller SR, Montori VM, Seaquist ER, Service FJ & The Endocrine Society (2009). Evaluation and management of adult hypoglycemic disorders: an Endocrine Society Clinical Practice Guideline. *Journal of Clinical Endocrinology & Metabolism*, 94(3): 709–28.

12. Anderbro T, Amsberg S, Adamson U, Bolinder J, Lins P, Wredling R, Moberg E, Lisspers J & Johansson UB (2010). Fear of hypoglycaemia in adults with type 1 diabetes. *Diabetic Medicine*, 27(10): 1151–58.

13. Pearson T (2008). Glucagon as a treatment of severe hypoglycemia: safe and efficacious but underutilized. *The Diabetes Educator*, 34(1): 128–34.

14. DCCT Research Group (Diabetes Control and Complications Trial Research Group) (1991). Epidemiology of severe hypoglycemia in the diabetes control and complications trial. *American Journal of Medicine*, 90(4): 450–59.

15. UKPDS Study Group (1998). Intensive blood-glucose control with sulphonylureas or insulin compared with conventional treatment and risk of complications in patients with type 2 diabetes. (UKPDS 33). UK Prospective Diabetes Study (UKPDS) Group. *The Lancet*, 352(9131): 837–53.

16. Australian Bureau of Statistics (2009). Causes of death in Australia [Online]. Available: abs.gov.au/AUSSTATS/abs@.nsf/mf/3303.0/ [Accessed 14 December 2011].

17. Bierhaus A & Nawroth PP (2009). Multiple levels of regulation determine the role of the receptor for AGE (RAGE) as common soil in inflammation, immune responses and diabetes mellitus and its complications. *Diabetologia*, 52(11): 2251–63.

18. Twigg SM & Cooper ME (2004). The time has come to target connective tissue growth factor in diabetic complications. *Diabetologia*, 47(6): 965–68.

19. Twigg SM (2010). Mastering a mediator: blockade of CCN-2 shows early promise in human diabetic kidney disease. *Cell Communication and Signaling*, 4(4): 189–96.

20. Brownlee M (2001). Biochemistry and molecular cell biology of diabetic complications. *Nature*, 414(6865): 813–20.

21. Jeong IK & King GL (2011). New perspectives on diabetic vascular complications: the loss of endogenous protective factors induced by hyperglycemia. *Diabetes & Metabolism Journal*, 35(1): 8–11.

22. Yu Liu D, Min T, Bolton V, Nubé SM, Twigg, DK Yue & SV McLennan (2009). Increased matrix metalloproteinase-9 predicts poor wound healing in diabetic foot ulcers. *Diabetes Care*, 32(1): 117–19.

23. McLennan SV, Wang XY, Moreno V, Yue DK & Twigg SM (2004). Connective tissue growth factor mediates high glucose effects on matrix degradation through tissue inhibitor of matrix metalloproteinase type 1: implications for diabetic nephropathy. *Endocrinology*, 145(12): 5646–55.

24. Min D, Lyons JG, Bonner J, Twigg SM, Yue DK & McLennan SV (2009). Mesangial cell-derived factors alter monocyte activation and function through inflammatory pathways: possible pathogenic role in diabetic nephropathy. *American Journal of Physiology – Renal Physiology*, 297(5): F1229–37.

25. Freedman BI, Bostrom M, Daeihagh P & Bowden DW (2007). Genetic factors in diabetic nephropathy. *Clinical Journal of the American Society of Nephrology*, 2: 1306–16.

26. Fitzgerald AP & Jarrett RJ (1991). Are conventional risk factors for mortality relevant in type 2 diabetes? *Diabetic Medicine*, 8(5): 475–80.

27. Castellino P, Tuttle KR & DeFronzo RA (1994). Diabetic nephropathy. *Current Therapy in Endocrinology and Metabolism*, 5: 426–36.

28. McGill M, Molyneaux L, Twigg SM & Yue DK (2008). The metabolic syndrome in type 1 diabetes: does it exist and does it matter? *Journal of Diabetes and its Complications,* 22(1): 18–23.

29. Ray JG, O'Brien TE & Chan WS (2001). Preconception care and the risk of congenital anomalies in the offspring of women with diabetes mellitus: a meta-analysis. *Quarterly Journal of Medicine,* 94(8): 435–44.

30. Tieu J, Middleton P & Crowther CA (2010). Preconception care for diabetic women for improving maternal and fetal health. *Cochrane Database of Systematic Reviews,* 12: CD007776.

31. Crowther CA, Hiller JE, Moss JR, McPhee AJ, Jeffries WS & Robinson JS (2005). Effect of treatment of gestational diabetes mellitus on pregnancy outcomes. Australian Carbohydrate Intolerance Study in Pregnant Women (ACHOIS) Trial Group. *The New England Journal of Medicine,* 352(24): 2477–86.

32. Jacqueminet S & Jannot-Lamotte MF (2010). Therapeutic management of gestational diabetes. *Diabetes & Metabolism,* 36(6 Pt 2): 658–71.

33. Thomson SE, McLennan SV, Kirwan PD, Heffernan SJ, Hennessy A, Yue DK & Twigg SM (2008). Renal CTGF correlates with glomerular basement membrane thickness and prospective albuminuria in a non-human primate model of diabetes: possible predictive marker for incipient diabetic nephropathy. *Journal of Diabetes and its Complications,* 22(4): 284–94.

34. Australian Government Department of Health and Ageing (2008). *Guidelines for the management of diabetic retinopathy.* Canberra: Australian Government Department of Health and Ageing.

35. Australian Government Department of Health and Ageing (2009). Australian national diabetes information audit & benchmarking. Canberra: Australian Government Department of Health and Ageing.

36. Nathan DM, Zinman B, Cleary PA, Backlund JY, Genuth S, Miller R & Orchard TJ (2009). Modern-day clinical course of type 1 diabetes mellitus after 30 years' duration: the diabetes control and complications trial/epidemiology of diabetes interventions and complications and Pittsburgh epidemiology of diabetes complications experience (1983–2005). *Archives of Internal Medicine,* 169: 1307–16.

37. Lehmann R & Schleicher ED (2000). Molecular mechanism of diabetic nephropathy. *Clinica Chimica Acta,* 297: 135–44.

38. Tesfaye S, Boulton AJ, Dyck PJ, Freeman R, Horowitz M, Kempler P, Lauria G, Malik RA, Spallone V, Vinik A, Bernardi L, Valensi P & Toronto Diabetic Neuropathy Expert Group (2010). Diabetic neuropathies: update on definitions, diagnostic criteria, estimation of severity, and treatments. *Diabetes Care,* 33(10): 2285–93.

39. Ford ES (2011). Trends in the risk for coronary heart disease among adults with diagnosed diabetes in the US: findings from the National Health and Nutrition Examination Survey (1999–2008). *Diabetes Care,* 34(6): 1337–43.

40. Kothari V, Stevens RJ, Adler AI, Stratton IM, Manley SE, Neil HA & Holman RR (2002). UKPDS 60: risk of stroke in type 2 diabetes estimated by the UK Prospective Diabetes Study risk engine. *Stroke,* 33(7): 1776–81.

41. Adler AI, Stevens RJ, Neil A, Stratton IM, Boulton AJ & Holman RR (2002). UKPDS 59: hyperglycemia and other potentially modifiable risk factors for peripheral vascular disease in type 2 diabetes. *Diabetes Care*, 25(5): 894–99.

42. Australian Government Department of Health and Ageing (2011). *National evidence-based guideline: prevention, identification and management of foot complications in diabetes*. Canberra: Australian Government Department of Health and Ageing.

43. Hermans MP, Ahn SA & Rousseau MF (2009). Erectile dysfunction, microangiopathy and UKPDS risk in type 2 diabetes. *Diabetes & Metabolism*, 35(6): 484–89.

44. Kordonouri O, Maguire AM, Knip M, Schober E, Lorini R, Holl RW & Donaghue KC (2009). Other complications and associated conditions with diabetes in children and adolescents. *Pediatric Diabetes*, 10(Suppl. 12): 204–10.

45. Brooks BA, Franjic B, Ban CR, Swaraj K, Yue DK, Celermajer DS & Twigg SM. (2008). Diastolic dysfunction and abnormalities of the microcirculation in type 2 diabetes. *Diabetes, Obesity and Metabolism*, 10(9): 739–46

46. Lo L, McLennan SV, Williams PF, Bonner J, Chowdhury S, McCaughan GW, Gorrell MD, Yue DK & Twigg SM (2011). Diabetes is a progression factor for hepatic fibrosis in a high fat fed mouse obesity model of non-alcoholic steatohepatitis. *Journal of Hepatology*, 55(2): 435–44.

47. Clark JM (2006). The epidemiology of nonalcoholic fatty liver disease in adults. *Journal of Clinical Gastroenterology*, 40: S5–S10.

48. UKPDS Study Group (1998). Effect of intensive blood-glucose control with metformin on complications in overweight patients with type 2 diabetes. (UKPDS 34). *The Lancet*, 352(9131): 854–65.

49. UKPDS Study Group (1998). Intensive blood-glucose control with sulphonylureas or insulin compared with conventional treatment and risk of complications in patients with type 2 diabetes. (UKPDS 33). *The Lancet*, 352(9131): 837–53.

50. ADVANCE Collaborative Group (2008). Intensive blood glucose control and vascular outcomes in patients with type 2 diabetes. *New England Journal of Medicine*, 358(24): 2560–72.

51. ACCORD Study Group (2008). Effects of intensive glucose lowering in type 2 diabetes. *New England Journal of Medicine*, 358(24): 2545–59.

52. Duckworth W, Abraira C, Moritz T, Reda D, Emanuele N, Reaven PD, Zieve FJ, Marks J, Davis SN, Hayward R, Warren SR, Goldman S, McCarren M, Vitek ME, Henderson WG & Huang GD (2009). Glucose control and vascular complications in veterans with type 2 diabetes. *New England Journal of Medicine*, 360(2): 129–39.

53. Nathan DM, Cleary PA, Backlund JY, Genuth SM, Lachin JM, Orchard TJ, Raskin P, Zinman B & DCCT/EDIC Study Research Group (2005). Intensive diabetes treatment and cardiovascular disease in patients with type 1 diabetes, *New England Journal of Medicine*, 353(25): 2643–53.

54. Holman RR, Paul SK, Bethel MA, Matthews DR & Neil HA (2008). 10-year follow-up of intensive glucose control in type 2 diabetes. *New England Journal of Medicine*, 359(15): 1577–89.

55. Tonna S, El-Osta A, Cooper ME & Tikellis C (2010). Metabolic memory and diabetic nephropathy: potential role for epigenetic mechanisms. *Nature Reviews Nephrology*, 6: 332–41.

56. Cheung NW, Conn JJ, d'Emden MC, Gunton JE, Jenkins AJ, Ross GP, Sinha AK, Andrikopoulos S, Colagiuri S & Twigg SM (2009). Position statement of the Australian Diabetes Society: individualisation of glycated haemoglobin targets for adults with diabetes mellitus. *Medical Journal of Australia,* 191(6): 339–44.

57. Chobanian AV, Bakris GL, Black HR, Cushman WC, Green LA, Izzo JL Jr, Jones DW, Materson BJ, Oparil S, Wright JT Jr & Roccella EJ (2003). The seventh report of the Joint National Committee on Prevention, Detection, Evaluation, and Treatment of High Blood Pressure: the JNC 7 report. National Heart, Lung, and Blood Institute Joint National Committee on Prevention, Detection, Evaluation, and Treatment of High Blood Pressure; National High Blood Pressure Education Program Coordinating Committee. *Journal of the American Medical Association,* 289(19): 2560–72.

58. Colhoun HM, Betteridge DJ, Durrington PN, Hitman GA, Neil HA, Livingstone SJ, Thomason MJ, Mackness MI, Charlton-Menys V, Fuller JH & CARDS investigators (2004). Primary prevention of cardiovascular disease with atorvastatin in type 2 diabetes in the Collaborative Atorvastatin Diabetes Study (CARDS): multicentre randomised placebo-controlled trial. *The Lancet,* 364(9435): 685–96.

59. Gaede P, Vedel P, Larsen N, Jensen GV, Parving HH & Pedersen O (2003). Multifactorial intervention and cardiovascular disease in patients with type 2 diabetes. *New England Journal of Medicine*, 348(5): 383–93.

60. Colagiuri R, Girgis S, Eigenmann C, Gomez M & Griffiths R (2009). *National evidence based guideline for patient education in type 2 diabetes.* Canberra: Diabetes Australia and the NHMRC.

61. Han DJ & Sutherland DE (2010). Pancreas transplantation. *Gut Liver,* 4(4): 450–65.

62. Ismail-Beigi F, Craven T, Banerji MA, Basile J, Calles J, Cohen RM, Cuddihy R, Cushman WC, Genuth S, Grimm RH Jr, Hamilton BP, Hoogwerf B, Karl D, Katz L, Krikorian A, O'Connor P, Pop-Busui R, Schubart U, Simmons D, Taylor H, Thomas A, Weiss D, Hramiak I & ACCORD trial group (2010). Effect of intensive treatment of hyperglycaemia on microvascular outcomes in type 2 diabetes: an analysis of the ACCORD randomised trial. *The Lancet,* 376(9739): 419–30.

63. Secrest AM, Becker DJ, Kelsey SF, LaPorte RE & Orchard TJ (2010). All-cause mortality trends in a large population-based cohort with long-standing childhood-onset type 1 diabetes: the Allegheny County type 1 diabetes registry, *Diabetes Care*, 33(12): 2573–79.

64. Gu K, Cowie CC & Harris MI (1999). Diabetes and decline in heart disease mortality in US adults. *Journal of the American Medical Association,* 281(14): 1291–97.

65. Rajamani K, Colman PG, Li LP, Best JD, Voysey M, D'Emden MC, Laakso M, Baker JR, Keech AC & FIELD study investigators (2009). Effect of fenofibrate on amputation events in people with type 2 diabetes mellitus (FIELD study): a prespecified analysis of a randomised controlled trial. *The Lancet,* 373(9677): 1780–88.

66. Insulin for Life website: www.insulinforlife.org/

21

Obesity treatment for adults, adolescents and children

Ian Caterson,[1] Nick Finer,[2] Louise A Baur[3] and Kate Steinbeck[4]

Obesity treatment aims to produce weight loss and weight-loss maintenance, as well as risk reduction, disease prevention, amelioration or cure. Treatment needs to be designed according to the person's need. A small loss (5%–10% of initial body weight) may suffice for disease prevention, but greater weight loss is often needed for mobility or for disease cure in those with a greater degree of obesity. For children and adolescents, family involvement and a developmentally appropriate approach are vital. For example, for pre-pubertal children, who are still growing in height, reduction in the rate of weight gain, or weight stability, may be sufficient to achieve health improvement. Lifestyle interventions to achieve energy restriction and increase energy expenditure (through activity and exercise) are the initial approach. Pharmacotherapy can improve the efficacy of lifestyle interventions. Intragastric devices and bariatric surgery may be appropriate for those with more severe disease, including selected older adolescents. While weight loss can be achieved, the major issue in treatment of obesity remains weight maintenance and efforts need to be directed to this end.

Overweight and obesity are common in Australia, with approximately one in five adults being obese, two in five overweight and approximately one in four of our children being overweight or obese. This condition has essentially become the norm. As is discussed elsewhere in this volume, this increasing obesity prevalence has come with increasing health problems and diseases. Whilst many of these diseases can be treated directly (and at continuing expense) it would be better to prevent such obesity-associated diseases by treating their underlying cause, that is by managing overweight and obesity properly. In fact, it would be even better to prevent overweight and obesity occurring in our society!

Traditionally the health professionals have been pessimistic about their ability to treat obesity but with the new realisations of what successful treatment really is, and with the newer treatment modalities, obesity treatment can be, and is, successful. What is needed

1 Boden Institute of Obesity, Nutrition, Exercise and Eating Disorders, University of Sydney.

2 University College Hospital, London, UK.

3 Children's Hospital, Westmead Clinical School, University of Sydney.

4 Adolescent Medicine, University of Sydney.

is a practical approach, individual goals for each patient and a system which provides the appropriate intervention as well as continuing support and follow-up. These aspects of obesity management for adults, adolescents and children will be discussed in the chapter.

Management of obesity in adults: whom to treat and how to treat?

There are a number of modalities involved in the management of obesity, which should be delivered as an integrated program. These modalities include standard lifestyle interventions (eating and activity), behaviour and group therapy, adjunctive therapy (pharmacotherapy, meal replacement regimes), some special devices (intragastric balloons) and bariatric surgery. A suggested approach utilising the patient's body mass index (BMI, weight/height^2, kg/m^2), the presence of obesity-associated comorbidities, and a range of treatment options is outlined in Table 1.

Table 1. A management approach for obesity in adults.

BMI (kg/m^2)*	Lifestyle**	Obesity drugs	VLEDs	Devices: eg intragastric balloon	Bariatric surgery
25 to 26.9	Advice				
27 to 34.9	Lifestyle program	Consider	Possibly		
27 to 34.9 ±comorbidity	Lifestyle program	Consider	Probably	Possibly	
>35 ±comorbidity	Lifestyle program	Consider	Utilise	Possibly	Consider
>40 (if no comorbidities)	Lifestyle program	Consider	Utilise	Possibly	Consider

* If there is increased waist circumference (the importance of which is described elsewhere in this volume) then a more intensive therapeutic regimen may be utilised at a lower BMI range.

** All the components of the lifestyle program and other therapies are described below. Obesity pharmacotherapy may be utilised to help maintain weight after it is lost using other treatment modalities instead of just being used to produce weight loss. Very low energy diets (VLEDs) are useful for initiating and obtaining weight loss, in weight maintenance and prior to bariatric surgery.

It is important that healthcare practitioners recognise when a patient has a weight problem and for them to be able to prescribe an appropriate management plan for the patient's degree of obesity, life stage and situation.

Lifestyle management

A lifestyle-management program remains the basis of all obesity treatment [1]. Such a program has a number of components, the most obvious of which are eating and physical activity plans. Another major component is a behaviour-modification program. Other aspects include goal setting, psychological support (and counselling if necessary), proper medical management and a long-term plan for maintaining weight loss. Such lifestyle programs have been shown to be effective [2], and losses of 6% or more of initial body weight can be achieved and maintained. There is no reason for such programs to be delivered solely by health professionals [3]. For those with a BMI in the lower overweight and obesity range (ie BMI 27 to 34.9 kg/m²), and without major medical complications, such programs can be delivered effectively in the community setting.

Goal setting

This is often ignored, or not specifically discussed with the patient. The goals will vary from patient to patient. It is important to set realistic goals for weight loss, of course, but other goals may be individual and/or medical. Other than weight loss, goals may include prevention and control of disease (such as diabetes), better mobility, less medications, ability to have a joint replacement, or a specific goal that the patient wants to achieve. Such goals should be discussed, recorded and when reached the achievement should be noted and the patient congratulated.

Eating

It is better to use the term 'eating plan' rather than 'diet'. Diets tend to be seen as short term and there are many which are pushed by magazines, in books, and online, and there is a large industry producing these diet plans. This plethora of diets is confusing and unhelpful for someone attempting to lose and then maintain weight loss. It has been shown that the amount of weight loss obtained does not depend on the type of eating plan prescribed; most produce similar weight losses at six months with gradual weight regain thereafter [4, 5]. Compliance to the plan, not the type of plan, is what produces weight loss [6]. What is really necessary is a 500 to 600 kcal (2100 to 2500 kJ) energy deficit and a plan that starts by making small changes to a patient's habitual consumption. Such changes may include decreases in portion size, a reduction in fat (and in particular saturated fat), possibly an increase in mono-unsaturated fat, a reduction in sugar-sweetened beverages and a low glycaemic index diet. An increase in protein in the diet may increase satiety. Any changes must be made specifically in the context of the patient's habitual diet. It is useful to keep food logs at regular intervals to check compliance and to use as a tool to suggest further changes in intake or eating patterns.

Physical activity

The term 'physical activity plan' is preferred to 'exercise', because the prescribed plan will include both planned exercise as well as incidental activity. A formal prescription of such a plan does produce greater compliance. Activity helps maintain lean mass and because of the increased energy deficit it promotes weight (kg) and fat mass loss. A simple initial approach is to use a physical activity questionnaire, determine how much time is spent walking or in specific exercise and perhaps suggest the use of a pedometer to get an activity baseline.

The activity prescription itself should be specific to the patient. It may include increased time walking, more incidental activity (taking an active option), and/or specific exercises, gym programs or training, or involvement in sport. For diabetes prevention, supervised exercise sessions have been shown to be part of all-effective programs. It is good to remember that the greater the patient's weight, the fewer 'steps' they have to do to lose weight. Activity should be monitored and the amount done recorded. Again this will help in assessment of compliance and will also be a tool for increasing the amount of activity performed.

Increased activity alone (as a weight-loss program) does not produce a great deal of weight loss. It may affect fat distribution [7, 8] but, for reasonable weight loss to ensue, activity must be combined with an eating plan [9].

Behaviour modification

The use of food and activity logs is part of behaviour modification. Another log that may be useful is one for mood, particularly at time of eating, as well as general affect. Cognitive behaviour therapy may be useful, particularly for optimising weight maintenance. Other techniques are those of cognitive restructuring, motivational enhancement therapy, psychological support and counselling. There are many techniques that may be used but to describe these in any detail is beyond the scope of this chapter. The techniques utilised need to be individualised to the patient's situation and life stage, so there really is no 'standard' program – rather, a series of techniques used when necessary [10].

An effective lifestyle program must contain some or all of these elements, and though patient education alone is not effective in producing weight loss, it too is a part of a successful program. A multidisciplinary team providing care is essential. Regular visits (at least fortnightly initially and then at longer intervals) are important. Weight regain does tend to recur, particularly in the second year of a program and it is at this stage that there needs to be further research on the effect of repeated, brief acute interventions, the use of pharmacotherapy for maintenance, and/or the use of very low energy diets (VLEDs).

If the lifestyle program is not successful, with goals not being attained, then adjunctive therapy should be considered. Such consideration should begin early in any program, say at one month, with reconsideration at regular intervals.

Adjunctive therapy

Very low energy diets (VLEDs)

Such formulations are effective at producing early weight loss [11], although after a time (two to three years) they appear to produce no more weight loss than a standard lifestyle program. However if their use is continued (as one to two meal replacements per day) then significant weight loss can be both achieved and maintained [12]. These diets tend to contain 500 to 800 kcal/day and the necessary vitamins and micronutrients. Early formulations did not contain high-quality protein and a number of deaths ensued, but these difficulties have been addressed and current formulations are safe, provided they are used according to protocol, and preferably under medical supervision [13].

These formulations are available as shakes, soups and bars, and in most countries they are classified as 'Foods'. They may be used as a full meal replacement protocol (every meal a VLED) or as a partial protocol (one to two meals a day as a VLED). The full protocol is best performed under clinical supervision, particularly if the patient has diabetes or cardiac disease. The full protocol has been used as the 'control treatment' in randomised trials of bariatric surgery and quite reasonable weight losses, of the order of 15% or more of initial body weight, are obtained.

Initial full-meal replacement protocols usually run for 12 to 16 weeks though under supervised conditions there is no reason why they should not be used for longer. They can be used as one to two meals per day to help maintain weight loss. They are generally used prior to bariatric surgery [14] to reduce some weight and to reduce fat in the liver (which makes surgery easier).

Pharmacotherapy

The relatively limited success of lifestyle interventions has driven the search for effective anti-obesity drugs. Drug treatment of obesity is driven by similar principles for pharmacotherapy of other chronic diseases: it needs to be effective and safe (particularly as it will need to be used long term), acceptable to patients and affordable [15]. While the physiological control of body weight theoretically provides many targets (satiety, nutrient absorption and energy expenditure), in practice it has proven hard to find safe and effective drugs and regulatory authorities such as the Food and Drugs Administration in US, European Medicines Evaluation Agency and Therapeutics Goods Administration in Australia, have set guidelines and standards of evidence for efficacy and safety that have proven a barrier to new drug development.

Drugs available in the past 20 years but no longer licensed

Amphetamine-like drugs with predominant actions of enhancing brain dopamine pathways included phentermine and diethylpropion. They produced anorexia (rather than satiety) and had some CNS stimulant properties. Although they produced weight loss of about 5%–10% they were not evaluated according to contemporary standards for clinical trials. Phentermine is available and used short term in the US, Asia and Australia, but not in Europe. The fenfluramines developed in the 1980s were effective satiety-enhancing drugs that acted mainly through enhancing central serotoninergic neuronal transmission (by both release and reuptake inhibition of serotonin). However they were associated with pulmonary hypertension and cardiac valve abnormalities (especially when combined with phentermine) and withdrawn from use in 2004. The endocannaboid receptor (CB1 receptor) was identified as an attractive target since it had long been known that stimulation of this receptor led to hunger; a number of selective CB1 receptor blockers were developed in the early 2000s, with rimonabant being licensed in Europe on the basis of four clinical trials that showed it could produce weight loss of about 10% absolute, 5.6 kg placebo-subtracted, and that efficacy was maintained over at least two years. Furthermore rimonabant use was associated with metabolic improvements of lipids and glycaemic control. However shortly after approval it became clear that there was an unacceptable incidence of depression and suicidal ideation with the drug that led to its withdrawal [16].

Sibutramine, a selective serotonin and norepinephrine-uptake inhibitor had been licensed and in use worldwide since the 1990s. It produced placebo-subtracted weight loss of about 5% over one year, but appeared to have greater efficacy when combined with intensive lifestyle interventions: in one trial an average 12·1 kg weight loss compared to five kilograms with sibutramine alone. Concerns remained that the drug had unwanted and potentially dangerous sympathomimetic effects that could raise blood pressure and pulse, so at the demand of the European Medicines Agency the Sibutramine Cardiovascular Outcomes (SCOUT) trial assessed the efficacy of sibutramine in reducing myocardial infarction, stroke, and cardiovascular mortality in 11 000 obese and overweight patients. In order to produce enough cardiovascular endpoints, patients with existing cardiovascular disease and diabetes and at high risk for future events were recruited (a population that would have been excluded according to the drug licence). The trial reported that despite well-sustained weight loss, there was an excess of non-fatal cardiovascular events in the subjects receiving sibutramine for up to four years [17] and this led to the withdrawal of the drug.

Current drugs licensed for obesity treatment

In 2011 orlistat, a pancreatic and intestinal lipase inhibitor, was the major drug licensed for obesity treatment. It produces malabsorption of about 30% of ingested dietary fat. Its use is limited by gastro-intestinal side effects (steatorrhea, flatus, urgency of defecation and sometimes even faecal incontinence) such that unless subjects are on a low-fat diet (maximum 90 gm fat daily) it is unlikely to be tolerated. In this setting the drug can produce an approximate 300 kcal/day energy loss through undigested fat. In a meta-analysis of 11 placebo-controlled trials of one year in over 6000 overweight or obese patients, orlistat 120 mg thrice daily reduced weight by about 3% more than placebo, with 21% reaching a 5% loss, and 12% a 10% or greater weight loss. Orlistat has favourable effects on blood pressure, lipids and blood glucose. In some countries orlistat is available at a dose of 60 mg thrice daily either over the counter or through pharmacist prescription [18–20].

Phentermine is available in Australia, the US and Asia. It is an older drug with a central action on appetite. There are no long-term studies, but it has been shown to be effective short term and may be used to help produce or maintain weight loss. Further studies are really needed to define its place in obesity management.

Drugs producing weight loss licensed for other indications

The glucagon-like peptide 1 (GLP-1) incretin analogues exenatide and liraglutide are both licensed for use as hypoglycaemic drugs for treating type 2 diabetes, and they produce a weight loss of two to four kilograms. GLP-1 agonists have complex modes of action on weight loss that include delayed gastric emptying, and both direct, and indirect via the vagus nerve, stimulation of central nervous system satiety pathways. The drug has to be given by subcutaneous injection. Liraglutide given at higher doses than used to treat diabetes is in clinical trials as a weight-loss agent in non-diabetics. Early results have shown body weight losses of about 10% associated with marked metabolic and cardiovascular improvements sustained for two years [21].

Currently much focus is on combining drugs at low doses to produce synergistic weight-loss effects while minimising side and unwanted effects [22]. Combining naltrexone (an opioid receptor antagonist) with bupropion (an antidepressant) showed synergistic effects on the firing of hypothalamic pro-opiomelanocortin neurons in mice. In a trial of nearly 2000 overweight and obese subjects the highest dose combination produced weight loss of 6.1% at one year compared to 1.3% on placebo. Side effects were mainly gastrointestinal, but there were transient increases in blood pressure with less fall than might have been expected from the weight-loss achieved [23].

The anti-epilepsy drug topiramate has been combined with phentermine and also investigated in clinical trials. In nearly 2500 patients the highest dose combination produced a weight loss after 56 weeks of just under 10% compared to 1.2% of those on placebo. Dizziness, depression and anxiety were the most common side effects and will need further evaluation before the drug will be licensed.

Bariatric surgery

Bariatric procedures aim to produce and maintain weight loss by altering energy balance primarily by reducing food intake and mitigating the physiological changes that drive weight regain. Most guidelines recommend that bariatric surgery be considered for those with a BMI above 35 kg/m^2 with an obesity-related comorbidity, or above 40 kg/m^2 in those without. A multidisciplinary team including surgeon, anaesthetist, physician, dietitian, specialist nurse and psychologist or psychiatrist is needed to provide optimal care.

Four procedures are most commonly performed, in modern practice all laparascopically: Roux-en-Y gastric bypass, adjustable gastric banding, sleeve gastrectomy and biliopancreatic diversion (Figure 1), with considerable variation between countries in the preferred procedures.

Roux-en-Y gastric bypass creates a small gastric remnant that empties directly into the transposed jejunum, bypassing the main body of the stomach, duodenum and proximal jejunum. Although the procedure was initially thought to produce weight loss by both restriction and malabsorption of food intake, it is clear that the impact of food entering rapidly into the distal jejunum is associated with the rapid release of gastrointestinal peptide satiety hormones including GLP-1 and Peptide YY (PYY), as well as decreasing the orexigenic hormone ghrelin, released from the stomach. Other factors postulated to produce weight loss include altered bile salt secretion and altered gut microbiota. Patients require lifelong vitamin B12 and vitamin D replacement. Weight losses average 35%–40% at five years.

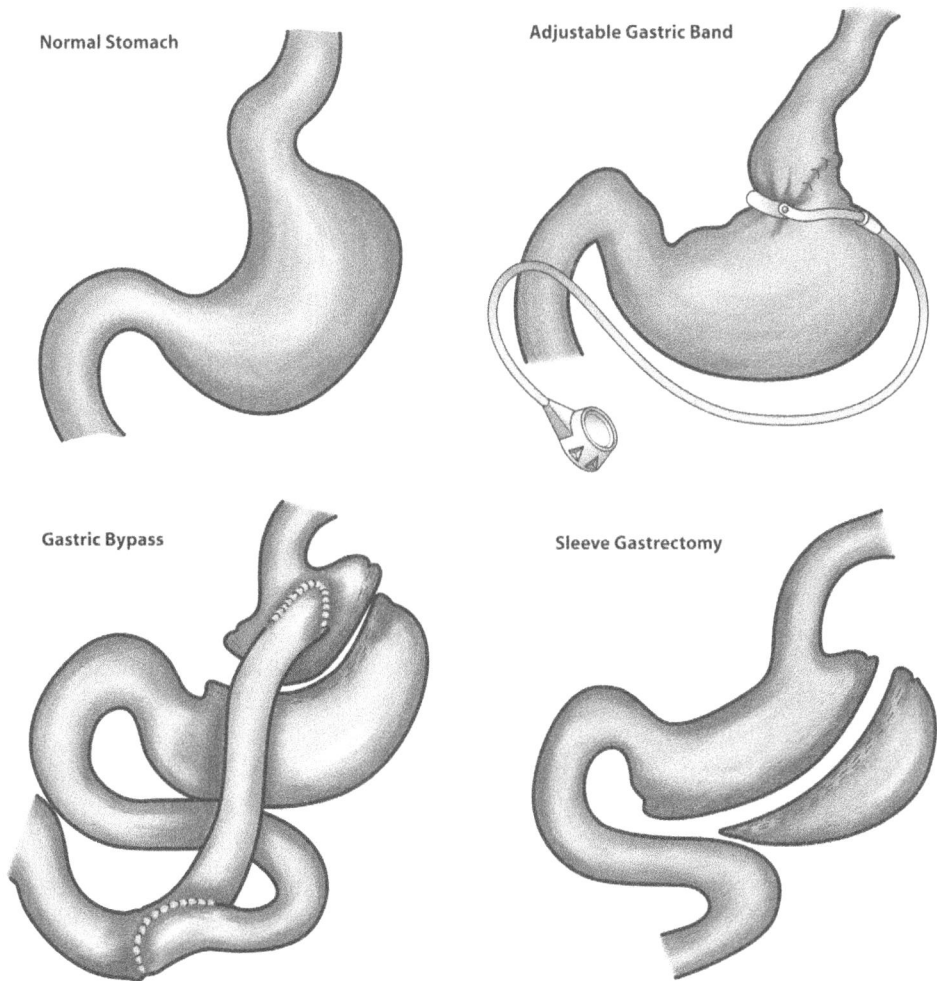

Figure 1. Types of bariatric surgery, shown schematically from top left to bottom right: normal stomach, adjustable gastric band, gastric bypass, sleeve gastrectomy.

Adjustable gastric bypass is a simpler procedure in which an adjustable silastic band is placedaround the proximal fundus of the stomach to leave a pouch of about 15 to 30 ccs. A tube leads from the band to a port positioned subcutaneously through which saline can be injected to tighten (or loosen) the band. Frequent adjustments of band filling are required and success is critically dependent on this process as well as the patient's willingness and ability to adapt their diet and respond to the sense of fullness that the band produces. Weight losses average 25%–30% at five years. Sleeve gastrectomy was originally introduced as a first step for patients at too high a surgical risk for a Roux-en-Y procedure, with the intention to convert the gastrectomy to a bypass at a second operation after the patient had lost some weight. The finding that sleeve gastrectomy led to similar weight loss and metabolic benefit as the full Roux-en-Y procedure led to enthusiasm for this technically simpler procedure, but more recent evaluation suggests weight-loss and metabolic improvement are less durable.

Bilio-pancreatic diversion with or without a duodenal switch procedure is a major malabsorptive procedure that is not widely performed and has been less well evaluated than other procedures. Although weight loss may be 40%–60%, nutritional complications are frequent.

The most compelling data for the success of bariatric surgery at producing weight loss and improving the clinical outcomes for obese patients comes from the 15-year follow-up data of the Swedish Obese Subjects study (SOS) [24]. This was a case controlled study, and the surgical techniques were not as advanced as performed nowadays. The persistent weight loss in the surgical groups was associated with a much reduced mortality: the unadjusted overall hazard ratio was 0.76 in the surgery group (P = 0.04), as compared with the control group, and the hazard ratio adjusted for sex, age and risk factors was 0.71 (P = 0.01). Other studies have confirmed that bariatric surgery is associated with reduced all-cause mortality including deaths from cardiovascular disease, diabetes and cancer.

Bariatric surgery has important benefits in patients with type 2 diabetes that extend beyond weight loss [14]. Up to 80% of people with type 2 diabetes may experience remission of their diabetes (normoglycaemia without the need for hypoglycaemic medication), the exact remission rate being determined by the type of surgery and the duration of diabetes prior to surgery. Systematic reviews suggest that about 60% will have remission after gastric banding (and that the remission is of slower onset and more closely related to weight loss) compared to 80% after Roux-en-Y bypass, and 95% after bilio-pancreatic diversion. The International Federation of Diabetes position statement in 2011 concludes that bariatric surgery: a) constitutes a powerful option to ameliorate diabetes in severely obese patients, often normalising blood glucose levels, reducing or avoiding the need for medications and providing a potentially cost-effective approach to treating the disease; b) is an appropriate treatment for people with type 2 diabetes and obesity not achieving recommended treatment targets with medical therapies; c) should be an accepted option in people who have type 2 diabetes and a BMI >35; and even d) an alternative treatment option in patients with a BMI between 30 and 35 when diabetes cannot be adequately controlled by optimal medical regimen, especially in the presence of other major cardiovascular disease risk factors [25].

Though it is effective for weight loss, the complications of bariatric surgery are significant [26]. The mortality risks of surgery itself are <0.5% overall, although the risks for those individuals with pre-existing cardiovascular disease or other morbidity may be substantially higher. Short-term complications are substantially lower with gastric banding compared to other procedures, but later complications are common. Re-operation rates for 'slipped' bands or erosion of the band through the stomach wall may occur in as many as 30% of banded patients after five years and a third may fail to lose or maintain weight loss [27]. Other longer-term complications in gastric bypass patients include strictures, excessive weight loss, and hypoglycaemic dumping. The latter appears to be driven by excessive incretin, and hence insulin responses to (inappropriate) high-carbohydrate meals.

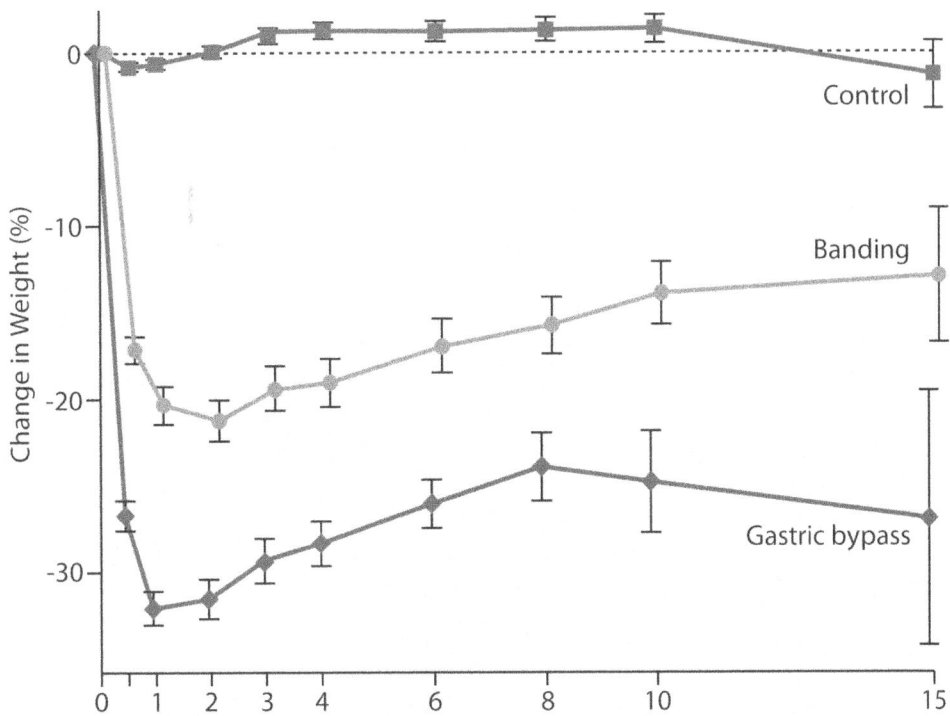

Figure 2. Weight trajectories from Swedish Obese Subjects study. Source: Sjöström L, Narbro K, Sjöström DC, Karason K, Larsson B, et al. (2007). Effects of bariatric surgery on mortality in Swedish obese subjects. *The New England Journal of Medicine*, 357(8): 747.

While bariatric surgery has much to offer, for optimal results highly experienced surgeons doing high volumes of surgery, in patients who have an adequate understanding that surgery is an aid not a 'quick fix' to weight loss, and with excellent nutritional support and more general psychological counseling are needed.

Devices

There are a number of devices which have been used to manage obesity. One in relatively common use is the intragastric balloon. This is placed endoscopically, inflated with fluid, and for the first week after placement the patient stays on VLEDs until the balloon becomes fixed. This device restricts eating and in a recent trial with obese subjects we have shown weight losses of 14% of initial body weight at six months compared to 4.8% in controls who were treated with a lifestyle program [28]. After the balloon is removed at the six month time point, there is some weight regain but at 12 months there is still more weight lost by the 'balloon' group (some 9% of initial weight), whilst those in the control group maintain their weight loss. There are side effects of the balloon, especially cramping and vomiting, but those treated this way have a significant increase in their measured quality of life. Other devices being investigated include endoduodenal sleeves (a plastic sleeve which lines the duodenum) and gastric pacemakers. These too need to be placed endoscopically.

General issues

Obviously many of those overweight or obese will already have an obesity-related comorbidity, either metabolic or mechanical (these are discussed elsewhere in this volume). These problems should be treated actively, but at the same time a weight-loss program should be instituted and conversely during a weight-loss program there should be active, effective treatment of such comorbidities. Weight loss can help improve these medical problems [29] and also reduce the medications required to treat them [30], as well as improving quality of life.

At the same time care should be taken to not use, or minimise the use and dose of, drugs which may cause weight gain. These include antipsychotics and antidepressants, steroid therapy, anticonvulsants (especially valproate) and medications used to manage diabetes. Where possible an alternate drug which has no effect on weight, or which can help weight loss should be chosen. For example, use of an SSRI such as fluoxetine in depression can promote weight loss, topiramate is an anti-epileptic which promotes weight loss [31], metformin may produce or assist with weight loss and some of the newer anti-diabetic agents, such as the GLP1 agonists, promote weight loss.

Maintenance of weight loss

This is a vexed issue. Within three to five years of completed and effective weight-loss programs most of the weight loss will have been regained, though there is increasing evidence these programs can be effective [32]. Even following bariatric surgery, where there is substantial weight loss which can be maintained for years, there tends to be a slow regain (though not to initial weight). This regain is due to 'relaxation' of the lifestyle program and is caused by underlying physiological drivers, such as elevated appetite hormones causing increased hunger, which force a reversion to old eating patterns (as an example).

There are some individuals who lose weight and do keep it off for years. These individuals undertake high levels of physical activity, eat breakfast and regular meals, a diet that is low in fat, and they self monitor which is a way of catching 'slips' early and correcting them. However, this type of response is not the common one.

Does that mean weight-loss programs are always failures and therefore should not really be attempted? The answer to this is a resounding 'no' on at least two counts. Firstly, weight loss does have an effect on many aspects: the control and prevention of disease, greater mobility, better quality of life and so on. There is even evidence from the diabetes prevention trials that a beneficial metabolic effect, the so-called metabolic memory, persists for years after the program has ceased and even if weight is regained.

Secondly, most of the reported weight-loss 'failures' are the follow-up of a single intervention. It is important that it is realised that the struggle against the issue of excess weight is a chronic, lifelong one. Programs need to be developed which include regular follow-up, which use pharmacotherapy to maintain loss, and have acute interventions if there is a small amount of regain (in our clinic we use a regain of three kilograms as the trigger for a more intense effort). The US-based Look AHEAD program in people with type 2 diabetes is one such example [32]. Multidisciplinary chronic care programs will become even more necessary as the cohort of those who have had bariatric surgery increases – this group will need such lifetime follow-up. With the development of these long-term programs there must be research on effectiveness and over time, long-term weight loss and maintenance will be achieved.

Management of obesity in children and adolescents: whom and when to treat?

Presentations to healthcare settings

Children and adolescents who are overweight or obese attend both primary and tertiary healthcare settings more frequently than might be expected from the background prevalence of this condition [33–36]. This is probably because of the health complications linked to their weight status. However, they rarely present to the doctor specifically for the problem of obesity. In a large random sample of Australian general practice surgeries, the BEACH study, 29.6% of two- to 18-year-olds were overweight or obese (11.4% overall were obese), compared with a background population prevalence of 23%–25% (5%–8% obese). Unfortunately, these patients are unlikely to have the problem of obesity addressed by the clinician. In the BEACH study, only 1:60 of those who were overweight or obese had any form of management provided for this issue [34].

Why might this situation be? While Australian general practitioners (GPs) state that they are committed to dealing with the consequences of obesity, they also cite a range of barriers to managing it, including inadequate time and reimbursement, an apparent lack of effective interventions and support services, low levels of parent or patient motivation, the complexity and sensitivity of the issue, and the need for further training [37]. Families themselves are somewhat circumspect about the role of GPs on this issue and do not see GPs as the primary source of advice about management of obesity in young people [38].

Indicators for treatment

So, should children and adolescents affected by obesity seek or receive treatment, and, if so, where? As a general principle, assessment and treatment is especially warranted for the following individuals [39–42]:

- Those who are moderately to severely obese
- Adolescents
- Those with obesity-associated complications, such as insulin resistance, obstructive sleep apnoea, psychosocial distress, fatty liver disease, cardio-metabolic risk factors, or orthopaedic complications
- Those with a high risk family history, such as parents, grandparents, siblings or aunts/ uncles with type 2 diabetes, premature heart disease, a history of bariatric surgery, obstructive sleep apnoea, hypertension or dyslipidaemia
- Those from a high-risk ethnic group, where cardio-metabolic complications are more

common, such as Aboriginal and Torres Strait Islanders, Maori and Pacific people, those from Mediterranean or Middle-Eastern countries or the Indian subcontinent, and native Americans.

Where should treatment be provided?

Given the high prevalence of child and adolescent obesity in most Westernised, and rapidly Westernising, countries, and its chronicity, coordinated models of care for health service delivery are needed. However, no country has yet established a cost-effective model of care for obesity management. One potential approach is that adapted from the UK National Health Service [43] and Kaiser Permanente [44] chronic disease pyramid of care. This is based upon a tiered level of service delivery relating to severity of disease.

Ideally, the vast majority of those affected by the problem of obesity should be managed via self-care or family-based care, with support from GPs or community-based health service providers. Such patients should be offered healthy lifestyle counselling or community-based group programs. The next stage of management involves more targeted recommendations for behavioural change, supported by involvement of allied health professionals, such as dietitians, or, indeed, a multidisciplinary team of therapists. The final stage, which is offered to children and adolescents with severe obesity, is provided by a specialist team and may include provision of pharmacotherapy, very low energy diets, or even bariatric surgery. The patient's age, severity of obesity and obesity-associated complications, and level of engagement with, and success of, previous interventions, should determine which stage of therapy is offered.

Unfortunately, such a staged approach to care is yet to be resourced or implemented widely in countries such as Australia. In reality, most children and adolescents who are affected by obesity will be managed by their GP, possibly with some involvement of a practice nurse or dietitian. Certainly, those children or adolescents who have severe obesity should be assessed, and have their care coordinated, by a paediatrician or adolescent physician, ideally with involvement of a multidisciplinary team of other therapists.

Lifestyle treatment

The mainstay of treatment of obesity in this age-group, as in adults, is lifestyle change. What is the evidence for this?

The 2009 Cochrane review on the treatment of child and adolescent obesity included 64 randomised controlled trials [45]. No one specific treatment program was recommended over another; however, positive outcomes were identified in several studies. A meta-analysis of several studies showed that family-targeted lifestyle intervention, involving various combinations of dietary, physical activity and behaviour modification, led to a significantly greater reduction in BMI or BMI z-score (ie BMI adjusted for age and sex) at six months than 'standard care'. For children aged less than 12 years there was a modest average reduction of 0.06 in BMI z-score, and in adolescents there was an average reduction of just over three BMI units.

However, many published studies are limited by varying attrition rates, small sample sizes, different measures of change in body size, and lack of assessment of other outcomes (for example, broader medical, psychosocial and behavioural outcomes). And they have typically involved fairly homogeneous patient samples managed in a tertiary care setting. Although recent trials are addressing some of these issues, much of the evidence to support effective intervention may not be readily generalisable to other clinical settings. For example, 'real-world' obesity clinics are usually less well resourced than programs in clinical trials, and patients seen in such clinics may be quite different from those who volunteer for trials. They may have more social disadvantage, or have psychosocial complications and other problems that make adherence to treatment more difficult. Not surprisingly, therefore, studies in clinical practice have demonstrated poorer results than in formal clinical trials [46]. Nevertheless, the broad principles of management are well recognised and are outlined in Box 1.

Box 1. Principles of obesity management in children and adolescents

- management of obesity-associated comorbidities
- family involvement
- a developmentally appropriate approach
- long-term behaviour modification
- dietary change
- increased physical activity
- decreased sedentary behaviours
- consideration of the use of pharmacotherapy and other forms of non-conventional therapy
- plan for longer-term weight maintenance strategies.

Effective management of obesity-associated comorbidities, such as sleep apnoea, dyslipidaemia, hypertension, non-alcoholic fatty liver disease or type 2 diabetes mellitus, is vital. Ideally, patients should be co-managed, in a coordinated way, by relevant specialist teams. In all cases, effective weight management should be a key element of the treatment of the comorbidity. Further discussion of the management of these comorbidities is beyond the scope of this review.

Family focus

Many clinical trials show that family-based interventions can lead to long-term relative weight loss (that is, from two to ten years) [45, 47–50]. Parental involvement is vital when managing obese younger children in particular [45, 48, 51–53]. This makes sense, as parents are normally the people in the family who are responsible for the food and physical activity environment, such as buying and cooking food, the types of routines around meals and meal times, rules around TV viewing and bed-time, role-modelling of eating and activity behaviours, and the use of the family car.

A developmentally appropriate approach

The developmental age of the patient – whether they are pre-adolescent, or adolescent, or, indeed, whether they have a developmental disability – will influence whether the patient per se is involved in treatment, and the type of parental engagement. A different approach is usually needed for pre-adolescent children compared to adolescents.

Pre-adolescent children

When managing pre-adolescent children, a parent-focused intervention, without direct engagement of the child, appears to have better outcomes to a child-centred approach [50, 54]. Obese children aged six to 11 years and their parents were randomly assigned to either parent-only group sessions (with an emphasis on general parenting skills), or child-only group sessions. At one and seven years follow-up from baseline, a significant reduction in overweight was observed in the parent-only group compared with the child-only group. At one year, there was a 14.6% reduction in overweight in the parent-only group versus 8.1% in the child-only group (p <0.03), with a nine times greater dropout rate in the child-only group [50]. At the seven-year follow-up, 60% of the children in the parent-only group, versus 31% of those in the child-only group, were classified as non-obese [54]. These and other studies suggest that when treating pre-adolescent children with obesity, therapy sessions involving the parent or parents alone, without the young child being present, could be the most effective.

Adolescents

There are fewer studies looking specifically at treatment of adolescents affected by obesity. The previously mentioned 2009 Cochrane review included 27 trials involving participants aged 12 years and older [45]. Twelve studies used behavioural lifestyle modification, ten involved drug therapy, three used physical activity, and two involved diet. Most included studies were of high intensity and were offered in secondary or tertiary level care settings. Many offered separate sessions for adolescents and parents. In clinical practice, it may be useful to have at least some of the session time just involving the adolescent and therapist, engaging the parent later.

Behaviour modification

Behaviour modification in weight management includes a set of techniques employed to change thought processes and actions associated with eating, physical activity and sedentary behaviours [55]. Many trials of obesity management in children and adolescents have included a behavioural component, although these are often poorly described. In general, the greater the range of behaviour change techniques used, the better the weight outcomes [48]. Goal setting, stimulus control and self-monitoring are three key behaviour change techniques used.

Goal setting can include performance goals (such as changing eating or activity behaviours) or outcome goals (such as specific weight loss). An example of a well-specified goal is:

> I will not buy any biscuits, chocolates or other high-fat foods during the weekly shopping. In order to make this easier, I will leave the children at home and shop on my own. If the children ask for junk food, then I will offer yoghurt or fruit instead.

Considerable session time may be required to set and review behaviour change strategies with families and young people [56].

Stimulus control refers to modifying or restricting environmental influences to aid weight control. The broader environment, whether at home, school or beyond, has a profound influence on a person's decisions around eating, physical activity or sedentary behaviours. Although many of these environmental influences are beyond the scope of an individual or family to change (for example, food marketing or food pricing), many opportunities exist for families to implement stimulus control in the everyday environment. Examples include: not eating in front of the television; not having television or other screens in bedrooms; using smaller plates, bowls and spoons; and not storing unhealthy food choices in the house [47].

Self-monitoring is the detailed recording of a specific behaviour and can contribute to better weight control in children and adolescents [57]. This self-monitoring can take several forms: use of a food diary, television use diary, daily pedometer measurement of physical activity, or weekly weighing, as examples [58].

Motivational interviewing is a 'client-centred, directive method for enhancing intrinsic motivation to change by exploring and resolving ambivalence' that is increasingly being used in obesity management [59]. It requires an empathetic and collaborative therapist who responds to the patient's (or parent's) ambivalence to change in a nonjudgmental fashion. In addition, the therapist uses open-ended questions and reflective listening techniques to help direct communication toward change in behaviour [41, 59, 60].

Dietary change and eating behaviours

A 2006 systematic review of paediatric obesity trials showed that interventions containing a dietary component were effective in achieving relative weight loss [61]. The Traffic Light (also known as the Stop Light) diet was the most commonly used diet intervention. Briefly, in the Traffic Light diet, foods are colour-coded to indicate those to be eaten freely (green) and those to be eaten more cautiously (amber and especially red) [55]. Although food or kilojoule exchange programs were also identified as common dietary interventions in the above review, only one trial compared diets of varying macronutrient composition. Since then, a substantial body of evidence has accumulated on the effects of diets with different macronutrient profiles on weight loss or maintenance, especially in adults, with results tending to favour diets proportionately higher in protein relative to carbohydrate and with a low glycaemic index [62–66]. For example, results published in 2010 from the DiOGenes randomised controlled trial compared the effect of five *ad libitum* diets (with variations in glycaemic index and protein content) on body composition in European children: a low protein–high glycaemic index diet increased body fat, whereas overweight or obesity decreased in the high protein–low glycaemic index diet group [65].

What recommendations should currently be given? Dietary interventions should follow national nutrition guidelines and have an emphasis on the following [47, 52, 66–68]:

- regular meals
- eating together as a family
- choosing nutrient-rich foods that are lower in energy and glycaemic index
- increased vegetable and fruit intake
- healthier snack food options
- decreased portion sizes
- promotion of water as the main beverage, and a reduction in sugary drink intake
- involvement of the entire family in making the change to a sustainable and healthy food intake.

In advising patients and families on dietary change, is there a potential risk of an eating disorder developing? Although most people with obesity do not have binge-eating disorder, the more severe the obesity, the more likely the patient is to have binge-eating disorder [69]. In addition, obesity in childhood, or parental obesity, is a risk factor for later bulimia, and overweight adolescents are more likely to use a range of unhealthy behaviours to binge-eat [70]. On the other hand, evidence indicates that professionally run paediatric obesity programs do not increase the risk of disordered eating and might, indeed, improve psychological wellbeing [71]. For these reasons, Hill has highlighted the need for 'properly and expertly managed' weight-control interventions to avoid the risk of an eating disorder [72].

Physical activity and sedentary behaviours

Physical activity

Involvement of children in a lifestyle program (for example, walking, running, cycling or swimming, based on the family's preference) leads to greater reductions in percentage overweight at six months and 17 months when compared with a program of organised aerobic exercise involving the same prescribed level of energy expenditure [73]. A study of similar design, but including a third control group involved in calisthenics, and with follow-up for ten years, showed that the lifestyle and aerobic exercise programs were superior in terms of percentage overweight reduction to the calisthenics control group [74].

A systematic review and meta-analysis of exercise interventions in overweight children and adolescents indicated that 155 to 180 minutes per week of supervised moderate-to-high intensity physical activity (with or without an associated dietary intervention) was effective in reducing body fat, although the effects on body weight and abdominal fat were inconclusive [75]. In 2008, the effect of resistance training on metabolic fitness in children and adolescents was investigated in a systematic review of 12 trials, with eight of them targeting people who were overweight or obese [76]. Most of the interventions included in that review involved circuit-type resistance training (moderate–high velocity, low–moderate load) involving machine weights. Unfortunately, limitations in study design and reporting prohibited definitive conclusions being established, but the beneficial effect of resistance training on health outcomes in adults was noted by the study authors.

Sedentary behaviours

Several studies and clinical guidelines address the issue of targeting sedentary behaviours. For example, in one study, 90 families of children aged eight to 12 years with obesity were assigned to different arms of a behavioural weight-control program in which either sedentary behaviours or physical activity were targeted, with two different levels of behaviour change being required. At two-year follow-up, similar improvements in aerobic fitness, body-fat percentage and percentage overweight were observed for all treatment arms, indicating that modifying sedentary behaviour is as effective as changing physical activity levels [77].

What recommendations can be given in terms of physical activity and reduction of sedentary behaviour? [39, 41–43, 45, 68]

- Increased physical activity may best result from a change in incidental or unplanned activity; for example, walking or cycling for transport, household chores, and playing with friends or family.
- Organised exercise programs, such as playing sports, are also important.
- Encourage children or adolescents to choose activities that they enjoy as these activities are more likely to be sustainable.
- Limit television and other 'small screen' recreational viewing to less than two hours per day. This may be extremely challenging given the multiple types of screen-based activities available to young people.
- Parental involvement is crucial if an increase in physical activity or a decrease in sedentary behaviour is to occur, including monitoring and limiting television use, role-modelling of healthy behaviours, and providing access to recreation areas or recreational equipment.

The Children's Hospital Big Five

At the Children's Hospital at Westmead, in Sydney, five strategies are emphasised when initially managing families with obese children or adolescents:

- Eat breakfast
- Choose water as your main drink
- Eat together as a family once a day, without the TV being on
- Limit TV and other 'small screens' to less than two hours per day
- Play, or be active, outside for at least 60 minutes each day.

Adjunctive therapy

The evidence to guide the use of less orthodox treatment approaches – such as VLEDs, pharmacological therapy or bariatric surgery – in the treatment of severe obesity is more limited than for behavioural interventions. In general, such therapies should occur on the background of a behavioural weight-management program and be restricted to specialist centres with expertise in managing severe obesity.

Very low energy diets (VLEDs)

As noted above, in adults, VLEDs are used to achieve rapid weight-loss prior to, or in conjunction with, the use of other longer-term treatment interventions [78]. VLEDs can also be associated with safe and substantial rapid weight loss in adolescents, typically producing six to 15 kg weight loss over three to 12 weeks [79–81]. However, most studies have been based on small sample sizes (less than 20 participants) and have lacked a control group, with very few studies having long-term follow-up [82]. To date, no randomised controlled trials have examined the effectiveness of a weight-management program incorporating initial VLED treatment in obese adolescents. The US Expert Committee recommended that VLEDs should ideally be used with severely obese patients who are managed by a multidisciplinary team in a tertiary care setting. They are not appropriate for use in young children.

Pharmacology in the treatment of childhood and adolescent obesity

The use of most anti-obesity agents (whether previously or currently available, or in development) is off label for children and adolescents. These agents should not be used in children and younger adolescents, as the risk outweighs the benefit and weight management depends primarily on parental control of the environment. There will be exceptional cases when anti-obesity agents might be trialled, with the appropriate consents in place. This will usually be for secondary obesity, for example hypothalamic hyperphagia syndromes. Somatostatin analogues have also been used with some success in children in this situation [83].

The choice of anti-obesity agents is limited and these should be prescribed as part of a lifestyle intervention, with diet and activity modification and behavioural intervention [84]. These agents may also be prescribed as part of bariatric surgery considerations and to enhance weight maintenance after weight loss in the older adolescent. As with adults, adolescents are likely to have unrealistic expectations of the benefits of drug therapy and these expectations may be greater in mid-adolescence when cognitive developmental stage limits their ability to understand the degree of weight loss possible. Adolescents generally have a very low tolerance for side effects and are likely to discontinue medication for tenuous reasons, including the lack of instantaneous benefit.

There is some data on orlistat use in adolescents with greater weight loss compared to placebo [84, 85]. The side effects of flatulence, diarrhoea with urgency and faecal leakage are highly socially distressing and for most adolescents unacceptable. If they are prescribed orlistat they will simply not take it when they have a fatty meal away from home, which may be when most higher calorie meals are consumed. For those who persist, careful monitoring of, and supplementation of, fat-soluble vitamins is important as adolescents appear more prone to deficiencies than adults.

Phentermine remains available in some jurisdictions and also for use in those over 12 years old. It has adverse effects including palpitations, headaches, hypertension, insomnia and euphoric states. Phentermine also has the potential for abuse and should not be used in adolescents, many of whom already have binge-eating disorders and will be seeking medication to produce some anorexia. As depression is often present in this situation, fluoxetine might be beneficial as a centrally acting psychotropic which does not induce weight gain.

There is some evidence in children and adolescents that metformin may have a beneficial effect on body weight. It is the drug of choice in those with type 2 diabetes, who are invariably overweight, as it does not induce further weight gain. There is some evidence from small trials that metformin improves metabolic profile and reduces visceral fat in clinical scenarios where there is insulin resistance and weight gain, but not overt diabetes. These trials include the use of atypical anti-psychotics, such as risperidone, which are frequently prescribed for behavioural disturbances [86], and in medical conditions where physical activity is severely restricted [87]. The actual weight-loss results are less consistent. Metformin, also off label, may be advantageous in the obese adolescent female with the polycystic ovary syndrome and anovulatory bleeding or acanthosis nigricans. Both these conditions will improve and in some there may be a weight benefit, based on some small clinical trials. It is essential that a low start dose of metformin is chosen, 250 mg daily commencing with the evening meal. The dose should be built up to two grams over three to four weeks to minimise risk of the well-known side effects of abdominal pain and diarrhoea. Vitamin B12 levels should be monitored as the development of deficiency is not uncommon.

Puberty is a time where weight gain can accelerate in an overweight child or adolescent [88]. While it is clear from the previous discussion that there are no available pharmacotherapeutic agents to counter this, clinicians should carefully consider prescription of commonly used drugs which may further increase weight. Select if possible an oral contraceptive which contains one of the newer gestagens, such as desogestrel or drospirenone. Consider etonogestrel, rather than medroxyprogesterone acetate as a long-acting contraceptive preparation.

Bariatric surgery

Bariatric surgery is a well-recognised form of therapy for adults with severe obesity, especially if medical therapy has failed [89]. What about its role in adolescents? Almost all of the literature in this area is of case studies or case series, with only one published randomised controlled trial to date [90].

Evidence for bariatric surgery in adolescents

A 2008 systematic review of bariatric surgery for adolescent obesity included studies that reported outcome data for patients under the age of 21 years (average age 16.8 years, range nine to 21) who were followed up for at least 12 months [91]. Nineteen papers were included, including eight studies of laparoscopic gastric banding, six studies of Roux-en-Y gastric bypass, and five studies of other surgical procedures. The laparoscopic adjustable banding procedures, with one to three years follow-up, had 95% confidence intervals for weight loss of –13.7 to –10.6 BMI units. No perioperative deaths were reported, and the main complication reported was the need for re-operation (for band slippage), which occurred in 8% of patients. For Roux-en-Y gastric bypass procedures, the mean weight loss was greater, with 95% confidence intervals of –17.8 to –22.3 BMI units, albeit over a longer period of follow-up (as the procedure has been established for longer). Some deaths were reported after this type of surgery. The most frequently reported complications related to protein-energy malnutrition and micronutrient deficiency. Note that none of the included studies in this systematic review was a randomised controlled trial, and hence the strength of evidence could only be classed as moderate to weak. However, these findings are similar to those seen in comparisons of bariatric surgery in adults [89].

After this review was published, the results of the first randomised controlled trial of bariatric surgery in adolescents with severe obesity became available in 2010 [90]. This study was undertaken in Melbourne and included 50 adolescents with severe obesity (BMI >35 kg/m²) aged between 14 and 18 years who were randomly assigned to receive either a supervised lifestyle intervention, involving reduced energy intake, increased physical activity and behaviour modification, or laparascopic adjustable gastric banding. By 24 months, the surgical group had an average reduction in BMI of 12.7 units, versus 1.3 units in the lifestyle group. The surgical group also had marked improvements in both cardiometabolic status and quality of life. However, eight operations (33%) were required in seven patients for revisional procedures.

Guidelines on bariatric surgery

In 2009, Australian and New Zealand consensus recommendations for bariatric surgery in adolescents were published by the professional bodies representing paediatricians, paediatric surgeons and bariatric surgeons [92]. The recommendations included the following:

- Patient: A minimum age of 15 years (or 14 years in exceptional circumstances); post-pubertal; presence of severe obesity (a BMI >40 kg/m², although it should be considered in adolescents with a BMI >35 kg/m² in the presence of severe obesity-associated complications); presence of an associated severe comorbidity; persistence of obesity despite involvement in a formal multidisciplinary and supervised program of lifestyle modification and pharmacotherapy; the adolescent and family understand, and are motivated to participate in, the ongoing treatment, lifestyle change and review following surgery; the adolescent is able to provide informed consent for the surgery.

- Surgical expertise and facilities: Surgery should be performed by an experienced bariatric surgeon affiliated with a team experienced in the assessment and long-term follow-up of the metabolic and psychosocial needs of the adolescent bariatric patient and family; the working party strongly recommended that publicly funded bariatric surgery be made available to those in need.

- Type of surgery: The majority recommendation was that the primary bariatric surgical procedure of choice for adolescents in Australia and New Zealand is laparoscopic adjustable gastric banding as it has good weight-based outcomes, has a low complication rate and is potentially reversible.

- Post-operative management and follow-up: Patients should be managed in the immediate post-operative period by a surgeon and bariatric surgical team with experience in adolescent care; adolescents will need more frequent post-operative follow-up than adult patients (eg four to six on weekly basis initially); patients will need ongoing care by a multidisciplinary team; issues such as improved fertility following weight loss, and hence the need for contraception, need to be considered; follow-up needs to extend beyond ten years, and ideally for the whole life.

One of the major challenges in Australia, as elsewhere, is how to ensure equitable access to such services for affected adolescents.

Long-term weight maintenance

Few high-quality studies have reported long-term outcomes of treatment of childhood and adolescent obesity [45]. In those which have reported long-term outcomes, a high proportion of participants maintained a reduction in overweight from two to ten years from baseline without additional intervention after the initial treatment phase (weeks to months) [45, 67, 93, 94]. However, in those who have undergone initial weight-management intervention, a period of further therapeutic contact (varying from four to 12 months) seems to slow weight regain [95]. At present, there is only limited evidence to guide the nature and type of weight-maintenance interventions in the child and adolescent age group.

Conclusions

Obesity and overweight are common problems at most life stages. They produce many associated comorbidities and psychosocial issues contributing to substantial public health problems and costs.

Treatment can be, and is effective. A lifestyle program should be associated closely with the treatment. Such a multidisciplinary program includes appropriate healthy eating, increased activity (both planned and incidental), behavioural techniques and counselling to help overcome ingrained habits and issues which may lead to weight gain. For children, the involvement of family in treatment is absolutely necessary. Finally, the program should not just be a 'once-off' because weight is regained due to physiological systems which drive appetite after weight loss. The program should be reinstituted or reinforced at regular intervals and patients given a weight regain limit at which to return for a 'booster' program.

A single treatment may be effective for those who need to lose a few kilos (5% or so of their initial weight), but for those with higher grades of obesity or complications of obesity, appropriate adjunctive therapies should be utilised and consideration given, when necessary, to bariatric surgery.

References

1. Caterson I (2009). Medical management of obesity and its complications. *Annals Academy of Medicine Singapore,* 38: 22–27.

2. Bjorvell H & Rossner S (1992). A ten-year follow-up of weight change in severely obese subjects treated in a combined behavioural modification programme. *International Journal of Obesity,* 16(8): 623–25.

3. Jebb S, Ahern A, Olson A, Aston L, Holzapfel C, Stoll J, et al. (2011). Primary care referral to a commercial provider for weight loss treatment, relative to standard care: an international randomised controlled trial. *The Lancet,* 378(9801): 1485–92.

4. Sacks F, Bray G, Carey V, Smith S, Ryan D, Anton S, et al. (2009). Comparison of weight-loss diets with different compositions of fat, protein and carbohydrates. *New England Journal of Medicine,* 360: 859–73.

5. McMillan-Price J, Petocz P, Atkinson F, O'Neill K, Samman S, Steinbeck K, et al. (2006). Comparison of 4 diets of varying glycemic load on weight loss and cardiovascular risk reduction in overweight and obese young adults: a randomized controlled trial. *Archives of Internal Medicine,* 166: 1466–75.

6. Dansinger ML, Gleason JL, Griffith JL, Selker HP & Schaefer EJ (2005). Comparison of the Atkins, Ornish, Weight Watchers, and Zone diets for weight loss and heart disease risk reduction: a randomized trial. *Journal of the American Medical Association,* 293(1): 43–53.

7. Despres JP, Tremblay A, Nadeau A & Bouchard C (1988). Physical training and changes in regional adipose tissue distribution. *Acta Medica Scandinavica, Supplementum,* 723: 205–12.

8. Despres JP & Lamarche B (1993). Effects of diet and physical activity on adiposity and body fat distribution: implications for the prevention of cardiovascular disease. *Nutrition Research Reviews,* 6(1): 137–59.

9. Despres J-P, Pouliot M-C, Moorjani S, Nadeau A, Tremblay A, Lupien PJ, et al. (1991). Loss of abdominal fat and metabolic response to exercise training in obese women. *American Journal of Physiology,* 261(2): E159–E67.

10. Wadden TA & Clark VL (2005). Behavioural treatment of obesity: achievements and challenges. In PG Kopelman, ID Caterson & WH Dietz (Eds). *Clinical obesity in adults and children.* (pp350–62). 2nd edn. Malden Oxford Carlton: Blackwell.

11. Richman RM, Steinbeck KS & Caterson ID (1992). Severe obesity: the use of very low energy diets or standard kilojoule restriction. *Medical Journal of Australia,* 156(11): 768–70.

12. Flechtner-Mors M, Ditschuneit HH, Johnson TD, Suchard MA & Adler G (2000). Metabolic and

weight loss effects of long-term dietary intervention in obese patients: four-year results. *Obesity Research,* 8(5): 399–402.

13. Lau N & Caterson I (2011). Meal replacement products and very low calorie diets in adult obesity. *Royal College of Pathologists Bulletin,* 155: (172–74).

14. Dixon J, O'Brien PE, Playfair J, Chapman L, Schachter LM, Skinner S, et al. (2008). Adjustable gastric banding and conventional therapy for type 2 diabetes: a randomized controlled trial. *Journal of American Medical Association,* 299(3): 316–23.

15. Lean M & Finer N (2006). ABC of obesity. Management: Part II – Drugs. *British Medical Journal,* 333(7572): 794–97.

16. Padwal R & Majumdar S (2007). Drug treatments for obesity: orlistat, sibutramine, and rimonabant. *The Lancet,* 369(9555): 71–77.

17. James W, Caterson I, Coutinho W, Finer N, Van Gaal L, Maggioni A, et al. (2010). Effect of sibutramine on cardiovascular outcomes in overweight and obese subjects. *New England Journal of Medicine,* 363(10): 309–17.

18. Swinburn BA, Carey D, Hills AP, Hooper M, Marks S, Proietto J, et al. (2005). Effect of orlistat on cardiovascular disease in obese adults. *Diabetes Obesity and Metabolism,* 7(3): 254–62.

19. Caterson ID (1988). Overweight, obesity and the role of the pharmacist. *Australian Pharmacist,* 7: 13–16.

20. Wittert G, Caterson I & Finer N (2007). The clinical effectiveness of weight loss drugs. *Journal of Obesity Research and Clinical Practice,* 1(1): 1–5.

21. Astrup A, Carraro R, Finer N, Harper A, Kunesova M, Lean M, et al. (2011). Safety, tolerability and sustained weight loss over 2 years with the once-dail human GLP-1 analog, liraglutide. *International Journal of Obesity,* Advance online publication, 16 August 2011.

22. Gadde K & Allison D (2009). Combination therapy for obesity and metabolic disease. *Current Opinion in Endocrinology, Diabetes and Obesity,* 16(5): 353–58.

23. Greenway F, Fujioka K, Plodkowski R, Mudaliar S, Guttadauria M, Erickson J, et al. (2010). Effect of naltrexone plus bupropion on weight loss in overweight and obese adults (COR-I): a multicentre, randomised, double-blind, placebo-controlled, phase 3 trial. *The Lancet,* 376(9741): 595–605.

24. Sjostrom L, Narbro K, Sjostrom C, Karason K, Larsson B, Wedel H, et al. (2007). Effects of bariatric surgery on mortality in Swedish obese subjects. *New England Journal of Medicine,* 357: 741–52.

25. Panel IDFC (2011). Bariatric surgical and procedural interventions in the treatment of obese patients with type 2 diabetes: a position statement from the International Diabetes Federation Taskforce on Epidemiology and Prevention. September [Online]. Available: www.idf.org/webdata/Bariatric-Surgery-Press-Briefing.pdf [Accessed 24 October 2011].

26. Padwal R, Klarenbach S, Wiebe N, Birch D, Karmali S, Manns B, et al. (2011). Bariatric surgery: a systematic review and network meta-analysis of randomized trials. *Obesity Reviews,* 12: 602–21.

27. Tice J, Karliner L, Walsh J, Petersen A & Feldman M (2008). Gastric banding or bypass? A systematic review comparing the two most popular bariatric procedures. *American Journal of Medicine,* 121: 885–93.

28. Fuller N, Pearson S, Lau N, Markovic T, Steinbeck K, Chettiar R, et al. (2010). A prospective, randomized, controlled trial of the bioenterics intragastric balloon (BIB) in the treatment of obese individuals with the metabolic syndrome. *Obesity Reviews,* 11(Suppl. 1): 436.

29. Unick J, Beavers D, Jakicic J, Kitabachi A, Knowler W, Wadden T, et al. (2011). Effectiveness of lifestyle interventions with severe obesity and type 2 diabetes: results from the Look AHEAD trial. *Diabetes Care*: (Aug 11) epub ahead of print.

30. Group TLAR (2007). Reduction in weight and cardiovascular disease risk factors in individuals with type 2 diabetes: one-year results of the look AHEAD trial. *Diabetes Care,* 30: 1374–83.

31. Astrup A, Caterson I, Zelissen P, Guy-Grand B, Carruba M, Levy B, et al. (2004). Topiramate for long-term weight maintenance of weight loss induced by a low-calorie diet in obese subjects. *Obesity Research,* 12: 1658–69.

32. Wing R & Group LAR (2010). Long-term effects of a lifestyle intervention on weight and cardiovascular risk factors in individuals with type 2 diabetes mellitus: four-year results of the Look AHEAD trial. *Archives of Internal Medicine,* 170: 1566–75.

33. Benson L, Baer H & Kaelber D (2007). Trends in the diagnosis in overweight and obesity in children and adolescents: 1999–2007. *Pediatrics,* 123: e153–e8.

34. Cretikos M, Valenti L, Britt H & Baur L (2008). General practice management of overweight and obesity in children and adolescents in Australia. *Medical Care,* 4: 1163–69.

35. O'Connor J, Youde L, Allen J & Baur L (2004). Obesity and under-nutrition in a tertiary paediatric hospital. *Journal of Paediatrics and Child Health,* 40: 299–304.

36. Woo J, Zeller M, Wilson K & Inge T (2009). Obesity identified by discharge ICD-9 codes underestimates the true prevalence of obesity in hospitalised children. *Journal of Paediatrics,* 154: 327–31.

37. King L, Loss J, Wikenfeld, Pagnini D, Booth M & Booth S (2007). Australian GPs' perceptions about child and adolescent overweigth and obesity: the Weight of Opinion study. *British Journal of General Practice,* 57: 124–29.

38. Shrewsbury V, King L, Hattersley L, Howlett S, Hardy L & Baur L (2010). Adolescent-parent interactions and communication preferencesregarding body weight and weight management: a qualitative study. *The International Society of Behavioral Nutrition and Physical Activity,* 7: 16.

39. Barlow S & The Expert Committee (2007). Expert Committee recommendations regarding the prevention, assessment, and treatment of children and adolescent overweight and obesity: summary report. *Pediatrics,* 120(Suppl. 4): S164–S92.

40. Krebs N, Himes J, Jacobson D, Nicklas T, Guilday P & Styne D (2007). Assessment of child and adolescent overweight and obesity. *Pediatrics,* 120(Suppl. 4): S193–S228.

41. National Health and Medical Research Council (2003). Clinical practice guidelines for the management of overweight and obesity in children and adolescents. Canberra: NHMRC.

42. Network SIG (2007). Management of obesity: a national clinical guideline. Edinburgh: SIGN.

43. National Institute for Health and Clinical Excellence (2010). Obesity: guidance on the prevention, identification, assessment and management of overweight and obesity in adults and children. *National Health Service National Institute for Health and Clinical Excellence* [Online]. Available: guidance.nice.org. uk/CG43/NICEGuidance/pdf/English [Accessed 2011].

44. Feacham R, Sekhri N & White K (2002). Getting more for their dollar: a comparison of the NHS with California's Kaiser Permanente. *British Medical Journal,* 324: 135–41.

45. Luttikhuis HO, Baur L, Jansen H, Shrewsbury V, O'Malley C, Stolk R, et al. (2009). Interventions for treating obesity in children. *Cochrane Database of Systematic Reviews,* 1.

46. Reinehr T, Widhalm K, L'Allemand D, Wiegand S, Wabitsch M, Holl R, et al. (2009). Two-year follow-up in 21,784 overweight children and adolescents with lifestyle intervention. *Obesity,* 17: 1196–99.

47. Dietz W & Robinson T (2005). Clinical practice: overweight children and adolescents. *New England Journal of Medicine,* 352: 2100–09.

48. McLean N, Griffin S, Toney K & Hardeman W (2003). Family involvement in weight contril, weight maintenance and weight-loss interventions: a systematic review of randomised trials. *International Journal of Obesity,* 27: 987–1005.

49. Nuutinen O & Knip M (1992). Predictors of weight reduction in obese children. *European Journal of Clinical Nutrition,* 46: 785–94.

50. Golan M, Weizman A, Apter A & Fainaru M (1998). Parents as the exclusive agents of change in the treatment of childhood obesity. *American Journal of Clinical Nutrition,* 67: 1130–35.

51. Nowicka P & Flodmark C-E (2008). Family in pediatric obesity management: a literature review. *International Journal of Pediatric Obesity,* 3:(Suppl. 1): 44–50.

52. Young K, Northern J, Lister K, Drummond J & O'Brien W (2007). A meta-analysis of family-behavioural weight-loss treatments for children. *Clinical Psychology Reviews,* 27: 240–49.

53. Shrewsbury V, Steinbeck K, Torvaldsen S & Baur L (2011). The role of parents in pre-adolescent and adolescent overweight and obesity treatment: a systematic review of clinical recommendations. *Obesity Reviews,* 12(10): 759–69.

54. Golan M & Crow S (2004). Targeting parents exclusively in the treatment of childhood obesity: long-term results. *Obesity Research,* 12: 357–61.

55. Epstein L, Myers M, Raynor H & Saelens B (1998). Treatment of pediatric obesity. *Pediatrics,* 101(Suppl. 2): 554–70.

56. Brennan L, Walkley J, Lukeis S, Rsiteska A, Archer L, et al. (2009). A cognitive behavioural intervention for overweight and obese adolescents illustrated by four case studies. *Behaviour Change,* 26: 190–213.

57. Saelens B & McGrath A (2003). Self-monitoring adherence and adolescent weight control efficacy. *Child Health Care,* 32: 137–52.

58. Alm M, Neumark-Sztainer D, Story M & Boutelle K (2009). Self-weighing and weight control behaviors among adolescents with a history of overweight. *Journal of Adolescent Health,* 44: 424–30.

59. Miller W & Rollnick S (2002). *Motivational interviewing: preparing people for change.* 2nd edn. New York: Guildford Press.

60. Carels R, Darby L, Cacciapaglia H, Konrad K, Coit C, Harper J, et al. (2007). Using motivational interviewing as a supplement to obesity treatment: a stepped care approach. *Health Psychology,* 26: 369–74.

61. Collins C, Warren J, Neve M, McCoy P & Stokes B (2006). Measuring effectiveness of dietetic interventions in child obesity: a systematic review of randomised trials. *Archives of Pediatric and Adolescent Medicine,* 160(9): 906–22.

62. Abete I, Astrup A, Martinez J, Thorsdottir I & Zulet M (2010). Obesity and the metabolic syndrome: role of different dietary macronutrient distribution patterns and specific nutritional components on weight loss and maintenance. *Nutrition reviews,* 68(4): 214–31.

63. Hession M, Rolland C, Kulkarni U, Wise A & Broom J (2009). Systematic review of randomised controlled trials of low-carbohydrate vs. low fat/low-calorie diets in the management of obesity and its comorbidities. *Obesity Reviews,* 10(1): 36–50.

64. Thomas DE, Elliott EJ, Baur L (2007). Low glycaemic index or low glycaemic load diets for overweight and obesity Low glycaemic index or low glycaemic load diets for overweight and obesity. *Cochrane Database of Systematic Reviews.* Issue 3. Article number CD005105.

65. Papadaki A, Linardakis M, Larsen T, VanBaak M, Lindroos A, Pfeiffer A, et al. (2010). The effect of protein and glycemic index on children's body composition: the DIOGenes randomised study. *Pediatrics,* 126(5): E1143–E52.

66. Larsen T, Dalskov S, VanBaak M, Jebb S, Papadaki A, Pfeiffer A, et al. (2010). Diets with high or low protein content and glycemic index for weight loss maintenance. *New England Journal of Medicine,* 363(22): 2102–13.

67. Epstein L, Valoski A, Wing R & McCurley J (1990). Ten-year follow-up of behavioral, family based treatment for obese children. *Journal of the American Medical Association,* 264(19): 2519–23.

68. Whitaker R (2003). Obesity prevention in pediatric primary care: four behaviors to target. *Archives of Pediatric and Adolescent Medicine,* 157(8): 725–27.

69. Fairburn C, Welch S, Doll H, Davies B & O'Connor M (1997). Risk factors for bulimia nervosa: a community-based case-control study. *Archives of General Psychiatry,* 54(6): 509–17.

70. Patton C, Selzer R, Coffey C, Carlin J & Wolfe R (1999). Onset of adolescent eating disorders: population-based cohort study over 3 years. *British Medical Journal,* 318(7186): 765–68.

71. Butryn M & Wadden T (2005). Treatment of overweight in children and adolescents: does dieting increase the risk of eating disorders? *International Journal of Eating Disorders,* 37(4): 285–93.

72. Hill A (2007). Obesity and eating disorders. *Obesity Reviews,* 8(Suppl. 1): 151–55.

73. Epstein L, Wing R, Koeske R & Valoski A (1982). A comparison of lifestyle change and programmed exercise on weight and fitness in obese children. *Behavior Therapy,* 16(4): 345–56.

74. Epstein L, Valoski A, Wing R & McCurley J (1994). Ten year outcomes of behavioral family-based treatment for childhood obesity. *Health Psychology,* 13(5): 373–83.

75. Atlantis F, Barnes E & Singh M (2006). Efficacy of exercise for treating overweight in children and adolescents: a systematic review. *International Journal of Obesity,* 30(7): 1027–40.

76. Benson A, Torode M & FiataroneSingh M (2008). Effects of resistance training on metabolic fitness in children and adolescents: a systematic review. *Obesity Reviews,* 9(1): 43–66.

77. Epstein L, Paluch R, Gordy C & Dorn J (2000). Decreasing sedentary behaviors in treating pediatric obesity. *Archives of Pediatric and Adolescent Medicine,* 154(3): 220–26.

78. Tsai A & Wadden T (2005). Systematic review: an evaluation of major commercial weight loss programs in the United States. *Annals of Internal Medicine,* 142(1): 56–66.

79. Figueroa-Colon R, VonAlmen T, Franklin F, Schuftan C & Suskind R (1993). Comparison of two hypocaloric diets in obese children. *American Journal of Disease in Childhood,* 147(2): 160–66.

80. Suskind R, Sothern M, Farris R, VonAlmen T, Schumacher H, Carlisle L, et al. (1993). Recent advances in the treatment of childhood obesity. *Annals of the New York Academy of Sciences,* 699: 181–99.

81. Widhalm K & Zwiauer K (1987). Metabolic effects of a very low calorie diet in obese children and adolescents with special reference to nitrogen balance. *Journal of the American College of Nutrition,* 6(6): 467–74.

82. Sothern M, Udall J, Suskind R, Vargas A & Blecker U (2002). Weight loss and growth velocity in obese children after very low calorie diet, exercise and behavior modification. *Acta Paediatrica,* 89(9): 1036–43.

83. Tzotzas T, Papazisis K, Perros P & Krassas G (2008). Use of somatostatin analogues in obesity. *Drugs,* 68(14): 1963–73.

84. Greydanus D, Bricker L & Feucht C (2011). Pharmacotherapy for obese adolescents. *Pediatric Clinics of Noth America,* 58(1): 139–53.

85. Chanoine JP, Hampi S, Jensen C, Boldrin M & Hauptman J (2005). Effect of orlistat on weight and body composition in obese adolescents: a randomized controlled trial. *Journal of the American Medical Association,* 293(23): 2873–83.

86. Shin L, Bregman H, Breeze J, Noyes N & Frazier J (2009). Metformin for weight controlin pediatric patientson atypical antipsychotic medication. *Journal of Child and Adolescent Psychopharmacology,* 19(3): 275–79.

87. Casteels K, Fieuws S, VanHelvoirt M, Verpoorten C, Goermans N, Coudyzer W, et al. (2010). Metformin therapy to reduce weight gainand visceral adiposity in children and adolescents with neurogenic or myogenic motor deficit. *Pediatric Diabetes,* 11(1): 61–69.

88. Jasik C & Lustig R (2008). Adolescent obesity and puberty: the 'perfect storm'. *Annals of the New York Academy of Sciences,* 1135: 265–79.

89. Colquitt J, Picot J, Loveman E & Clegg A (2009). Surgery for obesity. *Cochrane Database of Systematic Reviews,* 2.

90. O'Brien P, Sawyer S, Laurie C, Brown W, Skinner S & Veit F (2010). Laparoscopic adjustable gastric

banding in severely obese adolescents: a randomized trial. *Journal of the American Medical Association,* 303(23): 519–26.

91. Treadwell J, Sun F & Schoelles K (2008). Systematic review and meta-analysis of bariatric surgery for pediatric obesity. *Annals Surgery,* 248(5): 763–76.

92. Baur L & Fitzgerald D (2010). Recommendations for bariatric surgery in adolescents in Australia and New Zealand. *Journal of Paediatrics and Child Health,* 46(12): 704–07.

93. Magarey A, Perry R, Baur L, Steinbeck K, Sawyer M, Hills A, et al. (2011). A parent-led family-focused treatment program for overweight 5–9 year olds: the PEACH RCT. *Pediatrics,* 127: 214–22.

94. Collins C, Okely A, Morgan P, Jones R, Burrows T, Cliff D, et al. (2011). Parent diet modification, child-centered activity or both in obese children: an RCT. *Pediatrics,* 127(4): 619–27.

95. Wilfley D, Stein R, Saelens B, Mockus D, Matt G, Hayden-Wade H, et al. (2007). Efficacy of maintenance treatment approaches for childhood overweight: a randomised controlled trial. *Journal of the American Medical Association,* 298(14): 1661–73.

22

A 'cure' for diabetes and its complications

Kim Donaghue,[1,2] Tony Keech,[3, 4] Maria Craig[1,2,5,6] and Philip O'Connell[3,7]

The new millennium has brought continued hope for a 'cure' with major developments in immunology and understanding of pathogenesis of diabetes and its complications. Intervention studies to slow the progression of beta-cell destruction by using insulin to induce immune tolerance have shown promise in some subsection analysis but without overall benefit for primary outcome. The ongoing INIT 11 study delivers insulin nasally. The TRIGR study eliminates cow milk in babies at risk with promising effect for antibody generation. Stem cells also offer promise. Islet cell transplantation from cadavers is minimally invasive and has shown great promise, but has been slowed due to lack of donors and immunosuppression needs. For those with established diabetes, randomised controlled trials have demonstrated minimising and slowing of progression of diabetes vascular complications. These interventions include intensive glycaemic treatment, blood pressure lowering and lipid lowering agents. Good randomised controlled clinical trials provide the best evidence of these benefits, which must then be followed by more research to better understand mechanisms of disease pathogenesis and treatment effects.

The elusive cure for diabetes is a dream of many individuals and their families who live with diabetes. Increasing numbers of children are now diagnosed with diabetes, with the prevalence in Australia recently reported to be one in 724 children aged less than 15 years, and one in 391 adolescents aged ten to 14 years [1]. Much clinical research is making this dream closer to delivery. Family members are enrolling in natural history and clinical intervention trials to help understand, delay and hopefully stop the disease.

Research to cure diabetes is now multipronged. A number of studies have focused on predicting risk, which then has allowed development of studies to intervene in the

1 Children's Hospital, Westmead.

2 Discipline of Paediatrics and Child Health, Sydney Medical School, University of Sydney.

3 Sydney Medical School, University of Sydney.

4 NHMRC Clinical Trials Centre, University of Sydney.

5 St George Hospital.

6 School of Women's and Children's Health, University of New South Wales.

7 Centre for Transplant and Renal Research, Westmead Millennium Institute for Medical Research.

prediabetes period, before the glucose levels are abnormal. Treatment within the first 100 days after the clinical diagnosis to switch off the immune process or boost the immune defenses is currently under investigation. Research aimed at curing established diabetes uses cell-based therapies including transplantation of islets, the insulin-producing beta cell. Such therapies currently require immunosuppression to prevent rejection and recurrence of the initial diabetogenic process.

Type 1 diabetes is an autoimmune disease, meaning that the body fights itself by activation of the immune system and not recognising the pancreas beta cells as 'self' but as 'foreign'. Our understanding of this loss of 'self-tolerance', is pivotal to development of a cure with many intervention trials now aimed at 'inducing self-tolerance'. In the development of diabetes there is activation of both arms of the immune system: humoral immunity (antibody production by B lymphocytes) and cellular immunity (T lymphocytes). We can measure antibodies with relative ease but measurement of T-cell function is more difficult. Most intervention studies use antibodies to identify the population at risk for diabetes, and use antibodies as a surrogate marker of progression. However T-cell activation precedes antibody production.

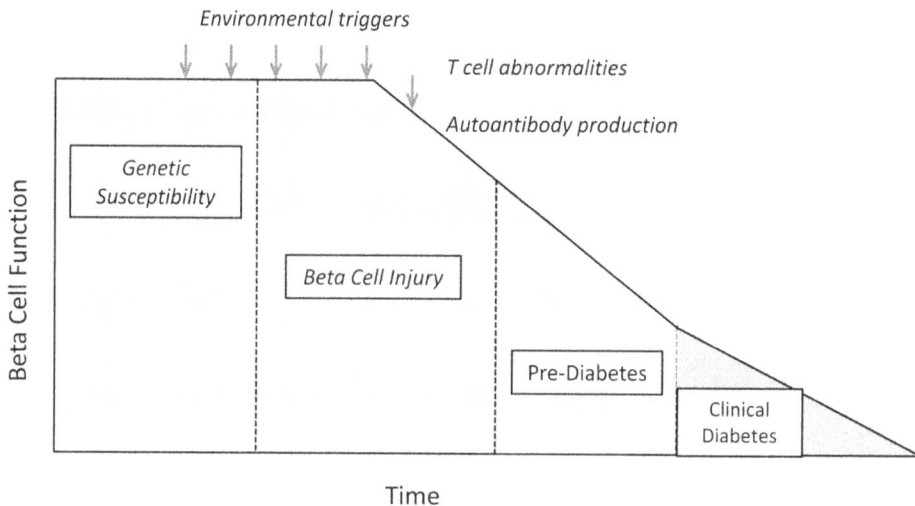

Figure 1. Progression of beta-cell failure in type 1 diabetes.

We now know that the autoimmune process occurs in individuals who are genetically predisposed and that this process appears to be triggered by environmental factors, including viral infection (Figure 1). The autoimmune reaction results in loss of beta-cell mass and hence function which occurs over months to years, during which time prevention may be possible (preclinical preservation). The insulin response to glucose given intravenously is a well-established method to measure beta-cell function in this preclinical phase, prior to abnormal glucose levels. After clinical diagnosis and/or presentation with hyperglycaemia, there is still some functioning pancreas or beta-cell function. This remaining function results in the well-recognised 'remission phase' during which exogenous insulin requirements can be reduced substantially. Clinical diabetes intervention aims to preserve beta-cell function. This can be measured by C peptide production in response to stimuli, as C peptide is secreted by the beta cell at the same time as insulin.

For those with established diabetes, as detailed in other chapters in diabetes complications (Twigg and McLennan), the risks of long-term end-organ diabetes complications can be reduced by risk factor minimisation targeted at modification of lipids, blood pressure as well as glucose (Figure 2).

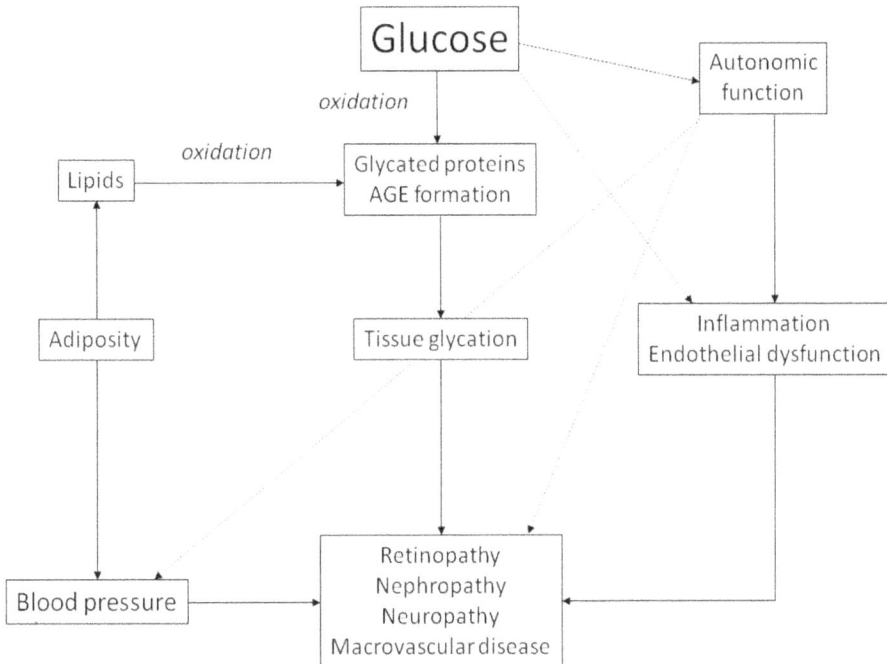

Figure 2. Overview of pathogenesis of long-term vascular complications and modifiers of glucose action.

Studies to understand the genetic and environmental risks

The Type 1 Diabetes Genetics Consortium (T1DGC) is an international project designed to identify genes that modify the risk of diabetes. Families with two or more members with type 1 diabetes have provided blood for this purpose, through four regional centres (Asia Pacific, Europe, UK and North America). More than 2500 families to date have contributed. It is sponsored by US National Institute for Diabetes and Digestive and Kidney Diseases (NIDDK) and the Juvenile Diabetes Research Foundation (JDRF) [2]. The major genetic risk is still located on the HLA region, but others genes have been identified, including other immunoregulatory genes [3]. The Australian National Health and Medical Research Council (NHMRC) is currently funding the Australian Childhood Diabetes DNA Repository (ACDDR), for family members with type 1 and type 2 diabetes, who contribute saliva from which genetic material is derived for subsequent analysis. Further the Type 1 Diabetes TrialNET is an international consortium aimed at understanding natural history, in particular antibodies, in family members and undertakes prevention and intervention trials. Family members can enroll for antibody screening at 200 sites worldwide, in North America, Australia and Europe.

The charmingly named TEDDY study (The Environmental Determinants of Diabetes in the Young) aims to determine infectious agents, dietary factors or other that may impact on diabetes development in children at high risk based on HLA genotyping. Recruitment has been from three centres in the US (Colorado, Washington and Georgia/Florida) and three centres in Europe (Finland, Germany and Sweden). Children from the general population as well as children from families placing them at high risk are recruited [4].

Infections have long been considered to be possible environmental triggers for the autoimmune process. Transmission of enteroviruses occurs by shedding from the respiratory or gastrointestinal tracts. A recent meta-analysis of 26 case-control studies showed a tenfold increase of enterovirus infection in patient at diabetes onset compared to controls [5]. In addition children were nearly four times more likely to have autoimmunity to the pancreas when there was molecular evidence of enterovirus (by finding RNA or viral protein in blood, stool or tissue). This meta-analysis was based on studies from 12 countries, mostly of children but some studies included adults up to the age of 53 years.

While there is a clear distinction between type 1 and type 2 diabetes in terms of pathogenesis, greater weight gain may also be an initiator and/accelerator for autoimmunity and type 1 diabetes. Younger age of diabetes onset is associated with higher body mass index (BMI) at diagnosis, particularly in very young children [6, 7]. Retrospective case control studies have demonstrated increased linear growth and weight gain in early childhood, independent of feeding, with type 1 diabetes [8–11]. The Australian BabyDiab study has followed babies with a first-degree relative with diabetes (parents or siblings) from birth to six years of age. Children with weight above average had more than twofold increase in antibody development than thinner children [12]. Those that gained the most weight during infancy also had an increased risk of islet autoimmunity. Insulin resistance, and associated inflammation, may underlie the role of overweight in the development of type 1 diabetes [13]. Insulin resistance predicted progression from islet autoimmunity to type 1 diabetes [14] and was greater in young children with islet autoimmunity in the German BabyDiab study [15]. Therefore, insulin resistance associated with overweight may be a key factor in both the development and progression of islet autoimmunity. The process may begin in utero; maternal weight before pregnancy and more than 15 kg weight gain during pregnancy predicted risk of islet autoimmunity in their offspring [16].

Vitamin D is an anti-inflammatory steroid with multiple immunomodulatory effects that can promote immune tolerance, however its role in type 1 diabetes remains controversial. A systematic review of observational studies examined whether vitamin D supplementation in infancy reduced the risk of type 1 diabetes in later life [17]. Infants who were supplemented with vitamin D had 29% lower risk of developing type 1 diabetes compared to those who were not supplemented. There was also some evidence of a dose–response effect, with those using larger amounts of vitamin D being at lower risk of developing type 1 diabetes. However, there are no randomised controlled trials examining the effect of vitamin D supplementation and type 1 diabetes risk.

Immunomodulatory trials

With most autoimmune diseases the main focus of therapy is to treat the abnormal immune response with immunosuppression. Diabetes, however, presents later in the autoimmune process when it is estimated more than 90% of islet function is destroyed, so immunosuppression may not be comparable to other autoimmune diseases some of which are relapsing. Nevertheless, recently a number of larger multicentre studies have reported the outcomes of short-term immunosuppression in new onset diabetes. Many of these treatments are currently marketed for the treatment of rheumatoid arthritis with good safety profiles. Therapy has aimed to modulate T-cell action, or reduce B cells with some success.

One TrialNET study used abatacept, which modulates T-cell co-stimulation, preventing full T-cell activation. In this study 112 newly diagnosed patients were randomised to either treatment or placebo injections at day 1, 14, 28 and then monthly for two years. There was a positive effect of the intervention with preservation of C peptide reserve for 9.6 months compared to the placebo treated group but this declined in parallel, meaning the effect was short term [18].

Another TrialNET used anti-CD20 monoclonal antibody, rituximab, which depletes B cells. In 78 newly diagnosed patients aged between eight and 40 years, the intervention compared to placebo showed positive effects for preservation of C-peptide production, glucose control and lower insulin dose [19].

The Protégé study used teplizumab, anti-CD3 therapy, which binds to T-cells and modulates their action. Enrolled were 516 subjects aged from eight to 35 years, within 12 weeks of diabetes onset in 83 centres across North America, Europe, India and Israel. The primary endpoint was a significant treatment effect at one year of insulin dose <0.5 units/kg/day with HbA1c <6.5%. Whilst this outcome was not achieved, a positive treatment effect was found in children aged from eight to 11 years, and earlier treatment within six weeks of diagnosis [20].

Inducing immune tolerance: antigen-based therapy

Glutamic acid decarboxylase (GAD) is a principle target (or antigen) for autoimmunity antibody production in diabetes. Consequently GAD therapy (two or three GAD injections or placebo) has been trialled after onset of clinical diabetes in patients aged three to 45 years. The initial pilot study in adolescents with two injections of GAD was promising, but the 15-site North American clinical trial was unsuccessful in preserving beta-cell function in the 145 participants [21].

For those in the prediabetes phase, the autoimmune process may be turned off by a process of 'immune tolerance'. Induction of immune tolerance has been sought by using GAD and by insulin itself to which antibodies are made in the prediabetes phase.

Prediction to progression of diabetes has focused on measurement of diabetes-associated antibodies in family members. Models are derived whereby there is a 26%–50% chance of progression to diabetes within five years based on the presence of positive antibodies.

The first trial to use insulin itself as the intervention was the Diabetes Prevention Trial – Type 1 Diabetes (DPT-1) [22]. In one arm low-dose insulin was given by injection to those at highest risk to progression (greater than 50%), and in the other arm insulin was given orally to those with moderate risk of progression. Unfortunately 241 of 670 developed diabetes at a mean age of 13.9 years. The numbers required to screen, in this case using the islet cell antibody, were very high: 103,000 relatives of T1 D patients. Whilst the analysis of the total group of participants did not show a positive effect of the intervention, subsequent analysis has provided evidence that insulin can induce 'self-tolerance' during prediabetes. Those with higher antibodies at baseline showed a significant treatment effect with a lower rate of developing diabetes than placebo treated individuals: 6% vs 10% per year, with a delay of 4.5 years, but after cessation the risk of developing diabetes reverted to that of the placebo treated group [23].

A better method of inducing tolerance potentially is delivering the treatment through the mucosa [24]. The Intranasal Insulin Trial 11 (INIT 11) is currently underway in 11 sites in Australia and New Zealand. The principal investigators are Len Harrison and Peter Colman in Melbourne, and the study is sponsored by Melbourne Health, funded by JDRF and NHMRC through the Diabetes Vaccine Development Centre (DVDC). Risk for diabetes is based on family members found to have two positive antibodies on screening. These individuals are then staged to determine sufficient beta-cell reserve: the insulin response to an intravenous glucose load. Prior to the onset of diabetes the first phase to be lost is the initial response to intravenous glucose. Those in the unsuccessful DIPP study had little insulin reserve, so the time to intervene in the disease process was probably too late, to salvage beta-cell function [25].

Better tests of T-cell function, in particular the T-cell regulatory (TReg) function, are required to help determine the early stages of the autoimmune process during which time intervention may be most successful. Screening of large numbers of family members is required to detect those at risk.

Dietary trials to modify the environment

Changing the environment may prevent the autoimmune process. Babies at high risk of developing diabetes may be amenable to dietary intervention. Cow milk has been investigated in observational studies and early introduction may be a trigger for the autoimmune process.

In Finland babies at risk of diabetes were randomised to delay in cow milk supplementation. This led to a delay in development of diabetes related autoantibodies [26]. This has led to the Trial to Reduce IDDM in Genetically at Risk (TRIGR), a multinational study, including Australia. Recruitment of 2160 infants is complete (enrolment 2002 to 2007) and the intervention completed mid 2007, with follow-up planned over ten years. Infants have been screened by cord blood or heel prick for HLA susceptibility, protection genotype and those without the protective genotype randomised to delay in introduction of cow milk protein [27].

Another possible triggering antigen may be gluten. In Germany delay in introduction of gluten has been investigated in a randomised control study (BABYDIET) of 150 infants: prior to two months of age, after six months and after 12 months. However recent outcome data have not shown a delay in onset of autoimmune markers, with 12% of children developing diabetes related antibodies at age of three years, seven developing diabetes, including four in the late exposure group [28]. This was a pilot study and compliance with the intervention was poor at 30%. Three times more infants are needed to properly examine this hypothesis.

Haemopoietic stem cell transplantation as a treatment for diabetes

Another more controversial form of therapy is haemopoietic stem cell transplantation (HSCT) to treat new onset T1D. HSCT involves mobilisation of haemopoetic stem cells (CD34+ cells) from the bone marrow, ablation of the recipients immune system followed by reinfusion of the autologous stem cells. The aim is to destroy the auto-reactive islet immune T-cells and to reconstruct the immune system without autoimmunity. The strategy has been used successfully in other autoimmune diseases where it is generally reserved for patients that are resistant to other treatments. In 2007 a study was undertaken in Brazil where HSCT was used to treat T1D within six weeks of diagnosis [29]. Twenty-three patients, aged between 13 and 33 years, were enrolled in the study. The investigators reported an improvement in diabetes with 20 of the 23 becoming insulin free for varying periods of time (one to 52 months). Eight of the 20 had relapsed during the time of reported follow-up. The remainder were still being followed at the time of the last report [30]. There was also evidence of improvement in C-peptide, and reduced HbA1c. There was a reduction but not an elimination of islet autoantibodies which suggests that the autoimmune disease was suppressed but not eliminated. This study, although instructive, needs to be interpreted with caution [31]. The authors themselves readily admit this. First, the study was an early-phase, proof-of-concept study, and was not a randomised controlled trial. The well-known honeymoon period that can occur at the onset of T1D complicates the interpretation of the results. The follow-up is relatively limited and the long-term benefits and side effects are unknown. We do know that a third of patients had relapsed and returned to insulin within three years, which is a relatively small gain for such aggressive therapy. Whilst there were no deaths, HSCT is not benign therapy. Two patients developed pneumonia and others developed endocrine abnormalities, including nine of 17 males developing oligospermia. A final point that makes investigations of this nature difficult in T1D is that all the recipients were young, which increases the anxiety and implications around long-term complications such as malignancy which may yet develop. Despite all these caveats the trial should be seen for what it is, the first of many attempts to cure T1D with cellular therapy rather spending a lifetime treating the consequences of islet destruction.

HSCT has been used as an adjunct to other treatments in T1D [32]. Not only is bone-marrow a source of haemopoetic progenitors, it is also a source of mesenchymal and endothelial stem cells. There is experimental evidence that these stem cells enhance immunomodulation and tolerance, as well as promote engraftment and enhance tissue repair. As a result HSCT is being evaluated in several autoimmune and degenerative conditions and has been proposed as adjunct therapy for other treatments in T1D. In fact there are more than 20 registered trials of HSCT in T1D. Several of these trials are using HSCT as a tolerising strategy to reduce or eliminate chronic immunosuppression in islet transplantation. In other studies HSCT is being trialled as a therapy to prevent progression of complications such as peripheral neuropathy. In all cases the study are exploratory proof-of-concept studies. While ongoing no study has conclusively demonstrated sustained benefit.

Clinical islet transplantation

Clinical human islet transplantation is a new and emerging therapy for a select group of patients with severe metabolic complications as a result of their diabetes. If successful it can provide near perfect blood glucose control without insulin injections and has brought forward the prospect of a cure for this debilitating chronic disease. Currently islet transplantation can be considered a novel therapy for a new indication and the objective benefits and potential risks remain to be fully established by clinical trials. At present the two main indications for islet transplantation are severe hypoglycaemia unawareness, refractory to conventional treatment and islet transplantation in conjunction with a kidney transplant. On the positive side, islet transplantation has been shown to abolish severe hypoglycaemic episodes and patients can expect to have an improved quality of life and reduced risk of end-organ complications. On the negative side, patients must take lifelong immunosuppression with all its short- and long-term complications. Despite these caveats, islet transplantation has created great interest amongst physicians as well as patient groups and several major clinical trials are ongoing. If nothing else, patient enthusiasm for these early trials has highlighted the lifelong burden and deficiencies of current insulin regimens.

Clinical islet transplantation is still a difficult procedure to perform. Islet isolation from a human pancreas requires a skilled laboratory team, a specialised GMP (good manufacturing practice) facility, and has been a limiting factor in the spread of the procedure beyond specialised institutions. Despite the fact that islet transplantation had been performed successfully in rodents, translation into the clinic has been difficult. Researchers in Edmonton were the first to develop islet transplantation into a reliable clinical therapy [33]. Their successes was based on the following principles:

• Selection of the appropriate group of patients for transplantation
• Using a non-toxic effective immunosuppressive regimen

- Isolating appropriate numbers of viable islets
- Transplanting sufficient numbers of islets to control blood glucose levels.

The basic premise of the Edmonton protocol has been that successful islet transplantation is dependent on the isolation and ongoing survival of the maximum number of islets possible. This has meant that most patients require two or more islet transplants to achieve insulin independence. Patients must not be overweight and therefore should be on a low-insulin dose compared to body weight. Once transplanted, islets face rejection and possibly autoimmune disease recurrence and hence islet recipients must take lifelong immunosuppression.

Added to this, pancreatic islets come from organ donors and there is a large mismatch between the number of people with type 1 diabetes and the number of organ donors. For instance in Australia there are 150,000 people suffering from type 1 diabetes and only 250 to 300 organ donors annually. Under the most optimistic of circumstances only 150 of these would be suitable or available for islet transplantation. For this reason definite sources of islet-cell replacement are being developed. These include pancreatic islets from pigs, so-called xenotransplantation, and stem cells. Although early phase I studies have been undertaken in humans, both these sources of islets remain in preclinical development.

Clearly human islet transplantation is not going to be an option for most people with diabetes. This and the current uncertainty has put pressure on transplant units to develop selection criteria that optimises the chances of a successful outcome whilst at the same time ensuring that the benefits of insulin independence are worth the long-term risks of life-long immunosuppression. The patients, who best satisfy these dual objectives, are those with severe hypoglycaemic unawareness. These patients no longer have warning signals of hypoglycaemia, and low blood sugar levels are not detected until they reach dangerously low levels. These patients require constant and intensive medical supervision. If it persists, it can lead to significant cognitive impairment and, in severe cases, can be fatal [34]. Not surprisingly patients who suffer from this problem have poor metabolic control with wide and sudden swings between hypo- and hyperglycaemia. In these circumstances successful islet transplantation will normalise blood glucose levels and prevent hypoglycaemic episodes [35].

Patients who have successfully achieved insulin independence following islet transplantation certainly have a life-changing experience. After many years of difficulty controlling diabetes with insulin, they find themselves insulin independent with perfect control and normal HbA1C. In our experience patients who were once housebound are able to return to active work. There is an obvious improvement in the patient's mood and quality of life. Even patients, who are not insulin independent but have documented evidence of islet graft function, achieve marked improvements in glycaemic control. Physiologic background basal insulin secretion appears to be sufficient to eliminate severe hypoglycaemia and often this is sufficient to dramatically improve the patient's quality of life. Furthermore, there is evidence that C-peptide secretion provides some protection against cardiac complications even in patients that still require exogenous insulin therapy. A study of kidney transplant recipients with type 1 diabetes who subsequently received an islet transplant, found that those that were C-peptide positive had improved cardiac outcomes compared to those with graft failure [36].

Thus far it would seem that the main negatives for patients are the side effects from immunosuppression. Despite this, there have been surprisingly few opportunistic infections and no deaths. Most immunosuppressive regimens include Tacrolimus and Sirolimus. Most transplanted patients suffer nagging complications such as mouth ulcers, ankle oedema and headaches. These are common side effects of Sirolimus and are often self-limiting although they have been serious enough to lead to withdrawal from the study in some cases. Many patients also need to commence lipid-lowering therapy for hypercholesterolaemia. More worrying are the side effects from Tacrolimus. In particular nephrotoxicity is a concern and it may be exacerbated by concomitant Sirolimus therapy. Many recipients have had a significant reduction in renal function, some even commencing dialysis therapy as a result. Many patients also need to start or increase anti-hypertensive medication [37].

For the islet transplantation to be really successful the majority of patient need to achieve long-term islet graft function. At the moment it is too early to determine whether this can be achieved easily. Many of the initial cohort of patients from Edmonton are back on insulin, although most have retained some graft function with good glycaemic control. This gradual loss of function has proven to be a difficult problem for investigators as it is not clear whether it is due to chronic rejection, disease recurrence or 'islet exhaustion'. This problem is exacerbated by the fact that there is no easy way to monitor graft function. Monitoring graft function by tissue biopsy has been a major reason for the improved survival of renal, liver and cardiac transplantation and the lack of a similar test for islet grafts is proving to be a major hurdle in determining the natural history of islet transplantation.

In 2002 the National Pancreas Transplant Unit at Westmead Hospital began a trial of pancreatic islet transplantation. Initially we are selecting patients with type 1 diabetes who suffer from severe hypoglycaemic unawareness that has failed to respond to intensive management by an endocrinologist. Of the six patients transplanted, three were able to cease insulin injections [38]. The good news for these patients is that they no longer suffer life-threatening 'hypos' and this has resulted in a substantial improvement in their quality of life. However, the immunosuppressive drugs cause significant side effects, and our view remains that this treatment should be reserved for those patients with the most severe metabolic complications from their diabetes. These promising findings led to the Australian Government funding a second multi-centre Australian trial which was led by the Westmead Hospital Centre. In this second trial 16 patients have been transplanted with measurable graft function in all patients bar one. Eight patients were insulin independent and all patients had abolition of their hypoglycaemic episodes. A new immunosuppressive regimen was evaluated which was beneficial at preventing rejection and better tolerated. These patients were compared with a similar cohort of patients who had severe hypoglycaemia and who were managed with intensive medical follow-up and insulin pumps. Those patients undergoing islet transplantation had improved blood glucose control and abolition of hypoglycaemia whereas those patients on insulin pumps had no reduction of hypoglycaemia.

These are early days in the development of this therapy and much needs to be done before this treatment can be offered to a wider group of patients. These trials are an important proof of principle and bring us a step closer to finding a cure for type 1 diabetes. We can help some patients but the treatment comes at a price. Areas requiring improvement include a need for more reliable islet isolation procedures, better and safer anti-rejection drugs and long-term studies to show that this treatment provides real benefits for patients. In addition to solving these technical problems, we need to develop alternative sources of donor islet tissue. Some researchers are developing stem cells. Our unit, in collaboration with others, is using gene therapy to develop pig islet cells for transplantation into humans. Over the past decade there has been substantial progress in cell-based therapy to treat type 1 diabetes. The current trials of human pancreatic islet transplantation have demonstrated that this type of approach can abolish the need for exogenous insulin and provide real benefits to patients. In addition the ongoing development of an indefinite source of islets provides hope that cell-based therapies could become the norm for type 1 diabetes rather than a life-changing therapy for a few.

Prevention of long-term complications

Both type 1 and type 2 diabetes lead to long-term complications of vascular disease affecting the eye, kidney, nerves and larger blood vessels of the heart and limbs. The biological contributors are similar but in type 2 diabetes there is possibly a greater impact of accompanying high blood pressure and abnormal lipids. For those with type 1 diabetes the features of the metabolic syndrome increase their risk of complications substantially, threefold in a recent study [39]. We are understanding more about the relative contributions to vascular disease and also the contribution of the autonomic nervous system which innervates the vasculature [40, 41].

Statins are of proven benefit to reduce vascular outcomes in line with the benefit demonstrated in those without diabetes [42], but its is unclear whether it is appropriate to initiate in all young people, especially when not considered safe during pregnancy. The Adolescent Type 1 Diabetes Cardiorenal Intervention Trial (AdDIT) will help determine whether adolescents at high risk to progression will benefit from Angiotensin converting enzyme inhibitors or statins [43]. This is a multinational study in the UK, Canada and Australia currently recruiting 500 at-risk adolescents as defined by the urinary concentration of the protein, albumin.

As well as statin therapy to reduce cholesterol, recent studies have examined triglyceride-lowering treatment in diabetes [44, 45]. The Fenofibrate Intervention and Event Lowering in Diabetes (FIELD) trial was a large randomised trial of fenofibrate to prevent vascular complications, in particular cardiovascular disease in T2DM patients. A total of 9795 T2DM subjects aged between 50 and 75 years were recruited from 63 centres in Australia, New Zealand and Finland between February 1998 and November 2000 and study closeout was early 2005. Subjects were randomised to receive either 200 mg co-micronised fenofibrate or matching placebo for an average of five years follow-up. The primary endpoint of non-fatal MI + CHD death was not significantly reduced by fenofibrate (HR =

0.89: 0.75 –1.05; p = 0.16), however, most other macrovascular endpoints were significantly reduced by treatment, including hospitalisation of ACS, non-fatal MI alone, coronary or carotid revascularisation [46]. Fenofibrate also profoundly reduced microvascular events, including eye complications (by 37%), albuminuria (18%) and loss of renal function (3.7 kidney-years saved), together with amputations (36%) [47–49].

Work is now underway exploring the blood biomarkers and genetic markers associated with both the cardiovascular and microvascular complications seen in the FIELD study, as well as with any predictors of benefit of treatment, supported by National Health and Medical Research Council (NHMRC) of Australia grants and the main study sponsor, Abbott, who market fenofibrate globally. Basic science (cellular and animal) research work is being conducted in parallel, in order to understand how fenofibrate might protect so powerfully against microvascular disease in type 2 diabetes. A better knowledge of how fenofibrate might mediate these large benefits may offer hope for even more potent treatments against diabetic complications in future.

Design of clinical trials for diabetes treatment and complications

Evaluations of potential new therapies for improving the treatment of type 1 or type 2 diabetes mellitus use classical methods of clinical trials design. This means that after short-term exposure trials in normal subjects (phase 1) and then patients (Phase 2) to establish the pharmacology of a new drug and then the activity of such an intervention and immediate safety of use, larger randomised trials, usually with placebo control are conducted in a parallel-group schema (Figure 3). Follow-up is over some months (Phase 2) in order to explore acceptance and compliance with planned dosing schedules, and more reliably establish the magnitude of benefits on glycaemic control, blood pressure, or similar. Thereafter, over some years usually (Phase 3), clinical trials designed to yield harder clinical endpoints such as changes in renal function, progression of retinopathy, or cardiovascular event reductions are conducted, to determine whether the sought benefits of the treatment are in fact borne out.

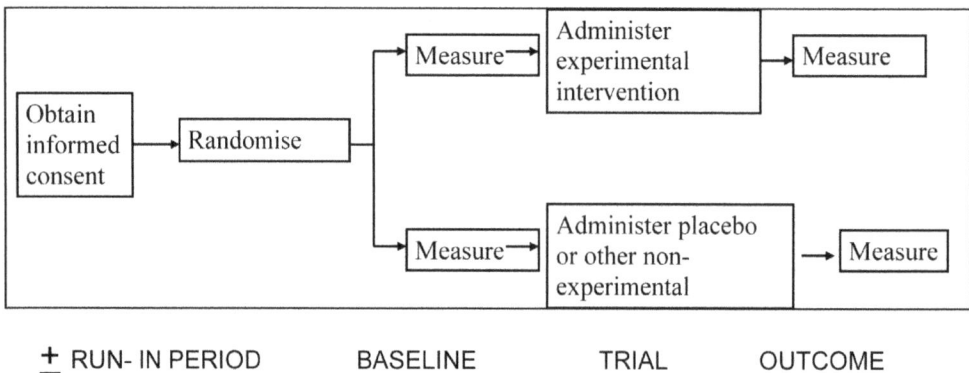

Figure 3. Parallel group randomised trial design

Table 1. Traditional clinical trial phases and their purposes.

Phase 1	Determines the action, distribution, metabolism and toxicity of different dosages of a drug in humans, healthy volunteers or patients with the disease being studied for whom alternative treatment options may have been exhausted. Only a few patients participate. Alternatively, it may be a small pilot study to establish safety and calibration of a device.
Phase 2	Determines the levels of efficacy and safety on a broader group of patients with the condition of interest.
Phase 3	Compares the intervention with the current standard treatment in a large number of patients (often hundreds or thousands) who suffer from the condition of interest. Patients are randomly allocated to either the new intervention or the standard treatment. A phase 3 trial usually determines whether the new intervention is sufficiently superior to the current or standard treatment to replace it or be a viable alternative. A phase 3 trial may also reveal further side effects of the intervention or identify subgroups for whom the intervention is particularly beneficial.
Phase 4	Long-term surveillance after drug approval may detect rare adverse effects or those that are apparent only over a long period. Unexpected benefits may also be identified, requiring further phase 3 trials for confirmation.

At the stage of a phase 3 trial, the results of which are of most direct potential applicability to clinician practice, most of the more common safety issues associated with an investigational treatment will have been identified. However, the possibility of previously unknown rarer side effects being recognised with longer exposure time, larger numbers or both remains, and it has not been uncommon for marketed products to be later withdrawn or more restricted in approved uses as more real-life experience becomes available, making these phase 3 trials, and after-market surveillance programs (phase 4) invaluable in identifying real advances for patient treatment policies [50, 51].

When large phase 3 trials of new drug therapy are designed, ideally they are set on a background of standard care, and the new therapy, or its matching placebo, are added to existing care. This often offers the advantage of more closely mimicking how the drug might be used in real life, and does not deny trial participants ongoing use of current best standard care. Occasionally, the new treatment might be proposed to replace an existing treatment, in which case a comparative trial of new versus established treatment may be conducted (in this instance a double-placebo or so-called double-dummy design would be needed in order to preserve blinding, if possible) [52].

Strong randomisation is pivotal to a good trial result, and ever more sophisticated methods to stratify a randomisation by important prognostic patient characteristics is making interpretation of trials results simpler, based on crude numbers of events. Randomisation ensures that the key variables influencing outcomes of interest are balanced between the group allocated to receive the active intervention and the control treatment. Processes used to randomise must be secure and unpredictable in advance, so as to ensure their integrity. This is often achieved by using a central web-based system [52].

Blinding or masking of treatments has become an important hallmark of good trials, when practicable. Because both trial participants or patients and their doctors may have in-built prejudices one way or another about the potential advantages of a new therapy under test, this can lead to inadvertent biases in assessing side effects, complications, outcomes and perceived links to study treatments. For that reason, great lengths are undertaken in order to try to avoid such biases from arising [52]. Part of this process is to mask study treatment with a placebo wherever possible, with matching colour, appearance, consistency, taste and so on, in order to avoid any party knowing which treatment is being received during the study. Of course, if an emergency clinical situation arises, then the opportunity to unmask immediately must be provided within the trial organisation, as the patients' best interests must remain foremost.

For the same reasons, outcome adjudication is also often set out to be performed at arms length from the trial apparatus, by a group of people with no other direct involvement in a study, so that decisions about the nature of outcome events or untoward complications can be judged impartially. Centres such as the NHMRC Clinical Trials Centre have decades of experience in helping investigators set up clinical trials with these considerations built in to the trial protocol and operational structures.

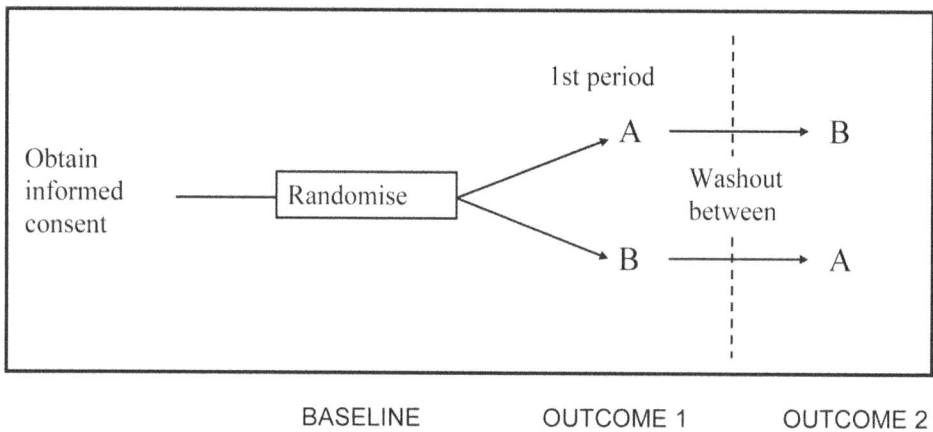

Figure 4. A two-period cross-over trial design.

When new devices are being tested, such as insulin pumps and continuous glucose monitors, blinding of the intervention is usually not possible. Some attempts can be made to reduce differences between groups, for example, whereby all subjects have devices installed, but not all are activated (early activation could be randomised), but generally in these circumstances, investigators rely on impartial assessments of outcomes being possible. This could include instances of hospitalisation or medical intervention being required for documented severe hypoglycaemia, in this example. This sort of trial might lend itself to a cross-over design whereby each subject experiences two phases of treatment with and without device support, each for sufficient time periods that reliable estimates of any advantages emerge (Figure 4). After pancreatic islet transplantation, insulin dosing requirements for glucose homeostasis may be the primary outcome studied.

There are many opportunities to enhance the design of phase 3 trials in practice. One way is to consider a run-in period prior to randomisation of patients into a trial. Most often, such a run-in period would be 'single-blind' meaning that only the patient would be unaware of what treatment was being offered to them, with study staff knowing that the patient was receiving (most commonly) a placebo at that point [52]. The potential advantages of a run-in period include (i) that the patient has already been entered into the trial routine; (ii) time is allowed to establish that subject characteristics meet all the inclusion criteria, including any special pathology results that are not immediately available; (iii) subjects have an opportunity to discuss trial participation with spouses and their usual doctors and to reflect on whether they wish to make what is often a long-term commitment to a tight schedule of follow-up visits (if they change their mind at this stage they have not upset the randomisation yet); (iv) subjects who are not likely to be good compliers can be identified in advance and excluded from randomisation if desired (though generalisability of final results may be affected if many subjects are excluded in this way); and (v) less commonly, the use of an active rather than placebo run-in period can characterise subjects in terms of their responsiveness to treatment, allowing later analyses identifying whether big-responders gain more benefit from treatment than small responders in some biomarker or other putative measure of treatment mechanism.

Another useful strategy might be to consider a washout period at the end of the study. Where a drug treatment may have exerted a potentially adverse effect in some way, it becomes important to know whether such an effect is reversible when the treatment is withdrawn. So, for example, a number of drugs developed for use in type 2 diabetes, including pan-PPAR agents, have shown renal injury in terms of increased proteinuria and loss of glomerular filtration rate (GFR) sufficient to prevent the drug development proceeding. In some cases, the renal injury has been permanent for some patients [53]. In the FIELD study, use of fenofibrate rapidly increased plasma creatinine levels by around 12%, a signal of some concern clinically, as this could potentially represent a small drop in GFR. Furthermore, the creatinine rise remained present for the duration of the five-year average treatment period, raising legitimate concerns about whether this could adversely affect cardiovascular risk. As it turned out, a washout study in over 600 patients showed that the increase in creatinine was fully reversible even after five years, and also unmasked a more favourable final GFR among subjects who had received fenofibrate rather than placebo during the trial [48].

Results of FIELD analysed by the extent of changes in creatinine during a six weeks active run-in period immediately prior to randomisation, among all 9795 patients further showed that cardiovascular events were reduced most by study treatment among subjects with a larger rise in creatinine (perhaps such an increase is a marker of greater drug bioactivity). Preservation of renal filtration function was no different according to the extent of the creatinine rise before randomisation during active run-in treatment [48].

Pre-specifying a number of secondary and tertiary outcomes in advance is important for how such results are perceived by the general community. Because 'data-dredging' can so easily lead to spurious findings, outcomes that have been planned out in detail before trial results are known carry much more weight both with journals and with peers. A significant time is required to set these out in a protocol ahead of trial commencement [52].

Uniquely in the disease area of type 2 diabetes, there are greater hurdles for new drug development and registration than in other disease domains. For products planning to be accessible in the US, the recently updated Food and Drug Administration (FDA) regulations mean that drugs intended for use in type 2 diabetes must prove their safety with respect to cardiovascular events. While drugs can reach market prior to the results of such trials being known, such trials must be planned or underway to ensure that a hazard from treatment exceeding a 30% increase in CVD risk (HR >1.3) can be ruled out at the end of such a study [53]. This has arisen after several drugs reaching routine clinical use in the market have been found to potentially give rise to CVD harm, most notably rosiglitazone, though the correct interpretation of the data from a number of relevant trials remains contested [54].

Conclusions

We are understanding more about the development of diabetes and its complications. Much exciting work has already been done but many critical studies are underway. We await the outcomes with hope that the increase in type 1 and type 2 diabetes may be reduced and diabetes complications minimised. Randomised clinical trials remain the best way to identify such advances, and must be well planned with clearly defined prespecified primary, secondary and tertiary outcomes to ensure the maximum scientific value is achieved.

References

1. Australian Institute of Health and Welfare (2011). *Prevalence of type 1 diabetes in Australian children, 2008* (14/06/11 edition). Canberra: Australian Institute of Health and Welfare.

2. Hilner JE, Perdue LH, Sides EG, Pierce JJ, Wägner AM, Aldrich A, et al. (2010). Designing and implementing sample and data collection for an international genetics study: the Type 1 Diabetes Genetics Consortium (T1DGC). *Clinical Trials*, 7(Suppl. 1): S5–S32.

3. Barrett JC, Clayton DG, Concannon P, Akolkar B, Cooper JD, Erlich HA, et al. (2009). Genome-wide association study and meta-analysis find that over 40 loci affect risk of type 1 diabetes. *Nature Genetics*, 41(6): 703–07.

4. Ziegler AG, Pflueger M, Winkler C, Achenbach P, Akolkar B, Krischer JP, et al. (2011). Accelerated progression from islet autoimmunity to diabetes is causing the escalating incidence of type 1 diabetes in young children. *Journal of Autoimmunity*, 37(1): 3–7.

5. Yeung W-CG, Rawlinson WD, Craig ME (2011). Enterovirus infection and type 1 diabetes mellitus: systematic review and meta-analysis of observational molecular studies. *British Medical Journal*, 342: d35.

6. Knerr I, Wolf J, Reinehr T, Stachow R, Grabert M, Schober E, et al. (2005). The 'accelerator hypothesis': relationship between weight, height, body mass index and age at diagnosis in a large cohort of 9248 German and Austrian children with type 1 diabetes mellitus. *Diabetologia*, 48(12): 2501–04.

7. Clarke SL, Craig ME, Garnett SP, Chan AK, Cowell CT, Cusumano JM, et al. (2006). Increased adiposity at diagnosis in younger children with type 1 diabetes does not persist. *Diabetes Care,* 29(7): 1651–53.

8. Hyppönen E, Virtanen SM, Kenward MG, Knip M & Akerblom HK (2000). Childhood diabetes in Finland Study Group: obesity, increased linear growth, and risk of type 1 diabetes in children. *Diabetes care,* 23(12): 1755–60.

9. Colman PG, Steele C, Couper JJ, Beresford SJ, Powell T, Kewming K, et al. (2000). Islet autoimmunity in infants with a type I diabetic relative is common but is frequently restricted to one autoantibody. *Diabetologia,* 43(2): 203–09.

10. Ziegler A-G, Schmid S, Huber D, Hummel M & Bonifacio E (2003). Early infant feeding and risk of developing type 1 diabetes-associated autoantibodies. *The Journal of the American Medical Association,* 290(13): 1721–28.

11. Virtanen SM, Kenward MG, Erkkola M, Kautiainen S, Kronberg-Kippilä C, Hakulinen T, et al. (2006). Age at introduction of new foods and advanced beta cell autoimmunity in young children with HLA-conferred susceptibility to type 1 diabetes. *Diabetologia,* 49(7): 1512–21.

12. Couper JJ, Beresford S, Hirte C, Baghurst PA, Pollard A, Tait BD, et al. (2009). Weight gain in early life predicts risk of islet autoimmunity in children with a first-degree relative with type 1 diabetes. *Diabetes Care*, 32(1): 94–99.

13. Couper J & Donaghue KC (2009). Phases of diabetes in children and adolescents. *Pediatric Diabetes*, 10(Suppl. 12):13–16.

14. Fourlanos S, Narendran P, Byrnes GB, Colman PG & Harrison LC (2004). Insulin resistance is a risk factor for progression to type 1 diabetes. *Diabetologia*, 47(10): 1661–67.

15. Winkler C, Marienfeld S, Zwilling M, Bonifacio E & Ziegler AG (2009). Is islet autoimmunity related to insulin sensitivity or body weight in children of parents with type 1 diabetes? *Diabetologia*, 52(10): 2072–78.

16. Rasmussen T, Stene LC, Samuelsen SO, Cinek O, Wetlesen T, Torjesen PA, et al. (2009). Maternal BMI before pregnancy, maternal weight gain during pregnancy, and risk of persistent positivity for multiple diabetes-associated autoantibodies in children with the high-risk HLA genotype: the MIDIA study. *Diabetes Care,* 32(10): 1904–06.

17. Zipitis CS & Akobeng AK (2008). Vitamin D supplementation in early childhood and risk of type 1 diabetes: a systematic review and meta-analysis. *Archives of Disease in Childhood*, 93(6): 512–17.

18. Orban T, Bundy B, Becker DJ, DiMeglio LA, Gitelman SE, Goland R, et al. (2011). Co-stimulation modulation with abatacept in patients with recent-onset type 1 diabetes: a randomised, double-blind, placebo-controlled trial. *The Lancet*, 378(9789): 412–19.

19. Pescovitz MD, Greenbaum CJ, Krause-Steinrauf H, Becker DJ, Gitelman SE, Goland R, et al. (2009).

Rituximab, B-lymphocyte depletion, and preservation of beta-cell function. *The New England Journal of Medicine*, 361(22): 2143–52.

20. Sherry N, Hagopian W, Ludvigsson J, Jain SM, Wahlen J, Ferry RJ, et al. (2011). Teplizumab for treatment of type 1 diabetes (Protégé study): 1-year results from a randomised, placebo-controlled trial. *The Lancet*, 378(9790): 487–97.

21. Wherrett DK, Bundy B, Becker DJ, DiMeglio LA, Gitelman SE, Goland R, et al. (2011). Antigen-based therapy with glutamic acid decarboxylase (GAD) vaccine in patients with recent-onset type 1 diabetes: a randomised double-blind trial. *The Lancet*, 378(9788): 319–27.

22. Diabetes Prevention Trial--Type 1 Diabetes Study Group (2002). Effects of insulin in relatives of patients with type 1 diabetes mellitus. *The New England Journal of Medicine*, 346(22): 1685–91.

23. Vehik K, Cuthbertson D, Ruhlig H, Schatz DA, Peakman M, Krischer JP, et al. (2011). Long-term outcome of individuals treated with oral insulin: Diabetes Prevention Trial-Type 1 (DPT-1) oral insulin trial. *Diabetes Care*, 34(7): 1585–90.

24. Fourlanos S, Perry C, Gellert SA, Martinuzzi E, Mallone R, Butler J, et al. (2011). Evidence that nasal insulin induces immune tolerance to insulin in adults with autoimmune diabetes. *Diabetes*, 60(4): 1237–45.

25. Ryhanen SJ, Harkonen T, Siljander H, Nanto-Salonen K, Simell T, Hyoty H, et al. (2011). Impact of intranasal insulin on insulin antibody affinity and isotypes in young children with HLA-conferred susceptibility to type 1 diabetes. *Diabetes Care*, 34(6): 1383–88.

26. Akerblom HK, Virtanen SM, Ilonen J, Savilahti E, Vaarala O, Reunanen A, et al. (2005). Dietary manipulation of beta cell autoimmunity in infants at increased risk of type 1 diabetes: a pilot study. *Diabetologia*, 48(5): 829–37.

27. TRIGR Study Group, Akerblom HK, Krischer J, Virtanen SM, Berseth C, Becker D, et al. (2011). The trial to reduce IDDM in the genetically at risk (TRIGR) study: recruitment, intervention and follow-up. *Diabetologia*, 54(3): 627–33.

28. Hummel S, Pfluger M, Hummel M, Bonifacio E & Ziegler AG (2011). Primary dietary intervention study to reduce the risk of islet autoimmunity in children at increased risk for type 1 diabetes: the BABYDIET study. *Diabetes Care*, 34(6): 1301–05.

29. Voltarelli JC, Couri CEB, Stracieri ABPL, Oliveira MC, Moraes DA, Pieroni F, et al. (2007). Autologous nonmyeloablative hematopoietic stem cell transplantation in newly diagnosed type 1 diabetes mellitus. *The Journal of the American Medical Association*, 297(14): 1568–76.

30. Couri CEB, Oliveira MCB, Stracieri ABPL, Moraes DA, Pieroni F, Barros GMN, et al. (2009). C-peptide levels and insulin independence following autologous nonmyeloablative hematopoietic stem cell transplantation in newly diagnosed type 1 diabetes mellitus.*The Journal of the American Medical Association*, 301(15): 1573–79.

31. Skyler JS (2007). Cellular therapy for type 1 diabetes: has the time come? *The Journal of the American Medical Association*, 297(14): 1599–600.

32. Fotino C, Ricordi C, Lauriola V, Alejandro R & Pileggi A (2010). Bone marrow-derived stem cell

transplantation for the treatment of insulin-dependent diabetes. *The Review of Diabetic Studies*, 7(2): 144–57.

33. Shapiro AM, Lakey JR, Ryan EA, Korbutt GS, Toth E, Warnock GL, et al. (2000). Islet transplantation in seven patients with type 1 diabetes mellitus using a glucocorticoid-free immunosuppressive regimen. *The New English Journal of Medicine,* 343(4): 230–38.

34. Cryer PE (2008). The barrier of hypoglycemia in diabetes. *Diabetes*, 57(12): 3169–76.

35. Ryan EA, Lakey JR, Rajotte RV, Korbutt GS, Kin T, Imes S, et al. (2001). Clinical outcomes and insulin secretion after islet transplantation with the Edmonton protocol. *Diabetes*, 50(4): 710–19.

36. Fiorina P, Folli F, Maffi P, Placidi C, Venturini M, Finzi G, et al. (2003). Islet transplantation improves vascular diabetic complications in patients with diabetes who underwent kidney transplantation: a comparison between kidney-pancreas and kidney-alone transplantation. *Transplantation*, 75(8):1296–01.

37. Shapiro AMJ, Ricordi C, Hering BJ, Auchincloss H, Lindblad R, Robertson RP, et al. (2006). International trial of the Edmonton protocol for islet transplantation. *The New English Journal of Medicine*, 355(13): 1318–30.

38. O'Connell PJ, Hawthorne WJ, Holmes-Walker DJ, Nankivell BJ, Gunton JE, Patel AT, et al. (2006). Clinical islet transplantation in type 1 diabetes mellitus: results of Australia's first trial. *The Medical Journal of Australia,* 184(5): 221–25.

39. McGill M, Molyneaux L, Twigg SM & Yue DK (2008). The metabolic syndrome in type 1 diabetes: does it exist and does it matter? *Journal of Diabetes and its Complications*, 22(1): 18–23.

40. Gallego PH, Wiltshire E & Donaghue KC (2007). Identifying children at particular risk of long-term diabetes complications. *Pediatric Diabetes,* Suppl. 6: 40–48.

41. Maguire AM, Craig ME, Craighead A, Chan AKF, Cusumano JM, Hing SJ, et al. (2007). Autonomic nerve testing predicts the development of complications: a 12-year follow-up study. *Diabetes Care,* 30(1): 77–82.

42. Cholesterol Treatment Trialists' Collaborators (2008). Efficacy of cholesterol-lowering therapy in 18,686 people with diabetes in 14 randomised trials of statins: a meta-analysis. *The Lancet*, 371(9607): 117–25.

43. Adolescent Type 1 Diabetes Cardio-renal Intervention Trial Research Group (2009). Adolescent type 1 Diabetes Cardio-renal Intervention Trial (AdDIT). *BMC Pediatrics*, 9: 79.

44. ACCORD Study Group, Ginsberg HN, Elam MB, Lovato LC, Crouse JR, Leiter LA, et al. (2010). Effects of combination lipid therapy in type 2 diabetes mellitus. *The New England Journal of Medicine*, 362(17): 1563–74.

45. ACCORD Study Group, ACCORD Eye Study Group, Chew EY, Ambrosius WT, Davis MD, Danis RP, et al. (2010). Effects of medical therapies on retinopathy progression in type 2 diabetes. *The New England Journal of Medicine,* 363(3): 233–44.

46. Keech A, Simes RJ, Barter P, Best J, Scott R, Taskinen M-R, et al. (2005). Effects of long-term fenofibrate therapy on cardiovascular events in 9795 people with type 2 diabetes mellitus (the FIELD study): randomised controlled trial. *The Lancet*, 366(9500): 1849–61.

47. Keech A, Mitchell P, Summanen P, O'Day J, Davis T, Moffitt M, et al. (2007). Effect of fenofibrate on the need for laser treatment for diabetic retinopathy (FIELD study): a randomised controlled trial. *The Lancet*, 370(9600): 1687–97.

48. Davis TME, Ting R, Best JD, Donoghoe MW, Drury PL, Sullivan DR, et al. (2011). Effects of fenofibrate on renal function in patients with type 2 diabetes mellitus: the Fenofibrate Intervention and Event Lowering in Diabetes (FIELD) Study. *Diabetologia*, 54(2):280–90.

49. Rajamani K, Colman PG, Li LP, Best JD, Voysey M, D'Emden MC, et al. (2009). Effect of fenofibrate on amputation events in people with type 2 diabetes mellitus (FIELD study): a prespecified analysis of a randomised controlled trial. *The Lancet*, 373(9677): 1780–88.

50. Furberg CD & Pitt B (2001). Withdrawal of cerivastatin from the world market. *Current Controlled Trials in Cardiovascular Medicine*, 2(5): 205–07.

51. Baron JA, Sandler RS, Bresalier RS, Lanas A, Morton DG, Riddell R, et al. (2008). Cardiovascular events associated with rofecoxib: final analysis of the APPROVe trial. *The Lancet*, 372(9651): 1756–64.

52. Keech A & Gebski V (2007). *Interpreting and reporting clinical trials: a guide to the consort statement and the principles of randomised controlled trials.* Sydney: Australasian Medical Publishing.

53. Ratner RE, Parikh S, Tou C & GALLANT 9 Study Group (2007). Efficacy, safety and tolerability of tesaglitazar when added to the therapeutic regimen of poorly controlled insulin-treated patients with type 2 diabetes. *Diabetes and Vascular Disease Research,* 4(3): 214–21.

54. Davis TM, Ting R, Best JD, Donoghoe MW, Drury PL, Sullivan DR, et al. (2011). Effects of fenofibrate on renal function in patients with type 2 diabetes mellitus: the Fenofibrate Intervention and Event Lowering in Diabetes (FIELD) Study. *Diabetologia*, 54(20): 280–90.

55. Furberg CD & Pitt B (2001). Withdrawal of cerivastatin from the world market. *Current Controlled Trials in Cardiovascular Medicine*, 2(5): 205–07.

56. Baron JA, Sandler RS, Bresalier RS, Lanas A, Morton DG, Riddell R, Iverson ER & Demets DL (2008). Cardiovascular events associated with rofecoxib: final analysis of the APPROVe trial. *The Lancet*, 372(9651): 1756–64.

57. Keech A, Gebski V & Pike R (2007). *Interpreting and reporting clinical trials: a guide to the CONSORT statement and the principles of randomised controlled trials.* Sydney: Australasian Medical Publishing Company.

58. Food and Drug Administration Center for Drug Evaluation and Research (CDER) (2008). Guidance for industry diabetes mellitus: evaluating cardiovascular risk in new antidiabetic therapies to treat type 2 diabetes [Online]. Available: www.fda.gov/Drugs/GuidanceComplianceRegulatoryInformation/ Guidances [Accessed 26 September 2011].

59. European Medicines Agency recommends suspension of Avandia, Avandamet and Avaglim [press release] (2010). London: European Medicines Agency; 23 Sep 2010 [Online]. Available: www.ema. europa.eu/ema/index.jsp?curl = pages/news_and_events/news/2010/09/news_detail_001119.jsp&mid = WC0b01ac058004d5c1&murl = menus/news_and_events/news_and_events.jsp [Accessed 24 October 2011).

Index

www.ingramcontent.com/pod-product-compliance
Lightning Source LLC
Chambersburg PA
CBHW080128270326
41926CB00021B/4393